FUNDAMENTALS OF NEUROANESTHESIA

FUNDAMENTALS OF NEUROANESTHESIA

A PHYSIOLOGIC APPROACH TO CLINICAL PRACTICE

EDITED BY

Keith J. Ruskin, MD

PROFESSOR OF ANESTHESIOLOGY AND NEUROSURGERY

DIRECTOR, NEUROANESTHESIA

DEPARTMENT OF ANESTHESIOLOGY

YALE SCHOOL OF MEDICINE

NEW HAVEN, CONNECTICUT

Stanley H. Rosenbaum, MD

PROFESSOR OF ANESTHESIOLOGY, MEDICINE

AND SURGERY

VICE CHAIR, ACADEMIC AFFAIRS

DIRECTOR, PERIOPERATIVE AND ADULT ANESTHESIA

DEPARTMENT OF ANESTHESIOLOGY

YALE SCHOOL OF MEDICINE

NEW HAVEN, CONNECTICUT

Ira J. Rampil, MD

PROFESSOR OF ANESTHESIOLOGY AND NEUROLOGIC SURGERY

STATE UNIVERSITY OF NEW YORK AT STONY BROOK

STONY BROOK, NEW YORK

OXFORD
UNIVERSITY PRESS

OXFORD

UNIVERSITY PRESS

Oxford University Press is a department of the University of Oxford.
It furthers the University's objective of excellence in research, scholarship,
and education by publishing worldwide.

Oxford   New York

Auckland   Cape Town   Dar es Salaam   Hong Kong   Karachi
Kuala Lumpur   Madrid   Melbourne   Mexico City   Nairobi
New Delhi   Shanghai   Taipei   Toronto

With offices in

Argentina   Austria   Brazil   Chile   Czech Republic   France   Greece
Guatemala   Hungary   Italy   Japan   Poland   Portugal   Singapore
South Korea   Switzerland   Thailand   Turkey   Ukraine   Vietnam

Oxford is a registered trademark of Oxford University Press
in the UK and certain other countries.

Published in the United States of America by
Oxford University Press
198 Madison Avenue, New York, NY 10016

Library of Congress Cataloging-in-Publication Data
Fundamentals of neuroanesthesia : a physiologic approach to clinical practice / edited by
Keith J. Ruskin, Stanley H. Rosenbaum, Ira J. Rampil.
p. ; cm.
Includes bibliographical references and index.
ISBN 978–0–19–975598–1 (alk. paper)
I. Ruskin, Keith.—   II. Rosenbaum, Stanley H.—   III. Rampil, Ira J.
[DNLM: 1. Anesthesia.—   2. Neurosurgical Procedures. WO 200]
RD87.3.N47
617.9′6748—dc23
2013009160

This material is not intended to be, and should not be considered, a substitute for medical or other professional advice. Treatment for the
conditions described in this material is highly dependent on the individual circumstances. And, while this material is designed to offer accurate
information with respect to the subject matter covered and to be current as of the time it was written, research and knowledge about
medical and health issues is constantly evolving and dose schedules for medications are being revised continually, with new side effects recognized and accounted for regularly. Readers must therefore always check the product information and clinical procedures with the most
up-to-date published product information and data sheets provided by the manufacturers and the most recent codes of conduct and safety regulation. The publisher and the authors make no representations or warranties to readers, express or implied, as to the accuracy or completeness
of this material. Without limiting the foregoing, the publisher and the authors make no representations or warranties as to the accuracy or efficacy of the drug dosages mentioned in the material. The authors and the publisher do not accept, and expressly disclaim, any responsibility for
any liability, loss or risk that may be claimed or incurred as a consequence of the use and/or application of any of the contents of this material.

1 3 5 7 9 8 6 4 2

Printed in China

CONTENTS

PREFACE

The practice of neurosurgery has fundamentally changed over the past few years. Recent accomplishments in neuroscience have provided increased opportunities to treat patients suffering from acute injuries to the nervous system, such as stroke, subarachnoid hemorrhage, and trauma. For example, there have been many significant advances in the management of patients with both ischemic and hemorrhagic stroke. Patients who would have once been considered to have an untreatable neurologic injury are now routinely being scheduled for interventional or surgical procedures, and a campaign has begun to educate the general public about the urgency of seeking treatment when they experience the symptoms of a stroke.

Until very recently, craniotomies, spinal instrumentation, and interventional procedures were limited to academic medical centers or tertiary care hospitals, but these procedures and many others are offered at community hospitals. Anesthesiologists who work in these hospitals and who may not have subspecialty training are being asked to care for patients who require a neurosurgical procedure. At the same time, emerging data suggest that the choices that we make in the operating room can improve the patient's ultimate outcome. A clear, concise textbook that covers the physiologic underpinnings of neurosurgical anesthesia while also providing practical information for the anesthesiologist who in general practice is a relatively new need.

Fundamentals of Neurosurgical Anesthesiology is written to help an anesthesia provider deal with planned neurosurgical procedures and the unforeseen emergencies that may occur during the perioperative period. As we were developing the specifications for this book, we decided on two goals: This book should provide the critical information that all anesthesia providers should have when caring for the neurosurgical patient, and it should contain a thorough and user-friendly review of the anesthetic management of neurosurgical patients. The first part of the book reviews physiology and pharmacology from the perspective of the neurosurgical patient while the remaining chapters cover the aspects of subspecialty practice. All chapters concentrate on the practical aspects of the practice of neurosurgical anesthesia. The chapter authors are all recognized experts and are extensively published in the field of neurosurgical anesthesia. Each contributor was asked to write a comprehensive discussion of the subject that also offered clear, practical recommendations for clinical practice. In addition to references to basic science literature, an effort has been made to include references to clinical studies or review articles that will provide additional information.

This book would not have been possible without the support of many people. The authors wish to thank Andrea Seils and Rebecca Suzan for patiently answering all of our questions and for their help with every aspect of this project. We would also like to thank the many members of our departments who reviewed chapters and offered thoughtful advice. Most importantly, we thank our families for their support and understanding while each of us spent many late nights in front of a computer or with printed chapters spread out around the house.

ACKNOWLEDGMENTS

This book would not have been possible without the help of many people. The authors would first like to thank their families for their constant support.

We would like to thank our editors, Andrea Seils and Rebecca Suzan, for their advice and guidance.

We also thank our authors, who produced outstanding manuscripts and turned them in on time.

Last, we thank the residents and faculty of the Yale University School of Medicine, Department of Anesthesiology, for their critical reviews of the manuscript and their thoughtful comments.

CONTRIBUTORS

Brooke Albright, MD, Major
United States Air Force
Adjunct Assistant Professor of Anesthesiology
Uniformed Services University of Health Sciences
Critical Care Air Transport Team
Landstuhl Regional Medical Center, Germany

John Ard, MD
Assistant Professor, Co-Director of Neuroanesthesia
Department of Anesthesiology
New York University Langone Medical Center
New York, New York

Joshua H. Atkins, MD, PhD
Assistant Professor of Anesthesiology and Critical Care
Assistant Professor of Otorhinolaryngology, Head
and Neck Surgery
Department of Anesthesiology and Critical Care
University of Pennsylvania
Philadelphia, Pennsylvania

Jess Brallier, MD
Assistant Professor of Anesthesiology
Mount Sinai Hospital
New York, New York

Ketan R. Bulsara, MD
Associate Professor of Neurosurgery
Director of Neuroendovascular and Skull Base
Surgery Programs
Yale School of Medicine
New Haven, Connecticut

Maria Bustillo, MD
Associate Director of Neuroanesthesiology
Department of Anesthesiology
Albert Einstein College of Medicine
Montefiore Medical Center
New York, New York

Veronica Chiang, MD
Associate Professor of Neurosurgery and
Therapeutic Radiology
Director, Stereotactic Radiosurgery
Medical Director, Yale New Haven Hospital Gamma
Knife Center
Yale School of Medicine
New Haven, Connecticut

Armagan Dagal, MD, FRCA
Acting Assistant Professor
Department of Anesthesiology and Pain Medicine
University of Washington
Seattle, Washington

Stacie Deiner, MD
Associate Professor of Anesthesiology, Neurosurgery
and Geriatrics & Palliative Care
Department of Anesthesiology
Icahn School of Medicine at Mount Sinai
New York, New York

Jeremy S. Dority, MD
Assistant Professor of Anesthesiology
University of Kentucky Medical Center
Durham, North Carolina

Jessica Dworet, MD, PhD
Assistant Professor
Department of Anesthesiology
Westchester Medical Center
Valhalla, New York

Patricia Fogarty-Mack, MD
Associate Professor of Clinical Anesthesiology
Department of Anesthesiology
Weill Cornell Medical College, Cornell University
New York, New York

Thomas M. Fuhrman, MD
Chief, Division of Neuroanesthesia
Professor of Clinical Anesthesiology
University of Miami Miller School of Medicine
Miami, Florida

Ryan A. Grant, MD, MS
Resident in Neurosurgery
Department of Neurosurgery
Yale-New Haven Hospital
Yale University School of Medicine
New Haven, Connecticut

Eric A. Harris, MD, MBA
Associate Professor of Clinical Anesthesiology
University of Miami Miller School of Medicine
Miami, Florida

Ryan Hakimi, DO, MS
Director, Critical Care Neurology
Assistant Professor
Department of Neurology
University of Oklahoma Health Sciences Center
Oklahoma City, Oklahoma

Ryan Hebert
Resident in Neurosurgery
Department of Neurosurgery
Yale-New Haven Hospital
Yale University School of Medicine
New Haven, Connecticut

James G. Hecker, MD, PhD
Associate Professor at Harborview Medical Center
Department of Anesthesiology and Pain Medicine
University of Washington
Seattle, Washington

Leslie C. Jameson, MD
University of Colorado, Anschutz Medical Campus
School of Medicine
Department of Anesthesiology
Aurora, Colorado

Markus Klimek, MD, PhD, DEAA, EDIC
Vice-Chairman
Department of Anesthesiology
Erasmus MC, University Medical Center
Rotterdam, The Netherlands

Avinash B. Kumar, MD, FCCM, FCCP
Associate Professor Anesthesia and Critical Care
Vanderbilt University
Nashville, Tennessee

Robert Lagasse, MD
Professor of Anesthesiology
Director, Quality Management and Perioperative Safety
Department of Anesthesiology
Yale School of Medicine
New Haven, Connecticut

Arthur M. Lam, MD, FRCPC
Medical Director of Neuroanesthesia and
Neurocritical Care
Swedish Neuroscience Institute
Clinical Professor
Department of Anesthesiology and Pain Medicine
University of Washington
Seattle, Washington

Maxwell S. Laurans, MD
Assistant Professor of Neurosurgery
Department of Neurosurgery
Yale School of Medicine
New Haven, Connecticut

Peter D. Le Roux, MD, FACS
Associate Professor
Department of Neurosurgery
University of Pennsylvania
Philadelphia, Pennsylvania

Vinod Malhotra, MB, BS
Professor of Clinical Anesthesiology
Professor of Anesthesiology in Clinical Urology
Department of Anesthesiology
Weill Cornell Medical College, Cornell University
New York, New York

Adrian A. Maung, MD
Assistant Professor of Surgery (Trauma)
Department of Surgery
Yale School of Medicine
New Haven, Connecticut

Craig D. McClain, MD
Assistant Professor of Anaesthesia
Harvard Medical School
Senior Associate, Department of Anesthesiology,
Perioperative and Pain Medicine
Boston Children's Hospital
Boston, Massachusetts

David L. McDonagh, MD
Associate Professor of Anesthesiology & Medicine
(Neurology)
Chief, Division of Neuroanesthesiology
Duke University Medical Center

Colleen M. Moran, MD
Assistant Professor
University of Pittsburgh
Department of Anesthesiology
Pittsburgh, Pennsylvania

Rashmi N. Mueller, MD
Clinical Associate Professor
Director of Neuroanesthesia, Department of Anesthesia
University of Iowa, Carver College of Medicine
Iowa City, Iowa

Thomas H. Ottens, MD, MSc
Resident in Anesthesiology
Department of Anesthesiology
University Medical Center Utrecht
Utrecht, The Netherlands

Anup Pamnani, MD
Assistant Professor of Anesthesiology
Weill Cornell Medical College, Cornell University
New York, New York

Stephen Probst, MD
Assistant Professor of Anesthesiology
University at Stony Brook
Stony Brook, New York

Ramachandran Ramani, MD, MBBS
Associate Professor of Anesthesiology
Department of Anesthesiology
Yale School of Medicine
New Haven, Connecticut

Ira J. Rampil, MS, MD
Professor of Anesthesiology and Neurological Surgery
State University of New York at Stony Brook
Stony Brook, New York

Stanley H. Rosenbaum, MD
Professor of Anesthesiology, Medicine
and Surgery
Vice Chair, Academic Affairs
Director, Perioperative and Adult Anesthesia
Department of Anesthesiology
Yale School of Medicine
New Haven, Connecticut

Ariane Rossi, MD
Department of Anesthesia
University Hospital and University of Lausanne
Lausanne, Switzerland

Keith J. Ruskin, MD
Professor of Anesthesiology and Neurosurgery
Director, Neuroanesthesia
Department of Anesthesiology
Yale School of Medicine
New Haven, Connecticut

Christoph N. Seubert, MD, PhD, DABNM
Associate Professor of Anesthesiology
Chief, Division of Neuroanesthesia
Department of Anesthesiology
University of Florida College of Medicine
Gainesville, Florida

Richard B. Silverman, MD
Assistant Professor of Clinical Anesthesiology
University of Miami Miller School of Medicine
Miami, Florida

Sulpicio G. Soriano, MD, FAAP
Endowed Chair in Pediatric Neuroanesthesia
Boston Children's Hospital
Professor of Anaesthesia
Harvard Medical School
Boston, Massachusetts

Luzius A. Steiner, MD, PhD
Professor and Chairman
Anesthesiology
University Hospital Basel
Basel, Switzerland

Lorenz G. Theiler, MD
Staff Anesthesiologist
Division of Neuroanesthesia
Department of Anesthesiology and Pain Therapy
University Hospital Inselspital and University of Bern,
Switzerland

Joss J. Thomas, MD, MPH, FCCP
Clinical Associate Professor of Anesthesia
Department of Anesthesia
University of Iowa, Carver College of Medicine
Iowa City, Iowa

Robyn S. Weisman, MD
Assistant Professor of Anesthesiology
Division of Regional Anesthesiology and
Acute Perioperative Pain Management
University of Miami - Jackson Memorial Hospital
Miami, Florida

1.

CENTRAL NERVOUS SYSTEM ANATOMY

Maxwell S. Laurans, Brooke Albright, and Ryan A. Grant

There are in the human mind a group of faculties, and in the brain groups of convolutions, and the facts assembled by science so far allow to state, as I said before, that the great regions of the mind correspond to the great regions of the brain.

—Paul Broca [1]

Dr. Pierre Paul Broca stated many years ago that our greatest attributes and our inner selves exist in a three-pound gelatinous organ of unparalleled complexity. Neuroanatomy is among the most complicated anatomy in the body, but it is essential for the neuroanesthetist to understand so that he or she can speak the same language as the neurosurgeon. This chapter puts central nervous system (CNS) anatomy into context by correlating structure with physiologic function. We begin with a review of basic terminology and orientation, followed by a study of each section of the brain, brainstem, and spinal cord, with special emphasis on anatomical compartments as they relate to surgical approaches.

BASIC TERMINOLOGY

The nervous system is composed of neurons, which are responsible for signaling, and the supportive glial cells. A neuron consists of a cell body (soma), dendrites (which receive information), and a long axon (which transmits information). Most neurons have several dendrites and several axons (i.e., they are *multipolar*), allowing for a complex signaling network. Communication occurs at a synapse, at which an electrical signal traveling as an action potential is transformed into a chemical neurotransmitter that relays the message to the target neuron. Synapses occur in every imaginable combination: axodendritic (most common), axoaxonic, dendro-dendritic, and dendroaxonal (reverse communication). The majority of these synaptic connections occur in the gray matter (neuronal cell bodies), with the white matter (myelinated axons) transmitting the signals over vast distances. The glial cells provide support and protection for neurons, help form the foundation of the blood–brain barrier [2], and deposit myelin, which insulates the axons and increases the velocity of the action potential. Interestingly, glial cells have now been implicated in learning, memory, and even direct signaling [3]. In the CNS, myelin is derived from the glial oligodendrocytes, whereas the supportive insulating glial cells in the peripheral nervous system (PNS) are called Schwann cells. Afferent fibers bring input to a given neural structure—that

is, they "arrive," and efferent fibers carry output from a neural structure—that is, they "exit." Last, ganglia refer to a group of cell bodies found in the PNS, whereas nuclei are a group of cell bodies found in the CNS (e.g., cranial nerve [CN] nuclei, basal ganglia, and thalami).

ORIENTATION PLANES

Anatomical terms for orientation are based on the long axis of a quadruped animal, which is parallel to the plane of the ground. However, humans have an upright posture, with the nervous system making a bend of approximately 90° at the midbrain–diencephalic junction. This means that structures above the midbrain have the same orientation of a quadruped animal (or a human on all fours), and below the midbrain the plane of structures is perpendicular to the ground. Rostral is toward the nose (Latin: beak), caudal is toward the tail (Latin), ventral is toward the belly (Latin), dorsal is toward the back (Latin). In the forebrain, anterior is rostral (toward the front of the head), posterior is caudal (toward the back of the head), superior is dorsal (toward the top of the head), and inferior is ventral (toward the bottom of the head). Below the midbrain, anterior is ventral (toward the front), posterior is dorsal (toward the back), superior is rostral (toward the nose), and inferior is caudal (toward the tail). Pathologists and radiologists use slightly different terminology: axial (i.e., horizontal or transverse) sections are parallel to the floor in an upright individual and orthogonal to the superior-inferior axis, sagittal sections are perpendicular to the left-right axis in an upright individual, and the coronal plane is orthogonal to the anterior-posterior axis.

MENINGES, VENTRICLES, AND CEREBROSPINAL FLUID

MENINGES

Within the cranial cavity, the brain is surrounded by the *meninges*: the dura mater, arachnoid mater, and pia mater. The dura mater is the toughest of the meninges (Latin: tough mother) and is firmly attached to the skull. The space between the skull and dura is known as the epidural space, which is a potential space that can become enlarged when it fills with hemorrhage producing an epidural hematoma, usually caused by laceration of the middle meningeal artery as it transverses the temporal bone of the skull. This anatomy explains why these bleeds appear as lenticular (lens-shaped) on computed tomography or magnetic resonance imaging because the dura mater is forced away from the skull at the site of hemorrhage, with the edge of the hemorrhage often stopping where the dura is most adhered at the cranial sutures. The dura becomes the falx cerebri when it dives between the hemispheres, separating the brain into two halves and then splitting superiorly and inferiorly to form the major venous drainage of the brain: the superior and inferior sagittal sinuses. The sagittal sinuses are critical venous structures, and operating near them entails the possibility of rapid blood loss and the possibility of air embolism. The two horizontal pieces of dura that separate the cerebellum from the remainder of the brain is the tentorium cerebelli ("tent over the cerebellum"), which separates the posterior fossa from the remainder of the intracranial compartment. During surgery in the posterior fossa, pressure can be transmitted to the brainstem, causing abrupt hypotension or bradycardia.

Beneath the dura mater is the thin, translucent *arachnoid mater*, which encloses the entire CNS. The space between the dura and arachnoid can fill with blood, causing a subdural hematoma, which is crescent shaped on computed tomography or magnetic resonance imaging. The arachnoid is spread over the sulci (inward grooves and valleys) of the cerebral cortex but does not enter them. The superior sagittal sinus has connections with the arachnoid mater via the arachnoid granulations, which are lined by arachnoid cap cells and are responsible for returning cerebrospinal fluid (CSF) to the venous system. The arachnoid granulations are the origin of meningiomas. The CSF flows in the subarachnoid space, between the arachnoid and pia mater, as do the largest blood vessels (i.e., middle cerebral, anterior cerebral, and posterior cerebral arteries [MCA, ACA, and PCA, respectively]). When these vessels bleed, the blood accumulates in the subarachnoid space, producing a subarachnoid hemorrhage (SAH). The *pia mater*, which is only a few cells thick, is the last meningeal layer and follows all contours of the brain, enclosing all except the largest blood vessels.

CEREBROSPINAL FLUID

CSF is mainly produced by ependymal cells of the choroid plexus, which are found throughout the ventricular system except for the cerebral aqueduct of Sylvius and the anterior/posterior horns of the lateral ventricles. The total volume of CSF is approximately 150 mL and is overturned approximately three times per day, yielding a daily production of 450 mL in the adult. In some parts of the CNS, the arachnoid and pia are widely separated, leaving large CSF-filled spaces known as cisterns.

VENTRICLES

The ventricular system is a set of cavities within the brain in which CSF is produced. The brain has four ventricles: one lateral ventricle in each hemisphere, a midline third ventricle, and a fourth ventricle. The lateral ventricles are relatively large and C-shaped, each connecting to the third ventricle via the interventricular foramen (of Monro). The third ventricle is connected to the fourth ventricle by the cerebral aqueduct (of Sylvius), which passes through the midbrain. The pons and medulla form the floor of the fourth ventricle and the cerebellum forms the roof. The fourth ventricle is connected to the subarachnoid space by the median aperture (foramen of Magendie), and two lateral apertures (foramina of Luschka), permitting CSF produced in the ventricles to bathe the surrounding brainstem, cerebellum, cerebral cortex, and spinal cord, ultimately flowing to the cauda equina. The CSF is eventually reabsorbed via the arachnoid villi into the superior sagittal sinus and via diffusion into the small vessels in the pia, ventricular walls, or other large veins draining the brain and spinal cord [4]. Obstruction to CSF outflow within the cranium can cause hydrocephalus, increasing intracranial pressure and rapidly causing impaired consciousness. CSF diversion via external ventriculostomy, ventricular shunt, or endoscopic third ventriculostomy can relieve the signs and symptoms of obstructive hydrocephalus. Endoscopic third ventriculostomy allows CSF to be resorbed by providing a direct connection between the floor of the third ventricle and the subarachnoid space. A ventricular shunt allows CSF to drain to the peritoneum, pleura, atrium, or externally in the terms of the ventriculostomy.

CEREBRAL CORTEX

Beneath the pia lies the cerebral cortex (telencephalon). The brain has numerous infoldings or valleys termed sulci that increase the amount of brain surface area inside the skull and allow more neurons to occupy the relatively small cranial space. The outward folds between these sulci are called gyri. The cerebral cortex consists of a right and a left hemisphere that are separated by a deep sulcus in the midline called the longitudinal fissure, in which the falx cerebri resides. Just beneath the bottom of the falx cerebri, in the depths of the longitudinal fissure, is a large band of white matter connecting the two hemispheres that is known as the corpus callosum. The corpus callosum connects homologous cortical areas between the two hemispheres and is subdivided into four parts: the *rostrum* (anterior part), *genu*

(Latin: knee), *body*, and *splenium*. The anterior and posterior commissures are also white matter tracts that connect the two hemispheres.

The cerebral hemispheres are subdivided into four major lobes: frontal, parietal, temporal, and occipital. The frontal lobes extend from the most rostral part of the brain to the central sulcus. The central (Rolandic) sulcus can be found as it starts from the highest point along the superior curvature of the hemispheres and then runs inferiorly toward the Sylvian (lateral) fissure. Posterior to the central sulcus is the parietal lobe, and inferior to the Sylvian fissure is the temporal lobe. The most posterior part of the cerebral cortex is the occipital lobe. When viewing the lateral side of the brain, there is no sharp demarcation between the parietal, temporal, or occipital lobes, but when viewed from a sagittal (medial) section, there is a parieto-occipital sulcus that separates the parietal and occipital lobes. Each lobe has multiple regions that support specific functions, such as language, sensation, memory, and thought. Although neuroanatomists frequently use the German anatomist Korbinian Brodmann's numerical architecture to identify areas of the brain (Brodmann areas), here we use the more commonplace neuroscience terms.

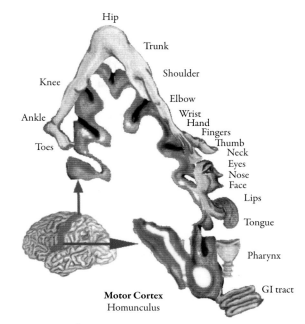

Figure 1.1 *Homunculus, Motor Cortex.* GI, *gastrointestinal.*

FRONTAL LOBE

The frontal lobes form the largest region of the brain and contain higher-order thought processes.

Most anterior is the prefrontal cortex, which is involved in executive function, decision making, personality, values, ethics, morals, love, and more basic functions such as hunger or fear. There are three major divisions of the prefrontal cortex: *dorsolateral*, *ventromedial*, and *orbitofrontal*. The most inferior of these divisions, located on top of the orbital ridges of the eyes, is the orbitofrontal gyri, which is connected to the limbic system and helps to make decisions based on primitive urges. The olfactory sulcus, which contains the olfactory bulb, is medial to the orbitofrontal gyri, allowing the sense of smell to synapse in the CNS. The gyrus rectus ("straight gyrus") is located at the midline and has no known specific function, but resection is sometimes used to increase visualization when working at the skull base, such as to improve exposure to clip an anterior communicating artery (AComm) aneurysm.

The most posterior portion of the frontal lobe contains the primary motor cortex (precentral gyrus), which is just anterior to the central sulcus. Neurons from this area produce movement by sending action potentials through axons to the brainstem and spinal cord via white matter tracts. The homunculus (Latin for "little human") is used to describe the part of the human body part controlled by each area of the motor cortex (Figure 1.1). The areas that control the lips, hands, feet, and sexual organs occupy the largest portions of the homunculus, correlating with the intensity with which humans interact with their environments. The most medial part of the primary motor cortex controls movements of the legs, feet, and genitals, whereas motor representations of the face and hands are more lateral.

Understanding the somatotopic organization of the homunculus allows neurologists and neurosurgeons to more specifically localize lesions of the motor cortex based on a patient's clinical presentation. For example, a midline parafalcine meningioma may produce contralateral leg weakness given mass effect on the medial portion of the motor cortex. Accompanying vasogenic edema may additionally produce contralateral face and arm weakness, as well as, potentially, speech difficulty depending on the patient's handedness and localization of the speech centers. Last, the ACA supplies the medial portion of the motor cortex (area controlling legs), and the MCA supplies the lateral portion (face and arms); therefore, a vascular insult to the ACA would be expected to cause contralateral leg weakness, and an MCA vasculature insult would yield weakness of the face and arm, as well as speech difficulty depending on cerebral hemisphere dominance.

The supplementary motor and premotor cortices are anterior to the primary motor cortex. These areas are responsible for modulating and planning movements (i.e., they determine whether motion is fast, slow, smooth, or spastic). Damage to the premotor cortex can result in transient paralysis or paraplegia that almost always improves, most likely due to cerebral plasticity [5]. Just anterior to the primary motor cortex, in the dominant hemisphere (most consistently determined by handedness), is Broca's area, which is responsible for speech production. Broca's area is located adjacent to the primary motor cortex, close to the face, tongue, and pharynx areas of the motor homunculus. Damage to Broca's area results in nonfluent aphasia

(Broca's aphasia), in which the patient has difficulty producing speech but can usually understand speech. Emphasis needs to be placed on this aphasia being a *language* deficit, as patients have difficulty with both speech and writing. Of note, language representation is almost always found in the left hemisphere, even in left-handed individuals. Surgical procedures in and around these eloquent structures are often performed with the patient awake so that he or she can participate in functional localization, allowing preservation of the appropriate faculties [6].

PARIETAL LOBE

The parietal lobe is located posterior to the central sulcus and is responsible for sensory integration, including spatial, auditory, and visual information (Figure 1.2). Sensory signals travel to the opposite primary somatosensory cortex (postcentral gyrus) via the thalamus; the postcentral gyrus has a homuncular representation similar to that of the precentral gyrus.

The supramarginal and angular gyri can be found by following the Sylvian fissure until it ends, with these gyri located looping over the fissure termination. These areas are important for language comprehension and processing and are usually considered two of the three parts of Wernicke's area. The superior temporal gyrus, in the temporal lobe, is the last part of Wernicke's area, with injury to these areas resulting in a fluent aphasia (Wernicke's aphasia), in which comprehension or meaningful speech is impaired. Patients speak with normal fluency, prosody

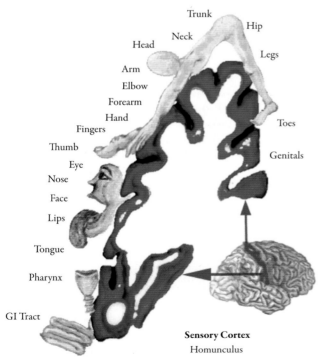

Sensory Cortex
Homunculus

Figure 1.2 *Homunculus, Sensory Cortex.* GI, *gastrointestinal.*

(stress and intonation), and grammatical structure but without meaning (nonsensical paraphasic errors known as "word salad"). The corresponding cortex for language on the nondominant side of the brain is involved in the emotional quality of language, allowing listeners to know if speech is happy, sad, angry, sarcastic, or mean. Interestingly, a language deficit in multilingual individuals may be limited to only one of their languages, suggesting that each language is stored in a distinct neuroanatomical location [7].

OCCIPITAL LOBE

The occipital lobe, which is primarily involved in vision, is located in the most posterior part of the cerebral hemisphere. The preoccipital notch, located on the ventral surface, separates the temporal and parietal lobes from the occipital lobe. On a medial cortex section, the calcarine fissure can be seen in the midline that divides the occipital lobe into superior and inferior portions. The primary visual cortex is found on the superior and inferior banks of the calcarine fissure and receives visual information from the lateral geniculate nucleus (LGN) of the thalamus—remember, "L" for light.

TEMPORAL LOBE

The temporal lobe is located ventral to the Sylvian fissure and is involved in memory, language, visual object association, and smell. The first gyrus ventral to the Sylvian fissure is the superior temporal gyrus, which processes auditory information and language comprehension (i.e., it is part of Wernicke's area). The middle and inferior temporal gyri, just beneath the superior temporal gyrus, are visual association areas and help to refine visual information in terms of object recognition. On the ventral surface of the temporal lobe, just beneath the inferior temporal gyrus, are the fusiform gyri, which are also responsible for visual association. On the ventromedial aspect of the temporal lobe is the parahippocompal gyrus, named because it overlies the hippocampus (Latin for "seahorse"), an important structure involved in memory formation. The most medial part of the temporal lobes is a small structure termed the uncus (Latin for "hook"). It has a projection of the olfactory tract and is one of the first structures to herniate in the setting of intracranial hypertension (i.e., uncal herniation). When this happens, it compresses the oculomotor nerve (CN III) against the tentorium and PCA, first dilating the pupil ("blown pupil") and then causing paralysis of medial and superior eye movements leading the eye to be deviated "down and out." Compression of the PCA can also produce posterior circulation infarcts. Last, inside the Sylvian fissure on the superior surface of each temporal lobe, running almost perpendicular toward the insula, is the primary auditory cortex (Heschl's gyrus).

INSULA

The insula (insular cortex or lobe), involved in taste processing, is found by gently increasing the separation of the Sylvian fissure—that is, pulling the temporal lobe inferiorly and the frontal-parietal lobes superiorly. Some authorities refer to this lobe as the fifth central lobe. The parts of the frontal, parietal, and temporal lobe that overly the insula are called the operculum. Damage to the operculum can result in Foix-Chavany-Marie syndrome (bilateral anterior opercular syndrome) with partial paralysis of the face, pharynx, and jaw. Characteristically, involuntary movements are preserved; that is, the patient can blink, yawn, and laugh but cannot open his or her mouth to command, nor close his or her eyes to command.

MAJOR WHITE MATTER TRACTS

Tracts are large groups of projection fibers, and they are named from their origin to their termination. The most important motor pathway is called the corticospinal tract, which begins in the precentral gyrus and projects down to the brainstem and spinal cord. The majority of fibers (approximately 85%) cross to control the opposite side of the body at the pyramidal decussation, which is located at the junction of the medulla and spinal cord. As a result, lesions in the primary motor cortex cause contralateral weakness (hemiparesis) or paralysis (hemiplegia). The somatosensory cortex receives information from ascending projection fibers of the spinal cord, including the dorsal columns (proprioception, vibration, fine touch) and anterolateral pathways—also known as the spinothalamic tract—(pain, temperature, crude touch). Commissural fibers relay information between the two hemispheres, with the largest being the corpus callosum (which connects homologous cortical area in the cerebral hemispheres). The two other commissural tracts are the anterior and posterior commissures. The anterior commissure connects the anterior part of the temporal lobes, traveling through the globus pallidus to get to the opposite side. The posterior commissure interconnects brainstem nuclei associated with eye movements and papillary constriction. Wernicke's and Broca's areas are connected by the arcuate fasciculus, with lesions leading to a disconnection between speech comprehension and motor output, resulting in an inability to repeat words or phrases (conduction aphasia).

The centrum semiovale (toward the dorsal cortex) and corona radiata (radiating crown) are axons that run *within* the cerebral cortex but do not have a distinct name (Figure 1.3). Axons running into or out of the cortex use the internal capsule, which is divided into three parts: the *anterior limb*, the *genu*, and the *posterior limb*. The anterior limb contains the anterior thalamocortical tracts and frontopontine tracts. The genu contains the corticobulbar tract ("cortex to brainstem"), which controls facial movement.

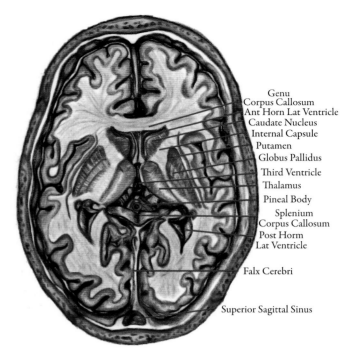

Genu
Corpus Callosum
Ant Horn Lat Ventricle
Caudate Nucleus
Internal Capsule
Putamen
Globus Pallidus
Third Ventricle
Thalamus
Pineal Body
Splenium
Corpus Callosum
Post Horn
Lat Ventricle

Falx Cerebri

Superior Sagittal Sinus

Figure 1.3   *Axial Cross Section.*

The posterior limb contains the corticospinal tract, rubrospinal tract, thalamocortical tracts, and occipitopontine tracts. The visual system uses a distinct white matter pathway that originates from the lateral geniculate nucleus of the thalamus. From here, visual information enters the primary visual cortex of the occipital lobe via the optic radiations. There are two sets of projections: one set runs in the temporal lobe (Meyer's loop) and terminates on the inferior bank of the calcarine fissure of the occipital lobe, and the other set runs in the parietal lobe and terminates on the superior bank of the calcarine fissure. Because the image on the retina is inverted, the superior bank of the calcarine fissure receives information from the inferior visual field and the inferior bank receives information for the superior visual field.

Other projection fibers include the uncinate fasciculus, which connects the temporal and frontal lobes, networking parts of the limbic system (i.e., hippocampi and amygdala) with the orbitofrontal cortex. The exact function of this system is unclear, but lesions have been implicated in anxiety, schizophrenia, depression, and Alzheimer's disease. The cingulum is a group of white matter association fibers that runs just beneath the gray matter of the cingulate gyrus and connects with the parahippocampal gyrus; lesions cause memory impairment and impaired emotional responsiveness.

DEEP CEREBRAL STRUCTURES

Subcortical gray structures include all nuclei that are not in the cerebral cortex or brainstem. The basal ganglia, basal forebrain, limbic system, memory systems, and diencephalon will be discussed here.

BASAL GANGLIA

The basal ganglia are a collection of nuclei that are located deep within the cerebral hemispheres and are associated with learning, movement, emotions, and cognition. The basal ganglia have five main components: the caudate, the putamen, the globus pallidus interna (GPi) and globus pallidus externa (GPe), the subthalamic nucleus (STN), and the substantia nigra. The caudate and putamen together are termed the striatum and are separated only by the internal capsule. The caudate is divided into a head, body, and tail, with the head located in the frontal lobe and extending posteriorly along the lateral wall of the lateral ventricle. It is a C-shaped structure that curves back and dives into the temporal lobe, where it becomes the tail. Degeneration of the caudate is implicated in Huntington's disease and responsible for the motor tics of Tourette syndrome. Degeneration of the caudate and putamen causes abnormal dance-like movements known as chorea.

The putamen is a dopaminergic structure that regulates movements and influences learning. It is the outermost portion of the basal ganglia, found lateral to the internal capsule. The putamen receives direct input from the cortex and other areas and projects to the globus pallidus. The globus pallidus (Latin for "pale globe") is found lateral to the internal capsule but medial to the putamen. It has two parts: the external part and the internal part, with projections extending to the substantia nigra. Neurons in the substantia nigra project to the putamen to activate dopamine receptors, thereby modulating movement. Two other important structures are the STN and the substantia nigra. The STN lies just inferior to the thalamus, is associated with hemiballismus (flailing arm movements), and is a common target for deep brain stimulation for Parkinson's disease and obsessive-compulsive disorder [8]. The substantia nigra is located in the brainstem with degeneration being responsible for Parkinson's disease. Like the cerebellum, the basal ganglia has no direct connections with the spinal cord and thus cannot initiate movement but instead can only modulate movement.

BASAL FOREBRAIN

The basal forebrain consists of multiple nuclei within the ventromedial frontal lobe that are responsible for memory, inspiration, and emotion. Some authors include the nucleus accumbens and ventral pallidum (reward circuitry), as part of the basal ganglia. The nucleus accumbens is a small nucleus within the striatum, located where the caudate and putamen are not divided by the internal capsule. It is a reward center that contains many opioid receptors and plays an important role in pleasure (e.g., food, sex, drugs), addiction, laughter, aggression, and fear. The nucleus basalis of Meynert, located ventral to the anterior commissure, has wide projections to the cortex and is rich in acetylcholine.

It is extremely important for memory, and its degeneration causes Alzheimer's disease. The septal nuclei are located anterior to the anterior commissure at the bottom of the septum pellucidum. The lateral septal nuclei receive input from limbic structures (i.e., amygdala), and the medial septal nuclei are associated with memory structures (i.e., hippocampus). Impairment, which commonly occurs during hemorrhage of an Acomm aneurysm, can lead to disinhibited behavior—what some describe as a patient being "Acommish."

LIMBIC SYSTEM AND MEMORY

The limbic system forms the inner border of cortex. It helps to control mood and performs internal evaluation of the environment. It denotes significance to experience and controls the emotional aspects of memories. Multiple areas are associated with the limbic system, including the amygdala, hippocampus, hypothalamus, cingulated gyrus, and nuclei within the basal forebrain. The amygdala (Latin for "almond") is composed of many small nuclei located at the most anterior portion of the inferior temporal horn of the lateral ventricle. It lies just anterior to the hippocampus in the temporal lobe and communicates with the hypothalamus and basal forebrain. The amyglala has a primary role in the processing, motivation, and emotional response of memory, particularly those related to reward and fear. Lesions of the amygdala result in Kluver-Bucy syndrome, which leave patients placid, hyperoral, hyperphagic, hypersexual, and with visual, tactile, and auditory agnosia (inability to recognize objects).

The hippocampus is required for memory consolidation (formation of long-term memories) and is located in the temporal lobe along the medial wall of the temporal horn of the lateral ventricle, just posterior to the amygdala. An axon bundle (the fornix) travels posteriorly and in a C-shaped pattern along the medial wall and floor of the lateral ventricle, eventually becoming attached to the bottom of the septum pellucidum. The fornix then splits at the anterior commissure and connects to the medial septal nuclei and the mamillary bodies of the hypothalamus. The majority of the fibers synapse at the mamillary bodies, which are two bumps posterior to the pituitary stalk (infundibulum), located on the undersurface of the brain. They can be seen clearly during endoscopic intraventricular surgery, such as the already mentioned endoscopic third ventriculostomy. Axons leaving the mammillary bodies become the mammillothalamic tract and synapse in the anterior nucleus of the thalamus and amygdala, with this circuit loop known as the Papez circuit because of its crucial role in storing memory. Damage to the mammillary bodies can result from thiamine (vitamin B1) deficiency and is implicated in the pathogenesis of Wernicke-Korsakoff syndrome. It may also cause anterograde amnesia (inability to lay down new memories), visual changes, and ataxia.

Removal of both hippocampi can also lead to permanent anterograde amnesia. This was first reported in a man (patient H.M.) who had both hippocampi resected during a temporal lobe operation for epilepsy [9]. After the operation, he could no longer lay down new memories, but remote memories were intact. Short-term memory was intact, but he could not consolidate his short-term memory into long-term memory. He could acquire new procedural memory, in which he would become more proficient at difficult motor tasks, but he could not recall being taught these aptitudes. Additional limbic structures include the parahippocampal gyri (spatial memory formation), cingulate gyrus (memory function, attention, autonomic functions), entorhinal cortex (memory formation and consolidation), piriform cortex (involved in smell), and the pituitary, hypothalamus, and thalamus, which will be discussed later.

DIENCEPHALON

The diencephalon is divided into four major nuclei: the thalamus, the hypothalamus, the subthalamus, and the epithalamus.

The thalamus is composed of a variety of nuclei and is thought to be a large relay station because nearly all pathways that project to the cerebral cortex synapse here. Pathways that connect through the thalamus include motor inputs, limbic inputs, sensory inputs, and all other inputs. The anterior nucleus, found at the rostral end of the dorsal thalamus, receives input from the mammillary bodies via the mamillothalamic tract, which in turn projects to the cingulate gyrus. These nuclei are involved in alertness, learning, and memory. The cingulate gyrus is located just superior to the corpus callosum and is important for memory consolidation. The ventral anterior/ventral lateral nucleus is located in the anterior and lateral portions of the thalamus and helps to coordinate and plan movement and to learn movements. It receives input from the basal ganglia and cerebellum and sends output to the precentral gyrus and motor association cortices. The ventral posterolateral nucleus is located in the posterior and lateral portion of the thalamus and relays somatosensory spinal cord input to the cerebral cortex. The ventral posteromedial nucleus (VPM) receives sensory information from the face via the trigeminal nerve (CN V). The medial geniculate nucleus is located at the posterior and medial portions of the thalamus and is involved in auditory processing—remember "M" for music. The LGN is found just lateral and slightly more posterior to the medial geniculate nucleus and is the synapse of the optic tracts—recall "L" for light. The two thalami communicate with each other via the massa intermedia (interthalamic adhesion), which crosses within the third ventricle. Lesions in the thalamus may result in contralateral sensory deficits or thalamic pain syndrome, which is characterized by hypersensitivity to pain. This is usually caused by disruption of the PCA, which is the dominant vascular supply to the thalamus. Bilateral lesions, or a unilateral lesion that exerts a mass effect on the other thalamus, may render the patient comatose either directly or from midbrain involvement. Lesions may also render patients akinetic or mute.

The hypothalamus, located just beneath the thalamus and above the brainstem, forms the most rostroventral portion of the diencephalon. It is responsible for maintaining homeostatic functions that include body temperature, hunger, sleep, fatigue, circadian rhythms, and sex drive. Some use the mnemonic of the "4 Fs" to remember its functions: feeding, fighting, fleeing, and sex. The hypothalamus is composed of many small nuclei and links the CNS to the endocrine system via the pituitary gland by synthesizing secreting neurohormones (hypothalamic-releasing hormones) that then either stimulate or inhibit secretion of pituitary hormones. A distinct groove along the wall of the third ventricle, known as the hypothalamic sulcus, separates the rostral hypothalamus and caudal subthalamus from the thalamus and epithalamus. The ventral surface of the hypothalamus is composed of the optic chiasm, infundibulum (pituitary stalk that connects the hypothalamus with the pituitary), and mammillary bodies.

As mentioned earlier, the subthalamus contains many different nuclei, but the most important is the STN. The STN is located beneath the thalamus in the most caudoventral portion of the diencephalon. It communicates with the globus pallidus to modulate movement. Lesions in this nucleus produce hemiballismus (contralateral flailing arm and leg movements). For these reasons, it is commonly targeted when deep brain stimulation is used for the treatment of patients with Parkinson's disease.

The epithalamus is located at the most dorsal and posterior portion of the diencephalon. It includes a small protuberance under the splenium of the corpus callosum (the pineal gland) that produces melatonin. The epithalamus also contains the posterior commissure, which is located between the pineal gland and the most anterior portion of the cerebral aqueduct, and connects midbrain nuclei. A tumor within the pineal gland can produce mass effect on the brainstem near the superior colliculus, leading to Parinaud's syndrome (upgaze paralysis, loss of convergence, and nystagmus). Intracranial hypertension can also exert pressure on these nuclei and cause impaired upgaze or forced downgaze. Additionally, a mass lesion in the region can block the cerebral aqueduct, causing obstructive hydrocephalus.

CRANIAL NERVES

Cranial nerves emerge directly from the brain. There are 12 pairs of CNs; CNs I and II emerge from the cerebrum, and the remainder emerge from the brainstem in a rostral to caudal orientation. The purely motor CNs are III, IV, VI, XI, and XII; the purely sensory are I, II, and VIII; and the mixed are V, VII, IX, and X. Motor CN nuclei are located more ventrally and sensory CN nuclei are located more dorsally. Each nerve will be individually discussed next.

CN I (OLFACTORY NERVE)

The primary olfactory neurons are purely sensory and are located in the nasal cavity. Their axons form the olfactory nerves, which pass through the cribiform plate and make synaptic connections with second-order neurons in the olfactory bulb. From the olfactory bulbs, fibers project via the olfactory tracts, which run in the olfactory sulcus between the gyrus rectus and orbital frontal gyri, as it courses into the temporal lobe. Lesions of the olfactory nerves result in anosmia, but unilateral loss is usually unnoticed and bilateral loss may be perceived as decreased taste. Head trauma that damages the cribiform plate can lacerate the nerve, as can intracranial lesions at the base of the frontal lobes near the olfactory sulci. Additionally, a fracture of the cribiform plate is a common cause of CSF rhinorrhea, which usually requires surgical repair to prevent development of a permanent CSF fistula and/or meningitis. Foster-Kennedy syndrome, caused by injury to the olfactory sulcus (usually caused by a meningioma), results in anosmia, optic atrophy in one eye (from tumor compression), and papilledema (from elevated intracranial pressure)

CN II (OPTIC NERVE AND CHIASM)

The optic nerve is another purely sensory nerve that originates from the retinal ganglion cells. The optic nerves enter the intracranial cavity from the orbit via the optic canal. Half of the axons cross to the contralateral side of the brain in the optic chiasm. Given the crossing of fibers, inferior compression of the chiasm from a superiorly growing sellar mass (e.g., pituitary tumor or craniopharyngioma), results in a slowly developing bilateral loss of peripheral vision (bitemporal hemianopsia—loss of the nasal retina fields). After the chiasm, the name of the visual pathways becomes the optic tracts, which eventually terminate in the LGN of the posterolateral thalamus.

CN III (OCULOMOTOR NERVE)

The oculomotor nerve is purely motor and controls four of the six extraocular muscles (superior rectus, inferior rectus, medial rectus, and inferior oblique), as well as the levator palpebrae (eyelid) and the parasympathetic portion of pupillary constriction. The oculomotor nerve is also involved in the accommodation of the lens for near vision. It exits between the interpeduncular fossa of the midbrain. The preganglionic parasympathetic neurons are located in the Edinger-Westphal nucleus of the midbrain, synapsing in the ciliary ganglion of the orbit with postganglionic parasympathetic fibers before passing to the papillary contrictors.

After leaving the midbrain, the oculomotor nerve transverses the cavernous sinus and then enters the orbit via the superior orbital fissure. Intracranial hypertension may cause compression of CN III, producing symptoms that include an eye that is deviated down and out (due to unopposed activity of the superior oblique and lateral rectus), a droopy eyelid (ptosis), and a dilated pupil (due to loss of parasympathetic innervation to the papillary sphincter muscles

CN IV (TROCHLEAR NERVE)

The trochlear nerve is the only nerve to exit from the dorsal brainstem (specifically the midbrain) and is located just caudal to the inferior colliculus. The trochlear nerve controls the superior oblique muscles, which depresses and internally rotates the eye. It is a purely motor nerve and because it innervates only one muscle, is the smallest of the nerves. The nerve travels around the brainstem to exit near the posterior region of the cavernous sinus. After traversing the cavernous sinus, it enters the orbit via the superior orbital fissure. The long and tortuous course of the trochlear nerve makes it susceptible to injury during surgery. The trochlear nerve is exquisitely sensitive to manipulation and patients often experience at least a transient 4th nerve palsy following a transtentorial approach to the posterior fossa. Trochlear palsy causes vertical diplopia, which the patient can improve by tilting the head away from the affected side.

CN V (TRIGEMINAL NERVE)

The trigeminal nerve is a mixed motor and sensory nerve that mediates cutaneous and proprioceptive sensations from the skin, muscles, joints in the face and mouth, and sensory innervation of the teeth. It is the afferent limb of the corneal ("blink") reflex and also mediates the jaw jerk reflex. The trigeminal nerve exits from the middle of the lateral pons, innervating the muscles of mastication and providing sensory input from the face. It has three major branches, termed the ophthalmic (V1), maxillary (V2), and mandibular (V3) divisions. After exiting the pons, the nerve enters Meckel's cave (a small fossa near the cavernous sinus) where the trigeminal ganglion is located. V1 travels through the cavernous sinus and exits the skull via the superior orbital fissure. V2 exits the skull via the foramen rotundum and V3 via the foramen ovale. Some authors use the mnemonic *Standing, Room, Only* to recall the three skull foramina that the trigeminal nerve exits through.

The trigeminal nuclei run from the midbrain to the upper cervical cord. Sensory fibers mediating fine touch and pressure enter the pons and synapse in the chief (principal) sensory nucleus, which is analogous to the posterior columns of the spinal cord. From here, the fibers cross via the trigeminal lemniscus to synapse in the VPM of the thalamus, and from there to the primary somatosensory cortex. Touch and pressure sensation from the oral cavity remains ipsilateral. Pain and temperature sensory fibers for the face enter the pons, travel through the spinal trigeminal tract, and then synapse in the spinal trigeminal nucleus, which is analogous to the anterolateral pathway of the spinal cord. From here, the pathway crosses as the trigeminothalamic tract and ascends to the VPM of the thalamus and then to the primary somatosensory cortex. The mesencephalic trigeminal nucleus and tract convey proprioception from the muscles of mastication, tongue, and extraocular muscles. The motor root of the trigeminal nerve joins V3 to exit the skull via the foramen ovale and then innervates the muscles of mastication. Sensory loss can be caused by mass lesions, trauma, or infection (i.e., herpes zoster). Lesions of the trigeminal brainstem nuclei results in ipsilateral facial sensory loss.

CN VI (ABDUCENS NERVE)

The abducens nerve innervates the lateral rectus and abducts the eye. It is a purely motor nerve that emerges at the caudal edge of the pons at the pontomedullary junction, close to the midline. It then traverses the cavernous sinus and enters the orbit through the superior orbital fissure. The abducens nuclei are located in the pons, and injury results in horizontal diplopia. Intracranial hypertension may cause a sixth nerve palsy and diplopia. Of all the CNs that traverse the cavernous sinus, it is the most medial.

CN VII (FACIAL NERVE)

The anatomy of the facial nerve is extremely complicated. It is a mixed nerve that innervates the muscles of facial expression, the orbicularis occuli, and forms the efferent limb of the corneal reflex. It also is the parasympathetic innervation for the salivary glands and lacrimal glands via the nervus intermedius. It mediates taste sensation from the anterior two-thirds of the tongue (via the chorda tympani), and innervates the skin of the external ear. Of note, nontaste sensation of the tongue is supplied by V3 of the trigeminal nerve. Taste and nontaste sensation to the posterior third of the tongue is supplied by the glossopharyngeal nerve (CN IX). Taste for the palate, posterior pharynx, and epiglottis is from the vagus nerve (CN X). The taste fibers enter the solitary tract of the medulla and synapse in the solitary nucleus, and ascend to thalamus via the central tegmental tract.

The facial nucleus is located in the pons, with its efferent fibers located dorsally around the abducens nuclei, forming the facial colliculus on the floor of the fourth ventricle. Lesions of the primary motor cortex (or corticobulbar tract) cause contralateral face weakness with sparing of the forehead. Ipsilateral weakness of the entire face is caused by peripheral nerve lesions (i.e., Bell's palsy) or lesions of the facial nucleus. The facial nerve is found far laterally in the cerebellopontine angle (CPA), adjacent to CN VIII. It then enters the internal auditory meatus and travels through the

auditory canal, giving off branches before it eventually exits the skull at the stylomastoid foramen. After passing through the parotid gland, it divides into five major branches: temporal, zygomatic, buccal, mandibular, and cervical (mnemonic = "To Zanzibar By Motor Car").

CN VIII
(VESTIBULOCOCHLEAR NERVE)

The vestibulocochlear nerve is a purely sensory nerve that is responsible for hearing, balance, postural reflexes, and orientation of the head in space. It often appears as one nerve with two ridges, which represent the auditory and vestibular portions of the nerve. It emerges far laterally, in the cerebellopontine angle, where it is closely associated with CN VII. This concept of CNs VII and VIII running in close association is extremely important during resections of vestibular schwannomas (also known by their older name of acoustic neuromas) because identification of the facial nerve is of utmost significance to prevent the patient from having an ipsilateral, peripheral facial palsy. The vestibulocochlear nerve with the facial nerve travels through the auditory canal to reach the cochlea and vestibular organs. The hearing pathways ascend through the brainstem bilaterally and synapse in the obligatory inferior colliculi, then the medial geniculate nuclei, and eventually the primary auditory cortex, via multiple decussations. For this reason, lesions in the CNS proximal to the cochlear nuclei will not result in unilateral hearing loss. Injury to CN VIII can cause unilateral hearing loss or dizziness and vertigo, depending upon the lesion.

The vestibular nuclei are responsible for posture, maintenance of eye position in response to movements, and muscle tone. They have multiple connections with the brainstem, cerebellum, spinal cord, and extraocular systems. The medial longitudinal fasciculus (MLF) is responsible for coordinating eye movements together and receives major contributions from the vestibular nuclei. It interconnects the abducens and oculomotor nuclei in horizontal gaze. For example, looking to the left activates the left abducens nerve and the corresponding right occulomotor nerve, so that both eyes look left together. Because this is a heavily myelinated pathway, patients with multiple sclerosis may have an MLF lesion, which causes an internuclear ophthalmoplegia (INO) in which the eyes do not move together during horizontal gaze.

CN IX (GLOSSOPHARYNGEAL NERVE)

The glossopharyngeal nerve is a mixed nerve with autonomic fibers that innervate the parotid gland and sensory fibers that mediates visceral sensations from the palate and posterior one-third of the tongue. The glossopharyngeal nerve also innervates the carotid body and is the sensory afferent limb for the gag reflex. The glossopharyngeal nerve has no real nucleus, but shares one with CNs VII and X. Because of its unclear demarcations in the brainstem, this shared nucleus is called the nucleus ambiguous. The nerve exits exclusively from the medulla and then leaves the skull via the jugular foramen.

CN X (VAGUS)

The vagus nerve is a mixed nerve with autonomic fibers that innervate smooth muscle in the heart, blood vessels, trachea, bronchi, esophagus, stomach, and intestine. The motor fibers originate in the nucleus ambiguous and innervate the striated muscles in the larynx and pharynx, which are responsible for swallowing and speech. The sensory component mediates visceral sensation from the pharynx, larynx, thorax, and abdomen and innervates taste buds in the epiglottis. The dorsal nucleus of the vagus contains secretomotor parasympathetic fibers that stimulate glands. The last nucleus is the solitary nucleus, which receives taste sensation, and information from blood pressure receptors and chemoreceptors. Injury to the recurrent laryngeal nerve during carotid endarterectomy, thyroid surgery, and anterior cervical disc surgery may cause unilateral vocal cord paralysis resulting in hoarseness.

CN XI (SPINAL ACCESSORY NERVE)

The spinal accessory nerve is a motor nerve that innervates the trapezius and sternocleidomastoid muscles. It emerges as a series of rootlets from the lateral sides of the first five cervical spinal cord segments, which then join to form the nerve before passing through the foramen magnum to enter the cranial cavity. The spinal accessory nerve finally exits the cranial cavity along with CNs IX and X.

CN XII (HYPOGLOSSAL NERVE)

The hypoglossal nerve is a motor nerve that innervates the intrinsic muscles of the tongue. It emerges from the medulla as a series of fine rootlets between the pyramid and the olive. Injury to the hypoglossal nerve causes the tongue to deviate towards the injured nerve.

BRAINSTEM

The brainstem is divided into three major regions: the midbrain, the pons, and the medulla. The brainstem contains the ascending and descending tracts that connect the spinal cord to the cerebrum, the CN nuclei, and connections to and from the cerebellum via three pairs of cerebellar peduncles. It is also responsible for motor and sensory innervation of the face and neck. The brainstem also regulates cardiac and respiratory function.

The corticospinal tract, posterior-column/medial lemniscus pathway, the spinothalamic tracts (anterolateral tract), descending hypothalamic axons, the medial longitudinal fasciculus (MLF), and the central tegmental tract travel through the brainstem. The corticospinal tract runs through the internal capsule, then through the cerebral peduncles (midbrain), then as the longitudinal fibers of the pons, and eventually the pyramids of the medulla before decussating on entry into the spinal cord. The medial lemniscus (the posterior column axons) is seen in all brainstem sections. The spinothalamic tract (pain and temperature) travels throughout the brainstem and is intermingled with the descending hypothalamic axons. The hypothalamic axons arise in the hypothalamus, coursing through the brainstem to exert control on preganglionic sympathetic and parasympathetic neurons in the brainstem and spinal cord. The preganglionic sympathetic neurons are located in the thoracic and lumbar spinal cord; hence the hypothalamic axons descend through the lateral portion of the brainstem (and run with the spinothalamic tracts) before they synapse on the intermediate horns of the spinal cord gray matter.

The reticular activating system (RAS) is located throughout the brainstem and is responsible for maintaining consciousness and regulating the sleep cycle. This is one of the reasons that increased intracranial pressure or downward herniation affects consciousness.

MIDBRAIN (MESENCEPHALON)

The midbrain is located between the diencephalon and the pons. The cerebral aqueduct is contained within the midbrain. Midbrain compression (e.g., herniation) can cause oculomotor nerve palsy, flexor (decorticate) posturing, and impaired consciousness. Two thick bands of white matter, known as the cerebral peduncles, are located at the most superior aspect of the midbrain and contain axons that are continuous with the internal capsule. Profound increases in intracranial pressure can cause uncal herniation, which compresses these peduncles and produces descending contralateral motor deficits. The space between the two cerebral peduncles is called the interpeduncular fossa, where the oculomotor nerve (CN III) exits the brainstem. The two superior colliculi are located on the dorsal surface of the midbrain, in addition to CN IV (trochlear nerve), which is just caudal to the inferior colliculus. The lateral lemniscus, located caudal to the interior colliculi, is a main auditory tract that carries information from cochlear nuclei and the superior olive on its way to the inferior colliculi. The superior colliculus (tectum) is involved in head and eye movement that occurs reflexively in response to visual stimuli. For example, when one sees something out of the corner of the eye, one reflexively turns the head to look at it. Similarly, the inferior colliculus sends axons to the superior colliculus that mediate reflexive orienting movements to sounds.

For example, when one hears a loud sound, one reflexively turns the head toward the sound. The inferior colliculus is also an obligatory relay nucleus in the auditory pathway and sends fibers to the thalamus and then to the primary auditory cortex.

The two red nuclei are located on each side of the brainstem. The red nucleus is involved in gross flexion of the upper body and has sparse control over the hands. Axons from the red nucleus relay information from the motor strip to the cerebellum through the inferior olive. Although the red nucleus is less important to motor function than the corticospinal tract, it coordinates crawling in infants. It facilitates flexion and inhibits extension of the upper extremities; thus, a lesion above the red nucleus results in disinhibition leading to flexion of the upper extremities in response to stimulation (decorticate posturing).

The cerebral aqueduct courses through the midbrain and is surrounded by the periaqueductal gray. The periaqueductal gray contains neurons that project to the raphe nuclei in the brainstem and are responsible for pain modulation and consciousness [10]. This is of clinical significance for neurosurgical procedures involving midbrain resections of tumors and cavernous malformations, as injury to the periaqueductal gray can result in a permanent coma. In terms of analgesia, opioids produce pain relief by binding to receptors located in the periaqueductal gray. Lateral to the periaqueductal gray is the mesencephalic tract of the trigeminal nerve, which courses through the brainstem. This nucleus is the only sensory ganglion that exists in the CNS and contains proprioceptive fibers from the jaw and mechanoreceptor fibers from the teeth. Some fibers go on to synapse in the motor nucleus of CN V (e.g., those responsible for the jaw jerk reflex).

PONS

The pons is located superior to the medulla, inferior to the midbrain, and anterior to the cerebellum. The fourth ventricle lies above the entire length of the pons. The pons is involved with regulation of rapid eye movement sleep, dreams, swallowing, facial expressions and sensation, posture, eye movements, balance, sexual arousal, and breathing (the pneumotaxic center controls the change from inspiration to expiration). The pons is divided into two parts: the basis pontis (a broad anterior bulge containing substantial pontine nuclei) and the pontine tegmentum (floor). Extending dorsolaterally from either side of the pons are large white matter tracts known as the superior, middle, and inferior cerebellar peduncles. As the corticospinal tracts travel through the pons, their name changes to the *longitudinal pontine fibers*. The pons also contains many discrete nuclei (pontine nuclei). The trigeminal nerve exits from the lateral pons and innervates the muscles of mastication and also carries sensation from the face. The facial motor nucleus is located in the pons with the axons curving dorsally and

rostrally to encircle the abducens nucleus. This bend to the facial nerve is called the *internal genu* with the axons wrapping around the abducens nuclei; the resultant bulge can be seen in the fourth ventricle as the facial colliculus. Injury to the facial colliculus will result in a ipsilateral peripheral facial palsy, and usually a concomitant abducens/horizontal gaze palsy given the close proximity of the facial nerve to the abducens nucleus. After the genu, the facial nerve exits just medial to the vestibulocochlear nerve at the pontomedullary junction. The abducens nerve exits ventrally from the nuclei, medial to the facial nerve.

MEDULLA

The medulla oblongata is the most caudal portion of the brainstem and is located between the pons and spinal cord. It contains the autonomic centers responsible for cardiac and respiratory functions. The chemoreceptor trigger zone (area postrema), which is also part of the medulla, is located in the floor of the fourth ventricle and is responsible for inducing vomiting. The junction of the medulla and spinal cord is located at the level of the foramen magnum. The medulla can be further divided into rostral (open) and caudal (closed) portions; the rostral medulla contains the fourth ventricle, which then closes off to become the central canal in the caudal medulla. The rostral medulla has prominent bulges known as the inferior olivary nuclei, which are associated with the cerebellum (overlying vermis and nodulus) and coordinate movements. On the ventral surface of the medulla are the pyramids, which are two longitudinal white matter elevations that descend the length of the medulla and eventually decussate. The pyramids are a continuation of the cerebral peduncles and contain the corticospinal tract. The dorsal column nuclei (soft touch) send axons that cross the medulla as internal arcuate fibers that form the medial lemniscus.

Many of the brainstem nuclei are located in the medulla. The hypoglossal nucleus is located in the ventrolateral portion of the central canal, with the nerve roots of the CN emerging from the medulla between the pyramids and olive. The nucleus of CNs IX, X, and XI is called the nucleus ambiguus and is located within the medullary reticular formation ventromedial to the nucleus and spinal tract of the trigeminal nerve. Dorsolateral to the hypoglossal nucleus is the dorsal motor nucleus of the vagus nerve (CN X). The solitary tract and nucleus are also located in the medulla and relay visceral sensation and taste from the facial, glossopharyngeal, and vagus nerves. The two vestibular nuclei can be seen at the medulla. The spinal trigeminal nucleus and the spinal tract of V are also located throughout the medulla, in a position analogous to the dorsal horn of the spinal cord. The spinothalamic (part of anterolateral system) and the dorsal and ventral spinocerebellar tracts continue their trajectory from the spinal cord. The inferior salivatory nucleus is close to the pontomedullary junction and controls the parasympathetic input to the parotid gland through the glossopharyngeal nerve. Both cochlear nuclei are located on the dorsolateral aspect of the inferior cerebellar peduncle.

CEREBELLUM

The cerebellum is responsible for modulating movement, including speed and force, learning of motor skills, and detection of movement errors. Like the basal ganglia, it modulates only upper motor neurons; there are no direct connections with lower motor neurons. The cerebellum is divided into three functional regions: the vestibulocerebellum, the spinocerebellum, and the cerebrocerebellum. The vestibulocerebellum is further subdivided into the flocculus and the nodulus, which assist in maintaining balance and equilibrium. The flocculi are found just caudal to the middle cerebellar peduncles, at the junction of the pons and medulla, and the nodulus is inside the fourth ventricle near the midline.

The spinocerebellum is made up of the vermis, which is located at the midline, and the paravermis, which is more lateral. The vermis modulates muscle movements in axial muscles (i.e., trunk and limbs) and the paravermis modulates movement in the distal gross muscles (i.e., the legs). On the inferior portion of the paravermis are two swellings called the tonsils, which may herniate through the base of the skull in the setting of intracranial hypertension. Congenital low-lying tonsils (i.e., Chiari malformation) can impair CSF outflow and lead to headaches or neurologic deficits if a syrinx develops in the spinal cord. Decompressive surgeries are aimed at treating the tonsilar herniation with a goal of restoring normal CSF dynamics. The cerebrocerebellum consists of the lateral portions of each cerebellar hemisphere, which regulate fine, complex movements (e.g., typing, piano playing).

VASCULATURE

Blood flow to the brain is supplied by two pairs of arteries: the internal carotid arteries (ICAs) and the vertebral arteries. The vertebral arteries enter the cranial cavity through the foramen magnum and join to become the basilar artery, which supplies blood to the posterior portion of the circle of Willis. The internal carotid arteries enter the skull through the carotid canals and supply the anterior circulation of the brain.

ANTERIOR CIRCULATION AND THE CIRCLE OF WILLIS

The ICAs travel along either side of the optic chiasm and then branch to form part of the circle of Willis (Figure 1.4). The circle of Willis is a circle of blood vessels on the ventral

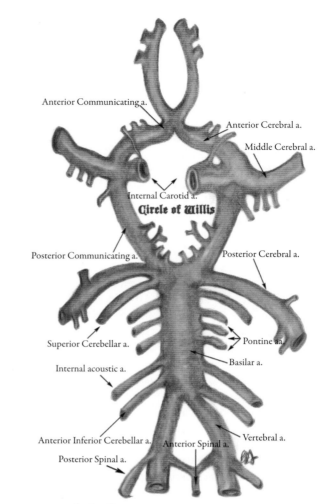

Figure 1.4   *Circle of Willis.*

surface of the brain that can, in theory, provide collateral circulation if flow through a vessel is damaged. It includes the PCA, posterior communicating artery (PComm), ACA, and the AComm. The PComms are small vessels that run posteriorly from the ICA to connect with the vertebrobasilar system. After entering the skull, the ICA branches into two main vessels: the ACA and MCA. The MCA supplies the lateral surface of the brain, traveling in the Sylvian fissure as it branches course over the lateral surface of the frontal, temporal, and parietal lobes. The lenticulostriate arteries are small penetrating branches off from the MCA that supply the putamen, globus pallidus, and internal capsule. The lenticulostriates are sensitive to blood pressure changes and can rupture in the setting of uncontrolled hypertension, causing a hemorrhagic stroke. The lenticulostriates are end arteries with no significant collateral circulation; the area that they perfuse will lose flow during profound hypotension, resulting in motor and sensory deficits. The medial lenticulostriate arteries arise from the ACAs and the lateral lenticulostriate arteries arise from the MCAs. Of note, some authors actually classify the perforating branches off the ACAs as "perforators" instead of lenticulostriates. Regardless, the largest branch off the ACA in this region is the recurrent artery of Heubner (medial striate artery), which supplies the head of the caudate and anterior limb of the internal capsule. The ACAs also originate from the ICA and run anterior and medially towards the midline, coursing over the corpus callosum, between the hemispheres in the longitudinal fissure, and supplying the medial aspect of the hemispheres as far back as the splenium. An ACA stroke can result in paralysis or sensory loss of the legs, whereas a MCA stroke can result in loss of paralysis or sensory loss of the face and/or arms. A MCA stroke of the dominant hemisphere may injure the language centers and produce aphasia.

VERTEBROBASILAR SYSTEM

The two vertebral arteries lie on either side of the medulla and join anteriorly at the caudal border of the pons to form the basilar artery. The vertebral arteries supply the medulla via small, penetrating branches. Basilar artery strokes usually are fatal because they cause the loss of cardiac, respiratory, and reticular activating function. Patients who survive may have a clinical syndrome known as locked-in syndrome in which the patient cannot move as the ventral brainstem tracts (motor) are destroyed, but the sensory tracts (more dorsal) may be left intact. These patients are unable to move, speak, or communicate with the world, except by blinking and possibly through upgaze. The anterior spinal artery branches off from the superior vertebral arteries, near the formation of the basilar artery, and runs caudally towards the spinal cord. The posterior inferior cerebellar artery (PICA) is the first major branch off the vertebral arteries and courses laterally, superiorly, and posteriorly, supplying the choroid plexus of the fourth ventricle, the inferior surface of the cerebellum, as well as the lateral medulla. The basilar artery supplies the pons through small penetrating vessels. The anterior inferior cerebellar artery (AICA) branches from the basilar artery and supplies the anterior and inferior portions of the cerebellum and the lateral pons. At the tip of the basilar artery are two bifurcations: the superior cerebellar arteries (SCAs), which supply the superior and dorsal portion of the cerebellum, and the PCAs, which supply the occipital lobe. Both the SCA and PCA help supply the lateral midbrain. The PCA runs above the tentorium cerebelli and the SCA courses below the tentorium cerebelli. The thalamoperforators originate from the tip of the basilar artery and the proximal PCA, entering the brain via the interpeduncular fossa before supplying parts of the thalamus and subthalamus.

VENOUS DRAINAGE

The septal vein is the primary drainage from the forebrain. It travels through the anterior septum pellucidum, joining the thalamostriate vein at the Foramen of Monro to become the internal cerebral veins. The internal cerebral veins then run along the roof of the third ventricle, eventually forming the great vein of Galen (great cerebral vein) under the splenium of the corpus callosum. This one central vein serves as the main drainage for all of the veins coming from the internal aspects of the cerebrum. The superior sagittal sinus is embedded in the superior aspect of the dura and drains the superior aspect of the brain. It is also responsible for recycling CSF. The superior sagittal sinus terminates at the confluence of the sinuses (torcular herophili) at the most posterior portion of the brain. The inferior sagittal sinus travels along the bottom of the falx cerebri and joins with the vein of Galen to become the straight sinus. The straight sinus then joins the superior sagittal sinus at the confluence, which then bifurcates to form the transverse sinuses. The transverse sinuses then makes as "S" turn in the posterior fossa to become the sigmoid sinuses before exiting the jugular foramen as the jugular vein.

SPINAL COLUMN

The spinal cord is a long tubular structure that contains a butterfly-shaped area of central gray matter that is surrounded by white matter and protected by a bony vertebral column. The anatomy of the spinal cord is nearly the obverse of the brain, in which gray matter is on the outside and white matter is on the inside. The spinal cord transmits information between the brain and the rest of the body, and mediates numerous reflexes. It extends from the medulla and continues through the conus medullaris to approximately the L1-L2 vertebrae, where it terminates as the filum terminale—a fibrous extension of meninges. The central gray matter is composed of a posterior (dorsal) horn that processes sensory information, an anterior (ventral) horn containing motor neurons, and an intermediate zone containing interneurons. The white matter is made up of posterior (dorsal) columns, anterior (ventral) columns, and lateral columns. The spinal cord varies in width; it is thickest in the cervical region because of the neural structures that run to and from the upper extremities. Like the brain, the spinal cord is also protected by meninges: the dura mater, the arachnoid mater, and the pia mater. The epidural space is filled with adipose tissue and contains a network of blood vessels. The subarachnoid space contains CSF and is in continuity with the brain. The spinal cord floats in the spinal column and is stabilized by denticulate ligaments, which are parts of pia that attach to the arachnoid and dura mater. The filum terminale provides longitudinal support, anchoring the cord to the coccyx.

The spinal cord is divided into 31 different segments, with spinal nerves exiting from each side of the cord. There are 8 cervical spine nerve pairs (C1-C8), 12 thoracic (T1-T12), 5 lumbar (L1-L5), 5 sacral (S1-S5), and 1 coccygeal pair; all nerve roots are, by definition, part of the peripheral nervous system. Spinal nerves are formed by the combination of dorsal and ventral roots exiting the cord and are mixed nerves, carrying motor, sensory, and autonomic information. Like the gray matter, the dorsal roots carry afferent sensory information and the ventral roots carry efferent motor axons. All of the spinal nerves except for C1 and C2 exit the spinal column through the intervertebral foramen, located between adjacent vertebrae. The C1 spinal nerves exit between the occiput and the atlas (first vertebra) and C2 spinal nerves exit between the posterior arch of the C1 vertebra and the lamina of the C2 vertebra. The conus medullaris is the terminal portion of the spinal cord and typically ends at approximately L1/2. Distal to this run the remaining peripheral nerve roots called the cauda equina. Each nerve roots goes on to supply muscles and skin, with each nerve's muscle area known as a myotome, and the sensory map the dermatome. After leaving the intervertebral foramen, the nerve branches into dorsal and ventral rami, which go on to innervate the muscles and skin of the posterior trunk and the remaining anterior parts of the trunk and the limbs. Some ventral rami combine with adjacent ventral rami to form a nerve plexus, such as the cervical, brachial, lumbar, and sacral plexi.

There are 33 vertebral segments: 8 cervical, 12 thoracic, 5 lumbar, 5 sacral (some authors count this as only 1 because it is fused), and 3 coccygeal segments. As the vertebral column grows longer than the spinal cord, the spinal cord level and bony vertebral segments do not correspond anatomically. For example, the lumbar and sacral spinal cord segments are found in the lower thoracic and upper lumbar spine. The spinal nerves for each segment exit at the level of the corresponding vertebrae, meaning that some nerves must travel a significant distance before exiting the canal. All spinal nerves exit below the corresponding vertebrae (e.g., the L5 spinal nerve exits below the L5 vertebrae), except in the cervical spine where there are 8 spinal nerves and only 7 vertebrae. Here, C1-C7 spinal nerves exit above the corresponding vertebrae and the C8 spinal nerve exits between the C7 and T1 vertebrae.

VASCULAR SUPPLY

The blood supply of the spinal cord arises from branches of the vertebral arteries and the spinal radicular arteries. The anterior spinal artery arises from the vertebral arteries near the formation of the basilar artery and travels along the ventral surface of the cord. The anterior spinal artery supplies approximately the anterior two thirds of the cord (the anterior horns and anterior-lateral columns). The dorsal surface of the cord is supplied by the posterior spinal arteries, which arise from the vertebral or posterior inferior cerebellar arteries. The posterior spinal arteries supply the posterior third of the cord, which includes the posterior columns and horns. As there are 31 bony spinal segments, 31 segmental arterial branches arise from the aorta and enter the spinal canal, with the majority of these vessels supplying the meninges.

Between six and ten branches actually supply the cord itself as radicular arteries. The most prominent of these vessels, the great radicular artery of Adamkiewicz, arises from the left side somewhere between T5 and L3, but most often between T9 and T12, and supplies the major portion of the lumbar and sacral cord. These radicular arteries can be injured during repair of a thoracic aortic aneurysm, resulting in loss of lower extremity motor function. In addition, a watershed zone exists from approximately T4 through T8, between the vertebral and lumbar arterial blood supplies. This region of the spinal cord is susceptible to infarction during periods of hypotension, especially when combined with external compression which impairs perfusion of this segment of the spinal cord (as with a tumor or herniated disc). The venous drainage of the spinal cord is through a plexus of epidural veins (Batson's plexus), which then drain into the systemic venous system. Epidural veins have no valves, meaning that infections and metastatic tumors can reflux into the spinal column (especially from the abdomen when intraabdominal pressure is increased). Additionally, increased thoracic pressure will lead to substantial reflux venous hemorrhage.

SPINAL CORD TRACTS

Sensory information is transmitted via the dorsal (posterior) column-medial lemniscus tract (touch, vibration, proprioception), the anterolateral (spinothalamic) system (pain and temperature), and the spinocerebellar tract. For the dorsal columns, the primary neuron enters the spinal cord and travels in these columns up to the lower medulla, and synapses with a secondary neuron in the dorsal column nuclei. If the first nerve enters below the spinal level of T6, it travels medially in the fasciculus gracilis (lower extremities), and if above T6, it travels laterally in the fasciculus cuneatus (upper extremities), with the first synapse in the respective nucleus gracilis or nucleus cuneatus.

The spinothalamic tract (anterolateral) first order neuron enters the spinal cord, ascends a few levels in Lissauer's tract, and synpases in the substantia gelatinosa. Second order axons from here decussate immediately in the spinal cord and ascend in the anterior lateral portion of the spinal cord, where it synapses in the ventral posterolateral nucleus of the thalamus. Thus, if you have a hemisection of the spinal cord, you will have ipsilateral loss of touch, proprioception, and vibration below the lesion, and contralateral loss of pain and temperature—clinically known as Brown-Sequard syndrome.

Proprioception, via the ventral and dorsal spinocerebellar tracts, ascends up the spinal cord to the cerebellum, with the primary neurons located in the dorsal root ganglia (DRG). These pathways involve two neurons, with the ventral spinocerebellar tract sending sensory information to synapse in the dorsal horn. Second order neurons then transverse to the ventral side in order to ascend to the cerebellum via the superior cerebellar peduncle. The dorsal spinocerebellar tract's first order neuron again is located in the DRG, which then synapses with the second order neurons in Clarke's nucleus, which then convey proprioceptive information to the cerebellum ipsilaterally via the inferior cerebellar peduncle. The last proprioceptive tract is the cuneocerebellar tract, which ascends ipsilaterally in the cervical spine to the cerebellum via the inferior cerebellar peduncle.

The motor fibers (corticospinal tract) use a two-neuron signaling pathway originating in the precentral gyrus. This pathway descends in the posterior limb of the internal capsule, through the cerebral peduncles, then down the pons as longitudinal fibers to become the medullary pyramids before decussating. The majority of fibers cross to the contralateral side as the lateral corticospinal tract and those that do not cross descend ipsilaterally as the ventral corticospinal tract. The axons of both pathways synapse on lower motor neurons in the ventral horns throughout the cord.

CONCLUSION

Through this chapter, we have sought to review basic terminology and orientation, the cerebral cortex, brainstem, and spinal cord, with selected emphasis on relating some of the anatomy to surgical approaches. By no means was this an exhaustive review, but only the tip of the iceberg. We hope this aids the anesthesiologist's understanding of anatomy. To close, we remind our readers of Dr. Paul Broca's quote: "There are in the human mind a group of faculties, and in the brain groups of convolutions, and the facts assembled by science so far allow to state, as I said before, that the great regions of the mind correspond to the great regions of the brain."

REFERENCES

1. Gerhardt von Bonin. *Essay on the Cerebral Cortex*. Charles C. Thomas, Springfield, Ill. 1950.
2. Benarroch EE. Blood-brain barrier: recent developments and clinical correlations. *Neurology*. 2012;78(16):1268–1276.
3. Ashton R, Conway A, Conway A, et al. Astrocytes regulate adult hippocampal neurogenesis through ephrin-B signaling. *Nat Neurosci*. 2012; 15(10):1399–1406.
4. Johnston M. The importance of lymphatics in cerebrospinal fluid transport. *Lymphat Res Biol*. 2003;1(1):41–44.
5. Bannur U, Rajshekhar V, Rajshekhar V. Post operative supplementary motor area syndrome: clinical features and outcome. *Br J Neurosurg*. 2000;14(3):204–210.
6. Brydges G, Atkinson R, Perry MJ, et al. Awake craniotomy: a practice overview. *AANA J*. 2012;80(1):61–68.
7. Larner AJ. Progressive non-fluent aphasia in a bilingual subject: relative preservation of "mother tongue." *J Neuropsychiatry Clin Neurosci*. 2012;24(1):E9–E10.
8. Mallet L, Polosan M, Jaafari N, et al. Subthalamic nucleus stimulation in severe obsessive-compulsive disorder. *N Engl J Med*. 2008;359(20):2121–2134.
9. Corkin S, Amaral DG, Gonzalez RG, et al. H.M.'s medial temporal lobe lesion: findings from magnetic resonance imaging. *J Neurosci*. 1997;17(10):3964–3979.
10. Hsieh K, Gvilia I, Kumar S, et al. c-Fos expression in neurons projecting from the preoptic and lateral hypothalamic areas to the ventrolateral periaqueductal gray in relation to sleep states. *Neuroscience*. 2011;188:55–67.

2.
THERAPEUTIC CONTROL OF BRAIN VOLUME

Leslie C. Jameson

The brain and the spinal cord are encased in a bony structure to support and protect them from the everyday trauma, but this protection has significant implications in the management of central nervous system (CNS) volume. In the cranium, the expansion of the primitive brain to a complex structure with a large cerebrum and cerebellum required significant additional structural support, which was accomplished by creating two relatively fixed dura-defined compartments. In the spinal cord, space occupying lesions compress normal parenchymal tissue causing damage to neurologic function in excess of the damage caused by the infiltrative lesion. Disruptions of spinal structures are major contributors to parenchymal tissue injury. The established volume imposed by these structures, dura and bony cranium, restricts the brain's ability to expand when the volume in one compartment exceeds the imposed limits and increased compartmental pressure occurs. Neurologic change, and often damage, ensues with parenchymal shift to another compartment, herniation. Common causes of volume expansion are local swelling, hemorrhage, tumor expansion, or cerebrospinal fluid (CSF) outflow obstruction. This inability to expand increases intracranial pressure (ICP) in either the affected compartment or throughout the cranium. Intracranial hypertension (ICH) causes cellular compression and decreased perfusion and may ultimately result in neuronal death.

The intracranial contents are composed of brain parenchyma (80% of intracranial volume [ICV]), CSF (8% to 12% of the ICV), and venous and arterial blood volume (6% to 8% and 2% to 4% of the ICV, respectively). These ranges represent normal fluctuations and the relative volume contributions. With normal ICV, physiologic events that can transiently increase both ICV and, potentially, ICP are of little consequence. When cerebral blood volume (CBV) increases (eg, Valsalva maneuver), for example, the CSF flows out of the cranium and its volume decreases. This results in no overall increase in ICP.

Although transient physiologic events produce brief, largely inconsequential changes in ICV and ICP

(Table 2.1), pathology has a significant impact on ICV and ICP. As with all closed containers, if a component volume increases *beyond* the ability of the other components' ability to compensate by decreasing their volume, the pressure in the container will increase. Measurement of ICP is therefore the most commonly used indirect method to detect changes in total ICV. Therapeutic decisions are often based on ICP as a surrogate for dynamic changes in ICV, while primarily computed tomography (CT) or occasionally magnetic resonance imaging (MRI) is used to accurately assess static volume [1].

The relationship between cranial volume and ICP is expressed as (1) *elastance*, the change in pressure in response to a change in volume ($\Delta P/\Delta V$), or (2) *compliance*, the change in volume in response to a change in pressure. The first studies that measured intracranial and intraspinal compliance used pressure as the independent variable (x axis) and volume as the dependent variable (y axis) [2]. Most studies published in the anesthesia literature and most of the classic anesthesia textbooks have therefore referred to compliance when they are actually discussing elastance (y-axis pressure, x-axis volume) [3]. Despite the confusion between elastance and compliance, the important issue is that a large increase in ICP can occur in response to a small increase in ICV. A clinician need only remember that a significant decrease in compliance or a significant increase in elastance indicates a condition that requires immediate attention.

BASIC PHYSIOLOGY

A brief overview of the basic physiology of the ICV components provides the knowledge that the practitioner needs to manipulate ICP. An in-depth discussion of these issues including physiologic mechanisms can be found in other chapters (see Chapters 1 and 3).

While CBV is the most dynamic component of brain contents, it contributes only a very small amount, 8% to

Table 2.1 CAUSES OF INTRACRANIAL PRESSURE INCREASES

PHYSIOLOGIC CAUSES	PATHOLOGIC CAUSES	
	Acute	*Chronic*
<ul><li>Increased abdominal/thoracic pressure (Valsalva, cough)</li><li>Relative hypoventilation (sleep, sedation)</li><li>Drug effect(general anesthetics, limited antibiotics)</li><li>Increased metabolic demands (seizures, fever)</li><li>Hypervolemia (fluid overload, head-down position)</li><li>Hypoperfusion (anemia, cerebral ischemia)</li></ul>	<ul><li>Intraparenchymal hemorrhage (hemorrhagic stroke, aneurysm rupture, postoperative intracranial hemorrhage)</li><li>Traumatic hemorrhage(epidural hematoma, acute subdural hematoma)</li><li>Acute cerebral edema (acute hyponatremia, hepatic coma, Reye's syndrome, cerebral contusion from traumatic brain injury [TBI], severe hypertension)</li></ul>	<ul><li>Slow-growing lesion (brain tumor—primary, metastatic, abscess)</li><li>Disturbance in CSF absorption, production, or flow (hydrocephalus, idiopathic intracranial hypertension)</li><li>Chronic subdural hematoma</li><li>Congenital anomalies (Arnold Chiari malformation, stenosis of aqueduct of Sylvius)</li></ul>

12%, to the total volume. Changes in blood pressure (BP), central venous pressure (CVP), arterial carbon dioxide ($PaCO_2$), oxygen content, and cellular activity produce rapid change by causing arterial vasoconstriction and vasodilation or restriction of venous outflow.

Four major vessels deliver arterial blood to the brain, the right and left vertebral and carotid arteries. The vertebral arteries combine to form the basilar artery and together perfuse the brainstem via the pontine arteries. The basilar artery becomes the posterior cerebral arteries and contributes to supratentorial blood supply via the circle of Willis. Likewise, the carotid artery becomes the middle cerebral artery and joins the circle of Willis. Thus, the supratentorial circulation includes the middle cerebral arteries but is dominated by the Circle of Willis, which distributes arterial blood flow to the cerebrum via anterior cerebral, posterior cerebral, and anterior and posterior communicating arteries.

The redundant arterial blood supply permits an on-demand response to cerebral metabolic requirements in normal brain: a rapid increase or decrease arterial in blood flow (CBF) and regional CBV in response to changes in regional brain activity. Alterations in regional or global CBF (mL/min) do not necessarily affect global arterial blood volume. Although increased metabolic demands may cause arterial vasodilation and therefore increased volume, redistribution of arterial flow or a decrease in venous volume may also occur. Cerebral perfusion CT can provide a rapid qualitative and truly quantitative evaluation of CBF [1] and is used primarily for estimating adequacy of region and global perfusion. In reality, however, there is no easy method to measure intracranial arterial or venous volume, and the safest clinical assumption is that increased demand means increased volume.

The brain has a very high metabolic rate, and to meet this demand, it requires approximately 15% of the cardiac output. Because the noncompliant cranium restricts total CBV and CBF, perfusion is tightly regulated through elaborate mechanisms that include chemical, myogenic, and neurogenic means. Chemical factors that rapidly alter CBF and CBV include alkalosis (vasoconstriction), acidosis (vasodilation), hypoxia (vasodilation), and local tissue factors (see Chapter 3).

Alterations in minute ventilation are the most rapid and readily available method to change arterial pH (pHa) and in turn modify CBF and CBV. Hypoventilation ($PaCO_2$ >45 mm Hg in healthy patients) causes respiratory acidosis and vasodilation, which then increases CBV. Alternately, hyperventilation ($PaCO_2$ <35 mm Hg in healthy patients) causes a respiratory alkalosis, which then causes cerebral vasoconstriction and decreases CBV in most settings. CBF/CBV varies directly with arterial carbon dioxide between 25 and 70 mm Hg with about a 2% CBF change for each 1–mm Hg change in $PaCO_2$. There is a prompt renal response to the respiratory alteration in pHa and more gradual correction of the change in pHa by the choroid plexus to correct the pHa toward normal and eliminate alkalosis or acidosis. If minute ventilation remains unchanged, pHa will return to normal (7.4) in approximately 6 to 12 hours [4–6]. Changes in cerebral perfusion and CBV are present only if pHa is abnormal. Thus hyperventilation produces arterial vasoconstriction for a relatively brief time. Within 8 hours of a $PaCO_2$ of 30 mm Hg, the pHa will be 7.4 due to this metabolic compensation. Allowing $PaCO_2$ to subsequently increase 10 mm Hg to 40 mm Hg will produce an acidosis and vasodilation, increasing CBF and CBV.

Cerebrovascular tone is not affected by hypoxia until PaO_2 falls below 60 mm Hg. At this point, rapid vasodilation occurs, which causes a marked increase in CBF/CBV. CBF may increase by 20% as PaO_2 falls from approximately 60 to 45 mm Hg [7].

It is, therefore, essential to maintain PaO_2 above 60 mm Hg threshold in patients with ICH who do not have preexisting pulmonary disease. Under normal circumstances, hypoxia is not an isolated respiratory finding since patients initially respond to hypoxia with hyperventilation. In high-altitude research after 3 to 4 weeks of chronic hypoxia, CBF has returned to normal. In patients with chronic hypoxia due to comorbid conditions, their PaO_2 response curve has shifted toward normal CBF at lower PaO_2 values [8].

Increased global or regional cerebral metabolic requirement for O_2 ($CMRo_2$) increases CBF/CBV. Agitation, seizures, rapid eye movement sleep, mental or physical activity and fever all increase $CMRo_2$ and, by implication, CBV/CBF. Temperature change has a direct effect on cerebral metabolic demand, with lower temperatures decreasing basal neuronal activity and $CMRo_2$. At 18°C, the CMR is about 10% of normal, which results a significant reduction in CBF and CBV. As the brain temperature increases, $CMRo_2$ increases with a concomitant increase in CBF and CBV to support changing cellular metabolic requirements. Mild hypothermia has been shown to decrease $CMRo_2$ and ICP [9].

Cerebral autoregulation, the capacity of the circulation to maintain a constant CBF over a wide range of cerebral perfusion pressures (CPPs), prevents major changes in cerebral perfusion in normal brain. During autoregulation, the cerebral vessels dilate and constrict to maintain perfusion at the required level. In the setting of brain injury or tumor, however, CBF/CBV can become directly related to CPP since the ability to appropriately alter vessel diameter is impaired. Increased BP independently increases CBF and CBV in abnormal but not normal brain, while decreased BP independently decreases CBF and CBV in abnormal but not normal brain. The range of systemic pressure over which cerebral autoregulation occurs varies with the patient. In general, maintaining the mean arterial pressure within ±30% of a patient's normal mean arterial pressure will keep CPP within the autoregulatory range. Many experts consider the lower limit of cerebral autoregulation to be 70 mm Hg in most adult patients [7, 10]. This is significantly higher than 55 to 60 mm Hg [10] that older studies considered to be acceptable. Exceeding the upper limit of autoregulation has a less well-defined effect on CBV. Interstitial fluid (tissue edema) is known to increase as a result of disruption of the blood–brain barrier (BBB), but the pressure threshold is unclear; eventually, hemorrhagic stroke may occur. Early studies in animal models and later studies in humans with a traumatic brain injury (TBI) found that when mean BP rose above 140 to 150 mm Hg, CBF, CBF, and ICP increased with each incremental increase in systemic pressure in patients without preexisting brain pathology [11, 12]. Maintaining mean arterial pressure near the normal value for each patient will maintain the status quo in terms of CBF/CBV.

Although most therapeutic interventions involve manipulation of the arterial component of blood volume, the venous component occupies 6% to 8% of the total ICV. The major veins include the superior sagittal sinus, the right and left inferior sagittal sinuses, transverse sigmoid sinuses, and, finally, the internal jugular veins. These vessels are often overlooked in the management of intravascular volume since their size is restricted by the dura and cranium. Venous drainage is passive, so any obstruction (eg, increased CVP), mechanical compression (eg, swelling, hemorrhage),

or reduction in diameter (eg, head turned, tumor compression) of these vessels will increase ICV. Maintaining adequate venous outflow will help to reduce ICP in most patients. To accomplish this, the head is maintained in a neutral position and elevated approximately 30 degrees, and actions that will increase CVP are avoided. Table 2.2 outlines general relationship between a variety of perturbations and CBF/CBV and, by inference, ICP. Pathologic states, such as cerebral venous thrombosis, can cause significant cerebral edema and elevated ICP [13].

CSF constitutes approximately 8% to 12% of the ICV; CSF volume is regulated by manipulating the ratio of production to resorption. Production is via passive filtration and active transport of the noncellular components of blood at the choroid plexus, while absorption occurs at arachnoid villa in dural sinusoids [14]. The CNS has about 150 mL of CSF, of which approximately 50% is in the cranium. CSF is produced at the rate of 450 to 600 mL/d [15]. Metabolic acids do not pass through the BBB and have little effect on the brain or CSF pH. Any intervention that increases the total CSF volume (increasing production, decreasing resorption, or obstructing outflow) can cause ICH. The effects of volatile anesthetics on CSF equilibrium are discussed elsewhere (see Chapters 9 and 10) but they are very small and have only been studied in animal models [16]. The only effective way to modulate CSF volume is through placement of a ventriculoperitoneal shunt, lumbar drain, or ventriculostomy. Changes in CSF volume are rapid and are one of the most effective methods used by the brain to maintain a stable ICP. Much of the intracranial elastance or compliance comes from changing CSF volume. Once this mechanism has been exhausted, very small increases in volume produce substantial increases in ICP.

Brain parenchyma, which occupies about 80% of the cranial volume, is composed of intracellular and extracellular components. The constituents of extracellular fluid and intracellular contents are maintained by the BBB, a combination of glial cells and vascular tight junctions. The BBB tightly controls the exchange of fluid, electrolytes, and glucose; it normally allows only small molecules (eg, Na^+, K^+) to enter the extracellular fluid space, where it is available to the cellular components. Glucose enters through active transport, but very large molecules (eg, albumin) are generally excluded.

Parenchymal edema is usually due to failure of the BBB. When the BBB fails, excess extracellular fluid and intracellular fluid accumulate, usually in the white matter [17]. Fluid leak can be caused by traumatic or pathologic disruption of the BBB (e.g., traumatic brain injury, tumor), severe systemic hypertension [18], passive fluid passage with reduced osmotic pressure, hyperglycemia, elevated venous pressure (compressive edema), and elevated CSF pressure (hydrocephalic edema). The threshold for BBB failure varies and is lower in abnormal vessels. Expansion of extracellular or intracellular volume is the most common cause of ICH. While CSF and

Table 2.2 THE EFFECT OF COMMON MEDICAL AND SURGICAL ACTIONS ON INTRACRANIAL PRESSURE

ACTION	EFFECT ON BRAIN	ICP RESPONSE
Physiologic		
↓ Paco₂ 25–30 mm Hg (<8 h)	Arterial vasoconstriction	↓
↓ Paco₂ 25–30 mm Hg (>8 h)	None	↔↑
↓ Pao₂ (<50 mm Hg)	↑ CBF/volume	↑
↑ BP	↓ Vascular volume	↔↓
↓ BP	↑ Vascular volume	↑
↑ CVP	↑ Venous volume	↑
Jugular venous obstruction	↑ Venous volume	↑
Head elevation	↓ Venous volume	↓
Agitation/seizures	↑ CMR/CBF/CBV	↑
Drugs to Reduce Parenchyma Volume		
Mannitol	↓ Interstitial fluid	↓
Hypertonic saline (3%)	↓ Interstitial fluid	↓
Furosemide	↓ CSF production, cellular edema	↓
Dexamethasone—TBI	No effect—TBI ↓ interstitial fluid	↔
Tumor intraoperative		↓*
Drugs used for Anesthesia or Sedation Effects		
Volatile anesthetics (>0.75 MAC)	↑ Arterial/venous volume	↑
Nitrous oxide	↑↔ CMR	↔↑
Intravenous Anesthetics		
Propofol	↓ CBF/CMR	↓
Barbiturate	↓ CBF/CMR	↓
Dexmedetomidine	↓ CBF	↓
Ketamine	↑ CBF, ↑ CMR	↑↔
Narcotics	↓ CBF/CMR	↔
Benzodiazepines	↓ CBF	↓↔
Muscle relaxants	↔	↔
Nondepolarizing	None	↔
Succinylcholine	↑ CVP	↑ (brief)
Cardiovascular Drugs		
Vasodilators	↑ Vascular volume	↑
Vasoconstrictors	↔↓ Vascular volume	↔↓
Surgical Interventions		
Intraventricular catheter	Removal of CSF	↓
Remove space occupying lesion (tumor, hematoma)	Removal parenchymal tissue	↓
Decompressive craniectomy	Removal parenchymal tissue	↓

*Late effect by reducing interstitial fluid and inflammation.

BP, blood pressure; CBF, cerebral blood flow; CBV, cerebral blood volume; CMR, cerebral metabolic rate; CVP, central venous pressure; TBI, traumatic brain injury.

blood can move into or out of the cranial vault in response to changes in volume and pressure, parenchymal tissue cannot. Once the compliance of CSF and CBV is exhausted, a small increase in volume from any source results in a large increase in ICP or a compartment pressure.

Tumors are the most common cause of increased parenchymal volume. Gradual displacement of functional brain with abnormal cells often remains asymptomatic until the patient presents with symptoms of ICH or neurologic impairment (eg, sensory or motor deficits, seizures). Studies using laser Doppler flowmetry suggest that tumors have lower CBF than normal brain tissue, but the autoregulatory response to Paco₂, Pao₂, or changes in BP is absent [19, 20]. Hyperventilation or hypertension may therefore shift local blood flow into the tumor, increasing its volume. Elevated ICP occurs when all compensatory mechanisms have been exhausted and is therefore a late finding in most patients with an intracranial tumor.

Rate of volume change significantly impacts the brain's ability to compensate. The more rapid the change in volume, the less likely it is that reductions in intravascular volume, CSF volume, or extracellular fluid volume will be effective at maintaining normal compartmental ICP. Thus, TBI, intraparenchymal hemorrhage (trauma or subarachnoid hemorrhage (SAH), and subdural or epidural hematoma all rapidly increase ICV and ICP. Attempts to estimate brain compliance (eg, midline shift, ventricle size, tumor edema, herniation of tissue outside compartment) using imaging are only modestly successful. The overall effects of changes in BP, $PaCO_2$, and PaO_2 on ICV/ICP are not completely predictable in any given patient with a parenchymal abnormality. Clinicians must be prepared to treat ICH and they must be aware that a physiologic response to a given intervention may not occur as expected.

MANAGEMENT OF ICP

ICP is altered by body position, clinical pathology (eg, tumor, chronic hydrocephalus), and age [21], In an adult, ICP is usually considered normal at between 7 and 15 mm Hg when the individual is supine; however, the mean ICP is negative (between –10 and –15 mm Hg) in the upright position [22]. ICH is defined as ICP >20 mm Hg.

The decision to treat ICH depends on the underlying pathophysiology. Although ICH is usually categorized as mild (20–29 mm Hg), moderate (30–40 mm Hg), or severe (>40 mm Hg), it is best to discuss with the neurosurgeon or neurointensivist the specific ICP goal for the patient [21]. In a patient with hydrocephalus, an ICP of 15 mm Hg may be abnormally high, especially if the patient has a ventriculoperitoneal (VP) shunt. Most VP shunts have a programmable pressure valve that allows the intracranial pressure to be adjusted to provide optimal relief of the patient's symptoms. In a patient with head injury, an ICP of <20 mm Hg is considered to be ideal, but an ICP of 25 mm Hg may need to be tolerated but managed aggressively.

Pathologic increases in ICP have the potential to cause brain injury, with the extent of the injury frequently depending on the cause as well as the rate of increase. A slow increase in ICP can be caused by a gradual increase in volume (eg, brain tumor, hydrocephalus) and may require little immediate therapeutic action. A rapid increase in ICP can require urgent therapy. *Critical ICP* is defined as a pressure that causes a critical reduction in CPP (mean systemic BP minus ICP) [23]. Older textbooks have defined critical CPP as <50 mm Hg, but recently the Brain Trauma Foundation has, based on their outcome data in head-injured patients, redefined critical CPP to be between 50 and 70 mm Hg depending on the age and comorbid conditions of the patient.

The clinical presentation of elevated ICP also depends to some extent on the rate at which ICP increases. If ICV increases slowly, an estimated 80-mL reduction [24] in the volume of normal cranial contents can occur before cranial elastance/compliance is exhausted and an elevation in ICP occurs. This accommodation occurs because of a reduction of CSF volume and extracellular fluid and movement of the brain tissue. If volume increases rapidly, compensatory mechanisms are markedly impaired with decreases in CSF and CBV the only possible mechanism. In general, increases in ICV become symptomatic when ICP begins to rise.

PATIENT ASSESEMENT

When evaluating a patient with the potential for increased ICP, it is important to estimate location of the patient's ICP on the compliance curve; this information will direct intraoperative management. Symptoms of mildly elevated ICP include a headache that worsens with lying flat, breath-holding, or a Valsalva maneuver (Table 2.3). Moderately elevated ICP produces symptoms that include nausea, vomiting, dizziness, blurred vision, difficulty concentrating, and memory lapses. Abnormal respiratory patterns may also occur. Neurologic symptoms that improve with steroid therapy suggest a previously significant elevation in ICP and the potential for ICH with any maneuver that increases cranial volume. The finding of papilledema on

Table 2.3 SIGNS AND SYMPTOMS OF INCREASED INTRACRANIAL PRESSURE

MILD ELEVATION (20–29 MM HG)	MODERATE ELEVATION (30–40 MM HG)	SEVERE ELEVATION (>40 MM HG)
• Unrelenting positional headache • Nausea and vomiting • Papilledema • Blurred vision • Loss of retinal venous pulsations	• Confusion and agitation • Drowsiness progressing to lethargy • Decreased papillary response (constriction, dilation), sluggish • Seizures • Spontaneous hyperventilation • Focal motor weakness	• Progressive decreased consciousness • Anisocoria (asymmetrical pupils) • Tonic eye deviation • Seizures • Decerebrate posturing • Cushing's reflex • Abnormal respiratory pattern • Hypotension • Death

a funduscopic examination is a very nonspecific sign. In one study, only 3.5% of patients with TBI and elevated ICP had papilledema when examined by a qualified ophthalmologist [25]. New-onset systemic hypertension may occur in the setting of increased ICP and is caused by autoregulatory mechanism attempts to maintain adequate CPP [12, 26].

The definitive diagnosis of ICH is made using an intraventricular ICP monitor or CT. Due to the invasive nature of ICP monitoring, CT has become the "gold standard" imaging technique to determine ICP. It is easily available and rapidly obtained and provides a high-resolution image. CT is routinely used for diagnosis and monitoring in patients with head trauma, basilar skull fracture, epidural or subdural hematoma, intraparenchymal and subarachnoid hemorrhage, cerebral edema, and cerebral contusion. Characteristic CT findings suggestive of elevated ICP include a decrease in ventricle size, decreased CSF around the basal cisterns, midline shift, loss of CSF between the cranium and brain, perifocal edema, and loss of definition of gyri or other brain structures. Brain herniation, the shift of intracranial contents into another compartment, may be present. MRI is useful in selected situation patients such as presurgical imaging of brain tumors or stereotaxic navigation but is not routinely performed for evaluating ICP [27].

Observations found on a neurologic examination usually depend on the location of the lesion or injury. As an example, a subdural hematoma on the left produces motor weakness on the right. Likewise, the signs and symptoms of brain herniation depend on the affected area of brain; the classic description is presented in Figure 2.1 [28]. Herniation often produces permanent neurologic sequelae and may be fatal. Nonspecific symptoms of herniation include obtundation, posturing, and Cushing's triad (also called Cushing response). Cushing's triad is usually described as severe systemic hypertension and bradycardia in the setting of increased ICP. Both bradycardia and tachycardia have been associated with ICH and systemic hypertension [26]. The absence of bradycardia should not delay treatment of critical ICP. Even in the absence of classic symptoms (Figure 2.1), the suspicion of brain herniation should trigger treatment.

Symptoms of brainstem herniation include third and sixth cranial nerve palsy, spontaneous hyperventilation progressing to an abnormal respiratory pattern (irregular, apneustic or apnea), and ultimately hypotension and death (Figure 2.1). Patients may exhibit decorticate posturing in which the arms are flexed or bent inward on the chest, the hands are clenched into fists, and the legs are extended and feet turned inward. Decorticate posturing is an ominous sign of severe brain damage that usually indicates injury of the cerebral hemispheres, the internal capsule, thalamus, and midbrain. Decerebrate posturing includes rigid extension of arms, legs, arching of the back, clenched teeth, and downward pointing toes. Decerebrate posturing can occur with any brainstem injury but is often associated with central transtentorial herniation. Decerebrate posturing usually suggests more severe injury than does decorticate posturing. Both require immediate treatment and, if surgery is indicated, the anesthetic technique must not risk further increases in ICP (Table 2.2) [29, 30].

The Brain Trauma Foundation published guidelines in 2007 for placement of an ICP monitor in patients with TBI (Table 2.4) [23, 30], and these guidelines are generally followed in all patients who experience a rapid increase in ICV (eg, SAH, stroke). Patients who meet the criteria for ICP monitoring during their preoperative assessment should be assumed to have ICH. To determine who will benefit from ICP monitoring, a careful neurologic assessment that combines the Glasgow Coma Scale (GCS), a directed neurologic exam, patient characteristics, and CT imaging must be performed. None of these characteristics alone predict who is at risk for developing ICH. Approximately 60% of patients with TBI who have an abnormal CT have ICH.

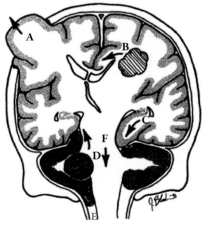

Category by Label	Symptoms
A. Transclival	Dependent on area of herniation
B. Subfalcine	Headache, Contralateral leg weakness
C. Transtentorial (Uncal)	Ipsilateral dilated pupil, contralateral hemiparesis, contralateral visual field loss, decorticate posture, decreased heart rate, respiratory abnormalities. (Ipsilateral hemiparesis possible with Kernohan's Notch, false localizer)
D. Transtentorial "Upward"	Nausea, vomiting, obtundation
E. Tonsillar	Headache to brainstem compression (heart rate and respiratory abnormalities)
F. Transtentorial Central	Bilateral arm dysesthesia, obtundation

Figure 2.1   Brain Herniation Syndromes. Brain contents protrude across dura to compartments with lower intracranial pressure. This results in six classically described syndromes. Many, if not most, brain herniation syndromes occur in combination or in combination with specific brain injuries. (Adapted from Fishman RA, Brain edema).

Table 2.4 **INDICATIONS FOR INTRACRANIAL PRESSURE MONITORING**

- **Glasgow Coma Scale (GCS) score <8 after resuscitation**
- **Abnormal head CT with evidence of brain edema/mass lesion effect**
- **Rapid neurologic deterioration plus clinical signs of increased intracranial pressure**
- **GCS score >8 but unable to follow serial neurologic examination due to**
  - **Drugs, anesthesia, prolonged non-neurologic surgery**
  - **Prolonged ventilation or use of positive end-expiratory pressure (eg, acute respiratory distress syndrome)**
- **Postneurosurgery for removal of intracranial hematoma**
- **Normal CT scan + 2 of the following**
  - **Age >40 y**
  - **Decerebrate or decorticate posturing**
  - **Systolic blood pressure <90 mm Hg**

Adapted from the text (2007; Brain Trauma, American Association of Neurological et al. 2007)

Only 4% of patients with a normal CT scan and no additional risk factors will develop ICH, but 60% of patients with a normal CT *and* two risk factors will develop ICH. ICP monitoring should be used in all patients with (1) an abnormal CT scan, (2) a normal CT scan plus two risk factors, or (3) a head injury who are going to receive a prolonged general anesthetic, especially when the surgery is not intended to treat the underlying cause of ICH.

ICP can be monitored with using a ventricular catheter or a transducer placed in the parenchyma, subdural space, or epidural space [32]. A ventricular catheter inserted into the lateral ventricle provides the most accurate pressure tracing and is therefore the preferred technique. It can measure elastance by showing ICP changes with vascular pulsations [22, 33] and can also be used to drain CSF to reduce ICV and ICP. When the lateral ventricle is compressed, CSF drainage becomes difficult and accurate pressure measurement can be lost. A saline-filled hollow screw can also be placed through the skull into the subdural/epidural space to measure ICP. This technique is associated with a lower risk of brain injury than the ventricular catheter, but it is considered to be less reliable and does not permit CSF drainage. It is ineffective if it becomes compressed between the brain and the cranium or if it is occluded by blood. An intraparenchymal fiberoptic microtransducer can be surgically inserted into the brain to monitor ICP. This device has several disadvantages: (1) it cannot be used to drain CSF, (2) device calibration may drift over time, and (3) when disconnected from the monitor it is impossible to recalibrate. All ICP monitors measure only the local pressure and may not reflect ICP elsewhere in the brain [22].

ICP is usually monitored continuously in patients with acute pathology. Until the cranium is opened, continuous ICP monitoring allows the clinician to observe pressure patterns and waveforms. Therapeutic decisions using patterns of ICP change require monitoring over extended periods of time (at least several hours) unless critical increases in ICP occur. Low and stable ICP (≤20 mm Hg) may be present following uncomplicated injury such as a mild TBI or a small SAH, but ICP may increase abruptly if significant cerebral edema develops [34]. High but stable ICP values are common in TBI, SAH, and parenchymal hemorrhage but should be aggressively treated. Ranges are discussed previously. A return to normal ICP is usually associated with an improved patient outcome.

Although anesthesiologists are rarely called on to interpret abnormal ICP patterns, understanding their significance allows appropriate modification perioperative management. Abnormal ICP patterns include vasogenic waves [35] ("B" waves), plateau waves, and "spikes" associated with a change in systemic BP. B waves are spontaneous slow waves (0.5 to 2 Hz) with an amplitude of about 20 mm Hg; they act as a warning sign of decreasing intracranial compliance and the exhaustion of the ability of the CSF to compensate for additional volume increase. Plateau waves are described as a sudden and rapid ICP elevation to >40 mm Hg that last for 5 to 20 minutes followed by an abrupt ICP decrease, usually to a value below baseline. Plateau waves are believed to be caused by the loss of effective autoregulation. The proposed cascade of events is active vasodilation that increases CBV. This in turn produces ICH and an associated decrease in CPP. Finally, active vasoconstriction reverses these events. Plateau waves have been associated with severe refractory ICH. More ominous are "spikey" waves that occur with changes in BP, even brief and temporary increases in mean systemic BP. Refractory ICH with ICP >100 mm Hg often leads to brain herniation and death. The anesthesiologist is most commonly confronted with this situation in the setting of a decompressive craniectomy and brain resection for refractory ICH.

INTERVENTION/TREATMENT

The specific strategy for decreasing ICP depends on the underlying cause. Correction of hyponatremia can reduce cerebral edema and return ICP to normal. Since interstitial and intercellular glucose mirrors serum glucose, rapid decreases in systemic glucose concentration can rapidly increase parenchymal volume and increase ICP as fluids enter the space to establish the new lower glucose concentration. During craniotomy, brain swelling may impair surgery or prevent dural closure. Treatment of cerebral edema may be required during the surgical procedure. Some studies recommend decompressive craniectomy to decrease life-threatening ICH.

Prevention or treatment of ICH or herniation consists of interventions that reduce ICV. In general, the therapeutic goals are to maintain ICP <20 to 25 mm Hg while maintaining CPP at ≥70 mm Hg (adult). Specific techniques that can be used to reduce the volume of specific intracranial components can be found in Table 2.2.

During a craniotomy, when the dura has been opened, the ICP is reduced to 0, but continued management of ICV is often necessary to provide good operative conditions. A longstanding, slight increase in ICP may require little change in medical management or anesthetic technique during surgery. Patients with indications of ICH, risk factors for impending ICP elevations, may require significant interventions to minimize increases in or reduce ICP.

The anesthesiologist has unique expertise to manage a patient with acutely elevated ICP. Acute medical management of a patient with increased or unstable ICP includes head of bed elevation to 30 degrees or as tolerated, hyperventilation, and the administration of osmotic agents and often propofol. Hyperventilation first by assisted mask ventilation, administration of propofol, followed by intubation will quickly reduce ICP. Fluid management for neurosurgical patients with or without elevated ICP emphasizes euvolemia and maintaining cerebral perfusion.

Administering a hyperosmotic solution such as mannitol or a 3% hypertonic saline solution can decrease brain volume. Furosemide may also be administered to reduce CSF production. The choice of osmotic agent is somewhat controversial. Hypertonic saline is being used at some centers, but mannitol remains the most commonly used osmotic agent. There is little evidence that hypertonic saline improves outcome [36]. Mannitol can cross into the interstitial space and may worsen brain edema. Hypertonic saline may also decrease ICP after a patient has become refractory to mannitol. The use of large amounts of hypertonic saline or normal saline may cause hypercholemic acidosis, which may in turn cause cerebral vasodilation and further increase ICP. Most clinicians are aware of these issues and choose to use mannitol for elevated ICP. Mannitol is typically administered in doses that range from 0.25 to 2 g/kg ideal body weight. Many neurosurgical teams have a "standard" dose between 70 to 100 g for all adult patients [37]. Mannitol should be administered as an infusion, not a bolus, over a minimum of 15 minutes. Bolus administration can lead to vasodilation and an impairment in the BBB [37]. Furosemide may also be used to reduce intravascular volume and reduce CSF production (see Chapter 10).

Hyperventilation will quickly reduce ICP until other interventions are effective. As discussed previously, the alkalosis produced by hyperventilation quickly diminishes. Studies in patients with TBI have firmly established that prolonged hyperventilation is associated with worse outcomes [4, 38, 39]. Although many neurosurgeons still request intraoperative hyperventilation, its use in this situation is designed to briefly improve operative conditions until a surgical solution is achieved. Minute ventilation is adjusted to produce a $PaCO_2$ of 28 to 30 mm Hg.

When the patient undergoes surgery, meticulous continuation of previous interventions and adoption of

Table 2.5 **CONSIDERATIONS TO REDUCE INTRACRANIAL PRESSURE IN THE OPERATING ROOM**

- **Patient positioning**
  - Maintain head elevation
  - Prevent increases in central venous pressure
  - Prevent jugular venous obstruction
- **Ventilation**
  - Use of minimum peak airway pressure,
  - Avoid of positive end-expiratory pressure,
  - Avoid $PaCO_2$, above preoperative levels
- **Fluids**
  - Administer modest amounts of fluid
  - Use isotonic solution when possible
  - Administer hyperosmotic solutions as an infusion

intraoperative anesthetic interventions are required. They are outlined in Table 2.5, but the physiologic responses discussed throughout this chapter can only be assumed to take place in normal brain tissue. Anesthetic drugs have a significant and complex effect on both $CMRo_2$ and CBF/CBV. Drugs that cause vasodilation increase ICV to a varying degree, while the opposite is true for vasoconstrictors. Potent volatile anesthetic agents cause vasodilation and increase CBV while decreasing $CMRo_2$; regional or global metabolic demands further increase CBF and CBV because autoregulation is maintained. The magnitude of the effects of volatile anesthetics is difficult to predict in a specific patient. Intravenous anesthetic agents generally have little effect on the cerebral vasculature may produce vasoconstriction. The effects of anesthetic agents and adjuvant drugs are discussed extensively in Chapters 9 and 10.

Careful attention to a patient's ICP status can direct therapeutic intervention and minimize further injury. An anesthetic technique should be chosen that is unlikely to increase ICP. It is generally acceptable to administer volatile anesthetics at a concentration below 0.75 MAC. Opioids produce minimal changes in as long as BP is maintained in the normal range. Intravenous anesthetics and sedatives, with the exception of ketamine, reduce CMR and arterial volume, potentially reducing ICP. A propofol-based TIVA is often advocated in patients with moderate to severe ICH, when the patient is at risk of herniation, or where brain volume impairs the surgery (especially when a decompressive craniectomy is planned). Most of the information about the use of dexmedetomidine is in the sedation or intensive care unit literature. There is no strong evidence against its use as a general anesthesia adjunct [40].

SUMMARY

Brain perfusion comes from the vertebral and carotid system with the circle of Willis providing means to ensure perfusion of the supratentorial structures even when one or more of the primary arteries is occluded. Elevated ICP results from an increase in intracranial contents in excess of the volume restriction placed on the brain by the bony cranium and dura supporting structures. The most common cause of elevated ICP is increased volume of the brain parenchyma, neurons, supporting structures, or interstitial fluid. Shifts in CSF volume and CBV are the most rapid and readily available means to alter ICV. All physiologic perturbations and drug administration that produce reductions in component volumes will decrease ICP. Normal responses to changing conditions only occur in normal areas of the brain that are not affected by tumor, vascular lesions, traumatic injury, and CSF obstruction. Anesthetic management must be adjusted to reduce intracranial contents with patients with suspected elevations of ICP.

REFERENCES

1. Hoeffner EG, Case I Jain R et al. Cerebral perfusion CT: technique and clinical applications. *Radiology.* 2004;231(3):632–644.
2. Marmarou A, Shulman K, LaMorgese J. Compartmental analysis of compliance and outflow resistance of the cerebrospinal fluid system. *J Neurosurg.* 1975;43(11):523–534.
3. Lanier W, Warner D. Intracranial elastance versus intracranial compliance: terminology should agree with that of other disciplines. *Anesthesiology.* 1992;77(11):403–404.
4. Akca O. Optimizing the intraoperative management of carbon dioxide concentration. *Curr Opin Anaesthesiol.* 2006;19(1):19–25.
5. Muizelaar JP, Poel HG., Li ZC, et al, Pial arteriolar vessel diameter and CO2 reactivity during prolonged hyperventilation in the rabbit. *J Neurosurg.* 1988;69:923–927.
6. Raichle ME, Posner JB, Plum F, Cerebral blood flow during and after hyperventilation. *Arch Neurol Psychiatry,* 1970;23:394–403.
7. Dagal A, Lam AM. Cerebral autoregulation and anesthesia. *Curr Opin Anaesthesiol.* 2009;22(5):547–552.
8. Ainslie PN, Ogoh S. Regulation of cerebral blood flow in mammals during hypoxia: a matter of balance. *Exp Physiol.* 2012;95(2):251–262.
9. Clifton GL, Miller ER, Choi SC, et al. Lack of effect of induction of hypothermia after acute brain injury. *N Engl J Med.* 2001;344:556–563.
10. Drummond JC. The lower limit of autoregulation: time to revise our thinking? *Anesthesiology.* 1997;86(6):1431–1433.
11. Strandgaard S, J.J., MacKenzie ET, Harper AM. Upper limit of cerebral blood flow autoregulation in experimental renovascular hypertension in the baboon. *Circ Res.* 1975;37:164–167.
12. Hlatky R, Valadka AB, Robertson CS. Intracranial pressure response to induced hypertension: role of dynamic pressure autoregulation. *Neurosurgery.* 2005;57:917–923.
13. Saposnik G, Barinagarrementeria F, Brown RD et al. Diagnosis and management of cerebral venous thrombosis: a statement for healthcare professionals from the American Heart Association/American Stroke Association. *Stroke.* 2011;42(4):1158–1192.
14. Bergsneider M. Evolving concepts of cerebrospinal fluid physiology. *Neurosurg Clin N Am.* 2001;12(4):631–638, vii.
15. Sullivan JT, Grouper S., Walker MT, et al. Lumbosacral cerebrospinal fluid volume in humans using three-dimensional magnetic resonance imaging. *Anesth Analg.* 2006;103:1306–1310.
16. Upton ML, Weller RO. The morphology of cerebrospinal fluid drainage pathways in human arachnoid granulations. *J Neurosurg.* 1985;63:867–875.
17. Stummer W. Mechanism of tumor-related brain edema. *Neurosurg Focus.* 2007;22:E8.
18. Hatashita S, Hoff JT, Ishii S. Focal brain edema associated with acute arterial hypertension. *J Neurosurg.* 1986;64:643–649.
19. Packard SD, M.J., Ichikawa T, et al. Functional response of tumor vasculature to Paco2: determination of total and microvascular blood volume by MRI. *Neoplasia.* 2003;5:330–338.
20. Arbit E, DiResta GR, Bedford RF, et al. Intraoperative measurement of cerebral and tumor blood flow with laser-Doppler flowmetry. *Neurosurgery.* 1989;24:166–170.
21. Jantzen JP, Jantzen Jen-Peter AH. Prevention and treatment of intracranial hypertension. *Best Pract Res Clin Anaesthesiol.* 2007;21(4):517–538.
22. Czosnyka M, Pickard JD. Monitoring and interpretation of intracranial pressure. *J Neurol Neurosurg Psychiatry.* 2004;75:813–821.
23. Brain Trauma F, et al. Guidelines for the management of severe traumatic brain injury. *J Neurotrauma.* 2007;24(Suppl 1):S1–106.
24. Han CY, Backous DD. Basic principles of cerebrospinal fluid metabolism and intracranial pressure homeostasis. *Otolaryngol Clin N Am.* 2005;38(4):569–576.
25. Steffen H, Eifert B, Aschoff A, et al. The diagnostic value of optic disc evaluation in acute elevated intracranial pressure. *Ophthalmology.* 1996;103(3):1229–1232.
26. Juul N, Morris GF, Marshall SB, et al. Intracranial hypertension and cerebral perfusion pressure: their influence on neurological deterioration and outcome in severe head injury. *J Neurosurg.* 2000;92:1–6.
27. Drummond JC, Patel PM. Neurosurgical anesthesia. In: Miller RD, E.L., Fleisher LA, et al, eds. *Miller's Anesthesia* vol 1 and 2, 7th edition. London: Elsevier; 2009:2046.
28. Fishman RA. Brain edema. *N Engl J Med.* 1975;293:706–711.
29. Fisher CM. Brain herniation: a revision of classical concepts. *Can J Neurol Sci.* 1995;22(2):83–91.
30. Singhi SC, Tiwari L. Management of intracranial hypertension. *Indian J Pediatr.* 2009;76(5):519–529.
31. Brain Trauma F, et al. Guidelines for the management of severe traumatic brain injury. VII. Intracranial pressure monitoring technology [erratum appears in *J Neurotrauma.* 2008;25:276–278. *J Neurotrauma.* 2007;24(Suppl 1):S45–S54.
32. Smith M. Monitoring intracranial pressure in traumatic brain injury. *Anesth Analg.* 2008;106(1):240–248.
33. Brain Trauma Foundation: American Association of Neurological Surgeons; Congress of Neurological Surgeons: Joint Section on Neurotrauma; Critical Care, Aans Cns Bratton SL, Chestnut RM, Ghajar J et. al. Guidelines for the management of severe traumatic brain injury. VII. Intracranial pressure monitoring technology. *J Neurotrauma.* 2007;24(Suppl 1):S45–S54.
34. Farhvar A, Huang JH, Papadakos PJ. Intracranial monitoring in traumatic brain injury. *Curr Opin Anaesthesiol.* 2011;24(2):209–213.
35. Balestreri M, et al. Association between outcome, cerebral pressure reactivity and slow ICP waves following head injury. *Acta Neurochir Suppl.* 2005;95:25–28.
36. Rozrt I, Tontisirin N, Muangman S, et al. Effect of equiosmolar solutions of mannitol versus hypertonic saline on intraoperative brain relaxation and electrolyte balance. *Anesthesiology.* 2007;107(5):697–704.
37. Rudehill A, Gordon E, Ohman G, et al. Pharmacokinetics and effects of mannitol on hemodynamics, blood and cerebrospinal fluid electrolytes, and osmolality during intracranial surgery. *J Neurosurg Anesthesiol.* 1993;5:4–12.
38. Curley G, Kavanagh BP, Laffey JG. Hypocapnia and the injured brain: more harm than benefit. *Crit Care Med.* 2010;38(5):1348–1359.
39. Brain Trauma F, et al. Guidelines for the management of severe traumatic brain injury. XIV. Hyperventilation [erratum appears in *J Neurotrauma.* 2008;25:276–278]. *J Neurotrauma.* 2007;24(Suppl 1):S87–S90.
40. Yasemin G, Turktan M, Erman T, et al. Anesthesia for craniotomy: comparison of sevoflurane, desflurane, or isoflurane anesthesia supplemented with an infusion of dexmedetomidine during supratentorial craniotomy. *Neurosurg Q* 2009;19(2):110–115.

3.

MONITORING CEREBRAL BLOOD FLOW AND METABOLISM

Peter D. Le Roux and Arthur M. Lam

INTRODUCTION

The human brain weighs about 2% of total body mass but consumes 20% of the oxygen and 25% of the glucose used by the whole body at rest. This high metabolic function is devoted to synaptic activity (50%), maintenance of ionic gradient (25%), and biosynthesis (25%). The oxygen and energy reserves in the brain are, however, very limited, and its survival and function depend on a steady supply of the cardiac output (15% to 20%) and a constant supply of oxygen and energy-rich substrate. Functional evaluation of cerebral blood flow (CBF) and metabolism are therefore important in the management of many diseases, including both acute brain injury, where the prevention and management of secondary brain injury through early detection with a variety of monitors are central to modern intensive care unit (ICU) care, and more delayed or chronic disorders where cerebral ischemia endangers patient outcome. In this chapter we will review: (1) CBF physiology and pathophysiology and (2) CBF monitors. CBF monitors can be considered in two broad categories: (1) radiologic techniques that provide a snapshot in time and (2) bedside monitors that, in turn, may be subdivided into monitors that are (a) invasive or noninvasive, (b) continuous or non-continuous, or (c) monitors that provide direct or indirect CBF measurements.

PHYSIOLOGY

Normal CBF in the human brain is approximately 50 mL/100 g brain tissue/min [1]. CBF in the gray matter (80 mL/100 g/min) is greater than that of the white matter CBF (20 mL/100 g/min). Mean arterial pressure (MAP), intracranial pressure (ICP), $Paco_2$, and Pao_2 are the main physiologic variables that influence CBF. The most important relationship is *flow–metabolism coupling,* whereby the cerebral metabolic rate of oxygen consumption ($CMRo_2$) is directly related to CBF and the arteriovenous difference of oxygen ($AVDo_2$) [2]. Normal and abnormal values of CBF and $CMRO_2$ are described in Table 3.1.

Blood flow within the brain is regulated to provide substrates according to neural tissue needs. This coupling occurs via several mechanisms: neurogenic, humoral, and myogenic. It is thought that local metabolic factors are of primary importance. In normal conditions, vasoactive substances are released in areas of increased cerebral activity that alter vascular tone and local perfusion. The compensatory increase in perfusion then creates a local washout effect, which then reduces perfusion. Key local metabolites include, among other substances, CO_2, potassium, adenosine, nitric oxide, histamine, and prostaglandins [3].

Several basic physical principles can be used to help describe CBF. Ohm's law predicts that flow (Q) is proportional to the pressure gradient between inflow and outflow (ΔP) divided by flow resistance (R): $Q = \Delta P/R$. Cerebral perfusion pressure (CPP) is the difference between arterial inflow (MAP) and venous outflow pressure and is the "driving pressure" for CBF. Because the pressure in the thin-walled veins cannot be measured, CPP is described by the equation: $CPP = MAP - ICP$.

Poiseulle's law is represented mathematically as $Q = (\pi r^4 \Delta P)/8\eta L$, where CPP is ΔP, blood viscosity is η, vessel radius is r, CBF is Q, and vessel length is L. Poiseulle's law shows that CPP, blood viscosity, and vessel radius are important determinants of CBF. Vessel length usually is not measured in physiologic systems. Direct measurement of viscosity (the internal friction that resists blood flow) is difficult. Viscosity can vary with hematocrit or other processes that alter the blood's cellular composition and also varies inversely with vessel diameter. This results from the increased velocity gradient of laminar flow as vessel size decreases, a parameter known as the shear rate [4]. For a given blood velocity, shear rates are greater in smaller vessels and apparent viscosity is consequently lower in the microcirculation. This effect is known as the Fahraeus-Lindquist

Table 3.1 NORMAL AND ABNORMAL VALUES FOR CBF AND CEREBRAL METABOLISM

Normal CBF human brain: 50 mL/100 g/min

Gray matter CBF: 80 mL/100 g/min

White matter CBF: 20 mL/100 g/min

CBF thresholds for ischemic and irreversible injury: ≤18 mL/100 g/min

- $CMRO_2$ 1.5 μmol/g/min (3.4 mL/100 g/min)

     $AVDo_2$ 6.5 mL/dL

     O_2ER 35%

- CMRG 0.325 μmol/g/min

     90% aerobic, 10% anaerobic metabolism

- CMRL −0.02 μmol/g/min

Oxygen consumption thresholds for ischemic and irreversible injury: 1.0 mL/100 g/min

O_2ER, oxygen extraction; CMRG, cerebral metabolic rate of glucose consumption; CMRL, cerebral metabolic rate of lactate consumption.

effect [5]. The most powerful factor in Poiseulle's law is vessel radius. For example, the maximum constriction of a vessel that can be obtained by hyperventilation is about 20% from baseline, but this relatively small amount of vasoconstriction decreases CBF by approximately 60% [6]. From a practical standpoint, the bulk of this change takes place in the microcirculation.

$CMRO_2$ can be calculated by knowing how much blood is flowing to the brain and how much oxygen the brain extracts from this blood ($AVDo_2$) and is described by the equation:

$$CMRO_2 = CBF \times AVDo_2$$

CEREBRAL BLOOD VOLUME

The average cerebral blood volume (CBV) is 3 to 4 mL/100 g and is determined by CBF and the diameter of the small veins and venules within the brain (the *capacitance vessels*). CBV therefore increases with vasodilatation and decreases with vasoconstriction, but the relationship between CBF and CBV is complex and these variables may be inversely related in both normal and pathologic states. Blood volume also is not equally distributed throughout the brain; there is a greater volume per unit weight in gray matter than in white matter. The central volume principle relates CBV (i.e., the volume of intravascular blood in the brain in milliliters) and CBF (the volume of blood that passes through the brain per unit time in mL/min) [7]:

$$CBF = CBV/\tau$$

This equation implies that change in vascular diameter will affect CBV but not necessarily CBF if mean transit time (τ)

also is altered. Normally, CBV increases are managed in two ways: (1) constriction of major feeding arteries to restrict inflow and (2) increased venous outflow. It is unclear whether CBV is itself regulated or simply changes passively from CBF regulation, but changes in CBV are important: a 1-mL change in CBV can be associated with a 7–mm Hg in pressure if the intracranial compliance is poor.

CEREBRAL AUTOREGULATION

The brain regulates its own blood flow through several mechanisms: *Metabolic autoregulation* produces changes in CBF that are proportional to changes in $CMRo_2$ (i.e., oxygen demand). *Pressure autoregulation* allows CBF to remain constant despite alterations in CPP. The mechanisms responsible for autoregulation have only recently been understood. The myogenic hypothesis states that smooth muscle in resistance arteries responds directly to CPP alterations [8]. The metabolic hypothesis states that CBF reduction stimulates vasoactive substance release from the brain that then stimulates cerebral vessel dilatation. There also appears to be a role for sympathetic nervous system modulation that can move the upper and lower limits of autoregulation to higher perfusion pressures.

In the healthy brain, CBF is actively controlled by increases or decreases in arterial diameter, which maintains constant flow over a range of perfusion pressures. When CPP exceeds the limits of the brain's ability to autoregulate, cerebral resistance vessels respond passively to further changes in pressure. Thus, CBF changes passively with increases or decreases in perfusion pressure after the limits of autoregulation are exceeded (Figure 3.1). In addition, oxygen extraction from the blood can increase to reduce the likelihood of cellular hypoxia associated with CBF reduction. Clinical symptoms develop only if the decrease in CPP exceeds the brain's ability to extract enough oxygen

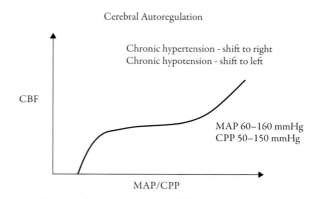

Cerebral Autoregulation

Chronic hypertension - shift to right
Chronic hypotension - shift to left

CBF

MAP 60–160 mmHg
CPP 50–150 mmHg

MAP/CPP

Figure 3.1   Relationship between cerebral blood flow (CBF) and mean arterial pressure (MAP). Pressure autoregulation, when normal, maintains a constant CBF even when MAP is altered (flat part of the curve).

to satisfy its metabolic demands. When the upper limits of autoregulation are exceeded, arteries passively dilate and breakdown occurs in the blood–brain barrier (BBB) and vascular endothelium, which in turn causes cerebral edema and/or hemorrhage.

PATHOPHYSIOLOGY

CBF and oxygen consumption thresholds identified for ischemic and irreversible injuries are 18 mL/100 g/min and 1.0 mL/100 g/min, respectively. When CBF is less than 25 mL/100 g/min, there is electroencephalographic (EEG) slowing, and at 20 mL/100 g/min, loss of consciousness occurs. Cellular homeostasis is endangered and neurons convert to anaerobic metabolism when CBF is less than 18 mL/100 g/min [9, 10], and once CBF is less than 10 mL/100 g/min, membrane integrity is compromised and irreversible brain damage occurs.

The amount of brain infarction, however, is related not only to CBF but also to time, both onset and duration [9], as well as to the extent of collaterals that can compensate for the hypoperfused region and by the subsequent neuronal loss from secondary injury. Secondary injury may be initiated or aggravated by (1) systemic insults such as arterial hypotension, hypoxemia, or altered glucose or temperature regulation, (2) flow–metabolism uncoupling in the brain, and (3) the metabolic, immunologic, and biochemical changes (local inflammatory changes, calcium and excitatory amino acid imbalances, and apoptosis) initiated by the original insult [11, 12]. Delayed brain ischemia often is the major common pathway of secondary brain damage. However, reperfusion injury also may occur: this hyperemia can lead to elevated ICP and decreased CPP and eventually impair regional CBF.

CBF MONITORING

A variety of CBF monitors are in clinical use (Table 3.2), but the "ideal" CBF monitor does not yet exist (Table 3.3). These monitors can be broadly classified as those that provide a single value at a specified point in time (e.g., radiographic or tomographic techniques), devices that can be used daily (e.g., transcranial Doppler [TCD] examination), or monitors that continuously display CBF information. These continuous monitors may be further classified as invasive (laser Doppler flowmetry [LDF], thermal diffusion [TD], jugular oximetry, direct brain oxygen, microdialysis) or noninvasive (e.g., TCD, near-infrared spectroscopy [NIRS], EEG). In turn, these continuous monitors may provide direct CBF data, indirect CBF data, or surrogate measurements to suggest cellular health to which CBF contributes (e.g., glucose metabolism using microdialysis, direct brain oxygen,

Table 3.2 **POTENTIAL METHODS TO ASSESS CBF**

- Clinical evaluation, serial assessment
- Systemic: BP, O_2 saturation, $EtCO_2$, temperature
- Hydraulic: ICP/CPP
- Electrophysiology: EEG, SSEP, BAER
- Radiographic/tomographic: PET, SPECT, CT-P, stable Xe-CT (^{133}Xe), MRI
- CBF: TCD, laser Doppler, thermal diffusion probe, transcranial cerebral oximetry
- Metabolic: Microdialysis, jugular venous oximetry, direct brain oxygen, NIRS

$EtCO_2$, end tidal carbon dioxide; SSEP, somatosensory evoked potential; BAER, brainstem auditory evoked potential.

NIRS, or EEG). Finally, the various monitors may be broadly divided into those that provide quantitative data or qualitative or trend data.

Two important concepts relevant to CBF monitoring have emerged in recent years: (1) the concept of "flow–metabolism coupling" that refers to the tight relationship between CBF and the $CMRO_2$ and (2) multimodality monitoring. These two concepts are interwoven particularly for patients in a critical care environment. *Multimodality monitoring* is defined as the use of more than one complementary method of monitoring a single organ when no one single method can provide complete information. It is also defined as the simultaneous collection of data from multiple diverse sources associated with a single patient coupled with the ability to view the data in an integrated and time-synchronized manner. This concept is very important when monitoring the brain, which is a complex system with interrelated hemodynamic, metabolic, and electrical subsystems. This type of analysis is essential when monitoring CBF or $CMRo_2$ because an increase in $CMRo_2$ is matched with an increase in CBF in normal brain. When blood supply is limited, there is

Table 3.3 **THE IDEAL CBF MONITOR**

- Portable
- Provides point-of-care measurement
- High spatial resolution
- High temporal resolution
- Continuous or frequently repeatable
- Does not interfere with patient care
- Noninvasive
- Reliable and reproducible quantitative data
- Not operator dependent
- Easy to perform; requires little training to use
- Suggest a cause and appropriate treatment

a compensatory increase in oxygen extraction, but this mechanism is limited, especially in the setting of brain injury. Simply measuring CBF, therefore, is not sufficient without some measure of metabolism. It is also important to realize that more monitoring does not mean better patient outcomes; it is what is done with the information that is important.

POINT-IN-TIME ASSESSMENT OF CBF AND METABOLISM

Radiographic or tomographic methods provide a snapshot view of CBF that can be quantitative, such as positron emission tomography (PET), stable xenon computed tomography (Xe-CT), quantitative magnetic resonance angiography (qMRA), or qualitative (e.g., single-photon emission computed tomography [SPECT] or CT perfusion [CT-P]). These methods can be useful in the treatment of both acute and chronic cerebral ischemia and also may be used in an outpatient setting. Patients with disorders such as subarachnoid hemorrhage (SAH), particularly those with vasospasm or head trauma or those who require therapeutic carotid occlusion or a bypass, can all be assessed with these techniques either alone or supplemented by other studies, such as conventional angiography. In acute stroke management, point-in-time assessment can be used to distinguish infarcted tissue from ischemic but potentially salvageable tissue (the *ischemic penumbra*) and help to select patients for thrombolytic therapy (Table 3.4).

PET

PET is a technique that measures the accumulation of positron-emitting radioisotopes within a three-dimensional object. These radioisotopes (or tracers) distribute to different compartments, according to their pharmacokinetic proprieties, and because specific radioisotopes are used, specific pathophysiologic processes can be targeted. Positron emitters have a short half-life, so PET studies require a nearby cyclotron. This increases costs; PET is available in only a few major medical centers.

PET often is considered the gold standard in physiologic or metabolic imaging and has excellent spatial resolution in three dimensions [13]. It is, however, most commonly used for research since the data often cannot be returned to the clinician in a timely manner for therapeutic decision-making. In addition, the accuracy of PET depends on the validity of kinetic models to derive quantitative measures of cerebral concentrations of the various radioligands. However, some of these kinetic models have not been tested in the injured brain.

PET can provide quantitative measurements of cerebral perfusion and metabolism including CBF, CBV, and $CMRo_2$. PET can also provide the only true measure of the *adequacy* of CBF: the oxygen extraction fraction (OEF)

Table 3.4 **RADIOLOGIC OR TOMOGRAPHIC METHODS TO ASSESS CBF**

MODALITY	ADVANTAGES	DISADVANTAGES
PET	Measures CBF, CBV, $CMRO_2$, CMRglu, OEF Quantitative	Patient transport Noncontinuous Radioactive compounds (^{15}O) Available in few centers
PWI	Measures CBF, CBV, MTT, TTP No radiation	Requires gadolinium IV contrast agent Transport Restrictions of MRI environment Semiquantitative Long scan time
Xe-CT	Measures CBF Quantitative Can be done with head CT	Transport Noncontinuous Research only (in U.S.) Lung disease may affect
SPECT	CBF	Transport Noncontinuous Radioactive compounds Semiquantitative
CT-P	Measure CBF, CBV, MTT, TTP Economical Rapid Quantitative	Transport Iodinated IV contrast agent

with only small amounts of tracer in a triple oxygen PET (using ^{15}O-labeled tracers in three separate scans: $H_2^{15}O$, $C^{15}O$, and $^{15}O_2$). To diagnose ischemia requires identification of areas with increased OEF [14]. The radioisotopes are distributed rapidly throughout the brain in proportion to CBF, and then rapidly washed out; this allows serial flows to be obtained. However, radiation limits the number of repeat studies that can be done. Following a stroke, PET can be used to identify a core of infarcted tissue (irreversible injury) with very low CBF, CBV, and oxidative metabolism [15] and to differentiate this from the surrounding penumbra where CBV is normal or elevated and CBF is preserved with increased OEF [16]. This tissue may be rescued and clinical studies have demonstrated that the extent of PET-identified penumbra is associated with outcome [17].

Although PET remains primarily a research tool, it has provided insights into the pathophysiology and therapy of several acute neurologic disorders. For example, PET studies have demonstrated the role of transfusion in SAH and its effects on Do_2 in the brain [18]. In traumatic brain injury (TBI), various PET studies have helped to better define ischemic thresholds after TBI and to assess the physiologic effect of therapies such as hyperventilation, CPP increase, and hyperoxia [19–21]. 18-Fluorodeoxyglucose (^{18}FDG)-PET can be used to estimate glucose metabolism and derive the oxygen-glucose ratio (OGR; $CMRo_2$/CMRglucose, both measured in μmol/100 g/min from triple oxygen and FDG-PET). PET studies also have shown that hypoxic cellular injury after TBI can be associated with diffusion rather than perfusion abnormalities [22] and that cellular injury may occur in the absence of ischemia (i.e., nonischemic metabolic crisis or hyperglycolysis) [23, 24].

PERFUSION-WEIGHTED MRI

In perfusion-weighted MRI (PWI), protons in arterial blood en route to the head are labeled with an inversion pulse and compared with a control image without an inversion pulse (arterial spin-labeling or time-of-flight PWI); this creates an intra-arterial contrast with the intracranial contents and so provides quantifiable and stable time series data that can be used to calculate quantitative CBF. Bolus-tracking, also called first-pass bolus method or susceptibility-based perfusion imaging, is another method to determine PWI but requires the intravenous injection of a paramagnetic contrast agent (i.e., gadolinium chelate). When PWI is used with diffusion-weighted MRI (DWI), the ischemic penumbra often can be identified, often within 30 minutes of symptom onset. It can assess vascular patency if MRA is added. No ionizing radiation is used, and there are usually fewer contraindications to gadolinium contrast agents than to iodinated contrast. PWI is relatively time consuming and generally less available and more expensive than CT, and it often can be a challenge to monitor critically ill patients in the MR scanner. The technique is not as fast as CT and requires that a potentially unstable ICU patient be transported to the MRI scanner. However, no pharmacologic contrast is required, and the results can be superimposed over the anatomic detail that accompanies the flow images with the structural MRI scans (Figures 3.2 and 3.3).

PWI can be used to calculate perfusion maps and the delay of mean transit time (MTT) to compare selected locations. Viable areas that lack adequate perfusion and are at risk for infarction can be identified with simultaneous PWI and DWI. Mismatched PWI/DWI has been used to assess the risk and benefit of thrombolysis in patients with acute stroke symptoms; however, absolute CBF and CBV values may be more accurate to evaluate the true perfusion deficit [25].

qMRA

Advances in phase contrast MRA (PCMR) permit noninvasive assessment of blood flow rates and flow direction in patients with complex cerebrovascular disorders [26, 27]. The technique is performed with a standard MRA and does not require contrast medium. Images from a two- or three-dimensional MRA are transferred to a noninvasive optimal vessel analysis (NOVA) workstation. The NOVA software uses proprietary computational algorithms to generate a detailed report of the quantitative flow rates in milliliters per minute and flow direction in each vessel. qMRA can be used to assess CBF and collateral circulation in stroke, transient ischemic attacks (TIAs), occlusive cerebral vascular disease, or subclavian steal syndrome or after bypass procedures (Figures 3.4a and 3.4b).

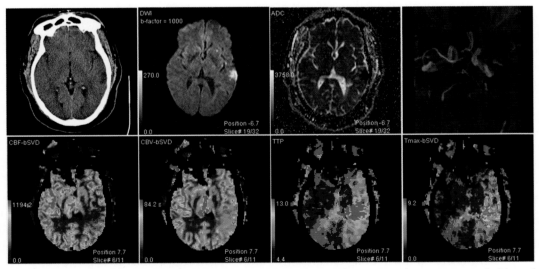

Figure 3.2   DSC perfusion MRI in acute ischemia: 56-year-old patient with gradual onset of expressive aphasia approximately 8 hours before imaging. Small CT and diffusion abnormalities (top row, first two images), and poor flow-related enhancement left MCA on MRA (top row, right image) are shown. Diffusion-perfusion mismatch is evident on left side (bottom row) with delay (prolonged TTP and T_{max} >5 seconds), decreased rCBF = 0.80, and increased rCBV = 1.15. Thrombolysis (IA-tPA) was performed with successful recanalization. *DSC perfusion maps were created for this figure using PMA image analysis software (copyright owner: Kohsuke Kudo) provided by ASIST-JAPAN.

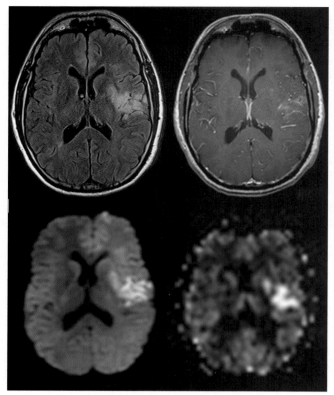

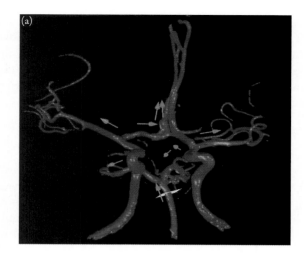

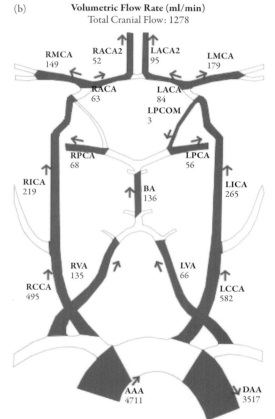

Figure 3.3 ASL perfusion MRI in luxury perfusion: subacute infarct left MCA branch territory is demonstrated on FLAIR (upper left), postcontrast T1-weighted (upper right), and diffusion weighted images (lower left). Pulsed ASL (PASL) perfusion MRI (lower right) shows increased blood flow in infarct that may indicate increased rate of hemorrhage and neuronal injury in the penumbra.

STABLE Xe-CT

Xe-CT scanning today is primarily a research technique in the United States that can be performed as part of a routine CT scan. Xe-CT uses inhaled nonradioactive xenon and the Kety–Schmidt equation to give regional CBF measurements in the cortex. Global CBF can also be measured. Patients inhale xenon, which is rapidly taken up into the blood and transported to the brain. End-tidal xenon is recorded continuously and is assumed to track arterial partial pressure. Xenon is radiopaque so changes in radiodensity with serial CT scans can be used to calculate CBF. Xe-CT studies can be repeated at 20-minute intervals; thus, reactivity challenge testing of therapies can be performed. For example, acetazolamide dilates cerebral blood vessels and can be used to assess cerebrovascular reserve (Figures 3.5a, 3.5b, and 3.6). Xe may potentially cause vasodilation and so augment CBF, although this may be partially counteracted by hyperventilation in spontaneously breathing subjects [28]. This effect can be eliminated by obtaining multiple early images and weighting calculations to the early portion of the wash-in curve [29–31]. Inert Xe also may have neuroprotective effects [32]. This technique requires that the patient inhale 26% to 33% stable Xe, making it impractical in patients who require a high F_{IO_2}.

Figure 3.4 qMRA illustrating vascular anatomy of circle of Willis (a) and flow map showing direction of flow and CBF value (b) (Courtesy of David Langer MD.).

SPECT

SPECT is widely available and relatively simple and inexpensive and relies on the imaging of gamma-emitting tracers that emit a single photon. ^{99m}Tc-hexamethylpropyleneamine oxide (HMPAO) is used to map CBF [33, 34]. This radioisotope crosses the blood–brain barrier and is distributed through the brain in proportion to flow. The tracer remains in the brain a long time and itself does not affect CBF. The tracer can be injected before the patient is transported to the

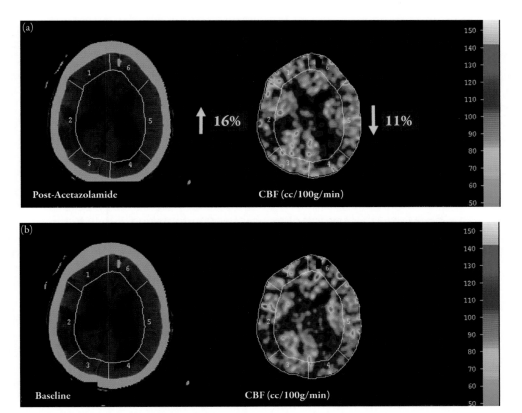

Figure 3.5 Stable xenon perfusion CT before and after acetazolamide: 47-year-old patient with severe intracranial carotid stenotic occlusive disease and Moyamoya collaterals. Baseline perfusion study (upper row) shows decreased cortical blood flow in anterior circulation territories, approximately 30 mL/100 g/min right MCA territory and 43 mL/100 g/min on left at level shown. After acetazolamide (lower row), mild augmentation by about 16% was apparent in the right MCA region of interest but decreased on left by about 11%, consistent with decreased cerebrovascular reserve on right and steal on left.

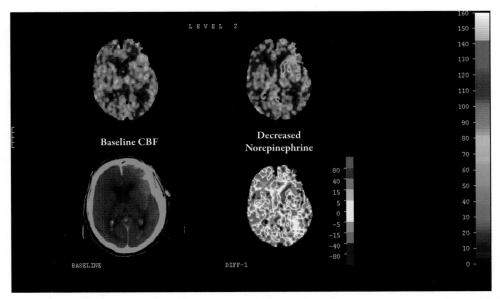

Figure 3.6 Stable xenon CT perfusion in a patient with vasospasm after subarachnoid hemorrhage to assess treatment efficacy. The baseline perfusion study (left) showed global decreased cortical blood flow on right a little more than on the left. Pressor levels were then decreased and the perfusion study repeated after 15 minutes at new MAP. Cortical blood flow decreased slightly on right, but there was a more prominent increase in blood flow on left, a paradoxical response to the decrease in pressor levels.

nuclear scanner, but the study cannot be easily repeated to assess the effects of therapeutic interventions. CBF measured by SPECT is semiquantitative (i.e., relative CBF is measured with this technique and images are relatively low resolution). For example, in suspected ischemia, the area with reduced flow needs to be compared with a presumably normal area in the contralateral cerebral hemisphere or the unaffected cerebellum. Clinical applications include assessment of acute stroke, cerebral vasospasm, and occlusive vascular disease. Functional reserve capacity also can be assessed after vasodilation is induced with acetazolamide or CO_2 [35]. SPECT also has been used to measure CBF several months after mild or moderate TBI. Reduced CBF is found in about half of the patients with TBI and is associated with unfavorable outcome and poor performance on neuropsychological testing [36, 37].

CT-BASED IMAGING (CT-ANGIOGRAPHY AND CT-P)

CT is the primary imaging modality for critically ill patients. Noncontrast head CT shows anatomic intracranial injury (e.g., hemorrhage, hydrocephalus, mass effect and shift, or ischemia/infarction, among others). Contrast-enhanced head CT can help identify some vascular abnormalities, masses, and blood–brain barrier disruption. CT-P and CT-angiography (CTA) can be used to assess CBF. CT-P measures intracranial blood flow and shows areas of abnormal CBF, whereas CTA provides anatomic information and may show vascular pathology (e.g., an aneurysm, stenosis, occlusion, or vasospasm). These studies all can be done on most commonly used CT scanners with commercially available software.

CT-P

Changes in tissue attenuation that occur in the brain over time can be measured during the infusion of iodinated contrast and the simultaneous acquisition of images using a helical CT multislice scanner in cine mode. Postprocessing of the data generates color-coded maps and quantification of various perfusion parameters, including CBF, CBV, MTT, and time-to-peak (TTP, the time from the start of contrast agent injection to the time of maximum enhancement). CT-P calculations are based on the central volume principle, described by the following equation:

$$CBF = CBV/MTT$$

where

CBF is measured in mL/100 g/min), CBV is measured in mL/100 g, and

MTT is measured in seconds (time of the bolus passing through a volume of tissue).
MTT is calculated from the arterial input time–density curve, CBV is calculated as the area under time–density

curve in the tissue of interest, and CBF is determined using the central volume principle [38, 39]. Hence, both global and regional CBF can be determined and are particularly useful to determine vasomotor reactivity or functional reserve.

CT-P is an evolving technology but has been used to help manage several clinical disorders including SAH and TBI (Figure 3.7). CT-P uses include diagnosis of acute infarction, vasospasm, autoregulation, cerebral vascular reserve in patients with chronic vascular occlusions, and evaluation of tumor vascularity. Blood–brain barrier permeability can be assessed in acute infarction to predict the risk of hemorrhagic transformation [40]. In addition, early imaging of the patient with an acute ischemic infarct can differentiate tissue at risk of infarction from tissue with irreversible injury (penumbra versus core). This may help to predict clinical outcome and which patients may benefit from thrombolytic therapy [41–43]. The parameters that define penumbra versus ischemic core in CT-P are controversial. In most series, the penumbra is considered to have reduced CBF, normal or elevated CBV due to cerebral autoregulatory response, and elevated MTT. A 34% CBF decrease relative to clinically normal areas is considered a threshold for ischemia and infarction, whereas a CBV threshold of 2.5 mL/100 g helps differentiate infarction from penumbra. Whether threshold perfusion values might be used in other disorders, such as TBI, is unclear.

CT-P can be obtained on any multislice CT scanner with appropriate software, meaning that it is widely available and relatively inexpensive. CT-P does have several disadvantages, however. It provides only limited anatomic coverage of the brain using current 16- to 128-slice scanners, so the regions of interest must be predetermined before the scan. CT-P studies are of limited spatial resolution in the posterior fossa and assume that the blood–brain barrier is intact. The reliability of absolute flow values determined by CT-P has been questioned. CT-P requires a dose of radiation and contrast load that are several times greater than those required for conventional head CT [44, 45], which may be a problem in patients with compromised renal function [46, 47].

CTA shows the anatomy of the vascular tree (Figure 3.8). CTA scans follow the first pass of contrast as it moves through the vascular tree of the imaged area. The scan acquisition typically is timed to be 1 to 2 seconds behind the arterial peak of the contrast bolus. The smallest available slice is used to acquire the scan; this helps detect small vascular abnormalities and improves the quality of the reconstructed image. Scans can be viewed as the initial acquisition (source images), as maximum intensity projections (MIPS) that are often thicker than the initial scan acquisition, or as true three-dimensional images. Interpretation of CTA should include the source images as well as the MIPS and the three-dimensional reconstructions. The common artifacts in a CTA examination arise from patient motion, which causes

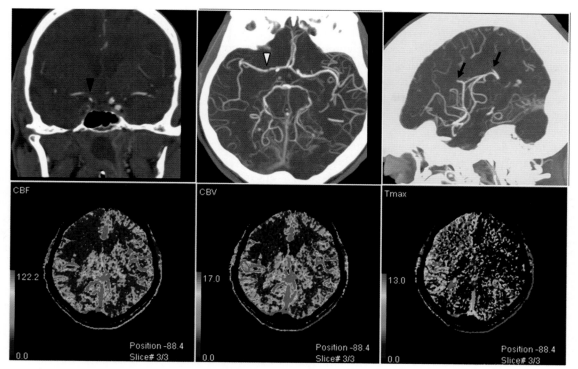

Figure 3.7   CTA and CT-P in acute ischemia: 85-year-old patient with right hemisphere ischemia 6 hours after onset. Coronal reformat of CTA (top left) shows occlusive thrombus in the supraclinoid right ICA (black arrowhead), and the rest of the intracranial and cervical ICA occluded as well. Some cross filling to right MCA was evident from left anterior circulation (top middle, white arrowhead) but occlusions where evident in distal branches (top right, black arrows). Perfusion deficits are nearly matched on right (T_{max} versus CBV and CBF) in MCA and ACA territories with prolonged T_{max} >5 seconds, decreased rCBF <0.30, decreased rCBV <0.40. IV-tPA had already been administered without improvement; IA-tPA was not administered due to time since onset, large infarct, large thrombus burden, and relatively matched defect. *DSC perfusion results were created for this figure using PMA image analysis software (copyright owner: Kohsuke Kudo) provided by ASIST-JAPAN.

misregistration in the MIPS and in the three-dimensional recontructions. Inadequate contrast caused by a mistimed contrast injection or poor cardiac output is less common.

CTA can be used to diagnose and evaluate intracranial aneurysms and to determine the underlying pathology in a patient with acute intracranial hemorrhage. CTA is generally used along with TCD, which is performed at the bedside. The two studies complement each other. It can also be used to evaluate cerebral vasospasm, intracranial vascular malformations, and venous thrombosis. CTA permits the assessment of extracranial and intracranial vascular structures in a patient with ischemic infarct or chronic cerebrovascular disease. CTA is also used to assess vascular injury following blunt or penetrating trauma. Numerous studies have

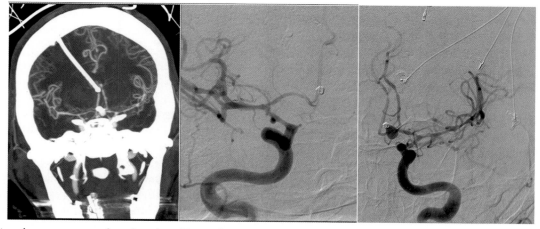

Figure 3.8   CTA to detect vasospasm after subarachnoid hemorrhage. Coronal MIP from CTA head (leftmost image) shows moderate to marked vasospasm left greater than right anterior circulation, confirmed on right (middle image) and left (rightmost image) carotid injections from conventional angiogram. Partially coiled anterior communicating artery aneurysm can be seen as well.

documented the accuracy of CTA for aneurysms greater than 4 to 5 mm in diameter. In various studies, CTA detects cerebral vasospasm with 75% to 90% accuracy compared with catheter angiography. CTA accuracy is much greater in the setting of either absent or severe vasospasm and is less accurate when vasospasm is mild or moderate [48, 49]. CTA cannot demonstrate changes in flow dynamics that are visible with catheter angiography.

The equipment required for CT imaging is usually located outside the Neurocritical Care Unit (NCCU), which requires that a critically ill patient be transported to a remote location. Portable CT scanners can be brought to the ICU, decreasing the risk associated with transport while producing quality images (including Xe-CT or CT-P) of adequate quality [50, 51].

BEDSIDE CBF AND ICP MEASUREMENTS

PET, SPECT, CT-P, Xe-CT, and MRI are noninvasive methods that assess the global cerebral perfusion and metabolism, although in some instances regional CBF measurements can be obtained. Imaging provides a comprehensive evaluation of cerebral perfusion at only one point in time (i.e., a single snapshot). However, cerebral autoregulation is a dynamic process, and in all disease processes, there are changes in CBF and metabolism that vary over time. Therefore, supplementation of global one-time assessment of CBF with continuous monitoring at the bedside is helpful.

There are several bedside methods (Table 3.5) that can be used to continuously monitor CBF or its surrogates. This permits detection of acute changes in CBF and metabolism and the effects of altered CBF on brain function and assessment of any therapeutic intervention. For the most part, these monitors provide regional information that complements radiologic measures of global CBF. Bedside monitors may be broadly divided into invasive or noninvasive monitors or monitors that provide direct CBF measurements or an indirect CBF or metabolism measurement through surrogates.

CPP AND ICP

CPP is an important driving force behind CBF and is a factor in the autoregulatory response of the cerebral vasculature. The principal determinants of CPP that can be measured in the ICU are MAP and ICP (i.e., patients require an ICP monitor). In addition, accurate MAP measurements require that an arterial pressure catheter be placed. The optimal position of the arterial pressure transducer (e.g., at the level of the foramen of Monroe or the heart) is controversial. In part, this may be determined by what type of ICP monitor is used. Under normal physiologic conditions, a MAP of

Table 3.5   BEDSIDE METHODS TO ASSESS CBF

MODALITY	ADVANTAGE	DISADVANTAGE
Invasive		
TDF	Direct Bedside monitoring Absolute CBF Regional flow	Invasive Regional flow only Data absent when temperature >39°C
LDF	Regional flow	Uses red cell flux as a surrogate Relative flow only
SjvO$_2$	Continuous monitoring Balance between flow and metabolism	Global and insensitive to regional changes Invasive Needs frequent recalibration
Pbto$_2$	Bedside measurement Continuous	Measures local O$_2$ tension Invasive
Microdialysis	Measures local biochemistry Early detection	Invasive Labor and time intensive Regional measures Indirect CBF measure
Noninvasive		
TCD	Noninvasive Real time with excellent temporal resolution Regional flow	Relative flow only Operator dependent 5%–10% failure rate
NIRS	Noninvasive Real time Bedside measurement	Extracranial blood contamination Ambient light interference Can only use in frontal location Depends on arbitrary derived algorithms
cEEG	Noninvasive Continuous Good spatial and temporal resolution	Prone to artifacts Resource intensive Nonspecific

CEA, carotid endarterectomy; cEEG, continuous electroencephalogram; ICH, intracranial hemorrhage.

These various bedside monitors can be used in several conditions (e.g., TBI, SAH, ICH, ischemic stroke) to guide therapy or assess risk, such as during carotid surgery, ICP management, for brain death determination, and to assess cerebral autoregulation or CO$_2$ reactivity.

80 to 100 mm Hg and an ICP of 5 to 10 mm Hg generate a CPP of 70 to 85 mm Hg, but true CPP may vary by up to 30 mm Hg from measurements with MAP [52–54].

Invasive ICP and CPP monitoring is a standard of care in many neurocritical care units when a patient is comatose. ICP may be measured using probes that are intraparenchymal, intraventricular, subdural, or epidural. Ventricular and parenchymal monitors are used most frequently. Intraventricular catheters connected to external pressure transducers are considered the "gold standard" ICP monitor but have more complications and the risk of infection is greater than with parenchymal monitors. Management and therapeutic targets remain controversial. In general, a minimum CPP threshold of 60 mm Hg is considered to be acceptable, but optimal CPP may vary in each patient and over time in an individual. Continuous monitoring permits values targeted to each individual at a given point in time [55]. In the setting of autoregulatory failure, CPP becomes the primary determinant of cerebral perfusion. On the other hand, evidence for brain hypoxia can be observed despite an adequate CPP or normal ICP in patients with TBI [56, 57]. In addition, once the CPP reaches the lower threshold of the autoregulatory breakthrough zone, hyperemia and secondary ICP increase may result [58]. Consequently, to best understand perfusion state (hypoperfusion or hyperperfusion), ICP and CPP monitoring can be supplemented with other monitors such as a jugular venous oxygen saturation monitor, microdialysis (e.g., lactate-pyruvate ratio), or brain tissue oxygen partial pressure.

ICP and CPP management remain central to neurocritical care, and treatment of patients with severe brain injury that results in intracranial hypertension should be directed at ICP and CPP management. Most management is threshold oriented (i.e., treat when ICP is >20 mm Hg or CPP is <60 mm Hg). Valuable information about compliance, CBF autoregulation, and CSF absorption capacity may also be obtained from waveform analysis or evaluation of derived indices of cerebrovascular reactivity (PRx) or cerebrospinal compensatory reserve (RAP) [52, 59]. These indices provide an approximation of the cerebrovascular autoregulatory reserve [53, 54, 60, 61]. Recent advances in data processing and computerized bedside monitoring have made it possible to perform online, real-time analysis of these indices and provide insight into a patient's compensatory reserve, as well as guide therapy even when the numerical value of ICP is normal.

TD FLOWMETRY

TD is based on thermal conductivity of brain tissue to measure quantitative blood flow: the temperature difference between the neutral plate and the heated element reflects local CBF [62]. In 1933, Gibbs [63] demonstrated that changes in CBF could be detected with a heated thermocouple, and in 1973, a mathematical model was developed to calculate absolute rCBF values. In 1973, TD was introduced to clinical practice, and validation studies showed that rCBF values obtained by TD agree with rCBF values obtained in Xe-CT studies and the hydrogen clearance method [64, 65].

TD probes can be placed on the brain surface during surgery (e.g., Flowtronics probe; Flowtronics, Phoenix, AZ). This has two gold disks that can be placed subdurally on the cortex to measure superficial rCBF. Alternatively, the probe may be positioned through a burr hole and secured with a metal bolt in the parenchyma (e.g., Hemedex Inc.,

Cambridge, MA). The Hemedex probe is placed approximately 25 mm below the dura in normal brain tissue that can be verified with a CT scan. Automatic recalibration occurs approximately every 30 minutes; this results in a loss of data for 2 to 5 minutes. When temperature is higher than 39°C, a safety mechanism interrupts cerebral perfusion monitoring during the fever. Together, these interruptions may lead to a loss of a third of measurements compared with other continuous monitors [66]. There are other limitations associated with TD probes: (1) it is invasive and so risks bleeding and/or infection, (2) it provides only a single focal CBF measurement from a small volume of tissue near the probe, and (3) when positioned near large vessels, it may produce inaccurate measurements. Loss of tissue contact and fever may also affect measurement reliability [62, 67].

Although TD CBF measures may not represent overall CBF, serial changes may aid in assessing therapeutic effects on ischemia or detection of early neurologic deterioration. Superficial (cortical) rCBF values between 40 and 70 mL/100 g/min are considered to be normal, whereas values less than 20 mL/100 g/min or greater than 70 mL/100 g/min represent ischemia and hyperemia, respectively [68]. The TD parenchymal microprobe (Hemedex) measures subcortical white matter perfusion, and a mean TD value of 18 to 25 mL/100 g/min is considered normal [65, 69]. In TBI, TD can be used to guide adequate perfusion and rCBF values can help predict outcome. Patients with a significant increase in rCBF from baseline values tend have a good outcome, whereas patients with initial very low values and those without an increase in baseline have a poor outcome [68, 70]. In SAH, TD can be used to detect vasospasm [69] (Figure 3.9). If correctly positioned, a CBF threshold of 15 mL/100 g/min and a cerebrovascular resistance of 10 can diagnose symptomatic vasospasm with a sensitivity of 90% and specificity of 75% [69]. Thermal diffusion also can be used intraoperatively to study hemodynamic changes in the surrounding brain tissue during aneurysm occlusion or removal of arteriovenous malformations or brain tumors [71, 72] (Figure 3.10).

LDF

LDF was introduced in 1977 to measure cutaneous blood flow. Today, the main manufacturers of laser Doppler instruments are Perimed AB (Stockholm, Sweden), Moor Instruments Ltd. (Axminster, UK), Vasamedics Inc. (St Paul, MN), Transonic Systems Inc. (Ithaca, NY), Oxford Optronix Ltd. (Oxford, UK), and LEA Medizintechnik (Giessen, Germany). In patients with neurologic disorders, LDF provides continuous, qualitative measurements of microvascular perfusion in a bedside monitoring device that can be used in the operating room or the ICU. Measurement is limited to regional blood flow [73], but LDF offers excellent temporal and dynamic resolution with ultra short time responses to fluctuations in CBF.

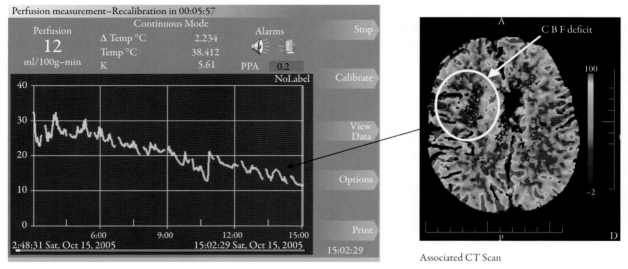

Figure 3.9 Thermal diffusion probe tracing that illustrates decline in CBF (left) and associated CT-P image (right) that confirms reduced CBF. (Courtesy of Frank Bowman and Stephen Lewis, MD, University of Florida.)

A small fiberoptic laser probe (diameter 0.5–1 mm) is applied to the brain surface during surgery [74] or placed in the brain parenchyma. This illuminates a tissue volume of about 1 mm³ with monochromatic laser light with a wavelength between 670 and 810 nm. When light strikes the brain tissue, photons are scattered and Doppler shifted in a random fashion through stationary tissue and moving red blood cells. To limit artifacts, the LDF probe should be placed in a relatively normal brain region without large vessels. A fraction of scattered shifted and nonshifted photons is detected by photoreceptors, which generates an electric signal that contains information about power and frequency proportional to the volume and velocity of red blood cells. The product of volume and velocity scales linearly with the perfusion (CBF) and is expressed in arbitrary units (AU) [75, 76], because LDF measures erythrocyte flux rather than actual CBF [77–80]. There is a high correlation between LDF and other blood flow–monitoring techniques such as

Xe clearance method, radioactive microspheres, hydrogen clearance technique, iodoantipyrine method, and thermal diffusion [81, 82].

LDF provides continuous measurement of rCBF and can be used in brain-injured patients to assess autoregulation and CO_2 reactivity, detect ischemic insults, and evaluate therapeutic responses [83, 84]. In TBI, preserved autoregulation determined with LDF is associated with a good outcome, whereas persistent loss of autoregulation is associated with a poor outcome [85]. Similarly, when the transient hyperemic response is assessed, patients with an unfavorable outcome after TBI have significantly lower LDF readings than do patients with a favorable outcome [86].

There are several limitations to LDF use: LDF is an invasive technique and measures CBF in a small brain volume in a semiquantitative manner. LDF probes require frequent calibration to obtain reproducible LDF data. External factors (e.g., room temperature, strong external light, and sound) or internal factors (e.g., microvascular heterogeneity, changes in hematocrit, or tissue or probe motion) may cause artifacts in measurement. Finally, LDF does not measure absolute CBF. LDF is best used as a trend monitor because it is difficult to determine a threshold LDF value that indicates cerebral ischemia.

TCD ULTRASONOGRAPHY

TCD ultrasonography uses reflected ultrasound from basal cerebral arteries and the Doppler principle to determine the velocity of blood in a single artery, usually the proximal arteries of the circle of Willis. TCD provides real-time dynamic information about blood flow velocity (BFV) and displays a continuous waveform similar to that obtained with intra-arterial blood pressure monitoring. TCD is a noninvasive technique that can be used in the ICU, operating

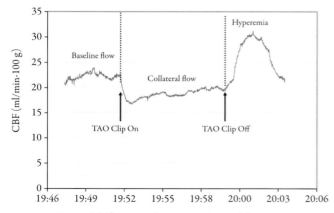

Figure 3.10 Thermal diffusion probe tracing obtained during cerebral aneurysm repair. The waveform illustrates typical CBF pattern before, during, and after temporary arterial occlusion (TAO). (Courtesy of Frank Bowman.)

room, or clinic [87]. It has several uses: (1) to help detect and guide management of patients who develop vasospasm after SAH, (2) to evaluate cerebral autoregulation in TBI and vasomotor reactivity in patients with occlusive vascular disease [88, 89–93], (3) to estimate noninvasive ICP (e.g., in coagulopathic patients) [94], (4) to help confirm brain death through demonstration of intracranial circulatory arrest [95], (5) to detect and monitor emboli [96], (6) to help diagnose hyperemia, and (7) to assess hemodynamic reserve after acetazolamide administration. Functional TCD (fTCD) has recently been developed to quantify the cerebrovascular response to cognitive and sensorimotor stimulation [97, 98].

TCD has several limitations: It is impossible to find a temporal ultrasonic window in 5% to 10% of patients. TCD ultrasonography is not a quantitative flow monitor. TCD provides information about the presence and character of flow, and can track relative changes when the diameter of the vessel is constant. The reproducibility of TCD recordings depends on a constant angle between the transducer and the insonated vessel. This is an important operator-dependent factor that is less likely to affect readings as the insonation angle becomes more parallel to the vessel being examined. Several other factors, including vessel diameter, hematocrit, P_{CO_2}, and blood pressure, affect BFV measurements [99]. For example, a decrease in vessel caliber can increase BFV despite a decrease in CBF (as in vasospasm). When vessel diameter stays constant, the flow characteristics in large conductance vessels can reflect the flow characteristics in the cerebral microcirculation [88].

Detection of Vasospasm After SAH

One of the most important uses of TCD is to monitor for and evaluate vasospasm after SAH (Table 3.6). Mean BFV is directly proportional to flow and inversely proportional to the cross-sectional area of the vessel. When vasospasm occurs, BFV increases. Several studies suggest TCD is most accurate for diagnosing middle cerebral artery (MCA) vasospasm. A mean MCA BFV that is less than 120 cm/s excludes clinically significant vasospasm, whereas a BFV greater than 180 cm/s is consistent with severe vasospasm. When the BFV is between 120 and 180 cm/s, the diagnosis of vasospasm becomes less accurate. Induced hyperemia is frequently used after SAH; this can paradoxically increase BFV. To help differentiate vasospasm from hyperemia, MCA BFV mean can be compared with extracranial carotid artery flow velocity (ECICA FV, which is unaffected by vasospasm). Vasospasm is likely if the ratio of MCA FV to ECICA FV (Lindegaard ratio) is greater than 3. A Lindegaard ratio greater than 6 is associated with severe angiographic vasospasm, whereas symptomatic vasospasm (delayed cerebral ischemia) has a ratio greater than 8 [100].

Table 3.6 **SUMMARY OF TCD USE TO DETECT VASOSPASM**

- Most reliable in MCA
- Age- and sex-corrected values
- Best coupled and interpreted with other techniques e.g. ICP, MABP, CO, ABG, hematocrit
- Changes in BFV reflect relative CBF changes
- Findings that suggest vasospasm
  - Early increase in MCA BFV
  - <120 cm/s—rules out clinically significant spasm
  - >200 cm/s—almost always indicates severe spasm
  - Rapid increase (>50 cm/s/day)
  - EC/IC ratio >6 = severe angiographic spasm; >8 = symptomatic
- Role of CO_2, acetazolamide, transient hyperemic response test (THRT)

BRAIN OXYGENATION

Monitoring cerebral oxygenation after brain injury may help to detect ischemia or other causes of secondary brain injury. Four methods are in current clinical use: jugular venous bulb oximetry, direct brain tissue oxygen tension measurement, near infrared spectroscopy, and ^{15}O PET. PET was discussed in the preceding section.

JUGULAR VENOUS OXIMETRY

Jugular venous oximetry relies on a sensor placed into the jugular bulb to assess global oxygenation. The jugular bulb is the final common pathway for venous blood draining from the cerebral hemispheres, cerebellum, and brain stem. Therefore, the oxygen saturation at the jugular bulb ($Sjvo_2$) reflects the balance between supply and oxygen consumption by the brain. Contribution of the extracranial circulation is estimated between 0% and 6.6% but can be greater if the catheter is placed below the facial vein, which joins the internal jugular vein a few centimeters below the jugular bulb.

$Sjvo_2$ can be measured by sampling blood intermittently or by using a fiberoptic oximeteric catheter to measure $Sjvo_2$ continuously. Serial or intermittent sampling is less expensive and allows calculation of $AVDo_2$, glucose, and lactate based on the Fick principle [101]. Two fiberoptic catheters are commercially available: the Oximetrix (Abbott Laboratories, North Chicago, IL) and the Edslab II (Baxter Healthcare Corporation, Irvine, CA). When cerebral metabolic rate is stable, changes in $AVDo_2$ will represent changes in CBF and global CBF adequacy [102]. However, jugular bulb catheters cannot be used to provide quantitative or regional CBF measurements and do not detect regional ischemia [103].

CMRo$_2$ is calculated from the CBF and the AVDo$_2$ using the following equation:

$$CMRO_2 = CBF \times (\text{arterial oxygen content} - \text{jugular venous bulb oxygen content})$$

Oxygen content can be determined using co-oximetry, or calculated using the following equations:

$$\text{Arterial oxygen content} = [(Hb \times 1.34 \times SaO_2) + (PaO_2 \times 0.0031)]$$

$$\text{Jugular venous oxygen content} = [(Hb \times 1.34 \times SjvO_2) + (PjvO_2 \times 0.0031)]$$

where Hb = hemoglobin in g/dL, Sao$_2$ = arterial saturation, Sjvo$_2$ = jugular venous bulb saturation, Pao$_2$ = oxygen partial pressure in arterial blood in mm Hg, and Pjvo$_2$ = oxygen partial pressure in jugular venous blood in mm Hg.

Because hemoglobin concentration should be the same in arterial and venous blood, and the amount of dissolved oxygen is minimal, cerebral metabolic rate for oxygen can be estimated from CBF and the difference in the arteriojugular bulb oxygen saturation.

$$CMRO_2 = CBF \times (SaO_2 - SjvO_2)$$

Therefore, the arteriovenous oxygen content (or saturation) difference can be used to compare changes in metabolism with alterations in CBF. Hypoperfusion and ischemia increase AVDo$_2$, while hyperemia will decrease AVDo$_2$. The same principle can be applied to other metabolites such as glucose and lactate (Table 3.7). Normal jugular venous oximetry (Sjvo$_2$) is between 55% and 75%. The ischemic threshold is an Sjvo$_2$ less than 50% for at least 10 minutes [104]. Low Sjvo$_2$ indicates either an increase in oxygen demand (e.g., fever or seizures) or reduced oxygen delivery (e.g., vasospasm or inadequate CPP). Increased Sjvo$_2$ (>70%) suggests that there is either more blood flow than the brain needs (hyperemia) or decreased metabolic demand.

Table 3.7 **JUGULAR BULB CATHETER VALUES**

- Sjvo$_2$ values
- Normal values: 60% (55%)–75% (80%)
- Ischemia: <50%–55%
- Hyperemic: >75%
- Ratios of serum to cerebral lactate and glucose levels
  - Arteriovenous difference of lactate (brain lactate divided by serum lactate) >0.08 = significant brain ischemia
- Arteriovenous difference of oxygen (AVDO$_2$)—relationship of flow to demand
  - AVDO$_2$ = CMRO$_2$/CBF (calculation – 1.39 (SAO$_2$ – SjO$_2$) × hemoglobinb/100
  - Normal = 5–7.5 vol%
  - Narrow AVDO$_2$ < 5 vol% = hyperemia (CBF > CMRO$_2$)
  - Wide AVDO$_2$ > 7.5 vol% = low flow (CBF < CMRO$_2$)

Sjvo$_2$ monitoring accurately reflects global cerebral oxygenation only when the dominant jugular bulb is cannulated. Studies have demonstrated as much as a 15% difference between right and left Sjvo$_2$ in patients with TBI [105]. Several methods may be used to determine which jugular bulb is dominant. Blood flow often is greater in the right jugular venous bulb [106]. Size of the jugular foramen will be larger on the dominant side. If ICP is being monitored, the dominant internal jugular vein can be determined by brief compression of each internal jugular vein: compression of the dominant jugular vein will cause a greater ICP increase.

Accurate positioning of the catheter is essential to avoid facial vein contamination Ultrasound can be used to ensure correct placement [107]. A lateral skull or cervical spine radiograph or an anteroposterior chest radiograph that includes a view of the neck should be obtained to confirm catheter position [108]. The catheter tip should lie at the level of and just medial to the mastoid bone above the lower border of C1. The catheter is then connected to a slow continuous infusion of 0.9% saline and flush system to maintain patency and reduce the incidence of wall artifacts [109]. For continuous monitoring, a fiberoptic catheter is passed through a 4F introducer into the jugular bulb. After the insertion and every 8 to 12 hours, the catheter must be recalibrated [110, 111].

Jugular bulb catheters should be used in conjunction with another monitor, such as an ICP monitor or EEG, and can provide serial assessments of CBF relative to cerebral metabolic rate at the bedside. This can be important because episodes of cerebral venous desaturation are common in comatose patients with TBI or SAH despite the use of invasive hemodynamic and ICP monitors [112, 113]. There is a well-described association between jugular venous desaturation (particularly Sjvo$_2$ <50% for >15 minutes) and poor neurologic outcome in TBI [113]. Jugular bulb catheters can help define treatment thresholds such as hyperventilation in patients with increased ICP [114]. This technique can also be used to detect intraoperative ischemia during surgical procedures such as cerebral aneurysm surgery, carotid endartrectomy, or cardiac surgery [102,115–117]. Jugular bulb oxygen desaturation has been associated with poor outcome in patients undergoing cardiac surgery, whereas a lactate oxygen index (LOI) less than 0.08 at any time during a cerebrovascular procedure is associated with a worse clinical outcome. Episodes of desaturation might not be identified without a jugular bulb catheter [102].

There are several potential limitations associated with jugular bulb catheters (Table 3.8). PET studies suggest that a relatively large brain volume (approximately 13%) must be affected before Sjvo$_2$ levels decrease less than 50% [78, 118], meaning that this technique has low sensitivity for ischemia. Heterogeneity in CBF or metabolic rate can lead to misleading information, especially when localized areas of hyperemia and ischemia exist. The reliability of this technique is limited by changes in arterial oxygen

Table 3.8 RETROGRADE JUGULAR CATHETERS: LIMITATIONS

- Changes in $SvjO_2$ associated with intracranial hypertension may only be observed after herniation
- Artifacts associated with catheter movement are common
- Incorrect placement can result in extracerebral contamination
- Single jugular bulb assessed
- Anemia may narrow $AVDO_2$
- Accuracy: 45%–50% sensitivity, 98%–100% specificity
- Recalibration at least every 12–24 hours with in vivo lab data
- Global measure—can miss regional hypoxia
- Risk of infection and thrombosis

content, hemodilution, jugular bulb catheter position, the necessity for frequent calibrations, or an increase in ICP. Complications of catheter insertion include arterial puncture, venous air embolism, and venous thrombosis [111]. The most common complications are carotid artery puncture and hematoma formation, which occur in about 1% to 4% of insertions and usually are self-limiting. Pneumothorax or damage to adjacent structures such as vagus and phrenic nerves, or the thoracic duct, is relatively rare. There is an increased risk of local and systemic infection with long-term placement.

BRAIN TISSUE OXYGEN MONITORING

Direct brain tissue oxygen ($PbtO_2$) monitors are the most frequently used technique in clinical practice to assess cerebral oxygenation. The two most frequently used systems are the Licox (Integra Neuroscience, Plainsboro, NJ) and the Neurotrend (Diametrics Medical, St. Paul, MN). The Licox system has been evaluated in more studies and is now more commonly used because the Neurotrend device is no longer commercially available in most countries. Less frequently used $PbtO_2$ monitors include the Neurovent-P Temp (Raumedic AG, Munchberg, Germany), which uses the same polagraphic technique as the Licox, and the OxyLab pO_2 (Oxford Optronix Ltd., Oxford, UK), which measures $PbtO_2$ using optical fluorescence technology.

The Licox $PbtO_2$ monitor uses a modified Clark electrode that depends on the electrochemical properties of noble metals to measure the oxygen content of tissue. This process is temperature dependent, so a temperature probe is provided with the $PbtO_2$ probe. $PbtO_2$ is displayed in units of tension (mm Hg). Oxygen content in units of mL O_2/100 mL can be derived using a simple conversion: 1 mm Hg = 0.003 mL O_2/100 g brain. The precise role of $PbtO_2$ in humans is only beginning to be elucidated, but most studies suggest that $PbtO_2$ does not simply indicate ischemia or blood flow. $PbtO_2$ varies not only with CBF (and factors

including CO_2 and MAP) but also with changes in arterial oxygen tension (PaO_2) [119–122]. $PbtO_2$ may therefore indicate the balance between regional oxygen supply and cellular oxygen consumption and may therefore describe the interaction between plasma oxygen tension and CBF [120]. Many factors influence $PbtO_2$ [123], including the suggestion that $PbtO_2$ may reflect oxygen diffusion rather than total oxygen delivery or cerebral oxygen metabolism [121, 122]. A $PbtO_2$ monitor differs from a jugular bulb catheter that indicates the balance between oxygen delivery and oxygen utilization because $SjvO_2$ measures the venous oxygen content in blood exiting the brain. $PbtO_2$ measures of the oxygen that accumulates in brain tissue and PET studies suggest that it may correlate inversely with OEF [19].

Brain oxygen monitors have been used in the clinical environment since 1993 and were first included in the treatment guidelines for severe TBI in 2007. Monitoring $PbtO_2$ has been validated against fiberoptic jugular oxygen saturation monitoring, Xe-enhanced CT scanning, and SPECT. Threshold values vary slightly depending on what type of $PbtO_2$ monitor is used, but values less than 20 mm Hg are considered worth treating and values less than 15 mm Hg indicate brain hypoxia or ischemia (Table 3.9) [110, 123–128]. In SPECT studies $PbtO_2$ averages 10 ± 5 mm Hg during episodes of cerebral ischemia and 37 ± 12 mm Hg in normal brain [127]. Decreases in $PbtO_2$ are not benign and are associated with independent chemical markers of brain ischemia [129] in microdialysis studies. The number, duration, and intensity of brain hypoxic episodes ($PbtO_2$ <15 mm Hg), and any $PbtO_2$ values 5 mm Hg or less are associated with poor outcome after TBI [126, 130–133]. Indeed, a $PbtO_2$ less than 10 mm Hg after TBI is associated with a significant increase in both mortality and unfavorable outcome [134]. The exact relationship with outcome, however, may vary depending on where the probe is placed (i.e., in normal white matter, in the penumbra, or in a contusion) [135].

Brain oxygen monitoring is useful in a variety of clinical situations where cerebral ischemia or secondary brain injury may occur [19, 136], and some studies suggest that $PbtO_2$ complements ICP monitoring. Episodes of brain hypoxia are common and may occur even when ICP and CPP are normal [56, 137], emphasizing the potential value of multimodal monitoring that integrates data from several physiologic monitors. A strong relationship is observed

Table 3.9 LICOX $PbtO_2$ VALUES

25–35 mm Hg	Normal
20 mm Hg	Compromised; begin treatment
15 mm Hg	Brain hypoxia
10 mm Hg	Severe brain hypoxia
5 mm Hg	Cell death

between PbtO$_2$ and several drivers of brain perfusion, such as MAP, CPP, and end-tidal CO$_2$ [110, 138, 139]. This can help clinicians to better understand the complex pathophysiology of the brain after an acute insult, evaluate autoregulation, and identify optimal physiologic targets and the utility of therapeutic interventions [138, 140–146]. Some, but not all, observational series suggest that the addition of PbtO$_2$-based care to conventional ICP- and CPP-based care is associated with improved outcome after severe TBI [147–150]; this question is now being evaluated in a multicenter clinical trial.

NEAR-INFRARED SPECTROSCOPY:

NIRS is a noninvasive technique that measures regional cerebral oxygen saturation (rSO$_2$). Commercially available monitors such as the INVOS Cerebral Oximeter (Somanetics, Troy, MI) and the Hamamatsu 100, 200 and 300 (Hamamatsu Photonics KK, Japan) are compact and portable and can detect changes in optical attenuation of a number of wavelengths of light. These devices provide bedside noninvasive measurements of cerebral oxygenation [151].

The technique is based on reflectance oximetry [152]. Briefly, NIRS relies on the concept that light of wavelengths of 680 to 1000 nm is able to penetrate human tissue and is absorbed by the chromophores oxyhemoglobin (HbO$_2$), deoxyhemoglobin (Hb), and cytochrome oxidase that vary according to tissue oxygenation and metabolism. The technique measures the light reflected from the chromophores and changes in the detected light levels can therefore represent concentration changes. NIRS reflects cerebral venous oxygen saturation. The change in total hemoglobin is directly related to the change in blood volume [153]. The INVOS system provides a numerical value for oxygen saturation using rSO$_2$: 60% to 80% has been reported as the normal range [154].

The noninvasive nature of NIRS made it particularly advantageous for monitoring cerebral oxygen of premature infants because their thin skull permitted transillumination. A reflectance mode is used in adults. Use of reflectance raises concerns about quantification, the volume and type of tissue being illuminated, and contamination of the signal by the extracranial tissue layers. The sampling volume of gray and white matter is unknown. A number of algorithms have been applied to overcome these issues, and techniques such as time resolved, phase resolved, and spatially resolved spectroscopy have been developed [155]. In any NIRS study, it is essential to consider whether the changes detected could be due, even in part, to extracerebral contamination including interference by ambient lighting. Other limitations include sample volume inaccuracies (increased signal path during cerebral edema following head injury), dependence on proprietary algorithms, and lack of MRI compatibility [156].

Whether the calculated cerebral oxygen saturation as a quantitative measure is accurate has yet to be established. There is no clear consensus value for NIRS-derived "thresholds" for ischemia–hypoxia [157], in part because factors including arterial oxygen saturation, systemic blood pressure, arterial carbon dioxide tension, hematocrit, regional CBV, and interindividual variation can influence cerebral tissue rSO$_2$. NIRS also does not resolve focal CBF abnormalities but may be useful as a monitor of general changes that indicate secondary brain injury. The use of NIRS to evaluate changes in regional cerebral oxygenation, CBF, and oxygen use in the brain is well described s [151, 158–161], particularly in patients with disturbed cerebral circulation such as TBI and intracranial hemorrhage, in patients undergoing carotid endarterectomy [161–164] or cardiac surgery [158, 159, 165, 166], in evaluation of a low cardiac output state [167], and in noninvasive cerebral autoregulation assessment [168]. For example, in TBI, oxyhemoglobin changes correlate with changes in jugular bulb SjvO$_2$, TCD, and laser Doppler [160]. Some studies suggest that NIRS can distinguish different cerebral oxygenation patterns that occur during different seizure types [169]. Finally, the combination of indocyanine green dye dilution and NIRS appears to help detect cerebral vasospasm and delayed cerebral ischemia after SAH [170] and to assess perfusion reductions in acute ischemic stroke.

Most NIRS systems are placed in the frontotemporal region in adults. For optimal performance, ambient light should be minimized, the skin surface should be clean and dry, and the optodes should be placed high on the forehead while avoiding the sagittal sinus in the midline and muscle (temporalis muscle). The optodes should be placed on a hairless part of the head because the hair follicles absorb light. The effect of extracranial signal contamination can be addressed in part by simultaneous measurement of arterial blood pressure and peripheral saturation.

CEREBRAL MICRODIALYSIS

Cerebral microdialysis (MD) is an in vivo technique to sample and collect low-molecular-weight substances from the interstitial space (i.e., brain extracellular fluid). It is a well-established laboratory tool that was introduced into the clinical neurosciences in the 1990s, where it can be used as a bedside monitor to analyze brain tissue biochemistry. Because MD measures changes at the cellular level, it is a useful technique to detect compromised brain function. Furthermore, because changes in microdialysis analytes may precede changes in other physiologic variables such as ICP [171, 172], it is possible to detect and treat adverse events before they cause irreversible injury. This can potentially widen the therapeutic window.

Microdialysis is not specifically a flow monitor; rather it measures changes in brain metabolism that may result from many causes, one of which is altered CBF. In clinical use,

MD is focused primarily on markers of cerebral energy metabolism (glucose, lactate, and pyruvate), neurotransmittors (glutamate), and cell damage (glycerol) through a bedside analyzer. In particular, measurements of glucose, pyruvate, and lactate provide information about the relative contributions of aerobic and anaerobic metabolism to bioenergetics. The lactate-pyruvate ratio (LPR) reflects cytoplasmatic redox state and thus gives information about tissue oxygenation and energetics. An elevated LPR (>40) frequently is interpreted as a sign of cerebral hypoxia or ischemia [173]. There also are several potential non–hypoxic–ischemic causes of an increased LPR [174], and in TBI, increases in markers of anaerobic metabolism can occur independent of CPP [175]. Microdialysis, therefore, can provide insight into both ischemic and nonischemic causes of cerebral distress. The role of microdialysis is described in several excellent reviews on MD and a consensus statement about its use [173, 176, 177].

The microdialysis catheter ideally should be placed in "at-risk" tissue since MD can only measure the local metabolic product in the catheter area. While threshold values for various MD markers are described (Table 3.10) [178, 179], there can be considerable patient variation and so trend interpretation is more useful than absolute measures. To date, MD has been used primarily in patients with TBI or SAH and has increased our understanding of the pathophysiology of these conditions, particularly when used with other monitors (e.g., PET, electrophysiology, and $Pbto_2$). In addition, MD can be used to identify optimal physiologic targets including CPP, hemoglobin, or temperature and the effects of various therapies including glycemic control, hyperventilation, induced normothermia, and surgery [21, 142, 180–185].

The most commonly assayed MD substances are associated with the aerobic and anerobic metabolism of glucose since tissue hypoxia is the final common pathway for cellular damage. Microdialysate glucose levels are reduced in

Table 3.10 **MICRODIALYSIS THRESHOLD VALUES**

DIALYSATE CONCENTRATION	REINSTRUP ET AL.	SCHULZ ET AL.	CLINICAL USE
Glucose (mmol/L)	1.7 (± 0.9)	2.1 (± 0.2)	<2.0
LPR	23 (± 4)	19 (± 2)	>25
Glycerol (μmol/L)	82 (± 44)	82 (± 12)	>100
Glutamate (μmol/L)	16 (± 16)	14 (± 3.3)	>15

Data from Reinstrup P, Ståhl N, Mellergård P, Uski T, Ungerstedt U, Nordström CH. Intracerebral microdialysis in clinical practice: baseline values for chemical markers during wakefulness, anesthesia, and neurosurgery. *Neurosurgery.* 2000;47(3):701–709; Schulz MK, Wang LP, Tange M, Bjerre P. Cerebral microdialysis monitoring: determination of normal and ischemic cerebral metabolisms in patients with aneurysmal subarachnoid hemorrhage. *J Neurosurg.* 2000;93(5):808–814.

patients with severe TBI and consistently low concentrations (<0.66 mmol/L) are associated with poor outcome [186]. Very low brain glucose is associated with reduced $Pbto_2$ and is observed during severe hypoxia or ischemia after TBI and SAH [187, 188]. The determinants of cerebral extracellular glucose concentration are complex, and in some patients, PET studies suggest low MD glucose is associated with hyperglycolysis rather than reduced supply of glucose and oxygen because of decreased cerebral perfusion [24]. Measurement of lactate and pyruvate concentrations provides further information about the state of anerobic glycolysis, but absolute brain lactate values alone do not always indicate the degree of anaerobic metabolism. The LPR and lactate-glucose ratios [179, 187, 189] therefore are considered better markers of anaerobic metabolism, and the LPR is the most commonly examined MD marker measured after brain injury. In humans, an LPR increase is associated with increased ICP [171], ischemia [190], vasospasm, or DIND after SAH [191]; reduced $Pbto_2$ [192]; increased OEF on PET [193]; and poor outcome after TBI and SAH [189, 194–197] (Figure 3.11).

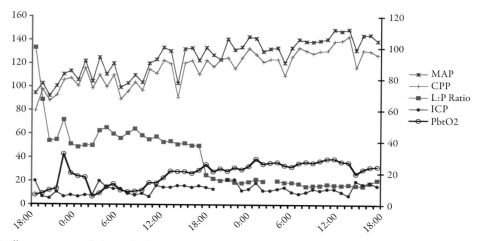

Figure 3.11   Line graphs illustrating microdialysis vales for the lactate-pyruvate ratio (LPR; red) and other physiologic values in a patient with SAH. When the MAP and CPP are increased through administration of vasopressor, there is a decline in the LPR and improvement in brain oxygen.

Less commonly assayed substances include glycerol and glutamate. Glycerol levels increase with membrane breakdown and consequently is a useful MD marker of tissue hypoxia and cell damage [198]. Four- to 8-fold glycerol increases are observed in severe or complete ischemia [179], and increased glycerol is associated with unfavorable outcome after TBI [199]. Increased glycerol can be observed when the blood–brain barrier is compromised, and so caution is needed to interpret an elevated brain glycerol unless there is an MD catheter placed in the abdominal subcutaneous adipose tissue for control comparisons [198]. Increased MD-glutamate concentrations have been associated with hypoxia, ischemia [200], and reduced $PbtO_2$ [201] or CPP [202]. In addition, increased MD glutamate is observed in patients with TBI or SAH with poor outcome [194, 195, 203]. In recent years, the role of glutamate in outcome has been challenged, and so its measurement is less frequently performed [204, 205].

EEG

The EEG provides a noninvasive method to assess brain function. Recent advances in computer technology have made continuous EEG (cEEG) monitoring practical, and its use is common in many NICUs. While cEEG most frequently is used for seizure detection and to guide pharmacologic treatment, cEEG also can be used to detect new or worsening brain ischemia because of the coupling between neuronal activity and CBF. cEEG is particularly useful in patients at high risk, especially those with SAH, when it can be used regardless of whether the patient is in a coma. In addition, EEG is an excellent intraoperative monitor of brain function.

EEG changes occur within seconds of CBF reduction [206, 207]. When CBF is less than 8 to 10 mL/100 g/min (i.e., sufficiently reduced to cause irreversible cell death), all EEG frequencies are suppressed [208, 209], but before that, different components of the EEG are altered depending on the amount of CBF decrease (Table 3.11). Therefore, EEG can detect a window when intervention may potentially prevent irreversible injury. Recent advances in computing now permit the real-time application of quantitative algorithms (qEEG). This allows a large amount of data over long time periods (raw EEG waveforms) to be examined and displayed in a summary as compressed spectral array, density spectral array, compressed EEG pattern analysis, or bandwidth power trends with ratios of power. Spectra or power ratios that are easy to interpret with scoring systems or alarms make quantitative cEEG a very useful NCCU or operating room monitor for ischemia and assessment of burst suppression and level of sedation monitor in real time [210–212]. Trend analysis of total power (1–30 Hz), variability of relative alpha (6–14 Hz/1–20 Hz), and post-stimulation alpha-delta ratio (8–13 Hz/1–4 Hz) [212–215] are associated with cerebral ischemia or angiographic

vasospasm after SAH, as well as with poor outcome after SAH and TBI. For example, Classen et al. (213, 214) found that a reduced poststimulation ratio of alpha-delta frequency power of greater than 10% relative to baseline in six consecutive cEEG measurements was 100% sensitive and 76% specific for DCI. These various EEG changes also may precede clinical changes by up to 2 days [216] (Figure 3.12).

In many respects, cEEG is an ideal monitor (Table 3.11). However, there are several technical (e.g., digital analysis and data reduction or electrical artifacts associated with a noisy NICU environment), patient-related (constant fixation of electrodes for patients who are agitated or who require transport; altered cranial anatomy such as monitoring devices, ventricular catheters, skull defects, or scalp edema), or system resource (e.g., availability of 24-hour coverage of experienced electroencephalographers, availability of networking with real-time and event respond access; automated alerting systems; and accessibility of remote online analysis resource) factors that can potentially limit the use of cEEG for immediate clinical decision-making [217].

MULTIMODALITY MONITORING AND THE FUTURE

The brain is highly dependent on a constant supply of oxygen and energy substrates. The relationship between metabolic supply and demand is changed in the injured brain because of disturbed autoregulation. In addition, a full understanding of how CBF is altered is important in the preoperative planning and the intraoperative phase and during ICU care of many neurologic disorders. Therefore, CBF monitoring is helpful to manage many diverse patients, including those with TBI, SAH, intracerebral hemorrhage, or ischemic stroke or those undergoing cardiac or cerebrovascular surgery, among others.

There are many techniques that can be used to assess CBF and $CMRo_2$, both directly and indirectly. A combination of monitoring techniques that can provide real-time information about the relative health or distress of the brain and adequacy of CBF is ideal (i.e., multimodality monitoring). Rather than simply using data from the monitors to indicate when critical deviations occur, the monitors should be used to guide goal-directed therapy through real-time physiologic end points. Long-term outcome is associated with appropriate integration of information from a variety of monitors, and the interpretation of this association between patient-centered outcomes and monitoring provides a rationale to use multimodal neuromonitoring for therapeutic end-points. However, currently there is no Level I evidence that demonstrates that any neuromonitoring makes a difference to patient outcome in disorders such as TBI or SAH among others, although recent systematic literature reviews suggest that goal-directed therapy based on information provided by a monitor

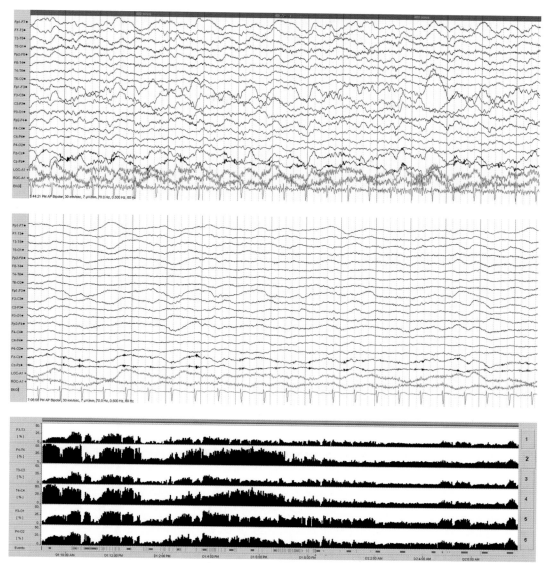

Figure 3.12   EEG can be used to detect ischemia. Top, EEG tracing with good alpha variability; middle, EEG tracing with poor alpha variability; bottom, graphical display illustrating poor alpha variability. (Courtesy Susan Herman, MD.)

may help improve outcome [150, 218, 219]. Further rigorous clinical evaluation is needed to determine whether goal-directed therapy based on monitoring is associated with better outcome. Alternatively, the information provided by monitors may be used as surrogate end points to evaluate other therapies.

Table 3.11   **EEG CHANGES AND DETECTION OF CEREBRAL ISCHEMIA**

CBF ML/100 G/MIN	EEG CHANGE	REVERSIBILITY
35–70	Normal	No injury
25–35	Loss of beta	Reversible
18–25	Theta slowing	Reversible
12–18	Delta slowing	Reversible
<8–10	Suppression	Irreversible

Heterogeneity among patients and pathologies make randomized clinical trials difficult [220, 221]. Monitoring indicators of cerebral oxygenation and perfusion makes sound physiologic sense, and it is this understanding that is valuable and allows therapy to be targeted to each individual. The true richness of multimodal neuromonitoring may still lie ahead; not in the development of new monitors or randomized clinical trials but in the analysis of relationships among the various parameters examined. When examining a patient in the ICU or in the operating room environment, particularly when a multitude of monitors are used, a physician may be confronted with up to 200 variables [222]. However, humans are not able to judge the relationship between more than two variables [223], and without this analysis, vital and important information may be lost [224]. Computer-assisted analysis with graphic analysis and decision support is now feasible and in the future will enhance the value of CBF and cerebral metabolic monitoring, in part because an understanding of the relationships between various monitored parameters should allow earlier identification of altered pathophysiology and thus create a wider therapeutic window to target therapy before irreversible injury occurs.

ACKNOWLEDGMENTS

The authors acknowledge Ronald Wolf, MD, Department of Radiology, University of Pennsylvania, for radiologic images.

REFERENCES

1. Sokoloff L. Metabolism of the central nervous system in vivo. In Field JMH, Hall VE, eds. *Handbook of physiology*. Washington, DC: American Physiological Society; 1960:1843–1864.
2. Butcher K, Emery D. Acute stroke imaging. Part II: the ischemic penumbra. *Can J Neurol Sci*. 2010;37:17–27.
3. Verweij BH, Amelink GJ, Muizelaar JP. Current concepts of cerebral oxygen transport and energy metabolism after severe traumatic brain injury. *Prog Brain Res*. 2007;161:111–124.
4. Chien S. Shear dependence of effective cell volume as a determinant of blood viscosity. *Science*. 1970;168:977–979.
5. Albrecht KH, Gaehtgens P, Pries A, et al. The Fahraeus effect in narrow capillaries (i.d. 3.3 to 11.0 micron). *Microvasc Res*. 1979;18:33–47.
6. Kontos HA, Raper AJ, Patterson JL. Analysis of vasoactivity of local pH, PCO2 and bicarbonate on pial vessels. *Stroke*. 1977;8:358–360.
7. Celsis P, Chan M, Marc-Vergnes JP, et al. Measurement of cerebral circulation time in man. *Eur J Nucl Med*. 1985;10:426–431.
8. Mitagvaria NP. Regulation of local cerebral blood flow. *Adv Exp Med Biol*. 1984;180:861–879.
9. Jones TH, Morawetz RB, Crowell RM, et al. Thresholds of focal cerebral ischemia in awake monkeys. *J Neurosurg*. 1981;54:773–782.
10. Schroder ML, Muizelaar JP, Kuta AJ, et al. Thresholds for cerebral ischemia after severe head injury: relationship with late CT findings and outcome. *J Neurotrauma*. 1996;13:17–23.
11. Chesnut RM. Management of brain and spine injuries. *Crit Care Clin*. 2004;20:25–55.
12. Springborg JB, Frederiksen HJ, Eskesen V, et al. Trends in monitoring patients with aneurysmal subarachnoid haemorrhage. *Br J Anaesth*. 2005;94:259–270.
13. Heiss WD, Herholz K. Brain receptor imaging. *J Nucl Med*. 2006;47:302–312.
14. Frackowiak RS, Lenzi GL, Jones T, et al. Quantitative measurement of regional cerebral blood flow and oxygen metabolism in man using 15O and positron emission tomography: theory, procedure, and normal values. *J Comput Assist Tomogr*. 1980;4:727–736.
15. Baron JC. Mapping the ischaemic penumbra with PET: implications for acute stroke treatment. *Cerebrovasc Dis*. 1999;9:193–201.
16. Moustafa RR, Baron JC. Clinical review: Imaging in ischaemic stroke—implications for acute management. *Crit Care*. 2007;11:227.
17. Heiss WD, Kracht LW, Thiel A, et al. Penumbral probability thresholds of cortical flumazenil binding and blood flow predicting tissue outcome in patients with cerebral ischaemia. *Brain*. 2001;124(Pt 1):20–29.
18. Dhar R, Zazulia AR, Videen TO, et al. Red blood cell transfusion increases cerebral oxygen delivery in anemic patients with subarachnoid hemorrhage. *Stroke*. 2009;40:3039–3044.
19. Johnston AJ, Steiner LA, Coles JP, et al. Effect of cerebral perfusion pressure augmentation on regional oxygenation and metabolism

after head injury. *Crit Care Med*. 2005;33:189–195; discussion 255–257.
20. Diringer MN, Videen TO, Yundt K, et al. Regional cerebrovascular and metabolic effects of hyperventilation after severe traumatic brain injury. *J Neurosurg*. 2002;96:103–108.
21. Nortje J, Coles JP, Timofeev I, et al. Effect of hyperoxia on regional oxygenation and metabolism after severe traumatic brain injury: preliminary findings. *Crit Care Med*. 2008;36:273–281.
22. Menon DK, Coles JP, Gupta AK, et al. Diffusion limited oxygen delivery following head injury. *Crit Care Med*. 2004;32:1384–1390.
23. Bergsneider M, Hovda DA, Shalmon E, et al. Cerebral hyperglycolysis following severe traumatic brain injury in humans: a positron emission tomography study. *J Neurosurg*. 1997;86:241–251.
24. Vespa P, Bergsneider M, Hattori N, et al. Metabolic crisis without brain ischemia is common after traumatic brain injury: a combined microdialysis and positron emission tomography study. *J Cereb Blood Flow Metab*. 2005;25:763–774.
25. Grandin CB. Assessment of brain perfusion with MRI: methodology and application to acute stroke. *Neuroradiology*. 2003;45:755–766.
26. Zhao M, Charbel FT, Alperin N, et al. Improved phase-contrast flow quantification by three-dimensional vessel localization. *Magn Res Imaging*. 2000;8:697–706.
27. Amin-Hanjani S, Charbel FT, Malisch T, et al. Use of quantitative magnetic resonance angiography to stratify stroke risk in symptomatic vertebrobasilar disease. *Stroke*. 2005;36:1140–1145.
28. Hartmann A, Dettmers C, Schuier FJ, et al. Effect of stable xenon on regional cerebral blood flow and the electroencephalogram in normal volunteers. *Stroke*. 1991;22:182–189.
29. Good WF, Gur D. Xenon-enhanced CT of the brain: effect of flow activation on derived cerebral blood flow measurements. *AJNR Am J Neuroradiol*. 1991;12:83–85.
30. Yonas H. Use of xenon and ultrafast CT to measure cerebral blood flow. *AJNR Am J Neuroradiol*. 1994;15:794–795.
31. Kashiwagi S, Yamashita T, Nakano S, et al. The wash-in/wash-out protocol in stable xenon CT cerebral blood flow studies. *AJNR Am J Neuroradiol*. 1992;13:49–53.
32. Luo Y, et al. Xenon and sevoflurane protect against brain injury in a neonatal asphyxia model. *Anesthesiology*. 2008;109:782–789.
33. Bullock R, Statham P, Patterson J, et al. The time course of vasogenic oedema after focal human head injury—evidence from SPECT mapping of blood brain barrier defects. *Acta Neurochir Suppl (Wien)*. 1990;51:286–288.
34. Murase K, Tanada S, Fujita H, et al. Kinetic behavior of technetium-99m-HMPAO in the human brain and quantification of cerebral blood flow using dynamic SPECT. *J Nucl Med*. 1992;33:135–143.
35. Bushnell DL, Gupta S, Barnes WE, et al. Evaluation of cerebral perfusion reserve using 5% CO2 and SPECT neuroperfusion imaging. *Clin Nucl Med*. 1991;16:263–267.
36. Bavetta S, Nimmon CC, White J, et al. A prospective study comparing SPET with MRI and CT as prognostic indicators following severe closed head injury. *Nucl Med Commun*. 1994;15:961–968.
37. Jacobs A, Put E, Ingels M, et al. Prospective evaluation of technetium-99m-HMPAO SPECT in mild and moderate traumatic brain injury. *J Nucl Med*. 1994;35:942–947.
38. Nabavi DG, C. A Craen RA, et al. Quantitative assessment of cerebral hemodynamics using computed tomography. Stability, accuracy, and precision studies in dogs. *J Comput Assist Tomogr*. 1999;23:506–515.
39. Wintermark M, M. P., Thiran JP, et al. Quantitative assessment of regional cerebral blood flow by perfusion CT studies at low injection rates: a critical review of the underlying theoretical models. *Eur Radiol*. 2001;11:1220–1230.
40. Hoeffner EG, Jain R, Gujar SK, et al. Cerebral perfusion CT: technique and clinical applications. *Radiology*. 2004;231:632–644.
41. Schaefer PW, R. L., Ledezma C, et al. First-pass quantitative CT perfusion identifies thresholds for salvageable penumbra in acute

stroke patients treated with Intra-arterial therapy. *Am J Neuroradiol.* 2006;27:20–25.

42. Silvennoinen HM, H. L., Lindsberg PJ, et al. CT perfusion identifies increased salvage of tissue in patients receiving intravenous recombinant tissue plasminogen activator within 3 hours of stroke onset. *Am J Neuroradiol.* 2008;29:1118–1123.

43. Knoepfli AS, S. L., Bonvin C, et al. Evaluation of perfusion CT and TIBI grade in acute stroke for predicting thrombolysis benefit and clinical outcome. *J Neuroradiol.* 2009;36:131–137.

44. Hirata M, S. Y., Fukutomi Y, et al. Measurement of radiation dose in cerebral CT perfusion study. *Radiat Med.* 2005;23:97–103.

45. Cohnen M, F. H., Hamacher J, et al. CT of the head by use of reduced current and kilovoltage: relationship between image quality and dose. *AJNR Am J Neuroradiol.* 2000;21:1654–1660.

46. Langner S, S. S., Kirsch M, et al. No increased risk for contrast-induced nephropathy after multiple CT perfusion studies of the brain with a nonionic, dimeric, iso-osmolal contrast medium. *Am J Neuroradiol.* 2008;29:1525–1529.

47. Newhouse JH, K. D., Qasim A, et al. Frequency of serum creatinine changes in the absence of iodinated contrast material: implications for studies of contrast nephrotoxicity. *Am J Radiol.* 2008;191:376–382.

48. Anderson GB, A. R., Steinke D, et al. CT angiography for the detection of cerebral vasospasm in patients with acute subarachnoid hemorrhage. *Am J Neuroradiol.* 2000;21:1011–1015.

49. Otawara Y, O. K., Ogawa A, et al. Evaluation of vasospasm after subarachnoid hemorrhage by use of multislice computed tomographic angiography. *Neurosurgery.* 2002;51:939–942.

50. Peace K, Maloney E, Frangos S, et al. The use of a portable head CT scanner in the ICU. *J Neurosci Nursing.* 2010;42:109–116.

51. Peace K, Wolfe R, Maloney E, et al. Portable head CT scan and its effect on intracranial pressure, cerebral perfusion pressure and brain oxygen. *J Neurosurg.* 2011;114:1479–1484.

52. Czosnyka M, Guazzo E, Whitehouse M, et al. Significance of intracranial pressure waveform analysis after head injury. *Acta Neurochir.* 1996;138:531–541; discussion 41–42.

53. Czosnyka M, Matta BF, Smielewski P, et al. Cerebral perfusion pressure in head-injured patients: a noninvasive assessment using transcranial Doppler ultrasonography. *J Neurosurg.* 1998;88:802–808.

54. Czosnyka M, Smielewski P, Kirkpatrick P, et al. Continuous monitoring of cerebrovascular pressure-reactivity in head injury. *Acta Neurochir Suppl.* 1998;71:74–77.

55. Robertson CS. Management of cerebral perfusion pressure after traumatic brain injury. *Anesthesiology.* 2001;95:1513–1517.

56. Stiefel MF, Udoetek J, Spiotta A, et al. Conventional neurocritical care and cerebral oxygenation after traumatic brain injury. *J Neurosurg.* 2006;105:568–575.

57. Le Roux P, Lam AM, Newell DW, et al. Cerebral arteriovenous difference of oxygen: a predictor of cerebral infarction and outcome in severe head injury. *J Neurosurg.* 1997;87:1–8.

58. Vespa P. What is the optimal threshold for cerebral perfusion pressure following traumatic brain injury? *Neurosurg Focus.* 2003;15:E4.

59. Steiner LA, Czosnyka M, Piechnik SK, et al. Continuous monitoring of cerebrovascular pressure reactivity allows determination of optimal cerebral perfusion pressure in patients with traumatic brain injury. *Crit Care Med.* 2002;30:733–738.

60. Lang EW, Czosnyka M, Mehdorn HM. Tissue oxygen reactivity and cerebral autoregulation after severe traumatic brain injury. *Crit Care Med.* 2003;31:267–271.

61. Lang EW, Lagopoulos J, Griffith J, et al. Cerebral vasomotor reactivity testing in head injury: the link between pressure and flow. *J Neurol Neurosurg Psychiatry.* 2003;74:1053–1059.

62. Lee SC, Chen JF, Lee ST. Continuous regional cerebral blood flow monitoring in the neurosurgical intensive care unit. *J Clin Neurosci.* 2005;12:520–523.

63. Gibbs FA. A thermoelectric blood flow recorder in the form of a needle. In: *Proceedings of the Society for Experimental Biology and Medicine, San Francisco.* 1933:141–146.

64. Gaines C, Carter LP, Crowell RM. Comparison of local cerebral blood flow determined by thermal and hydrogen clearance. *Stroke.* 1983;14:66–69.

65. Vajkoczy P, Roth H, Horn P, et al. Continuous monitoring of regional cerebral blood flow: experimental and clinical validation of a novel thermal diffusion microprobe. *J Neurosurg.* 2000;93:265–274.

66. Jaeger M, Soehle M, Schuhmann MU, et al. Correlation of continuously monitored regional cerebral blood flow and brain tissue oxygen. *Acta Neurochir.* 2005;147:51–56.

67. Rosenthal G, Sanchez-Mejia RO, Phan N, et al. Incorporating a parenchymal thermal diffusion cerebral blood flow probe in bedside assessment of cerebral autoregulation and vasoreactivity in patients with severe traumatic brain injury. *J Neurosurg.* 2011;114:62–70.

68. Sioutos PJ, Orozco JA, Carter LP, et al. Continuous regional cerebral cortical blood flow monitoring in head-injured patients. *Neurosurgery.* 1995;36:943–949.

69. Vajkoczy P, Horn P, Thome C, et al. Regional cerebral blood flow monitoring in the diagnosis of delayed ischemia following aneurysmal subarachnoid hemorrhage. *J Neurosurg.* 2003;98:1227–1234.

70. Miller JI, Chou MW, Capocelli A, et al. Continuous intracranial multimodality monitoring comparing local cerebral blood flow, cerebral perfusion pressure, and microvascular resistance. *Acta Neurochir Suppl.* 1998;71:82–84.

71. Nagao S, Veta K, Mino S, et al. Monitoring of cortical blood flow during excision of arteriovenous malformation by thermal diffusion method. *Surg Neurol.* 1989;32:137–143.

72. Ohmoto T, Nagao S, Mino S, et al. Monitoring of cortical blood flow during temporary arterial occlusion in aneurysm surgery by the thermal diffusion method. *Neurosurgery.* 1991;28:49–54.

73. Frerichs KU, Feuerstein GZ. Laser-Doppler flowmetry. A review of its application for measuring cerebral and spinal cord blood flow. *Mol Chem Neuropathol.* 1990;12:55–70.

74. Rosenblum BR, Bonner RF, Oldfield EH. Intraoperative measurement of cortical blood flow adjacent to cerebral AVM using laser Doppler velocimetry. *J Neurosurg.* 1987;66:396–399.

75. Bonner RF, Nossal R. Principles of laser-Doppler flowmetry. In Shepherd AP, Oberg PA eds. *Laser Doppler flowmetry.* Boston: Kluwer Academic; 1990:17–45.

76. Bolognese P, Miller JI, Heger IM, et al. Laser Doppler flowmetry in neurosurgery. *J Neurosurg Anesthesiol.* 1993;5:151–158.

77. Wright WL. Multimodal monitoring in the ICU: when could it be useful? *J Neurol Sci.* 2007;261:10–15.

78. DeGeorgia MA, Deogaonkar A. Multimodal monitoring in the neurological intensive care unit. *Neurologist.* 2005;11:45–54.

79. Bhatia A, Gupta AK. Neuromonitoring in the intensive care unit. I. Intracranial pressure and cerebral blood flow monitoring. *Intensive Care Med.* 2007;33:1263–1271.

80. Klaessens JHGM, Kolkman RGM, Hopman JCW, et al. Monitoring cerebral perfusion using near-infrared spectroscopy and laser Doppler flowmetry. *Physiol Meas.* 2003;24:N35–N40.

81. Eyre JA, Essex TJH, Flecknell PA, et al. A comparison of measurements of cerebral blood flow in the rabbit using laser Doppler spectroscopy and radionuclide labelled microspheres. *Clin Phys Physiol Meas.* 1988;9:65–74.

82. Fakuda O, Endo S, Kuwayama N, et al. The characteristics of laser-Doppler flowmetry for the measurement of regional cerebral blood flow. *Neurosurgery.* 1995;36:358–364.

83. Kirkpatrick PJ, Smielweski P, et al. Continuous monitoring of cortical perfusion by laser Doppler flowmetry in ventilated patients with head injury. *J Neurol Neurosurg Psychiatry.* 1994;57:1382–1388.

84. Kirkpatrick PJ, Smielweski P, et al. Early effects of mannitol in patients with head injuries assessed using bedside multimodality monitoring. *Neurosurgery.* 1996;39:714–720.

85. Lam JMK, Hsiang JNK, Poon WS. Monitoring of autoregulation using laser Doppler flowmetry in patients with head injury. *J Neurosurg.* 1997;86:438–445.

86. Smielewski P, Czosnyka M, Kirkpatrick P, et al. Evaluation of the transient hyperemic response test in head injured patients. *J Neurosurg.* 1997;86:773–778.

87. Eng CC, Lam AM, Byrd S, et al. The diagnosis and management of a perianesthetic cerebral aneurysmal rupture aided with transcranial Doppler ultrasonography. *Anesthesiology.* 1993;78:191–194.

88. Kincaid MS. Transcranial Doppler ultrasonography: a diagnostic tool of increasing utility. *Curr Opin Anaesthesiol.* 2008;21:552–559.

89. Molina CA, Alexandrov AV. Transcranial ultrasound in acute stroke: from diagnosis to therapy. *Cerebrovasc Dis.* 2007;24(Suppl 1):1–6.

90. Figaji AA, Zwane E, Fieggen AG, et al. Pressure autoregulation, intracranial pressure, and brain tissue oxygenation in children with severe traumatic brain injury. *J Neurosurg Pediatr.* 2009;4:420–428.

91. Stolz E, Cioli F, Allendoerfer J, et al. Can early neurosonology predict outcome in acute stroke? A metaanalysis of prognostic clinical effect sizes related to the vascular status. *Stroke.* 2008;39:3255–3261.

92. Martin KK, Wigginton JB, Babikian VL, et al. Intraoperative cerebral high intensity transient signals and postoperative cognitive function: a systematic review. *Am J Surg.* 2009;197:55–63.

93. Rigamonti A, Ackery A, Baker AJ. Transcranial Doppler monitoring in subarachnoid hemorrhage: a critical tool in critical care. *Can J Anaesth.* 2008;55:112–123.

94. Homburg AM, Jakobsen M, Enevoldsen E. Transcranial Doppler recordings in raised intracranial pressure. *Acta Neurol Scand.* 1993;87:488–493.

95. Sharma D, Souter MJ, Moore AE, et al. Clinical experience with transcranial Doppler ultrasonography as a confirmatory test for brain death: a retrospective analysis. *Neurocrit Care* 2011;14(3):370–376.

96. Poppert H, Sadikovic S, Sander K, et al. Embolic signals in unselected stroke patients: prevalence and diagnostic benefit. *Stroke.* 2006;37:2039–2043.

97. Dagal A, Lam AM. Cerebral autoregulation and anesthesia. *Curr Opin Anaesthesiol.* 2009;22:547–552.

98. Panerai RB. Transcranial Doppler for evaluation of cerebral autoregulation. *Clin Auton Res.* 2009;19:197–211.

99. Tegeler C, Eicke M. Physics and principles of transcranial Doppler ultrasonography. In Babikian V, Wechsler L, eds. *Transcranial Doppler ultrasonography.* St. Louis: Mosby; 1993.

100. Jahromi BS, MacDonald RL. Vasospasm: diagnosis and medical management. In Le Roux P, Winn HR, Newell DW, eds. *Management of cerebral aneurysms.* Philadelphia: Elsevier Science; 2004:455–487.

101. Ketty SS, Schmidt CF. The nitrous oxide method for the quantitative determination of cerebral blood flow in man: theory, procedure and normal values. *J Clin Investig.* 1948;27:476–483.

102. Matta BF, Lam AM, Mayberg TS, et al. A critique of the intraoperative use of jugular venous bulb catheters during neurosurgical procedures. *Anesth Analg.* 1994;79:745–750.

103. Feldman Z, Robertson CS. Monitoring of cerebral hemodynamics with jugular bulb catheters. *Crit Care Clin.* 1997;13:51–77.

104. Robertson CS, Gopinath SP, Goodman JC, et al. SjvO2 monitoring in head injured patients. *J Neurotrauma.* 1995;12:891–896.

105. Stocchetti N, Paparella A, Brindelli F, et al. Cerebral venous oxygen saturation studied with bilateral samples in the internal jugular veins. *Neurosurgery.* 1994;34:38–44.

106. Gibbs EL, Gibbs FA. The cross sectional areas of the vessels that form the torcular and the manner in which blood is distributed to the right and to the left lateral sinus. *Anat Rec.* 1934;54:419.

107. National Institute for Clinical Excellence. NICE technology appraisal guidance No 49: Guidance on the use of ultrasound locating devices for placing central venous catheters. 2002.London NICE. Available from www.nice.org.uk/pdf/ultrasound_49_GUIDANCE.pdf

108. Bankier AA, Fleischmann D, Windiscch A, et al. Position of jugular oxygen saturation catheter in patients with head trauma: assessment by use of plain films. *Am J Radiol.* 1995;164:437–441.

109. Gunn HC, Matta BF, Lam AM, et al. Accuracy of continuous jugular bulb venous oximetry during intracranial surgery. *J Neurosurg Anesthesiol.* 1995;7:174–177.

110. Gopinath SP, Valadka AB, Uzura M, et al. Comparison of jugular venous oxygen saturation and brain tissue PO2 as monitors of cerebral ischemia after head injury. *Crit Care Med.* 1999;27:2337–2345.

111. Goetting MG, Preston G. Jugular bulb catheterization: experience with 123 patients. *Crit Care Med.* 1990;18:1220–1223.

112. Sheinberg GM, Kanter MJ, Robertson CS, et al. Continuous monitoring of jugular venous oxygen saturation in head-injured patients. *J Neurosurg.* 1992;76:212–217.

113. Gopinath SP, Rogertson CS, Constant CF, et al. Jugular venous desaturation and outcome after head injury. *J Neurol Neurosurg Psychiatry.* 1994;57:717–723.

114. Thiagarajan A, Goverdhan P, Chari P, et al. The effect of hyperventilation and hyperoxia on cerebral venous oxygen saturation in patients with traumatic brain injury. *Anesth Analg.* 1998;87:850–853.

115. Moss E, Dearden NM, Berridge JC. Effects of changes in mean arterial pressure on SjO2 during cerebral aneurysm surgery. *Br J Anaesth.* 1995;75:527–530.

116. Croughwell ND, Newman MF, Blumenthal JA, et al. Jugular bulb saturation and cognitive dysfunction after cardiopulmonary bypass. *Ann Thorac Surg.* 1994;58:1702–1708.

117. Crossman J, Banister K, Bythell V, et al. Predicting clinical ischaemia during awake carotid endarterectomy: use of the SJVO2 probe as a guide to selective shunting. Physiol. Meas. 2003;24:347–335.

118. Artru F, Dailler F, Burel E, et al. Assessment of jugular blood oxygen and lactate indices for detection of cerebral ischemia and prognosis. *J Neurosurg Anesthesiol.* 2004;16:226–231.

119. Hemphill JC 3rd, Knudson MM, Derugin N, et al. Carbon dioxide reactivity and pressure autoregulation of brain tissue oxygen. *Neurosurgery.* 2001;48:377–383.

120. Rosenthal G, Hemphill JC III, Sorani M, et al. Brain tissue oxygen tension is more indicative of oxygen diffusion than oxygen delivery and metabolism in patients with traumatic brain injury. *Crit Care Med.* 2008;36:1917–1924.

121. Scheufler KM, Rohrborn HJ, Zentner J. Does tissue oxygen-tension reliably reflect cerebral oxygen delivery and consumption? *Anesth Analg.* 2002;95:1042–1048.

122. Scheufler K-M, Lehnert A, Rohrborn H-J, et al. Individual values of brain tissue oxygen pressure, microvascular oxygen saturation, cytochrome redox level and energy metabolites in detecting critically reduced cerebral energy state during acute changes in global cerebral perfusion. *J Neurosurg Anesthesiol.* 2004;16:210–219.

123. Maloney-Wilensky E, Le Roux P. The physiology behind direct brain oxygen monitors and practical aspects of their use. *Childs Nerv Syst.* 2010;26:419–430.

124. Doppenberg EM, Zauner A, Watson JC, et al. Determination of the ischemic threshold for brain oxygen tension. *Acta Neurochir Suppl.* 1998;71:166–169.

125. Bardt TF, Unterberg AW, Hartl R, et al. Monitoring of brain tissue PO2 in traumatic brain injury: effect of cerebral hypoxia on outcome. *Acta Neurochir Suppl.* 1998;71:153–156.

126. Kiening KL, Unterberg AW, Bardt TF, et al. Monitoring of cerebral oxygenation in patients with severe head injuries: brain tissue PO2 versus jugular vein oxygen saturation. *J Neurosurg.* 1996;85:751–757.

127. Hoffman WE, Charbel FT, Edelman G. Brain tissue oxygen, carbon dioxide, and pH in neurosurgical patients at risk for ischemia. *Anesth Analg.* 1996;82:582–586.

128. Chang JJ, Youn TS, Benson D, et al. Physiologic and functional outcome correlates of brain tissue hypoxia in traumatic brain injury. *Crit Care Med.* 2009;37:283–290.

129. Hlatky R, Valadka AB, Goodman JC, et al. Patterns of energy substrates during ischemia measured in the brain by microdialysis. *J Neurotrauma.* 2004;21:894–906.

130. Dings J, Meixensberger J, Jager A, et al. Clinical experience with 118 brain tissue oxygen partial pressure catheter probes. *Neurosurgery.* 1998;43:1082–1095.

131. van Santbrink H, Maas AIR, Avezaat CJJ. Continuous monitoring of partial pressure of brain tissue oxygen in patients with severe head injury. *Neurosurgery.* 1996;38:21–31.

132. van den Brink WA, van Santbrink H, Steyerberg EW, et al. Brain oxygen tension in severe head injury. *Neurosurgery.* 2000;46:868–878.

133. Bardt TF, Unterberg AW, Hartl R, et al. Monitoring of brain tissue PO2 in traumatic brain injury: effect of cerebral hypoxia on outcome. *Acta Neurochir Suppl.* 1998;71:153–156.

134. Maloney-Wilensky E, Gracias V, Itkin A, et al. Brain tissue oxygen and outcome after severe traumatic brain injury: a systematic review. *Crit Care Med.* 2009;37:2057–2063.

135. Longhi L, Valeriani V, Rossi S, et al. Effects of hyperoxia on brain tissue oxygen tension in cerebral focal lesions. *Acta Neurochir Suppl.* 2002;81:315–317.

136. Rose JC, Neill TA, Hemphill JC 3rd. Continuous monitoring of the microcirculation in neurocritical care: an update on brain tissue oxygenation. *Curr Opin Crit Care.* 2006;12:97–102.

137. Gracias VH, Guillamondegui OD, Stiefel MF, et al. Cerebral cortical oxygenation: a pilot study. *J Trauma.* 2004;56:469–474.

138. Tolias CM, Reinert M, Seiler R, et al. Normobaric hyperoxia-induced improvement in cerebral metabolism and reduction in intracranial pressure in patients with severe head injury: a prospective historical cohort-matched study. *J Neurosurg.* 2004;101:435–444.

139. Gupta AK, Hutchinson PJ, Fryer T, et al. Measurement of brain tissue oxygenation performed using positron emission tomography scanning to validate a novel monitoring method. *J Neurosurg.* 2002;96:263–268.

140. Al-Rawi PG, Hutchinson PJ, Gupta AK, et al. Multiparameter brain tissue monitoring correlation between parameters and identification of CPP thresholds. *Zentralbl Neurochir.* 2000;61:74–79.

141. Dohmen C, Bosche B, Graf R, et al. Identification and clinical impact of impaired cerebrovascular autoregulation in patients with malignant middle cerebral artery infarction. *Stroke.* 2007;38:56–61.

142. Oddo M, Frangos S, Maloney-Wilensky E, et al. Effect of shivering on brain tissue oxygenation during induced normothermia in patients with severe brain injury. *Neurocrit Care.* 2010;2:10–16.

143. Weiner GM, Lacey MR, Mackenzie L, et al. Decompressive craniectomy for elevated intracranial pressure and its effect on the cumulative ischemic burden and therapeutic intensity levels after sever traumatic brain injury. *Neurosurgery.* 2010;66:1111–1119.

144. Figaji AA, Zwane E, Fieggen AG, et al. Pressure autoregulation, intracranial pressure and brain tissue oxygenation in children with severe traumatic brain injury. *J Neurosurg Pediatr.* 2009;4:420–428.

145. Smith MJ, Maggee S, Stiefel M, et al. Packed red blood cell transfusion increases local cerebral oxygenation. *Crit Care Med.* 2005;33:1104–1108.

146. Muench E, Horn P, Bauhuf C, et al. Effects of hypervolemia and hypertension on regional cerebral blood flow, intracranial pressure, and brain tissue oxygenation after subarachnoid hemorrhage. *Crit Care Med.* 2007;35:1844–1851.

147. Spiotta AM, Stiefel MF, Gracias VH, et al. Brain tissue oxygen-directed management and outcome in patients with severe traumatic brain injury. *J Neurosurg.* 2010;113:571–580.

148. Narotam PK, Morrison JF, Nathoo N. Brain tissue oxygen monitoring in traumatic brain injury and major trauma: outcome analysis of a brain tissue oxygen-directed therapy. *J Neurosurg.* 2009;111:672–682.

149. Martini RP, Deem S, Yanez ND, et al. Management guided by brain tissue oxygen monitoring and outcome following severe traumatic brain injury. *J Neurosurg.* 2009;111:644–649.

150. Nangunoori R, Maloney-Wilensky E, Stiefel MD, et al. Brain tissue oxygen based therapy and outcome after severe traumatic brain injury: a systematic literature review. *Neurocrit Care.* 2012;17(1):131–138.

151. Al-Rawi PG, Kirkpatrick PJ. Tissue oxygen index (TOI): thresholds for cerebral ischaemia using near infrared spectroscopy. *Stroke.* 2006;37:2720–2725.

152. Wyatt JS, Cope M, Delpy DT, et al. Measurement of optical path length for cerebral near-infrared spectroscopy in newborn infants. *Dev Neurosci.* 1990;12:140–144.

153. Hebden JC, Gibson A, Austin T, et al. Imaging changes in blood volume and oxygenation in the newborn infant brain using three-dimensional optical tomography. *Phys Med Biol.* 2004;49:1117–1130.

154. Misra M, Stark J, Dujovny M, et al. Transcranial cerebral oximetry in random normal subjects. *Neurol Res.* 1998;20:137–141.

155. Al-Rawi PG, Smielewski P, Kirkpatrick PJ. Evaluation of a near-infrared spectrometer (NIRO 300) for the detection of intracranial oxygenation changes in the adult head. *Stroke.* 2001;32:2492–2500.

156. Calderon-Arnulphi M, Alaraj A, Slavin KV. Near infrared technology in neuroscience: past, present and future. *Neurol Res.* 2009;31:605–614.

157. Highton D, Elwell C, Smith M. Noninvasive cerebral oximetry: is there light at the end of the tunnel? *Curr Opin Anaesthiol.* 2010;23:576–581.

158. Al-Rawi PG, Smielewski P, Hobbiger H, et al. Assessment of spatially resolved spectroscopy during cardiopulmonary bypass. *J Biomed Opt.* 1999;4:208–216.

159. Nollert G, Jonas RA, Reichart B. Optimising cerebral oxygenation during cardiac surgery: a review of experimental and clinical investigations with near infrared spectrophotometry. *Thorac Cardiovasc Surg.* 2000;48:247–253.

160. Kirkpatrick PJ, Smielewski P, Czosnyka M, et al. Near infrared spectroscopy use in patients with head injury. *J Neurosurg.* 1995;83:963–970.

161. Kirkpatrick PJ, Smielewski P, Whitfield P, et al. An observational study of near infrared spectroscopy during carotid endarterectomy. *J Neurosurg.* 1995;82:756–763.

162. Gopinath SP, Robertson CS, Contant CF, et al. Early detection of delayed traumatic intracranial hematomas using near-infrared spectroscopy. *J Neurosurg.* 2001;83:438–444.

163. Pennekamp CW, Bots ML, Kappelle LJ, et al. The value of near-infrared spectroscopy measured cerebral oximetry during carotid endarterectomy in perioperative stroke prevention. A review. *Eur J Vasc Endovasc Surg.* 2009;38:539–545.

164. Giustiniano E, Alfano A, Battistini GM, et al. Cerebral oximetry during carotid clamping: is blood pressure raising necessary? *J Cardiovasc Med (Hagerstown).* 2010;11:522–528.

165. Vohra HA, Modi A, Ohri SK. Does use of intra-operative cerebral regional oxygen saturation monitoring during cardiac surgery lead to improved clinical outcomes? *Interact Cardiovasc Thorac Surg.* 2009;9:318–322.

166. Murkin JM, Arango M. Near-infrared spectroscopy as an index of brain and tissue oxygenation. *Br J Anaesth.* 2009;103(Suppl 1):i3–i13.

167. Hirsch JC, Charpie JR, Ohye RG, et al. Near infrared spectroscopy (NIRS) should not be standard of care for postoperative management. *Semin Thorac Cardiovasc Surg Pediatr Card Surg Annu.* 2010;13:51–54.

168. Lee JK, Kibler KK, Benni PB, et al. Cerebrovascular reactivity measured by near-infrared spectroscopy. *Stroke.* 2009;40:1820–1826.

169. Sokol DK, Markand ON, Daly EC, et al. Near infrared spectroscopy (NIRS) distinguishes seizure types. *Seizure.* 2000;9:323–327.

170. Keller E, Wolf M, Martin M, et al. Estimation of cerebral oxygenation and hemodynamics in cerebral vasospasm using indocyanin green dye dilution and near infrared spectroscopy: a case report. *J Neurosurg Anesthesiol.* 2001;13:43–48.

171. Belli A, Sen J, Petzold A, et al. Metabolic failure precedes intracranial pressure rises in traumatic brain injury: a microdialysis study. *Acta Neurochir (Wien).* 2008;150:461–469.

172. Adamides AA, Rosenfeldt FL, Winter CD, et al. Brain tissue lactate elevations predict episodes of intracranial hypertension in patients with traumatic brain injury. *J Am Coll Surg.* 2009;209:531–539.

173. Tisdall MM, Smith M. Cerebral microdialysis: research technique or clinical tool. *Br J Anaesth.* 2006;97:18–25.

174. Larach DB, Kofke WA, Le Roux P. Potential non-hypoxic/ischemic causes of increased cerebral interstitial fluid lactate/

pyruvate ratio (LPR): a review of available literature. *Neurocrit Care*. 2011;15(3):609–622.

175. Vespa PM, O'Phelan K, McArthur D, et al. Pericontusional brain tissue exhibits persistent elevation of lactate/pyruvate ratio independent of cerebral perfusion pressure. *Crit Care Med*. 2007;35:1153–1160.

176. Bellander BM, Cantais E, Enblad P, et al. Consensus meeting on microdialysis in neurointensive care. *Intensive Care Med*. 2004;30:2166–2169.

177. Goodman JC, Robertson CS. Microdialysis: is it ready for prime time? *Curr Opin Crit Care*. 2009;15:110–117.

178. Reinstrup P, Stahl N, Mellergard P, et al. Intracerebral microdialysis in clinical practice: baseline values for chemical markers during wakefulness, anesthesia, and neurosurgery. *Neurosurgery*. 2000;47:701–709.

179. Schulz MK, Wang LP, Tange M, et al. Cerebral microdialysis monitoring: determination of normal and ischemic cerebral metabolisms in patients with aneurysmal subarachnoid hemorrhage. *J Neurosurg*. 2000;93:808–814.

180. Oddo M, Schmidt JM, Carrera C, et al. Impact of tight glycemic control on cerebral glucose metabolism after severe brain injury: a microdialysis study. *Crit Care Med*. 2008;36:3233–3238.

181. Oddo M, Milby A, Chen I, et al. Hemoglobin concentration and cerebral metabolism in patients with aneurysmal subarachnoid hemorrhage: a microdialysis study. *Stroke*. 2009;40:1275–1281.

182. Nordstrom CH, Reinstrup P, Xu W, et al. Assessment of the lower limit for cerebral perfusion pressure in severe head injuries by bedside monitoring of regional energy metabolism. *Anesthesiology*. 2003;98:809–814.

183. Nordstrom CH. Assessment of critical thresholds for cerebral perfusion pressure by performing bedside monitoring of cerebral energy metabolism. *Neurosurg Focus*. 2003;15:E5.

184. Marion DW, Puccio A, Wisniewski SR, et al. Effect of hyperventilation on extracellular concentrations of glutamate, lactate, pyruvate, and local cerebral blood flow in patients with severe traumatic brain injury. *Crit Care Med*. 2002;30:2619–2625.

185. Nortje J, Gupta AK. The role of tissue oxygen monitoring in patients with acute brain injury. *Br J Anaesth*. 2006;97:95–106.

186. Vespa PM, McArthur D, O'Phelan K, et al. Persistently low extracellular glucose correlates with poor outcome 6 months after human traumatic brain injury despite a lack of increased lactate: a microdialysis study. *J Cereb Blood Flow Metab*. 2003;23:865–877.

187. Goodman JC, Valadka AB, Gopinath SP, et al. Extracellular lactate and glucose alterations in the brain after head injury measured by microdialysis. *Crit Care Med*. 1999;27:1965–1973.

188. Unterberg AW, Sakowitz OW, Sarrafzadeh AS, et al. Role of bedside microdialysis in the diagnosis of cerebral vasospasm following aneurysmal subarachnoid hemorrhage. *J Neurosurg*. 2001;94:740–749.

189. Persson L, Valtysson J, Enblad P, et al. Neurochemical monitoring using intracerebral microdialysis in patients with subarachnoid hemorrhage. *J Neurosurg*. 1996;84:606–616.

190. Stahl N, Mellergard P, Hallstrom A, et al. Intracerebral microdialysis and bedside biochemical analysis in patients with fatal traumatic brain lesions. *Acta Anaesthesiol Scand*. 2001;45:977–985.

191. Skjoth-Rasmussen J, Schulz M, Kristensen SR, et al. Delayed neurological deficits detected by an ischemic pattern in the extracellular cerebral metabolites in patients with aneurysmal subarachnoid hemorrhage. *J Neurosurg*. 2004;100:8–15.

192. Benveniste H. Brain microdialysis. *J Neurochem*. 1989;52:1667–1679.

193. Hutchinson PJ, Gupta AK, Fryer TF, et al. Correlation between cerebral blood flow, substrate delivery, and metabolism in head injury: a combined microdialysis and triple oxygen positron emission tomography study. *J Cereb Blood Flow Metab*. 2002;22:735–745.

194. Hutchinson PJ, Al-Rawi PG, O'Connell MT, et al. Head injury monitoring using cerebral microdialysis and paratrend multiparameter sensors. *Zentralbl Neurochir*. 2000;61:88–94.

195. Hutchinson PJ, Al-Rawi PG, O'Connell MT, et al. On-line monitoring of substrate delivery and brain metabolism in head injury. *Acta Neurochir Suppl*. 2000;76:431–435.

196. Zauner A, Doppenberg EM, Woodward JJ, et al. Continuous monitoring of cerebral substrate delivery and clearance: initial experience in 24 patients with severe acute brain injuries. *Neurosurgery*. 1997;41:1082–1091.

197. Kett-White R, Hutchinson PJ, Al-Rawi PG, et al. Adverse cerebral events detected after subarachnoid hemorrhage using brain oxygen and microdialysis probes. *Neurosurgery*. 2002;50:1213–1221.

198. Hillered L, Valtysson J, Enblad P, et al. Interstitial glycerol as a marker for membrane phospholipid degradation in the acutely injured human brain. *J Neurol Neurosurg Psychiatry*. 1998;64:486–491.

199. Peerdeman SM, Girbes AR, Polderman KH, et al. Changes in cerebral interstitial glycerol concentration in head-injured patients; correlation with secondary events. *Intensive Care Med*. 2003;29:1825–1828.

200. Nilsson OG, Brandt L, Ungerstedt U, et al. Bedside detection of brain ischemia using intracerebral microdialysis: subarachnoid hemorrhage and delayed ischemic deterioration. *Neurosurgery*. 1999;45:1176–1184.

201. Valadka AB, Goodman JC, Gopinath SP, et al. Comparison of brain tissue oxygen tension to microdialysis-based measures of cerebral ischemia in fatally head-injured humans. *J Neurotrauma*. 1998;15:509–519.

202. Vespa P, Prins M, Ronne-Engstrom E, et al. Increase in extracellular glutamate caused by reduced cerebral perfusion pressure and seizures after human traumatic brain injury: a microdialysis study. *J Neurosurg*. 1998;89:971–982.

203. Staub F, Graf R, Gabel P, et al. Multiple interstitial substances measured by microdialysis in patients with subarachnoid hemorrhage. *Neurosurgery*. 2000;47:1106–1115.

204. Obrenovitch TP, Urenjak J. Is high extracellular glutamate the key to excitotoxicity in traumatic brain injury? *J Neurotrauma*. 1997;14:677–698.

205. Hillered L, Vespa PM, Hovda DA. Translational neurochemical research in acute human brain injury: the current status and potential future for cerebral microdialysis. *J Neurotrauma*. 2005;22:3–41.

206. Sundt TM Jr, Sharbrough FW, Anderson RE, et al. Cerebral blood flow measurements and electroencephalograms during carotid endarterectomy. *J Neurosurg*. 1974;41:310–320.

207. Sundt TM Jr, Sharbrough FW, Piepgras DG, et al. Correlation of cerebral blood flow and electroencephalographic changes during carotid endarterectomy: with results of surgery and hemodynamics of cerebral ischemia. *Mayo Clin Proc*. 1981;56:533–543.

208. Astrup J, Siesjo BK, Symon L. Thresholds in cerebral ischemia: the ischemic penumbra. *Stroke*. 1981;12:723–725.

209. Jordan KG. Emergency EEG and continuous EEG monitoring in acute ischemic stroke. *J Clin Neurophysiol*. 2004;21:341–352.

210. Hirsch LJ. Continuous EEG monitoring in the intensive care unit: an overview. *J Clin Neurophysiol*. 2004;21:332–340.

211. Claassen J, Hirsch LJ, Emerson RG, et al. Treatment of refractory status epilepticus with pentobarbital, propofol, or midazolam: a systematic review. *Epilepsia*. 2002;43:146–153.

212. Hebb MO, McArthur DL, Alger J, et al. Impaired percent alpha variability on continuous electroencephalography is associated with thalamic injury and predicts poor long-term outcome after human traumatic brain injury. *J Neurotrauma*. 2007;24:579–590.

213. Claassen J, Hirsch LJ, Kreiter KT, et al. Quantitative continuous EEG for detecting delayed cerebral ischemia in patients with poor-grade subarachnoid hemorrhage. *Clin Neurophysiol*. 2004;115:2699–2710.

214. Claassen J, Mayer SA, Hirsch LJ. Continuous EEG monitoring in patients with subarachnoid hemorrhage. *J Clin Neurophysiol*. 2005;22:92–98.

215. Labar DR, Fisch BJ, Pedley TA, et al. Quantitative EEG monitoring for patients with subarachnoid hemorrhage. *Electroencephalogr Clin Neurophysiol*. 1991;78:325–332.

216. Vespa PM, Nuwer MR, Juhasz C, et al. Early detection of vasospasm after acute subarachnoid hemorrhage using continuous EEG ICU monitoring. *Electroencephalogr Clin Neurophysiol.* 1997;103:607–615.

217. Wittman JJ Jr, Hirsch LJ. Continuous electroencephalogram monitoring in the critically ill. *Neurocrit Care.* 2005;2:330–341.

218. Stein SC, Georgoff P, Meghan S, et al. Relationship of aggressive monitoring and treatment to improved outcomes in severe traumatic brain injury. *J Neurosurg.* 2010;112:1105–1112.

219. Stein SC, Georgoff P, Meghan S, et al. 150 Years of treating severe traumatic brain injury: a systematic review of progress in mortality. *J Neurotrauma.* 2010;27:1343–1353.

220. Narayan RK, Michel ME, Ansell B, et al. Clinical trials in head injury. *J Neurotrauma.* 2002;19:503–557.

221. Kofke WA. Incrementally applied multifaceted therapeutic bundles in neuroprotection clinical trials... time for change. *Neurocrit Care.* 2010;12:438–444.

222. Morris G, Gardner R. Computer applications. In Hall J, Schmidt G, Wood L, eds. *Principles of critical care.* New York: McGraw-Hill; 1992:500–514.

223. Jennings D, Amabile T, Ross L. Informal assessments: data-based versus theory-based judgments. In Kahnemann D, Slovic P, Tversky A, eds. *Judgments under uncertainty: heuristics and biases.* Cambridge, UK: Cambridge University Press; 1982:211–230.

224. Goldberger AL, Amaral LA, Hausdorff JM, et al. Fractal dynamics in physiology: alterations with disease and aging. *Proc Natl Acad Sci U S A.* 2002;99(Suppl 1):2466–2472.

4.
NEUROMONITORING BASICS: OPTIMIZING THE ANESTHETIC

Stacie Deiner

INTRODUCTION: THE EVOLUTION OF MONITORING FOR SPINE AND BRAIN SURGERY

The potential for neurologic injury during surgery of the brain and spinal cord has caused a strong interest in the early recognition of iatrogenic compromise. In 1973, Vauzelle and colleagues published a report on the practice of awakening patients during critical phase of their spine surgery (i.e., after the placement of rods during scoliosis surgery) and asking them to move their extremities [1]. If the patient was able to move, then the spinal cord was considered to be intact and surgery was allowed to proceed. If the patient did not move, then the hardware was removed and the surgery was terminated. This first attempt at intraoperative monitoring of the spinal cord had some obvious disadvantages: it was time consuming, it could cause physical or psychological harm to the patient, and it was impractical to perform multiple times. Hence, the need was recognized for a test of spinal cord integrity that was less dangerous and could be repeated throughout the surgery.

The ankle clonus reflex test addressed some of the issues of the wake-up test and was primarily used in children during scoliosis surgery [2]. This test assesses whether the lower extremity stretch reflex remains intact; passive dorsiflexion of the foot stimulates the stretch reflex and produces rhythmic contraction of the calf muscles (clonus). This reflex is absent in normal awake patient because of central reflex inhibition but is present during periods of light anesthesia in neurologically intact patients due to the return of lower motor neuron function before the appearance of inhibitory upper motor neuron impulses. Presence of the ankle clonus reflex signifies intact spinal cord pathway along the reflex arc. However, absence of the reflex may be due to an anesthesia plane that is too light or too deep or due to injury to the cord at the surgical site. This lack of specificity was proved in many studies, and the test has fallen out of favor [3–5].

In the late 1970s and early 1980s, studies in animal models suggested that changes in somatosensory evoked potentials (SSEPs) of the hindlimbs during distraction of the spinal cord correlate with loss of motor and sensory function [6, 7]. Subsequently SSEP signal changes have been found to correlate well with clinical outcomes and serum markers of cell damage [8, 9]. This information is the basis of modern intraoperative neuromonitoring. In this chapter, we will consider the major types of intraoperative neuromonitoring currently in use: SSEPs, motor evoked potentials (MEPs), electromyography (EMG), brainstem evoked auditory responses (BAER), and visual evoked potentials (VEPs). We will discuss the utility/indication, anesthetic considerations, and limitations of each modality. This chapter is not meant to be an exhaustive discussion of the techniques of monitoring. For a more in-depth discussion, the reader is referred to many excellent texts and review articles [10–12]. Rather, this chapter will discuss the fundamental basis of neuromonitoring for the purpose of helping anesthesia practitioners understand the rationale for choosing a particular test, suggestions of how to facilitate acquisition of signals through anesthetic technique, and the significance of intraoperative deterioration in evoked potentials.

SSEPS

DEFINITION

SSEP monitoring involves peripheral stimulation of a mixed motor/sensory nerve, which then initiates sensory and motor transmissions. These transmissions are recorded as an EEG response monitored by electrodes over the sensory cortex and peripherally as muscle contractions. The most commonly monitored nerves are superficial and large enough to be stimulated easily. Examples include the median (C6-T1), ulnar (C8-T1), common peroneal (L4-S1), and posterior tibial (L4-S2). A disturbance of transmission can be caused by an injury anywhere along the peripheral nerve, plexus, spinal cord, or cortex (Figure 4.1). The neural tract for the upper extremity ascends the ipsilateral dorsal column, synapses at the nucleus cuneatus, crosses at the cervicomedullary junction, continues to ascend via the medial lemniscus, and projects to the contralateral parietal sensory cortex. Sensory evoked responses from the lower extremity ascend along a similar path; in addition, some of the signal travels via the anterolateral spinocerebellar pathways. Signals are usually recorded at three or four sites along the sensory pathway from the periphery to the cortex. For example, in the upper extremity, a stimulus at the median nerve would be recorded over Erb's point, cervical vertebrae, and cortex (Figure 4.2).

UTILITY

In animal studies, depression of SSEP signals correlates with loss of sensory and motor function during spine distraction [7]. In the absence of malfunctioning monitoring equipment, these changes are caused by loss of blood supply to the cord from direct compression or disruption of the blood supply to the cord by secondary factors (e.g., low blood pressure). The largest study to examine the utility of SSEP responses included 51,000 patients with scoliosis and was conducted by the Scoliosis Research Society (SRS) and European Spinal Deformities Society. In this study, patients who underwent surgery with SSEP monitoring had a significantly lower (0.55%) incidence of neurologic injury than did patients who did not have SSEP monitoring (0.7% to 4%) [13]. Based on these data, the SRS issued a position statement that "neurophysiological monitoring can assist in the early detection of complications and possibly prevent

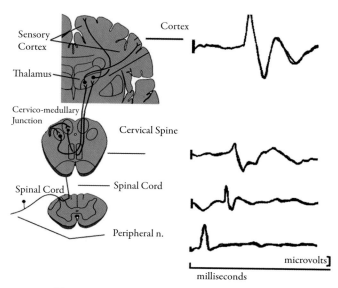

Figure 4.2   SSEP response recorded at different portions of the ascending somatosensory pathway.

postoperative morbidity in patients undergoing operations on the spine" [14]. Subsequently, surveys suggest that most surgeons in the United States use SSEP monitoring for most of their spine surgery cases [15].

SSEP monitoring has utility in many other types of surgery where direct injury to a neural structure is possible. For example, SSEPs can be used during resection of spinal cord tumors or to find the optimal area for transection during dorsal root entry zone lesioning. Some uses of SSEPs outside of spinal surgery include the prevention of positioning injuries through evaluation of peripheral nerves and brachial plexus. SSEPs can be used to identify areas for surgical repair when there has been nerve injury. In combination with auditory and cranial nerve monitoring, SSEPs may be used to assess the integrity of the brainstem during surgery on the posterior fossa. Direct monitoring of the sensory cortex using bipolar recording strips can be used to identify the gyri separating the motor and sensory strip.

Like EEG, SSEPs are sensitive to changes in blood flow below a threshold (20 mL/100 g/min) and are lost entirely during ischemia (15–18 mL/100 g/min). This information can be used to determine the critical threshold for induced hypotension or anemia, which may occur at unanticipated levels in predisposed individuals [16]. Systemic blood pressure is an imprecise surrogate marker of oxygen delivery to the spinal cord because of regional compromise of flow due to spinal pathology or surgical compression. Neural tissue sensitivity to changes in blood flow can be important in open craniotomy and interventional radiology procedures for arteriovenous malformations and intracranial aneurysms. SSEPs can also detect changes in blood flow during vascular surgery procedures such as carotid endarterectomy. Postoperatively, SSEPs can be used to identify cerebral vasospasm after subarachnoid hemorrhage.

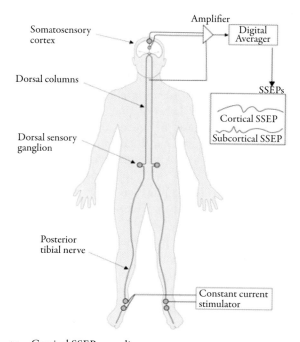

Figure 4.1   Cortical SSEP recording. Source: Devlin Schwartz, J American Academy of Orthopedic Surgeons. 15(9) Sept 2007, 549–60.

ANESTHETIC CONSIDERATIONS

All anesthetic agents affect conduction along neural pathways, as demonstrated by their effect on EEG, and will therefore affect the acquisition of evoked potentials to varying degrees. Anesthetic agents may affect the evoked responses by either direct inhibition of synaptic pathways or indirectly by changing the balance of inhibitory and excitatory influences. The magnitude of the effect increases with the number of synapses in the pathway.

Most anesthetic agents depress evoked response amplitude and increase latency (Figure 4.3). Inhaled anesthetics accomplish this by altering specific receptors or through nonspecific effects on cell membranes that alter the conformation structure of the receptor or ion channel. The effect of halogenated agents on SSEP signals directly correlates with potency: isoflurane > enflurane > halothane. Studies suggest that sevoflurane and desflurane are similar to isoflurane [17]. Nitrous oxide reduces SSEP cortical amplitude and increases latency alone or with halogenated inhalational agents or opioid agents. The greatest effect is seen in the waveforms recorded over the cortex and less in the Erb's point and cervical waveforms. Compared with equipotent halogenated anesthetic concentrations, nitrous oxide produces more profound changes in cortical SSEPs [17].

Intravenous agents have effects on evoked potentials on the basis of their affinity for neurotransmitter receptors (e.g., γ-aminobutyric acid, *N*-methyl-D-aspartate, glutamate, etc.). The effect varies with the specific receptor and pathways affected. Propofol, benzodiazepines, and barbiturates cause significant depression of the amplitude of the waveforms. Benzodiazepines and barbiturates infusions are no longer commonly used for maintenance anesthesia during spine surgery for various reasons, including their extremely long context-sensitive half-life, the potential of barbiturates to cause hyperalgesia, and prolonged

depression of the signals after a bolus induction dose. While an induction dose of propofol causes depression of SSEPs, its context-sensitive half-time is significantly shorter, and therefore its titratability makes it an important component of a maintenance anesthetic during a monitored spine surgery, especially in combination with other favorable drugs. Opioids affect SSEP signals less than do inhalational agents, making them an important component of evoked potential monitoring. Bolus doses of opioids can be associated with a mild decrease in amplitude and an increase in latency in responses recorded from the cortex. Opioid infusions are generally conducive to monitoring, and many neuroanesthesiologists have taken advantage of remifentanil, which has an extremely short half-life, to supplement an intravenous maintenance anesthetic. Some intravenous anesthetics that do not depress SSEP waveform amplitude include etomidate and ketamine. These drugs increase signal amplitude, potentially by attenuating inhibition [17]. In addition to its beneficial effects on neuromonitoring signals, ketamine is a powerful analgesic and may be especially helpful for controlling pain in opioid-tolerant patients [18]. Recent studies have examined the effect of dexmedetomidine on the acquisition of neuromonitoring signals. Several studies have found that the use of dexmedetomidine is compatible with the acquisition of SSEPs [19]. The effect of inhalational and intravenous agents on SSEP monitoring, with suggested dosage range, is summarized in Table 4.1.

Neuromuscular blocking agents have their affect at the neuromuscular junction and therefore do not negatively affect the acquisition of SSEP signals. If anything, this class of drugs improves the acquisition of signals by decreasing movement artifact.

LIMITATIONS

Although SSEPs are effective for monitoring the integrity of the dorsal columns, the technique is limited in its ability to predict overall clinical outcomes. Most important, the presence of SSEPs does not guarantee an intact motor pathway. This is because the motor and sensory tracts are located in different regions of the spinal cord and have distinct blood supplies. Although in early reports, SSEP preservation in patients with postoperative paraplegia was considered to be a failure of SSEP monitoring, this was inappropriate because preserved SSEPs are considered to be false negative only when there is a postoperative sensory deficit [20]. While it is likely that stretch injury, such as due to distraction during scoliosis surgery, might affect both pathways, it is possible that surgery may directly injure one of the tracts (e.g., placement of a strut graft during an anterior cervical discectomy). In patients undergoing scoliosis surgery Nuwer and colleagues found that 0.063% of patients with preserved SSEPs had permanent neurologic deficits [15]. In comparison, 0.983%

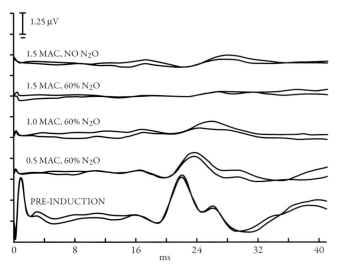

1.25 μV

1.5 MAC, NO N₂O

1.5 MAC, 60% N₂O

1.0 MAC, 60% N₂O

0.5 MAC, 60% N₂O

PRE-INDUCTION

0   8   16   24   32   40

ms

Figure 4.3   Effect of anesthetics on cortical SSEPs.

Table 4.1　**EFFECT OF ANESTHETIC AGENTS ON EVOKED POTENTIALS**

Drug	SSEPs		BAEPs		VEPs		Transcranial MEPs	
	LAT	*AMP*	*LAT*	*AMP*	*LAT*	*AMP*	*LAT*	*AMP*
Isoflurane	Yes	Yes	No	No	Yes	Yes	Yes	Yes
Enflurane	Yes	Yes	No	No	Yes	Yes	Yes	Yes
Halothane	Yes	Yes	No	No	Yes	Yes	Yes	Yes
Nitrous oxide*	Yes	Yes	No	No	Yes	Yes	Yes	Yes
Barbiturates	Yes	Yes	No	No	Yes	Yes	Yes	Yes
Etomidate	No	No	No	No	Yes	Yes	No	No
Propofol	Yes	Yes	No	No	Yes	Yes	Yes	Yes
Droperidol	No	No	No	No	—	—	Yes	Yes
Diazepam	Yes	Yes	No	No	Yes	Yes	Yes	Yes
Midazolam	Yes	Yes	No	No	Yes	Yes	Yes	Yes
Ketamine	No	No	No	No	Yes	Yes	No	No
Opiates	No	No	No	No	No	No	No	No
Dexmedetomidine	No	No	No	No	No	ND	ND	No

LAT, mean latency; AMP, amplitude.

---

of patients in the same study had SSEP changes without deficits (false positive). Therefore, the best use of SSEPs is either to detect injury to the sensory tracts when this is the primary concern or in combination with other modalities (e.g., MEPs).

MEPS

DEFINITION

MEPs refers to the use of direct electrical or magnetic stimulation of the motor cortex to produce electrical activity which can be recorded as D waves and I waves, or with epidural electrodes on the surgical field, or as compound muscle action potentials (CMAPs) measured by pairs of needles over the corresponding muscle (Figure 4.4). The electrical stimulation to evoke the response results in a volley of activity that descends the anterior horn of the corticospinal tract. After synapsing in the anterior horn, the impulse travels via peripheral nerve and crosses the neuromuscular junction, resulting in a muscle response.

As mentioned earlier, the sole use of SSEP monitoring to determine integrity of the spinal cord during surgery eventually gave rise to multiple reports of unchanged signals associated with postoperative motor deficit and normal sensory function. This indicated that the anatomic isolation of the motor tracts required the addition of a monitoring modality that would monitor them directly. The ventral portion of the spinal cord is particularly vulnerable to injury

because of its relatively tenuous blood supply: a single anterior spinal artery supplies 75% of the entire cord, which includes the motor tracts. Therefore, the anterior portion of the cord is more susceptible to hypoperfusion injury due to anemia, hypotension, and blood vessel compression.

MEPs can be recorded rapidly by a single brief stimulation or with several pulses to facilitate smaller responses; in

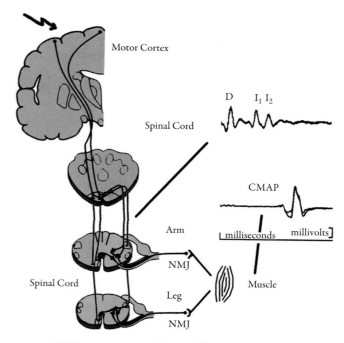

Figure 4.4　MEP responses recorded over different portions of the descending motor pathway.

comparison, SSEP requires multiple stimulations and signal averaging. Common muscles monitored include the adductor policis brevis, biceps, triceps, dorsal intraosseous, tibialis anterior, and anal sphincter. The required pattern of stimulation and milliamperes required for stimulation is highly variable between individuals and even within the same individual during an uncomplicated surgical procedure.

UTILITY

MEP monitoring can be used to detect injury whenever the motor portion of the cord or cortex may be at risk during a surgical procedure. A common use is during scoliosis surgery, when studies have suggested a high correlation of MEP recordings with neurologic outcome. In the largest study, transient changes were relatively common (11.3%); however, permanent MEP changes were associated with neurologic injury [21]. Another use of MEP monitoring is for spinal surgery when the anterior portion of the cord is particularly at risk, such as anterior cervical discectomy. Hildebrand and colleagues described several cases of anterior cervical surgery in which SSEPs were maintained while MEPs were decreased during the placement of an anterior strut graft. The MEPs recovered after removal of the graft [22]. MEPs are well validated for prevention of motor injury during resection of spinal cord tumors [23]. It has been demonstrated that MEPs are more sensitive to spinal cord ischemia than are SSEPs [24, 25]. However, in both surgery for deformities and surgery for tumors, several studies have demonstrated that no single modality monitors the entire spinal cord [26, 27]. When used in combination with SSEP, MEPs are associated with a higher sensitivity and specificity of motor tract injury than is single-modality monitoring [28].

MEP monitoring has been used in craniotomy to prevent injury to the motor cortex. For example, direct motor cortex stimulation can be used to define the edge of motor cortex tumors [29]. MEP is a sensitive indicator of hypoperfusion of the motor cortex, and permanent changes in MEPs during aneurysm clipping are associated with postoperative paresis [30]. Similar to monitoring of the spinal cord, multimodality monitoring is also recommended during craniotomy. Multiple studies have described cases of preserved responses of either SSEP or MEP without changes in the other modality. Brainstem surgery for tumor resection is a good example where multimodal monitoring is used; MEP may be used in combination with SSEP, EMG, and auditory responses to map anatomic landmarks and facilitate the surgical approach.

ANESTHETIC CONSIDERATIONS

MEPs are extremely sensitive to anesthetic agents at the level of the synaptic transmission to the alpha motor neurons to produce CMAP responses. However, responses recorded before this synapse (e.g., D and I waves) are relatively insensitive to anesthetic technique. While some stimulation techniques (e.g., multiple pulses of stimulation) are used to facilitate acquisition of signal, MEPs remain much more sensitive to anesthetic agents and are more difficult to obtain and maintain than are SSEPs [31].

All of the volatile agents are associated with a significant and dose-dependent depression of MEP responses. Inhaled anesthetics suppress pyramidal activation of spinal motor neurons at the level of the ventral horn. Studies suggest that relatively low doses of volatile anesthetics (0.25–0.5 MAC) suppress single pulse transcranial stimuli [32, 33]. While more aggressive stimulation patterns can produce CMAP responses in some patients, others are entirely unattainable [34]. This may be a function of preexisting myelopathy due to the spinal disease process, neuropathy secondary to diabetes, or, more insidiously, subclinical neuropathy associated with chronic hypertension [35]. When the concentration of inhaled anesthetic approaches 1 MAC, less than 10% of patients have appreciable signals [36]. It is controversial whether nitrous oxide is associated with less depression than other agents and can be supplemental to other agents (e.g., ketamine, opioid, or low-dose propofol). Up to 50% nitrous oxide has been shown to be compatible with an adequate myogenic response, especially when intravenous drugs with minimal effects are used (ketamine, opioid) [37, 38]. However, higher doses and use with propofol may be associated with significant (>50%) reduction in CMAP amplitude.

Barbiturates and propofol are associated with a dose-dependent decrease in CMAP amplitude and need for more aggressive stimulation patterns to produce similar CMAP waveforms. Propofol has become ubiquitous during surgery for which MEP monitoring is planned because of its more favorable context-sensitive half-time, titratability, and side effect profile. An exact dose–response curve plotting serum propofol concentrations and MEP signal strength has been difficult to determine due to heterogeneity of anesthetic technique across studies, lack of control for variation in blood pressure, and patient comorbidities. Opioids can suppress cortical excitation but have minimal effect when used as an infusion, and as such are often used in combination with propofol or low-dose inhalational agents. However, care must be taken because bolus doses of opioids can be associated with prolonged CMAP depression, with longer-acting narcotics having prolonged effects [39, 40]. Benzodiazepines can also cause CMAP amplitude depression but have been shown to have minimal effects when used for premedication or used as an infusion. Because of their less favorable context-sensitive half-life, benzodiazepines are generally not used as a maintenance anesthetic (see Table 4.1).

Etomidate causes minimal and transient suppression of CMAP amplitude without increasing latency, even with induction doses. It is likely that etomidate accomplishes this via disinhibition of subcortical structures, resulting in increased excitability of the motor system. Administration of etomidate may cause adrenocortical suppression. It also frequently causes nausea, which limits its utility as a maintenance anesthetic.

Ketamine can be a useful adjunct in the anesthetic of patients with chronic pain. Low- to moderate-dose ketamine (1 mg/kg or 0.25–0.5 mg/kg/hr) has a minimal effect on MEP responses, both as bolus dose and as an infusion. High-dose ketamine (4–8 mg/kg) can be associated with moderate depression of CMAP amplitudes. A recent study showed that a loading dose of 0.5 mg/kg followed by an infusion of 10 μg/kg/min was associated with a lower 48-hour postoperative narcotic consumption and no increase in side effects [18]. Previous studies have suggested that ketamine, when used with narcotic infusion and nitrous oxide, is associated with a 40% incidence of psychedelic side effects; however, another study suggested that this is significantly reduced with the addition of propofol [41].

Neuromuscular blockade, while not completely incompatible with MEP monitoring, is unpredictable and therefore not recommended. Studies suggest that use of neuromuscular blocking drugs when carefully monitored using single twitch M-responses to maintain twitch height 20% to 50% of baseline allows CMAP responses [42]. However, this may be difficult to perceive if clinically monitoring twitch height or if the patient has preexisting neurologic dysfunction [43]. If neuromuscular blockade is required, then the patient should not have any existing neurologic deficits and an accelerometer should be as an objective measure of twitch height. In general, if there is a question regarding whether the absence of an MEP signal in a patient who has received a neuromuscular blocking agent is due to neuromuscular blockade or neurologic injury, then the pattern (single limb versus complete loss of responses) and twitch height should be considered.

LIMITATIONS

Beyond its limitations as a single modality monitor, MEPs can be more technically difficult to obtain and maintain than SSEPs. Chen and colleagues studied more than 300 high-risk spine surgeries and found that the success rate for upper extremity MEP signals was 94.8%, but only two thirds of patients had consistent signals for the lower extremity [31]. The likelihood of success was lower in children under 7 years old and adults over 64 years of age, and this was compounded by the presence of preexisting neurologic deficits. In comparison the same study demonstrated SSEP success rates greater than 98% in the upper extremities, and 93% in the lower extremity. In children with cerebral palsy scheduled for scoliosis surgery, SSEPs are attainable in greater than 80% of patients, whereas MEPs are reliably present only in 40% to 60% [44]. MEPs are also exquisitely sensitive to anesthetic technique (see earlier) and the patient's neurophysiologic status. It has been demonstrated that MEPs cannot be reliably obtained in patients undergoing aortic aneurysm surgery that involves lumbar epidural cooling [45].

Use of MEPs have significant safety considerations, some of which are due to the inability to use neuromuscular blocking agents (i.e., the patient may move) and others that are inherent to the technique itself. The most common safety consideration is the possibility of bite injuries, which can occur because of direct activation of the temporalis muscle during cortical stimulation [46]. Bite injuries vary in severity and include a tongue hematoma, buccal lacerations, injury to the dentition, and jaw fracture. When MEP monitoring is planned, use of a bite block is mandatory. The bite block is placed between the molars on the side opposite to the endotracheal tube and secured in place. Oral airways are generally not large or solid enough to be sufficient for this purpose. In a patient without molars, it is acceptable to use a rolled gauze in the front of the oropharynx; however, it is important that the roll is not so bulky that it precludes venous drainage of the tongue [47].

Relative contraindications to MEP monitoring include a history of seizure disorder, increased intracranial pressure or cortical lesions, defects of the skull or skull convexity, implanted deep brain stimulator leads, cardiac pacemakers, or automated internal defibrillators. MEP monitoring should be used with caution in patients with epilepsy because pulses of electrical current delivered to the brain may cause seizures in susceptible patients. This phenomenon, called *kindling*, has been described a single case report [48]. While the most conservative approach is to avoid MEP in patients with seizure history, limited MEP testing may be used in certain high-risk procedures if the risk of a neurologic injury outweighs the relatively small possibility of inducing seizures. In this case, EEG activity is monitored during surgery, and use of total intravenous anesthesia generally serves to suppress seizure activity, which did resolve spontaneously with cessation of monitoring in the single report in which it was described.

The issue of electrical interference with implanted cardiac devices is somewhat more complex. The proximity of the stimulus to the device makes interference more likely than during SSEPs. However, the presence of a pacemaker or automated implanted cardioverter-defibrillator is a relative contraindication, and in procedures that carry a high risk of neurologic injury, MEP monitoring may be indicated. In this case, the patient, surgeon, monitoring team, and cardiologist should discuss the relative risks of MEP monitoring and decide on a plan in advance of the scheduled surgery. If MEPs are strongly indicated, pacemaker dependence should be assessed. If the patient has an implantable cardioverter-defibrillator, antitachyarrhythmia properties should be disabled and external pacing/defibrillation pads should be placed on the patient.

Pulse oximetry and invasive arterial monitoring should be used to throughout the procedure to allow continuous assessment of the patient's cardiac rhythm. The external pads should remain in place until the procedure is finished and the device has been interrogated, to ensure that it is fully active and functional. Placement of a magnet on the patient's chest is not recommended, especially during prone positioning, due to the potential for dislodgement and injury caused by compression of the skin between the device and the magnet.

EMG

DEFINITION

EMG is a measurement of electrical activity generated by muscle contraction. EMGs are recorded by two electrodes in or near a muscle. Two major types of EMG are recorded during surgery. *Passive,* or *free run,* EMGs reflect spontaneous activity and are continually recorded during the procedure. *Stimulated EMG* is generated by applying an electrical stimulus either directly to a nerve or in its immediate vicinity. The response is recorded as a waveform or an audible tone.

The pattern of EMG response can be used to determine the difference between normal muscle activity during light anesthesia, reversible insult, or injury. Normal EMG waveforms associated with light anesthesia are characteristically of low amplitude and high frequency. Extremely deep general anesthesia is associated with a lack of spontaneous activity and may even result in difficulty eliciting a stimulated response. Less ominous but abnormal activity is characterized by short asynchronous polyphasic waves called burst activity. This type of activity can be caused by fluid irrigation, nerve traction, or brief trauma. This type of activity is generally not sustained, resolves with cessation of the stimuli, and is not associated with permanent injury [11]. The presence of neurotonic activity, which consists of prolonged (minutes to hours) presence of synchronous waveforms, is more ominous [11]. This type of injury is associated with more significant stretch injury (spinal distraction with hardware placement) or compression with retractions. If this type of activity is not addressed by relieving the traction on the nerve, the likely result is a postoperative deficit.

UTILITY

While SSEP and MEP monitor the integrity of a tract, they may not be sensitive for injury of a single nerve root. EMG allows the identification of a single nerve, especially in cases where the anatomy is abnormal (e.g., scar tissue or tumor). EMG is extremely sensitive and can detect activation of only 1% to 2% of a muscle's fibers [49]. Commonly monitored nerves include cervical nerve roots during spine

surgery (C2-7), lumbrosacral (L2-S2) during spine surgery, facial nerve during acoustic neuroma surgery or parotid surgery, recurrent laryngeal nerve during anterior cervical surgery, and cranial nerves during brainstem surgery.

EMG monitoring is considered to be the standard of care for many surgical procedures in which the facial nerve is at risk. Examples include acoustic neuromas, parotid tumors, and cerebellar pontine angle tumors. The integrity of branches of the trigeminal nerve may also be identified with EMG recordings of the orbicularis oculi, oris, mentalis, and temporalis. Both the facial and trigeminal nerves may be monitored by intraoperative stimulation during decompression for trigeminal neuralgia with improved results [48, 50]. Cranial nerve monitoring has become commonplace during radical neck, thyroid, parotid, and auditory surgery and skull base tumor resection. In the lower extremity, free run EMG can be used to avoid sciatic nerve injury during hip arthroplasty.

During spine surgery, both free run and stimulated EMG can be useful to identify correct placement of pedicle screws. Without the use of EMG stimulation, the incidence of neurologic complications associated with pedicle screw placement is estimated to be 2% to 10% [51–53]. In one study using pedicle screw stimulation, this complication was avoided entirely [54]. To perform pedicle screw stimulation, an electrode is attached to a screw that has been placed into a pedicle (Figure 4.5). If the cortex has been breached, then the current required to cause the nerve root to fire and generate EMG activity is one-tenth less than if the bone is intact. In real terms, screw placements with thresholds greater than 10 mA are almost always in the correct position [54]. EMG response at less than 10 mA suggests the need for further inspection of the screw by the surgeon. Likelihood of false positive response correlates positively with stimulation intensity.

ANESTHETIC CONSIDERATIONS

EMG response is generally not dependent on anesthetic technique, except for extremely deep general anesthetics—beyond what is used in clinical practice. Since the response depends on

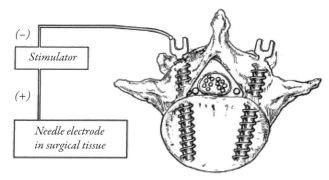

Figure 4.5 EMG stimulation technique used during pedicle screw placement.

muscle activity, paralytic administration should be avoided or titrated with care. Studies suggest that EMG activity can be recorded with as few as two train-of-four (TOF) responses [55]. However, this is assuming that the muscle recording TOF has the same sensitivity to muscle relaxant as the group where EMG monitoring is desired. Also, care must be taken that the TOF electrodes are over a nerve, and not causing direct muscle stimulation, which would cause an underestimation of the neuromuscular blockade.

LIMITATIONS

EMG activity may not be present in the face of real injury in the following cases: chronically compressed nerve roots (which may require much higher stimulation to fire), sharp complete transection of a nerve root, excessive pharmacologic blockade, and recording electrodes not placed into the myotome corresponding to the nerve in question. For these reasons, it is advisable to test a positive control (i.e., the exposed nerve root) before stimulating a screw [51].

BAERS

DEFINITION

Auditory evoked responses are generated by direct stimulation of the cochlea with click noises.

UTILITY

BAERs are used to monitor cranial nerve VIII function during acoustic neuroma surgery and is associated with better preservation of hearing in patients with good hearing before surgery [56]. BAER can also be used to monitor cranial nerve VIII during cerebellar pontine angle tumor resection, decompression of cranial nerves VII and V, and aneurysm clipping in the brainstem, where small case studies have suggested its ability to detect hypoperfusion [57]. It can also be used to detect brainstem function in comatose patients.

ANESTHETIC CONSIDERATIONS

There is minimal effect of anesthetic technique on BAER. Even planes of anesthesia causing an isoelectric EEG are compatible with BAER [57]. BAERs are mildly sensitive to extremes of physiology: temperature, hypoxia, and hypotension (see Table 4.1).

LIMITATIONS

Inadequate responses may be the result of soaking or dislodgement of the insert, which sits in the auditory canal, or the use of ultrasound aspiration devices [57]. Auditory evoked potentials are also unusable in patients who are deaf. They are affected by *auditory masking,* which occurs when there is a loud noise near the patient (i.e., drilling) that prevents the patient's brain from processing the auditory stimulus.

VEPS

DEFINITION

VEPs are elicited by flash stimulation of the retina via plastic goggles or contact lenses and recorded over the scalp centrally and over the occipital and parietal regions.

UTILITY

VEPs vary with stimulus, part of the retina stimulated, degree of pupil dilation, and the patient's attention level in awake patients. While VEPs are seldom used in the operating room, they are sensitive for compression of the optic nerve [58]. Outside of the operating room, this monitoring technique can be used to confirm a diagnosis of multiple sclerosis [59].

ANESTHETIC IMPLICATION

Similar to other potentials recorded over the cortex, VEPs are extremely sensitive to anesthetic agents (see Table 4.1).

LIMITATIONS

The technical aspect of performing VEPs can be difficult, and previously VEPs have been considered highly variable and therefore intraoperative changes are not specific for injury. Hence, VEPs represent the least commonly used evoked response monitoring technique intraoperatively. However, recent studies have asserted that VEPs may be more reliable than previously thought [58].

OTHER FACTORS AFFECTING MONITORING

Maintenance of a steady neurophysiologic condition is the primary way in which the anesthesiologist can facilitate neuromonitoring. Maintenance of blood flow is extremely important for SSEP and MEP monitoring. Similar to cortical EEG, signals are depressed at 20 mL/100 g/min and lost between 15 and 18 mL/100 g/min. In the operating room, the anesthesiologists generally do not directly measure blood flow or tissue oxygenation. Blood pressure is a crude surrogate of blood flow and may be influenced by systemic factors, like a right-shift of autoregulation curves secondary to poorly treated hypotension or local factors like compression by positioning (e.g., brachial plexus injury), spinal hardware, retractors, or clamps. Therefore, it is not always possible to define a "safe" intraoperative blood pressure. A decrement in MEP/SEP signals in the face of a decline in blood pressure without a change in anesthetic technique should be considered to be due to a clinically significant drop in blood flow. It these cases, the surgeon should be informed about the change, the blood pressure raised by use of vasopressors, patient positioning optimized, and any contributing surgical factors considered. Increased intracranial pressure is another reason for decrement of signals, which may be due to decrease in perfusion.

Evoked signals are also sensitive to anemia. Paradoxically, an increase in amplitude is observed in mild anemia; moderate anemia is associated with an additional mild prolongation in latency. Significant depression of SSEPs occurs at extremely low hematocrits (<10 mg/dL) [60]. Hypoxia results in signal decrement, as does hypocarbia through a mechanism involving vasoconstriction. The effects of hypothermia (increased latency, slowing of conduction) can be a result of systemic hypothermia or because of local irrigation with cold solution. Significant electrolyte disturbance could also change neural conduction, which would affect evoked potential signals.

CONCLUSION

Modern neuromonitoring may consist of multimodal use of SSEP, MEP, EMG, BAER, and VEP. Tests are generally chosen to monitor the structures at risk during a surgical procedure. Although not mandatory, use of intraoperative neuromonitoring is associated with improved surgical outcomes for many procedures. The anesthesiologist should strive to understand the indications for test selection, how to optimize signal attainment, and how to respond to an intraoperative change in signals (Table 4.2). Through communication with the neuromonitoring team and the surgeon, the anesthesiologist can play an important role in using these tests to maximize postsurgical outcomes.

Table 4.2 **RESPONDING TO AN INTRAOPERATIVE CHANGE IN EVOKED POTENTIALS**

Communication regarding surgical factors
Increase blood pressure
Check hematocrit, electrolytes
Encourage check of monitoring equipment
Discontinue inhalational agents
Review recent intravenous medications given via bolus
Wake-up test

REFERENCES

1. Vauzelle C, Stagnara P, Jouvinroux P. Functional monitoring of spinal cord activity during spinal surgery. *Clin Orthop Relat Res.* 1973;93:173–178.
2. Hoppenfeld S, Gross A, Andrews C, et al. The ankle clonus test for assessment of the integrity of the spinal cord during operations for scoliosis. *J Bone Joint Surg Am.* 1997;79:208–212.
3. Ewen A, Cox RG, Davies SA, et al. The ankle clonus test is not a clinically useful measure of spinal cord integrity in children. *Can J Anaesth.* 2005;52:524–529. doi:10.1007/BF03016533
4. McCulloch PR, Milne B. Neurological phenomena during emergence from enflurane or isoflurane anaesthesia. *Can J Anaesth.* 1990;37:739–742. doi:10.1007/BF03006531
5. Rosenberg H, Clofine R, Bialik O. Neurologic changes during awakening from anesthesia. *Anesthesiology.* 1981;54:125–130.
6. Jones SJ, Edgar MA, Ransford AO, et al. A system for the electrophysiological monitoring of the spinal cord during operations for scoliosis. *J Bone Joint Surg Br.* 1983;65:134–139.
7. Nordwall A, Axelgaard J, Harada Y, et al. Spinal cord monitoring using evoked potentials recorded from feline vertebral bone. *Spine (Phila Pa 1976).* 1979;4:486–494.
8. Schick U, Dohnert J, Meyer JJ, et al. Prognostic significance of SSEP, BAEP and serum S-100B monitoring after aneurysm surgery. *Acta Neurol Scand.* 2003;108:161–169.
9. Manninen P, Sarjeant R, Joshi M. Posterior tibial nerve and median nerve somatosensory evoked potential monitoring during carotid endarterectomy. *Can J Anaesth.* 2004;51:937–941. doi:10.1007/BF03018896.
10. Deletis V, Shils J. *Neurophysiology in neurosurgery.* Philadelphia: Academic Press; 2004.
11. Jameson LC, Sloan TB. Monitoring of the brain and spinal cord. *Anesthesiol Clin.* 2006;24:777–791.
12. Devlin VJ, Schwartz DM. Intraoperative neurophysiologic monitoring during spinal surgery. *J Am Acad Orthop Surg.* 2007;15:549–560.
13. Dawson EG, Sherman JE, Kanim LE, et al. Spinal cord monitoring. Results of the Scoliosis Research Society and the European Spinal Deformity Society survey. *Spine (Phila Pa 1976).* 1991;16(8 Suppl):S361–S364.
14. Scoliosis Research Society. Position statement: Somatosensory evoked potential monitoring of neurologic spinal cord function during spinal surgery. Scoliosis Research Society, September 1992. Available at http://www.srs.org/professionals/advocacy_and_public_policy/Position_Statement_on_Somatosensory_Evoked_Potential_Monitoring.htm
15. Nuwer MR, Dawson EG, Carlson LG, et al. Somatosensory evoked potential spinal cord monitoring reduces neurologic deficits after scoliosis surgery: results of a large multicenter survey. *Electroencephalogr Clin Neurophysiol.* 1995;96:6–11.
16. Horiuchi K, Suzuki K, Sasaki T, et al. Intraoperative monitoring of blood flow insufficiency during surgery of middle cerebral artery aneurysms. *J Neurosurg.* 2005;103:275–283. doi:10.3171/jns.2005.103.2.0275
17. Sloan TB, Heyer EJ. Anesthesia for intraoperative neurophysiologic monitoring of the spinal cord. *J Clin Neurophysiol.* 2002;19:430–443.
18. Loftus RW, Yeager MP, Clark JA, et al. Intraoperative ketamine reduces perioperative opiate consumption in opiate-dependent patients with chronic back pain undergoing back surgery. *Anesthesiology.* 2010;113:639–646. doi:10.1097/ALN.0b013e31819e90914
19. Anschel DJ, Aherne A, Soto RG, et al. Successful intraoperative spinal cord monitoring during scoliosis surgery using a total intravenous anesthetic regimen including dexmedetomidine. *J Clin Neurophysiol.* 2008;25:56–61. doi:10.1097/WNP.0b013e318163cca6
20. Lesser RP, Raudzens P, Luders H, et al. Postoperative neurological deficits may occur despite unchanged intraoperative somatosensory evoked potentials. *Ann Neurol.* 1986;19:22–25. doi:10.1002/ana.410190105

21. Langeloo DD, Lelivelt A, Louis Journee H, et al. Transcranial electrical motor-evoked potential monitoring during surgery for spinal deformity: a study of 145 patients. *Spine (Phila Pa 1976)*. 2003;28:1043–1050. doi:10.1097/01. BRS.0000061995.75709.78

22. Hilibrand AS, Schwartz DM, Sethuraman V, et al. Comparison of transcranial electric motor and somatosensory evoked potential monitoring during cervical spine surgery. *J Bone Joint Surg Am*. 2004;86-**A**:1248–1253.

23. Kothbauer KF, Deletis V, Epstein FJ. Motor-evoked potential monitoring for intramedullary spinal cord tumor surgery: correlation of clinical and neurophysiological data in a series of 100 consecutive procedures. *Neurosurg Focus*. 1998;4:e1.

24. Costa P, Bruno A, Bonzanino M, et al. Somatosensory- and motor-evoked potential monitoring during spine and spinal cord surgery. *Spinal Cord*. 2007;45:86–91. doi:10.1038/sj.sc.3101934

25. Deletis V, Sala F. Intraoperative neurophysiological monitoring of the spinal cord during spinal cord and spine surgery: a review focus on the corticospinal tracts. *Clin Neurophysiol*. 2008;119:248–264. doi:10.1016/j.clinph.2007.09.135

26. Tsirikos AI, Howitt SP, McMaster MJ. Segmental vessel ligation in patients undergoing surgery for anterior spinal deformity. *J Bone Joint Surg Br*. 2008;90:474–479. doi:10.1302/0301-620X. 90B4.20011

27. Sala F, Bricolo A, Faccioli F, et al. Surgery for intramedullary spinal cord tumors: the role of intraoperative (neurophysiological) monitoring. *Eur Spine J*. 2007;16(Suppl 2):S130–S139. doi:10.1007/s00586-007-0423-x

28. Hyun SJ, Rhim SC, Kang JK, et al. Combined motor- and somatosensory-evoked potential monitoring for spine and spinal cord surgery: correlation of clinical and neurophysiological data in 85 consecutive procedures. *Spinal Cord*. 2009;47:616–622. doi:10.1038/sc.2009.11

29. Neuloh G, Schramm J. Motor evoked potential monitoring for the surgery of brain tumours and vascular malformations. *Adv Tech Stand Neurosurg*. 2004;29:171–228.

30. Zhou HH, Kelly PJ. Transcranial electrical motor evoked potential monitoring for brain tumor resection. *Neurosurgery*. 2001;48:1075–1080; discussion 1080–1081.

31. Chen X, Sterio D, Ming X, et al. Success rate of motor evoked potentials for intraoperative neurophysiologic monitoring: effects of age, lesion location, and preoperative neurologic deficits. *J Clin Neurophysiol*. 2007;24:281–285. doi:10.1097/WNP.0b013e31802ed2d4

32. Haghighi SS, Sirintrapun SJ, Keller BP, et al. Effect of desflurane anesthesia on transcortical motor evoked potentials. *J Neurosurg Anesthesiol*. 1996;8:47–51.

33. Haghighi SS, Madsen R, Green KD, et al. Suppression of motor evoked potentials by inhalation anesthetics. *J Neurosurg Anesthesiol*. 1990;2:73–78.

34. Deiner SG, Kwatra SG, Lin HM, et al. Patient characteristics and anesthetic technique are additive but not synergistic predictors of successful motor evoked potential monitoring. *Anesth Analg*. 2010;111:421–425. doi:10.1213/ANE.0b013e3181e41804

35. Edwards L, Ring C, McIntyre D, et al. Cutaneous sensibility and peripheral nerve function in patients with unmedicated essential hypertension. *Psychophysiology*. 2008;45:141–147. doi:10.1111/j.1469-8986.2007.00608.x

36. Kawaguchi M, Sakamoto T, Ohnishi H, et al. Intraoperative myogenic motor evoked potentials induced by direct electrical stimulation of the exposed motor cortex under isoflurane and sevoflurane. *Anesth Analg*. 1996;82:593–599.

37. van Dongen EP, ter Beek HT, Schepens MA, et al. The influence of nitrous oxide to supplement fentanyl/low-dose propofol anesthesia on transcranial myogenic motor-evoked potentials during thoracic aortic surgery. *J Cardiothorac Vasc Anesth*. 1999;13:30–34.

38. Ubags LH, Kalkman CJ, Been HD, et al. Differential effects of nitrous oxide and propofol on myogenic transcranial motor evoked responses during sufentanil anaesthesia. *Br J Anaesth*. 1997;79:590–594.

39. Taniguchi M, Nadstawek J, Langenbach U, et al. Effects of four intravenous anesthetic agents on motor evoked potentials elicited by magnetic transcranial stimulation. *Neurosurgery*. 1993;33:407–415; discussion 415.

40. Schmid UD, Boll J, Liechti S, et al. Influence of some anesthetic agents on muscle responses to transcranial magnetic cortex stimulation: a pilot study in humans. *Neurosurgery*. 1992;30:85–92.

41. Kawaguchi M, Sakamoto T, Inoue S, et al. Low dose propofol as a supplement to ketamine-based anesthesia during intraoperative monitoring of motor-evoked potentials. *Spine (Phila Pa 1976)*. 2000;25:974–979.

42. van Dongen EP, ter Beek HT, Schepens MA, et al. Within-patient variability of myogenic motor-evoked potentials to multipulse transcranial electrical stimulation during two levels of partial neuromuscular blockade in aortic surgery. *Anesth Analg*. 1999;88:22–27.

43. Lang EW, Beutler AS, Chesnut RM, et al. Myogenic motor-evoked potential monitoring using partial neuromuscular blockade in surgery of the spine. *Spine (Phila Pa 1976)*. 1996;21:1676–1686.

44. Master DL, Thompson GH, Poe-Kochert C, et al. Spinal cord monitoring for scoliosis surgery in Rett syndrome: can these patients be accurately monitored? *J Pediatr Orthop*. 2008;28:342–346. doi:10.1097/BPO.0b013e318168d194

45. Shine TS, Harrison BA, De Ruyter ML, et al. Motor and somatosensory evoked potentials: their role in predicting spinal cord ischemia in patients undergoing thoracoabdominal aortic aneurysm repair with regional lumbar epidural cooling. *Anesthesiology*. 2008;108:580–587. doi:10.1097/ALN.0b013e318168d921

46. MacDonald DB. Safety of intraoperative transcranial electrical stimulation motor evoked potential monitoring. *J Clin Neurophysiol*. 2002;19:416–429.

47. Ellis SC, Bryan-Brown CW, Hyderally H. Massive swelling of the head and neck. *Anesthesiology*. 1975;42:102–103.

48. Mooij JJ, Mustafa MK, van Weerden TW. Hemifacial spasm: intraoperative electromyographic monitoring as a guide for microvascular decompression. *Neurosurgery*. 2001;49:1365–1370; discussion 1370–1371.

49. Leppanen RE, Abnm D, American Society of Neurophysiological M. Intraoperative monitoring of segmental spinal nerve root function with free-run and electrically-triggered electromyography and spinal cord function with reflexes and F-responses. A position statement by the American Society of Neurophysiological Monitoring. *J Clin Monit Comput*. 2005;19:437–461. doi:10.1007/s10877-005-0086-2

50. Edwards BM, Kileny PR. Intraoperative neurophysiologic monitoring: indications and techniques for common procedures in otolaryngology-head and neck surgery. *Otolaryngol Clin North Am*. 2005;38:631–642, viii. doi:10.1016/j.otc.2005.03.002

51. Holland NR. Intraoperative electromyography during thoracolumbar spinal surgery. *Spine (Phila Pa 1976)*. 1998;23:1915–1922.

52. Holland NR, Lukaczyk TA, Riley LH 3rd, et al. Higher electrical stimulus intensities are required to activate chronically compressed nerve roots. Implications for intraoperative electromyographic pedicle screw testing. *Spine (Phila Pa 1976)*. 1998;23:224–227.

53. Matsuzaki H, Tokuhashi Y, Matsumoto F, et al. Problems and solutions of pedicle screw plate fixation of lumbar spine. *Spine (Phila Pa 1976)*. 1990;15:1159–1165.

54. Toleikis JR, Skelly JP, Carlvin AO, et al. The usefulness of electrical stimulation for assessing pedicle screw placements. *J Spinal Disord*. 2000;13:283–289.

55. Owen JH, Kostuik JP, Gornet M, et al. The use of mechanically elicited electromyograms to protect nerve roots during surgery for spinal degeneration. *Spine (Phila Pa 1976)*. 1994;19:1704–1710.

56. Tonn JC, Schlake HP, Goldbrunner R, et al. Acoustic neuroma surgery as an interdisciplinary approach: a neurosurgical series of 508 patients. *J Neurol Neurosurg Psychiatry*. 2000;69:161–166.

57. Legatt AD. Mechanisms of intraoperative brainstem auditory evoked potential changes. *J Clin Neurophysiol*. 2002;19:396–408.

58. Ota T, Kawai K, Kamada K, et al. Intraoperative monitoring of cortically recorded visual response for posterior visual pathway. *J Neurosurg*. 2010;112:285–294. doi:10.3171/2009.6.JNS081272

59. Ko KF. The role of evoked potential and MR imaging in assessing multiple sclerosis: a comparative study. *Singapore Med J*. 2010;51:716–720.

60. Nagao S, Roccaforte P, Moody RA. The effects of isovolemic hemodilution and reinfusion of packed erythrocytes on somatosensory and visual evoked potentials. *J Surg Res*. 1978;25:530–537.

5.

CEREBRAL ISCHEMIA AND NEUROPROTECTION

James G. Hecker

The best hope for a good outcome after an ischemic event requires early recognition and the rapid implementation of appropriate therapies. This chapter discusses the clinical management of neurosurgical problems, with special emphasis on challenges that may be encountered in community practice as well as major academic medical centers. Wherever possible, algorithms or guidelines for management will be discussed, key points will be highlighted, and illustrations will be used. The subspecialty of neurosurgical anesthesiology requires that the anesthesiologist have an understanding of neuroanatomy, neurophysiology, and the surgical procedure. There must be close cooperation between the anesthesiologist and neurosurgeon and, as appropriate, with the neurologist and electrophysiologist.

After discussing existing treatments, we will then offer a summary of contemporary advances in knowledge about secondary injury. A discussion of novel strategies of postischemia resuscitation that attenuate secondary injury can be divided into those strategies proved to be effective and those that are probably effective or intuitive. Finally, we will explore exciting ideas that have the potential to provide a comprehensive model for the central nervous system (CNS) in normal physiology and pathophysiology and to offer the possibility of prophylactic therapies.

References will include scientific citations and review articles that will be provided in a separate section, Recommended Further Reading.

CEREBRAL ISCHEMIA

IMMEDIATE INJURY

Ischemia can occur from a variety of causes and mechanisms that range from global hypoperfusion to intracellular pathology. In 1997 [1, 2], Pedrizet reintroduced the concept of *"near lethal"* stressors, championed by Hans Selye,

that are usually ischemic but can be any near-lethal insult at a cellular or tissue level. It is important to consider neurophysiology and pathophysiologic processes in the context of global and local cerebral blood flow (CBF), cerebral metabolic rate (CMR), intracranial pressure (ICP), cerebral perfusion pressure (CPP), autoregulation, and normal and injured brain. We will define and discuss neuroprotection in the sense of "optimized physiologic parameters," in so far as we know them, both before and after ischemia or other "near-lethal" insults.

CNS injury is often ischemic (i.e., hypoxia, due to an embolic or thrombotic stroke) but can also be due to hemorrhage, trauma, or surgical injury, or it can be the result of a host of infectious, inflammatory, neurodegenerative, septic, immune, or drug insults. CNS injury in the *perioperative* period is primarily ischemic in nature, and this ischemic injury may be caused by the surgical procedure, positioning, or surgical retraction. These insults may be transient or permanent and may manifest as speech, motor, or sensory deficits; increases in ICP; CNS edema; new-onset seizures; nausea and vomiting; epidural, subdural, or parenchymal hematoma; or cranial nerve and brainstem injury. Surgical procedures that most commonly cause CNS injury include repair of a brain or spinal cord aneurysm or arteriovenous malformations; craniotomy for traumatic brain injury (TBI) or tumor; thoracic or, less commonly, abdominal aortic aneurysm resection (including thoracic endovascular aortic repair); carotid endarterectomy; coronary artery bypass graft surgery (especially including valve repair and aortic arch procedures); deep hypothermic circulatory arrest; and interventional neuroradiology (including thrombolysis, stents, coiling]. Any surgical procedure that involves massive blood loss (e.g., major spine procedures), sitting position, or prolonged hypotension can cause CNS ischemia. An initial ischemic insult can predispose cells and tissues of the CNS to secondary injury by triggering pathways via multiple mechanisms, which we will describe in more detail later.

ASSESSMENT POINTS

PREOPERATIVE ASSESSMENT

In addition to a standard preanesthesia assessment, evaluation of a patient scheduled to undergo a neurosurgical procedure should include the following:

CNS. The history should include seizures, transient ischemic attacks, and manifestations of intracranial hypertension such as nausea and vomiting. In patients who have already been admitted to the intensive care unit or emergency department, the flow sheet should be reviewed for mannitol or hypertonic saline. In patients who are intubated and mechanically ventilated, the respiratory flow sheet should be reviewed to determine whether the patient is being hyperventilated and for how long. The patient should be examined for focal neurological deficits or changes in mental status such as lethargy or severe headache due to trauma, intracranial hypertension, or drugs.

Head and Neck. A discussion with the patient or family members and a careful review of the chart may elicit a history of difficult intubation or difficult ventilation. The chart should be reviewed for the presence of intracranial hypertension. If the patient has a traumatic injury, the radiographs of the cervical spine should be reviewed. If the cervical spine is not cleared, airway management should include a strategy for protecting the spinal cord. The patient should be examined for any other head or neck injury that could interfere with airway management. The remainder of the airway examination should include assessment of the Mallampati score, dentition, neck range of motion, and other standard parameters. The presence ICP monitors, whether they are draining, and ICP should be noted.

Cardiac. The patient should be asked about a history of hypertension, cardiac disease, or carotid artery stenosis. A history of myocardial ischemia or infarction, cardiac failure, dysrhythmia (new-onset heart block or bradycardia) is also significant. If the patient has received diuretics for management of intracranial hypertension, his or her volume status should be carefully evaluated. If possible, a history of exercise tolerance and ability to climb stairs or perform household chores will indicate the patient's cardiopulmonary fitness. The physical examination should include jugular venous distention and peripheral edema. An electrocardiogram will demonstrate dysrhythmias and ST-segment changes, which may indicate the presence of cardiac complications of an intracranial bleed. If time permits and the patient has a significant cardiac history, a preoperative echocardiogram or intraoperative transesophageal echocardiogram may help to guide management.

Coexisting Disease. The history and physical examination should focus on the nature of any traumatic injury, the presence of cervical spine injury, traumatic brain injury (TBI), other fractures, intra-abdominal or intrathoracic injury, and blood loss. In diagnosing and managing intraoperative problems, a knowledge of smoking history, use of illicit inhaled or intravenous drug use, chest tube output, and mechanism of injury to determine the likelihood of crush injury, possible aspiration, and potential for cardiac or lung contusion injury are all extremely useful.

Angiographic or Radiographic Studies. If time permits, CT, MRI, and angiographic images should be reviewed with the neurosurgeon. Critical findings include intracranial hemorrhage (ICH), cerebral edema, and midline shift.

Drugs. If the patient is obtunded, a review of the chart will reveal previously administered sedatives or opioids. The medication history should also include a review of antiepileptic drugs.

Laboratory Studies. If time permits, laboratory studies should include a complete blood count with platelets, coagulation studies (prothrombin time and international normalized ratio), electrolytes, an ethanol level, and a toxicology screen to include cocaine, amphetamines, and sedatives.

PREOPERATIVE PREPARATION

Sedative drugs interfere with the care team's ability to follow the neurologic examination and may cause hypoventilation that can exacerbate intracranial hypertension. Sedatives should therefore be avoided if the clinical situation permits. If the patient is extremely anxious before surgery, small, divided doses of a reversible sedative (e.g., midazolam) can be administered if the patient is in a monitored setting. If there is any question as to the patient's ability to maintain a patent airway and adequate respirations, he or she should be intubated and mechanically ventilated. If ICP is elevated, the head should be elevated to 30 degrees whenever possible. Intracranial hypertension can be managed with hypertonic saline, mannitol, or a loop diuretic. If the patient requires anticonvulsant therapy, fosphenytoin is preferable to phenytoin because rapid administration of phenytoin may cause cardiovascular collapse. If the patient has received levetiracetam, the patient may be at increased risk for intraoperative seizures. Preoperative preparation may include an antisialogogue if awake fiberoptic intubation is anticipated. Sodium citrate–citric acid may be advisable for the patient who is not NPO.

Anesthetic Technique

Monitoring

Intraoperative monitors include those recommended by the American Society of Anesthesiologists's Standards for Basic Anesthetic Monitoring. Additional monitoring should include an intra-arterial catheter for most neurosurgical procedures. A central venous catheter should be considered for major vascular procedures and surgery that will be done in the sitting position. If the operative site will be positioned above the heart, continuous precordial Doppler should be used. If available, a multiorifice central venous catheter can be used to withdraw air from the right atrium, although the data that support it's utility are limited. The choice of neurophysiologic monitoring (e.g., electroencephalography [EEG], evoked potentials) depends on the surgeon and institution, but these techniques are becoming more common and may become the new standard of care in neurosurgery, interventional neuroradiology, and major spine procedures. If the surgeon requests titration of propofol or a barbiturate to burst suppression for an aneurysm or other intracranial vascular procedure, a processed EEG device (e.g., BIS, Covidien, Inc., Mansfield, MA) is an acceptable substitute if the raw waveforms can be displayed [3]. TBI patients often present with attenuated EEG. The surgeon may request a lumbar drain to improve surgical exposure or to decompress the spinal cord. Zoll pads or esophageal pacer should be placed preoperatively if the surgeons anticipate needing cardiac standstill for aneurysms.

Induction

The primary goal during induction is a smooth transition to anesthesia while maintaining hemodynamic stability. Even brief episodes of hypoxia and hypercapnia cause cerebral vasodilation and are especially deleterious in the neurosurgical patient. Wide swings in blood pressure during induction may exacerbate wall stress in and cause aneurysmal rebleeding. The choice of a specific agent is driven by the patient's underlying illness and comorbidities. Although propofol is used for most procedures, etomidate minimizes the risk of hypotension in patients with significant cardiac disease or hypovolemia due to polytrauma with hypotension. If etomidate is used for induction in normovolemic patients, however, the patient may develop hypertension during intubation. Ketamine is usually avoided because it may increase ICP. Short-acting antihypertensives that offer rapid onset and offset (e.g., esmolol and nicardipine) are particularly efficacious for tight blood pressure control.

Intraoperative

Sturgess and Matta [4] state, in the context of brain protection, "In the meantime attention to maintaining physiological normality is our best option" (p. 167). The goal of the anesthesiologist during the procedure is to optimize the patient's CNS physiology within the confines of surgical operating conditions and patient comorbidities. As during induction, this includes tight control of blood pressure, keeping it at a value that maintains cerebral perfusion without hypertension or swings in pressure. The use of propofol and barbiturates, along with diuretics (mannitol and furosemide), provides brain relaxation consistent with adequate perfusion. In general, less than 1 MAC of a potent volatile anesthetic is consistent with this goal. An infusion of propofol is also effective but will decrease CBF more than CMR. Adjust anesthetics to take into account a reduced potential for recall after TBI or intracranial procedures. Propofol should not be used to control blood pressure as it will delay a return to an alert patient and an adequate neurologic examination; an antihypertensive should be used instead. Surgeons may request burst suppression during periods of hypoperfusion (e.g., application of a temporary clip), although the evidence supporting this practice is not conclusive, particularly in human clinical trials based on better animal results [5]. Warner and colleagues [6] showed that EEG burst suppression in a focal model is not required for full neuroprotection. Further, not all anesthetics achieve equal neuroprotective effects despite EEG suppression, and the animal studies on which this technique is based did not look at extended behavioral outcomes that are now the standard for assessment of neuroprotection. Baugham [7] reviewed global versus focal ischemia models and the differences between barbiturates and other anesthetics for EEG silencing for focal neuroprotection, and suggests that other mechanisms are involved as well. Surgical retraction can cause local hypoperfusion and postoperative edema. If simultaneous somatosensory evoked potential (SSEP) and motor evoked potential (MEP) neurophysiologic monitoring is planned, with or without brainstem auditory evoked response (BAER)monitoring, then total intravenous anesthesia with propofol, remifentanil, and dexmedetomidine provides anesthesia and immobility while allowing adequate signals.

Anticipated Problems and Concerns

Airway edema may occur in the immediate postoperative period if the patient was positioned prone or the surgical site required extreme rotation, flexion, or extension of the neck. Brain edema, hemodynamic lability, and reperfusion syndrome (in patients who have undergone an intracranial vascular procedure) may occur in the postoperative period. Seizures may occur in patients who have undergone a surgical procedure involving the cerebral cortex. Surgical procedures involving the cerebellum or brainstem may cause delayed cardiopulmonary complications, and some neurosurgeons prefer that these patients remain intubated and sedated for 24 hours after surgery.

Postoperative Considerations

Whenever possible, the patient should be awakened immediately after the surgical procedure and should be able to cooperate with a neurologic examination. High infusion rates of propofol for extended periods of time may prevent this, particularly in the older patient. Delayed emergence is common in older patients, particularly after an intravenous anesthetic with propofol and remifentanil. Using dexmedetomidine as an adjunct allows the propofol infusion rate to be decreased and provides a smooth, rapid emergence and neurologic examination. If the patient was easy to ventilate via mask and is not at risk for aspiration, a deep extubation may be considered. Many neurosurgeons request an emergency CT scan if they are not able to perform a neurologic examination immediately after surgery. To control hypertension, divided doses of labetalol or a nicardipine infusion are usually effective.

AVOIDING ISCHEMIA

HYPOTENSION AND ISCHEMIA

CBF is normally 50 mL/100 g tissue/min and is proportional to CMR [8]. Blood flow of less than 15 mL/100 g/min will eventually lead to cell death. Surgical retraction can cause local ischemia even when global CBF is within normal limits. CPP can be calculated using the formula

$$\mathbf{CPP = MAP - ICP}$$

where MAP = mean arterial pressure.

In normal patients, CBF is autoregulated when CPP is between 50 and 150 mm Hg. This curve is, however, shifted toward the right (toward higher pressures) in patients with hypertension. Autoregulation may also be lost in patients with either local or global cerebral pathophysiology, and recent studies suggest that the lower boundary for MAP-dependent CBF may have a much wider range than has been previously thought. Keep CPP greater than 55 to 60 mm Hg, and even greater in patients with CNS injury or neuropathology such as TBI or increased ICP from tumor or hemorrhage. Strategies for monitoring and optimizing CBF are summarized in a recent review by Dagal and Lam [9]. They emphasize the importance of secondary injury after an initial insult, including hyperperfusion syndrome, and the value of flow–metabolism coupling. They review current methods to measure CBF with correlation to methods to also measure cerebral metabolic rate oxygen consumption ($CMRO_2$) [9]. These same authors also compared the effects of various anesthetics on cerebral autoregulation [10] and evaluated methods to measure autoregulation. They conclude that intravenous anesthesia with propofol and remifentanil, or sevoflurane as an alternative, preserves autoregulation with the least dose-dependence [10]. Oxygenation during severe hypoxia is preserved with cerebral arterial dilation, which increases CBF [11].

HYPERTENSION

Sustained hypertension can cause intracranial edema, increased ICP, blood–brain barrier breakdown, and hemorrhage. In the setting of a hemorrhagic stroke, *Cushing's response* may occur; this is a clinical triad that is usually defined as hypertension, bradycardia, and irregular respiration, or less commonly defined as widened pulse pressure (with elevated systolic and either elevated or normal diastolic blood pressure), irregular respiration, and bradycardia. This triad is a reflexive response to increased ICP. Increases in ICP lead to decreased CPP, and the initial hypertension and tachycardia is a sympathetic response to maintain cerebral perfusion. The increased systemic blood pressure stimulates carotid baroreceptors, which induces bradycardia. These hemodynamic changes, or the increased ICP, lead to the irregular respirations. Even a small amount of blood extravasation into the cerebrospinal fluid (CSF) can cause profound hypertension, and this appears to be a direct physiologic response as it occurs immediately and long before the onset of ICP increases. Severe hypertension can occur during interventional neuroradiology procedures when a coil perforates the wall of an aneurysm, causing a subarachnoid hemorrhage. The blood pressure should be decreased slowly while watching for signs of cerebral ischemia because an increased MAP may be necessary to maintain an adequate CBF in the setting of increased ICP and loss of autoregulation.

TACHYCARDIA

In patients with aneurysms, because aneurysm wall stress is the differential of pressure over time (dP/dT), wall stress on the vessel wall is a function of both fluid pressure and heart rate (how fast the pressure wave transverses the vessel wall) Therefore, heart rate is as important as absolute pressure.

ICP CHANGES

ICP is normally between 4 and 10 mm Hg. In general, increasing pressure causes CSF to flow into the spinal canal at an increased rate, with a concomitant decrease in the size of the ventricles. Elderly patients have more room for expansion because the brain atrophies with age. As ICP increases, however, cerebral ischemia may occur. Imaging reveals loss of the sulci and midline shifts if CSF outflow decreases unilaterally. CSF outflow obstruction may further increase the pressure. Intracranial hypertension can cause or exacerbate cerebral edema or brain herniation. One of the first signs of intracranial hypertension may be a persistent headache associated with nausea and vomiting. Intracranial hypertension can impair mental status and cognitive function. Cranial nerve impingement can cause focal neurologic signs. Markedly increased ICP can ultimately cause Cushing's triad: bradycardia, hypertension, and respiratory dysfunction. Physical examination may reveal asymmetric pupils, obtundation, and loss of eye reflexes, all of which are signs of herniation. Abrupt drainage of excessive amounts of CSF in patients with brain edema due to ICH or tumor may cause tentorial or tonsillar herniation. Bradycardia, a widened QRS complex, and sudden loss of consciousness may result. This is also in the differential for mental status changes after lumbar drain placement.

NAUSEA AND VOMITING

Nausea and vomiting can occur at any time in the perioperative period and is caused by a variety of factors including intracranial hypertension, surgical irritation during awake craniotomy, bleeding, and anesthetic agents. Vomiting can increase ICP and should be treated aggressively. Apfel and colleagues [12] developed a predictive risk score for nausea and vomiting after discharge, which also concludes that patients most at risk might benefit from aggressive prophylaxis, including use of propofol, dexamethasone, and ondansetron and avoidance of inhaled anesthetics, high-dose opioids, and neuromuscular blockade (NMB).

SEIZURES

Intraoperative seizures may be caused by dural irritation, a preexisting seizure disorder, tumors, and possibly medications (e.g., levetiracetam). If the brain is exposed, seizures may be rapidly stopped by irrigating the brain with cold saline. Pharmacologic management includes benzodiazepines or propofol; an antiepileptic such as phenytoin may also be of benefit. If the purpose of the surgery is to localize an epileptic focus, the surgeons should be consulted before administration of any medication that raises the seizure threshold.

HYPERVENTILATION AND HYPOVENTILATION

Elevated $PaCO_2$ increases CBF, which may in turn increase ICP. Some surgeons may request that end-tidal CO_2 ($EtCO_2$) be maintained at greater than 40 mm Hg during implantation of a ventriculoperitoneal shunt. Hypocapnia decreases CBF, which may produce cerebral ischemia. Hyperventilation should therefore be avoided unless it is necessary for increased ICP with impending herniation, and even then only as long as necessary as accommodation will occur and only as a bridge to definitive treatment. Hyperventilation may also be used to improve surgical conditions in conjunction with elevating the head of the bed, avoiding hypoxia, and the use of drugs such as mannitol and furosemide. The normal gradient between $PaCO_2$ and $EtCO_2$ is between 4 and 10 mm Hg. $PaCO_2$ may rarely also be less than $EtCO_2$ but should be correlated with an arterial blood gas.

ABRUPT CHANGE IN $ETCO_2$

Venous air embolism (VAE) may present with an abrupt decrease in $EtCO_2$. An arterial blood gas will show a simultaneous increase in $PaCO_2$ that is caused by the increased dead space in the lungs. A slow decrease in $EtCO_2$ may indicate falling cardiac output. Malignant hyperthermia (MH) should be considered in the setting of a rapid (but not abrupt) increase in CO_2 that is associated with other signs of a hypermetabolic state (e.g., sustained tachycardia and hypertension).

CMR VERSUS CBF

CMR is decreased after administration of thiopental, propofol, ketamine, or etomidate. Potent volatile anesthetics also decrease CMR and can cause uncoupling and increases in CBF at concentrations greater than 1 MAC [13]. Inhaled anesthetics may have both neuroprotective effects through anesthetic preconditioning as well as potentially neurotoxic effects. The mechanism of improved surgical operating conditions with propofol may be a greater decrease in CBF than CMR due to its CNS vasoconstricting properties. Volatile anesthetics may also interfere with neurophysiologic monitoring. These agents decrease MEPs and SSEPs significantly while BAERs are usually preserved.

RECALL

Neuronal activity is decreased during periods of reduced CBF. This occurs before energy stores are exhausted and may be a protective mechanism. Recall of intraoperative events is therefore markedly reduced after TBI, stroke, or intracranial neurosurgical procedures. It is possible, therefore, to separate the need for amnestic effects from hemodynamic considerations and the need to manage ICP and CPP.

ICP VERSUS CBF

The ultimate goal is to optimize oxygen delivery at lowest possible intracranial volume in the setting of decreased compliance (i.e., intracranial hypertension). Use of the internal jugular vein for central venous access should be avoided if possible because it may obstruct venous drainage, thereby increasing ICP. Hyperventilation should only be used acutely and sparingly to improve the surgical field, for impending herniation, or for rapid, large increases in ICP that cannot be treated by other means.

MILD/MODERATE HYPOTHERMIA

The use of hypothermia for global ischemia after a witnessed cardiac arrest is supported by Level 1 evidence. Although the Intraoperative Hypothermia for Aneurysm Surgery Trial (IHAST) did not demonstrate a therapeutic effect from mild hypothermia in patients undergoing aneurysm clipping, there are currently large clinical trials of hypothermia under way in Europe and Asia for patients with TBI, stroke, and ICH. Proposed flaws of IHAST include cooling the subjects too much, rewarming them too quickly, not maintaining hypothermia for a sufficient length of time, and a heterogeneous patient population. Mild to moderate hypothermia (33.5° to 35.5°C) provides most of the benefits of cooling with few of the complications and may be of benefit, although this is controversial. The number of clinical trials currently under way suggests a resurgence of interest in hypothermia for neuroprotection.

HYPERTHERMIA

Hyperthermia has been shown to be detrimental in patients with brain injury [14, 15]. If the patient is cold, he or she should be rewarmed only to 36°C because brain temperature is always approximately 1°C warmer than core temperature [16–19].

NEUROMONITORING

Intravenous anesthetics may alter neuromonitoring, particularly when administered as boluses at the beginning of the procedure. NMB may be used to facilitate airway management but must be discontinued well before MEP or EMG monitoring is required, although partial muscle relaxation is probably acceptable. The depth of anesthesia should be maintained at a constant level during neuromonitoring because the varying anesthetic depth or the technique used will produce a change in the signals. Dexmedetomidine may be used as an adjunct that will allow lower doses of propofol and achieve smooth, earlier emergence and an improved neurologic examination. Intraoperative angiography with intravenous dye and in–operating room portable CT scanners are now available.

HYPERGLYCEMIA AND HYPOGLYCEMIA

Avoid both extremes of blood glucose. Although outcomes after TBI, stroke, and sepsis and in the ICU are improved with tight glucose control, hyperglycemia after severe stress may be a biomarker for a more complicated stress response pathway.

PATHWAYS CONTRIBUTING TO CNS INJURY

NEUROPROTECTION VERSUS NEURORESUSCITATION

Neuroprotection, as the term is most commonly used, is the practice of preventing or minimizing the effects of the extensive secondary or tertiary injury that occurs after ischemic, surgical, or traumatic CNS insult. *Neuroprotection* is, however, more accurately defined as the ability to protect the CNS (or other organ systems) before the injury occurs. For example, Fukada and Warner [5] define *neuroprotection* as treatment initiated before an ischemic insult, with the goal of improving tolerance to ischemia or other significant ("near-lethal") stressors. They differentiate *neuroprotection* from *neuroresuscitation,* which they define as treatment(s) begun after a severe CNS insult with the goal of minimizing *secondary injury,* via whatever pathway, and of maximizing recovery [5]. Neuroresuscitation includes therapies or therapeutics after surgery, stroke, TBI, or spinal cord injury (SCI).

Anesthesiologists, alone among medical specialists, can predict when a patient might be exposed to an ischemic event and may therefore be able to protect to the CNS beforehand. Intraoperative ischemia may be inadvertent or may be an unavoidable consequence of the surgical procedure. Anesthetic neuroprotection at the present involves the acute anesthetic management of physiologic variables (i.e., MAP, CBF, ICP, O_2, CO_2) to ensure oxygenation, ventilation, and perfusion; to preserve autoregulation; and to appropriately match fluids to the clinical circumstances. Neuroprotection by anesthesiologists or other specialists may in the near future include the administration of prophylactic drugs, gene expression, or other cellular manipulation before a stressor.

NEUROPROTECTION: PHARMACOLOGIC AND PHYSIOLOGIC INTERVENTIONS—WHAT WORKS?

Early research focused on the possible benefit of thiopental-induced burst suppression and hypothermia. Baughman [7] reviewed the use of barbiturates as the gold standard for lowering the CMR for brain protection during focal ischemia. Barbiturates, or any other drug that suppresses CMR, were found to be protective against incomplete ischemia, but not complete cessation of CBF, as occurs in cardiac arrest. The effect was dose-dependent and an isoelectric EEG seemed to be necessary [3], but further research indicated that complete burst suppression is not necessary for neuroprotection [6] and that not all anesthetics are equal in effectiveness [20–23]. The dose-dependent reduction in CBF and CMR for the barbiturates appears to be roughly equal. Etomidate also decreases CMR and has less of an effect on blood pressure, but the ratio of CMR to CBF suppression may not be favorable, and etomidate is regionally variable and causes adrenal suppression. Propofol lowers CMR and may act as an antioxidant, or even as an *N*-methyl-D-aspartate (NMDA) antagonist, but has the same problematic effect on the CMR-CBF ratio as etomidate. Potent volatile anesthetics appear to be both neuroprotective (anesthetic preconditioning) and potentially neurotoxic, and all anesthetics elicit many other responses as well.

Anesthetic agents modulate excitatory and inhibitory circuits in the brain and spinal cord, which in turn leads to changes in perception and responses to stress, stimulation, and environmental cues. Anesthetics induce transcriptional and probably translational modifications that include Toll-like receptor (TLR) signaling in lipid rafts; this appears to play a key role in preconditioning and inflammatory responses. Normal immediate-early gene (IEG) responses (discussed further later) are altered by anesthetics in a drug-specific manner. Halogenated potent volatile anesthetics have been linked to postoperative cognitive dysfunction [24] and neurodegeneration in the developing brain [25, 26] but have paradoxically also shown neuroprotective effects in other models [27, 28]. Dose-dependent responses in autoregulation and CBF are different for the inhaled and intravenous anesthetic agents. Opioids and inhaled and intravenous anesthetics are reviewed in depth in Chapters 9 and 10.

Fukada and Warner [5] critically reviewed the available literature for neuroprotection, and divided strategies of clinical practice into *pharmacologic therapies*, which are limited to anesthetics, and *physiologic interventions*. Table 5.1 shows the evidence from animal and clinical studies for both preinjury and postinjury interventions and includes both physiologic manipulations and anesthetics [5].

Although a variety of interventions can reduce the extent of ischemic injury if they are given before the insult, only propofol and mild hypothermia show any efficacy postischemia in experimental animals. Moderate hypothermia, lidocaine, barbiturates, and normoglycemia are the only treatments shown to have benefit in humans when given before an ischemic event. Propofol has a "well defined absence of benefit" in human studies [5]. Normoglycemia, moderate hypothermia, and possibly hyperbaric oxygen are the only interventions backed by solid evidence in humans after an ischemic event. Sustained protection is achieved in experimental animals only with moderate hypothermia, normoglycemia, and isoflurane or sevoflurane but not desflurane. Only moderate hypothermia has shown to provide sustained protection in humans, both after global ischemia as well as after TBI [29], possibly by a heat shock protein (HSP) mechanism [30].

Sturgess and Matta [4] summarize similar observations and conclusions by stating that "Brain protection has traditionally focused on maintaining, as nearly as possible, normal physiological parameters." What little the clinician has to offer at present consists of attention to basic physiology, and in particular to optimizing CNS physiology, with the goal of minimizing the extent of secondary injury by

Table 5.1 EVIDENCE-BASED STATUS OF PLAUSIBLE INTERVENTIONS TO REDUCE PERIOPERATIVE ISCHEMIC BRAIN INJURY

INTERVENTION	PREISCHEMIC EFFICACY IN EXPERIMENTAL ANIMALS	POSTISCHEMIC EFFICACY IN EXPERIMENTAL ANIMALS	PREISCHEMIC EFFICACY IN HUMANS	POSTISCHEMIC EFFICACY IN HUMANS	SUSTAINED PROTECTION IN EXPERIMENTAL ANIMALS	SUSTAINED PROTECTION IN HUMANS
Moderate hypothermia	++	++	−/+	++*	++	++
Mild hyperthermia	− − −	− − −	− −	− −	− − −	− −
Hyperventilation	− −	− −	− −	− −	− −	− −
Normoglycemia	++	− −	+	+	++	− −
Hyperbaric oxygen	++	− −	− −	−/+	− −	− −
Barbiturates	++	−	+	−	− −	− −
Propofol	++	+	−	− −	− −	−
Etomidate	− − −	− −	− −	− −	− −	− −
Nitrous oxide	−	− −	− −	− −	− −	− −
Isoflurane	++	− −	− −	− −	++	− −
Sevoflurane		− −	− −	− −	++	− −
Desflurane	++	− −	− −	− −	− −	− −
Lidocaine	++	− −	+	− −	− −	− −
Ketamine	++	− −	− −	− −	− −	− −
Glucocorticoids	− − −	− −	− −	− −	− −	− −

++, Repeated physiologically controlled studies in animals/randomized, prospective, adequately powered clinical trials; +, consistent suggestion by case series/retrospective or prospective small sample size trials, or data extrapolated from other paradigms; −/+, inconsistent findings in clinical trials; may be dependent on characteristics of insult; −, well–defined absence of benefit; − −, absence of evidence in physiologically controlled studies in animals/randomized, prospective, adequately powered clinical trials; − − −, evidence of potential harm; *, out–of–hospital ventricular fibrillation cardiac arrest.

preventing exacerbation after cerebral ischemia. Providing a suitable surgical field may at times necessitate tradeoffs in the management of ICP, CPP, and CBF. It is now clear that neuroprotection is not simply a reduction in CMR [7]. This means that traditional methods of physiologic "neuroprotection" include maintaining normocapnia whenever possible, avoiding hypoxia, controlling ICP, minimizing aneurysmal wall stress, avoiding hyperthermia (and usually avoiding severe hypothermia), ensuring adequate cerebral venous drainage and proper positioning, and avoiding large swings in blood pressure during induction, emergence, and changes in the level of surgical stimulation.

Researchers and large pharmaceutical companies continue to try new drugs after stroke with the hope of finding a protective agent; these expensive efforts include numerous human clinical trials that show no benefits despite animal models showing efficacy at several different targets [31, 32]. These therapies should probably be called *neuro-resuscitation*, or perhaps secondary *neuroprotection*. Similar trials have also targeted the complications of Parkinson's disease, Alzheimer's disease, and amyotrophic lateral sclerosis (ALS). Reasons for these failures include a rush to market, insufficient validation in sufficient numbers of species, patient heterogeneity and comorbidities, lack of adequate outcomes measures and biomarkers, and, perhaps most importantly, the numerous mechanisms and pathways involved in a complicated and intertwined sequence and time course of secondary injury.

Molecular Biology of Ischemic Injury

Cessation or reduction of blood flow to a region of brain causes the initial insult to neurons and glial cells in white and gray matter. Intraoperative ischemia may be unintentional (e.g., using excessive force during retraction) or may be an unavoidable part of the surgery, such as temporary occlusion of a parent vessel during aneurysm surgery. The initial injury may consist of a severely ischemic core surrounded by a partially perfused region in which the initial injury is limited. This is a near-lethal insult at a cellular or tissue level and elicits a specific cellular stress response consisting of interleukins, CD (cluster of differentiation [cell surface molecules that often trigger a signal cascade]) cell markers, and TLRs on the cell surface and secreted into the extracellular space. *IEG* stress and immune responses are triggered immediately, before cell death, and lead to local and distant signaling. This stress response varies over time, and the specific stress response pattern is probably of prognostic and diagnostic value. In rough order of appearance (speculative), these pathways include the following:

- Energy depletion
- Transcription factor and *IEG* activation

- Translational arrest
- Loss of cellular polarization
- Loss of calcium and potassium channel integrity
- Excitotoxic neurotransmitter release
- NMDA complex activation
- Inflammatory cell activation and signaling
- Cytokine release
- Membrane fluidity and potential changes
- Nitric oxide and free radical release
- Loss of calcium homeostasis
- Excitatory amino acids release
- Release of proteases, endothelins, endonucleases, matrix metalloproteinases (MMPs), and lipases
- Mitochondrial breakdown and release
- Activation of apoptosis pathways [calpains, caspases, and poly(ADP) ribose]
- Cell necrosis, which releases further inflammatory mediators

Caspases, like the HSPs, are proenzymes that can be released even with translational arrest and are both pro-apoptotic and antiapoptotic. Apoptosis, a slower form of cell death that is controlled and less immunogenic, is a major part of cell pruning during development. After an ischemic event, it is subject to modulation and is triggered in cells that have a chance of rescue by trophic signals. For example, apoptosis is often touted as a target for prevention of further neuronal cell loss after CNS injury, but a live neuron is not necessarily a functional neuron [33]. Later events include macrophage infiltration, edema, and reperfusion injury, which includes further edema, free radical formation, membrane destabilization, essential amino acids, calcium dysregulation, mitochondrial failure, and protein unfolding.

The initial injury signals may lay the groundwork for recovery. The balance between recovery and survival, and death by necrosis or apoptosis reflects a balance between biochemical and physiologic reactions to ischemia. Stress responses lead to widespread secondary injury cascades that may also be a part of a recovery cascade. A response occurs, is regulated, and then a counterregulation balances and controls the initial and subsequent responses. The tipping point determining outcome will vary with the different pathways. This competition between cell death versus repair pathways determines whether a given local injury is irreversible. The physiologic responses to ischemia or to any severe stress (e.g, sepsis) is called the *acute phase response* (APR) and is tightly regulated at both transcriptional and translational levels through feedback pathways (tumor necrosis factor [TNF], TLRs, interleukins, kinases, phosphorylation, second messengers). Stress responses include acute and counter-regulatory generalized immunosuppression that is necessary for control of the acute pro-inflammatory responses, by mediating the acute counter-regulatory stress responses [34]. In this regard, the immune system, inflammatory responses, coagulation cascades, and excitatory/inhibitory neurotransmitters all have remarkable similarities. Both reactive (feed forward) and feedback inhibitory responses are simultaneously stimulated by any severe cellular, tissue, or organ stressor. These responses have probably evolved to facilitate acute survival after injury (i.e., coagulation, immune surveillance, and shunting of metabolic pathways for immediate and increased energy requirements). Feedback inhibitory mechanisms are induced simultaneously to ensure that if the organism survives the acute insult it is not overwhelmed by overactive immune, procoagulant, inflammatory, or excitatory pathways. Neuroexcitation, neuroprotection, and neurotoxicity may all be outcomes of different relative pathways of actions of the anesthetics. Minimizing anesthetic neurotoxicity may be a simple as the use of, or the avoidance of, certain anesthetic agents. For example, neuroexcitation may lead to neuroprotection after a recovery period by eliciting a stress response (preconditioning]. Overexcitation may induce an apoptotic or a necrotic cell death pathway.

The appropriate physiologic response to a severe stressor that follows the initial insult is thus tightly regulated. Loss of tight regulation can lead to diseases that include autoimmune disorders (e.g., multiple sclerosis, arthritis), coagulopathy (e.g., hypercoagulation or bleeding), sepsis, diabetes mellitus, and asthma. The elderly patient who survives severe trauma with the intervention of sophisticated medical care may have upregulated stress responses that are no longer beneficial after days or weeks in the intensive care unit. Protection from subsequent severe ischemia (preconditioning) may thus depend on the induction of regulatory feedback. Idiosyncratic immune function and robust survival responses may be linked to genetic susceptibilities and genetic variability.

The most important pathways of secondary injury have most likely been identified. An excellent summary of known mechanisms in signaling and triggers to individual pathways, injury, and apoptosis can be found in Kass and colleagues [35], or in Menon and Wheeler [32], which contains one of the most concise summaries of pathways in secondary injury after CNS ischemia. The pathophysiology of cerebral ischemia probably has considerable overlap with many of the pathways involved in TBI or SCI. Loane and Faden review translational and emerging therapies for TBI, concluding that in TBI, like ischemia, "Given the multifactoral nature of the secondary injury processes after trauma it is unlikely that targeting any single factor will result in

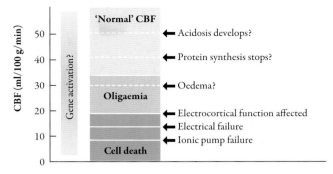

Thresholds of cerebral ischaemia

Figure 5.1   Review of evidence on which to base potential efficacy of interventions to reduce perioperative ischemic brain injury.

significant improvement in outcome after TBI in human injury" (p. 599) [36]. Figure 5.1 from Menon and Wheeler [32] illustrates an intuitive model for the spectrum of cellular consequences as CBF decreases, from acidosis and translational arrest, to edema, to neurocortical signaling impairment, and to membrane instability and ion pump failure.

The known cell mechanisms that are potentially affected by these cascades are listed in Figure 5.2 [32].

Finally, Figure 5.3 illustrates the proposed sequence of events, from immediately after the injury to weeks later. Although these figures depict the most important mechanisms and their time courses as they are currently understood, much remains unknown. It is not known which of these potential pathways are the most important at a given time after injury, which probably explains why clinical trials after stroke or TBI have been unsuccessful. The relative importance of individual mechanisms that contribute to secondary injury after an initial ischemic insult probably depends on severity and location of ischemia, is multimodal, and changes with time after injury. The relative importance or significance of any one mechanism is not known, and this is one of the major gaps in current understanding of secondary injury.

Investigators have developed experimental and computational models for individual pathways of injury after ischemia. But integrating multiple simultaneous pathways of injury, stress, and responses is not yet possible. Without the ability to do so, it is impossible to determine which are the important mechanisms as they evolve over time following the initial insults. For example, it may be useful to block secondary inflammation and cytokine release from necrotic cells to prevent a cascade of inflammation and edema. As seen in Figures 5.2 and 5.3 [32], modeling even one neuron or one neurovascular unit after ischemia is a daunting challenge [37], much less modeling a significant portion of the CNS within the niche environment. Iadecola and Anrather [38] suggest that the protective mechanisms that are rapidly induced by ischemic brain offer insights into a coordinated multipathway approach

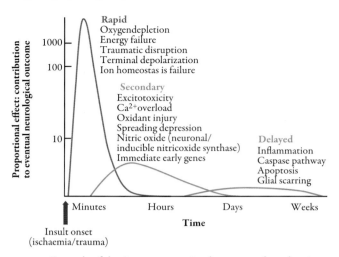

Rapid
Oxygendepletion
Energy failure
Traumatic disruption
Terminal depolarization
Ion homeostas is failure

Secondary
Excitotoxicity
Ca²⁺overload
Oxidant injury
Spreading depression
Nitric oxide (neuronal/
inducible nitricoxide synthase)
Immediate early genes

Delayed
Inflammation
Caspase pathway
Apoptosis
Glial scarring

Minutes   Hours   Days   Weeks
Time

Insult onset
(ischaemia/trauma)

Figure 5.2   Example of the time course or simultaneous and overlapping pathways of secondary injury after ischemia [Reprinted from Menon and Wheeler [32] with permission.)

that "relies on coordinated neurovascular programs" for endogenous neuroprotection and not just selected individual targets that have been unsuccessful in clinical trials. Because of the unique architecture of the CNS, function can be impaired at a site distant from the initial injury. This is termed *diaschisis* and is due to axonal disruption. For example, a crossed cerebellar diaschisis is a loss of function in the cerebellum that results from a cerebral injury to the opposite (contralateral) side or hemisphere. Numerous types of injuries can affect the corticopontocerebellar tracts, and cerebellar diaschisis may be correlated with poor outcomes after stroke.

Preoperative stress conditioning has been shown to prevent paralysis after aortic surgery in animal models [39], and this may hold promise for patients undergoing a repair of a thoracic aortic aneurysm repairs. The proposed mechanism is regulation and expression of inducible, protective members of the heat shock protein family. Gidday and colleagues have published many studies of ischemic tolerance and CNS preconditioning that show evidence for *transient ischemic preconditioning* [40, 41]. Preconditioning reprograms gene and protein expression and as a result changes the response to subsequent ischemia in the preconditioned brain. Animals that hibernate or stay underwater for prolonged periods, or at altitude, habituate to ischemia, and arousal of hibernating animals appears to model reperfusion after stroke but without the same injurious effects [40]. These examples of animals that survive prolonged ischemia provide insights and potential targets for similar preconditioning in humans. For example, heat shock protein 70 (Hsp70) is overexpressed in hibernating turtles and arctic ground squirrels [30], just as it is in cardiac tissue in humans with myocardial ischemia immediately before cardiac bypass surgery [42].

Strategies that target multiple or final common pathways, such as hypothermia and ischemic and immune preconditioning, are similar in concept to multimodal drug treatment strategies. Pharmacologic preconditioning is a novel approach in this category; Gidday reviews [41] a surprisingly long list of U.S. Food and Drug Administration–approved drugs that also show preconditioning effects, in addition to volatile anesthetics. These are drugs that "share a common, but limited, set of overlapping molecular signaling

Processes in secondary neuronal injury

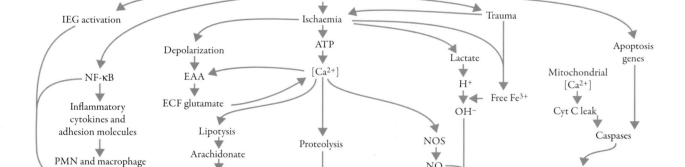

ATP, adenosine triphosphate; [Ca²⁺], cytosolic calcium concentration; cyt C, cytochrome C; EAA, excitatory aminoacid; ECF, extracellular fluid; IEG, immdiate early gene; LT, leukotrienes; NF-κB, nuclear factor κB; No, nitric oxide; NOS, nitric oxide synthase; ONOO⁻, peroxynitite; PMN, polymorphoruclear leukocytes; PGs, prostaglandins

Figure 5.3   Schematic example of pathways in secondary injury after CNS ischemia, as known currently [Reprinted from Menon and Wheeler [32] with permission.)

pathways" (p. 20) and induce a transcriptional and translational state that has many of the same features of ischemic tolerance [40]. Stenzel-Poole and colleagues [43] performed microarray analysis in mice of gene expression after ischemia, ischemia after preconditioning, and hibernation (hypoxia), which revealed three distinct gene expression patterns. They also performed a functional metabolic analysis, and conclude that "preconditioning is predisposed towards *dampening* [emphasis added] cellular activity" (p. 1033) [43]. Recent investigations of additional targets and pathways have identified hypoxia inducible factors. These studies suggest, for example, that patients at risk for stroke and who have a history of TIAs could undergo repetitive, noninjurious CNS or even limb ischemia. This would theoretically upregulate protective intracellular pathways that probably include the HSPs. Alternatively, delivery and integration using viral vectors of gene constructs with ischemia-inducible transcriptional sequences have been proposed for patients with a history of TIAs. In theory, genes that produced an intracellular protein that attenuated secondary injury after an ischemic insult would then only be triggered by ischemia.

HYPOTHERMIA

Although the use of hypothermia remains unproved except for witnessed cardiac arrest, therapeutic mild to moderate hypothermia may offer a way to favorably impact several of the injury mechanisms discussed earlier simultaneously. Sinclair and Andrews reviewed the use of hypothermia in TBI and provide a summary of possible mechanisms for beneficial effects of hypothermia in 12 secondary injury pathways [44], all of which overlap mechanisms previously discussed. Reasons for lack of efficacy in human clinical trials in TBI and intracranial hemorrhage include insufficient duration and too rapid rewarming and the heterogeneity of patients and standard therapies. Hypothermia, because it acts on multiple pathways, may be a therapy that is the equivalent of a multitarget therapeutic agent.

RESUSCITATION OF BRAIN AND OTHER ORGANS

No single intervention is likely to be successful in preventing secondary injury after CNS injury. The problem, and the promise, is illustrated by the hundreds of articles that describe proteins, antibodies, receptors, small RNAs, or genes, each of which provides a degree of neuroprotection either before or shortly after an ischemic insult. Examples of most promising approaches include calcium and sodium channels, mitochondria, reactive oxygen species, tight junctions, edema, membranes, and free radicals. But none of these single targets have proved to be successful. As an example of this, the mitogen-activated protein kinase pathway is a well-characterized cell death mechanism. Peptides targeting the c-jun N-terminal kinase (JNK) portion of this

pathway protect against excitotoxicity in vitro [45]. But this research is an example, chosen arbitrarily, of a negative result of this promising *single* target, protein kinase (JNK), despite animal and neuronal culture models showing efficacy. Instead, it is likely that multiple, perhaps sequentially timed, interventions will ultimately be needed to significantly attenuate neurotoxicity and secondary injury. This will likely be a combination of small molecules, trophic factors, antiapoptotic factors, HSPs, cytokines, small interfering RNA, nucleic acids, steroids, and possibly anesthetics. We must first understand the complex biology and most important injury pathways and the time course over which they occur. Small molecules targeting these pathways are logical first candidates for therapeutic drugs. But the advent of gene therapy also promises the potential to infuse nucleic acids that express free radical scavengers [46] or HSPs [47–49] or, indeed, any gene sequence for which the cDNA is known [46–49]. The techniques for measurement, modeling and delivery are improving; *it is the ability to determine which are the critical and dominant mechanisms at each time point that are lacking.*

The majority of strokes are embolic in etiology (Figure 5.4). While tissue plasminogen activator (tPA) is most effective if given within 4 hours, desmoteplase is fibrin specific and has a longer half-life of activity, and therefore potentially a longer window or therapeutic efficacy. The key is to identify patients in whom the cellular insult has not led to an *irreversible* injury already. Diffusion-weighted imaging has been suggested as a way to identify salvageable infarct territory. Perfusion-weighted MRI can also be used to show delayed perfusion, which may indicate territory with sufficient flow for some intact membrane potential and cell survival. Intra-arterial tPA or desmoteplase can be used for much longer, up to 9 hours after stroke onset, as can mechanical devices such as the Merci or Penumbra catheter systems, but with an increased risk of hemorrhage. A longer

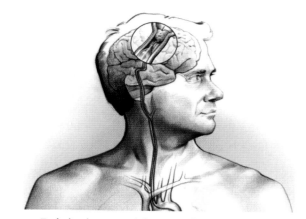

Figure 5.4 Embolic clot retrieval showing inflated balloon preventing uncontrolled reperfusion and clot being retrieved. After clot retrieval balloon can be reinflated and catheter distal to balloon can be used for controlled reperfusion to minimize secondary injury in ischemic and newly reperfused territory [Reprinted from Hartford Hospital Website, Hartford, CT.)

therapeutic window for reperfusion would be better, but this requires better ways to evaluate risks of hemorrhage as well as controlled reperfusion to minimize the secondary injury pathways by attacking multiple targets. Resuscitation with reperfusion "recipes" rather than single drugs may eventually salvage much more of the penumbra region after ischemia.

Trummer [50] reported successful resuscitation after 15 minutes of complete global ischemia (warm cardiac arrest) in juvenile pigs, achieved by careful and controlled reperfusion with a recipe of drugs that included lidocaine, barbiturate, cooling, low O_2 content [51], free radical and Ca^{2+} scavengers, and steroids for membrane stabilization. In the same way, after embolic stroke, a "reperfusion recipe" could be delivered intra-arterially to the ischemic and newly reperfused territory using percutaneous catheters in the interventional neuroradiology suite, with careful management of reperfusion parameters. Buckberg [52] suggests that controlled reperfusion has been convincingly demonstrated to salvage multiple organs, including brain, and may be the "unifying recovery denominator." Controlled reperfusion with a controlled reperfusate, first in the catheterization lab after stoke, will lead to broader applications after sudden death [52, 53]. The research reports described here have in common a theme of upregulation or downregulation of coordinated programs of proteins, genes, networks, stress responses, and cascades, rather than a focus on any one target [43].

SYSTEMS BIOLOGY AND PHYSIOLOGIC MODELING

Systems biology attempts to model complete physiologic systems, with boundary conditions set by normal physiologic limits [54]. Examples of individual components include neurovascular bundles, the "niche" environment, and immune and inflammatory function in the various stages of injury and repair after an initial ischemic insult [55]. A wide range of mediators, local and systemic, are produced, which can both exacerbate and modulate the subsequent innate and adaptive immunity. Effects are unclear and contradictory and depend on degree and timing, and they state that "although counteracting the inflammatory response to ischemic injury may ameliorate the tissue damage in the acute phase, it may also compromise repair mechanisms and worsen the long-term outcome of the injury" [55].

Despite improvements in systems biology, model complexity is at the stage of yeast and single-celled organisms. We are far from the ability to integrate and model steady state ensembles of cortical neurons. The complexity in integrating the multitude of cells and tracts in the brain is difficult to imagine, and the addition of an ischemic insult makes the problem even more challenging. Design of experiments to demonstrate clinical efficacy for multimodal therapies is challenging. It is, however, clear that secondary injury after stroke is not well understood, and it will be impossible to design the multimodal therapies above until these multipathway interactions are known. Most research funding has supported single-target, single-hypothesis experiments, even though secondary injury is local and ultimately depends on the integration of cellular and subcellular events that result from multiple overlapping, temporally related pathways. Neurovascular bundles and enervation are related to the "niche" environment, which is the complex and rich local environment of cells, matrix, local mediators, and interconnections. Just as it is for stem cells, the local niche is critical in determining outcomes to cellular perturbations. Researchers are beginning to understand and measure most of the key variables in determining how cells and systems survive, but measurement tools for CNS function are still rudimentary and do not have sufficient resolution (functional MRI or positron emission tomography, for example) to precisely measure the effects of a given intervention. Martin Smith and colleagues [56] recently reported the complex interactions of neural inputs, oscillatory electrical signaling in the CNS, and the effects of the neurovascular bundle in regulation of CBF and autoregulation. Other researchers can measure CBF and monitor autoregulation within a cerebrovascular bundle using near-infrared spectroscopy [57, 58]. Combined laser-Doppler flowmetry and photo spectrometry have also been used to measure autoregulation and microcirculation in real time during coronary artery bypass graft surgery and intracranial procedures [59,60]. Genomewide association studies (GWAS) are reporting correlations of multiple genes with various diseases, including many of direct interest to anesthesiologists, such as diabetes, drug interaction susceptibility, and control of blood pressure. These GWAS reports of genetic predispositions and susceptibilities are potentially of great value in determining risks of ischemia and individual patient responses to severe stressors [61]. A review of all of the proposed mechanisms and overlapping pathways makes it obvious that an approach using systems biology is necessary, in which all known interactions and pathways are modeled, compared with available experiments, and the most important mechanisms are determined at each point in time from minutes after initial near-lethal stressor through weeks or months after injury. This in turn requires a comprehensive, integrated, computational neurosciences approach to model these overlapping and widely interacting pathways [62]. Navlakha and Bar-Joseph describe shared principles between biological systems and computational systems, such as synchronization, coordination, and distribution. Biological systems have redundant gene and pathway backups, and it is no wonder that any one treatment (knock-out of one gene or one transcription factor) is seamlessly and easily compensated for in decentralized molecular systems [62].

MODELING STATES OF CONSCIOUSNESS AND ISCHEMIA

A variety of disciplines are making significant advances in modeling of complex behaviors and in technical measurement capabilities. Refined descriptions, models, and understanding of consciousness and anesthetic actions are critically important to modeling and understanding the impacts of ischemia. The ability to model states of consciousness is advancing rapidly (for example, the work of Emery Brown [63–66], George Mashour [67, 68], or Giulio Tononi [69–71]. These authors describe that "consciousness arises from the complex interaction of many kinds of activity… And emerges from the integration of information across large networks," while unconsciousness is disconnect or interference between different brain networks or regions [66]. Brown examined the different arousal states with five classes of intravenous anesthetics with a systems analysis and made the provocative statement that "general anesthesia is less mysterious than currently believed" [64]. Mashour and colleagues have described specifics of preferential inhibition of frontal parietal feedback connectivity underlying understanding anesthetic interferences with consciousness [67]. Tononi developed an integrated information theory of consciousness and used it to analyze pathological cognitive function, with obvious relevance in recovery after CNS ischemia [71].

The current state of knowledge of emerging mechanisms of disruptions in cellular signaling after CNS ischemia has recently been described [72], specifically mechanisms in signaling cascades that "mediate cross-talk between redundant pathways of cell death" an important concept in evaluating the multiple, redundant, overlapping, amplifying or antagonistic pathways in time and space. This discussion, however, was limited to glutamate, transient receptor potential (TRP), and acid sensing channels, and connexins. The historical focus on excitotoxicity does not account for CNS injury, but the analysis is not comprehensive. Lauritzen and colleagues [73] review the clinical relevance of cortical spreading depolarization (CSD) in the aftermath of stroke, migraines, TBI, and SAH and the potential role in significantly contributing to secondary injury due to impacts on excitatory amino acids, extracellular fluid microenvironment, neurovascular bundle, brain energy, and microperfusion. The role of CSD in multiple types of injury is puzzling, and it is unknown whether CSD is a response to, or a causal agent in, multiple pathways.

Of particular interest in CNS ischemia is the work of DeGracia, which includes numerous descriptions of molecular pathways of cerebral ischemia [74], including the HSPs [75]. He developed a bistable network-based framework for state analysis of stress responses and cell death damage mechanisms after ischemia [76–80]. In contrast to the classic ischemic cascade model of ischemic injury, DeGracia's model is a "non-linear Boolean system which depends on the mutual interactions of all of the disease-relevant alterations and the outcome of which cannot be predicted by superposition of the individual injury pathways" (p. 56) [76].

As more is learned about the importance of oscillatory networks in signaling, it may become possible to understand how the CNS achieves awareness or consciousness, and then how it can recover from ischemia. Siegel and colleagues [81] recently described spectral fingerprints of neuronal interactions, the large-scale, frequency-specific neuronal oscillatory patterns that appear to define consciousness. Perhaps apoptosis, for example, is a key factor in repairing the neural networks, just as it prunes neurons with insufficient connections. Electrophysiologist Henry Markham is currently attempting to build a supercomputer model called the Human Brain Project (HBP) beginning in 2012. HBP would integrate all 60,000 brain research articles each year and incorporate "everything, from the genetic level, the molecular level, the neurons and synapses, how microcircuits are formed, macrocircuits, mesocircuits, brain areas,. . . until we get to behavior and cognition" (p. 457) [82]. Although he has been successful in integrating all available rat cortex experiments into, first, a single neuron, then a cortical column model, and now a simulation of 100 interconnected neuronal columns, the HBP would require computing power of 10^{18} operations per second; computers with this speed will most likely not be available until the next decade [82]. Despite these encouraging advances, there are still basic questions about whether models of the human brain can be based on computer-based machine intelligence or whether empirical or cell-based models are needed [83].

CONCLUSION

The future of research in the fields of neuroresuscitation and neuroprotection is wide open, with controversial ideas and many unknowns. Baugham [7] states that "It is amazing that… there is a paucity of prospective randomized clinical trials comparing different treatments upon which to base cerebral protectant therapy." This is, perhaps, understandable given the current lack of understanding of the complex interactions of secondary injury pathways. If anesthesiologists are able to pursue this research, the next decade can be very exciting for neurosciences and neuroanesthesia research. Improvements in reperfusion resuscitation will lead to progress in resuscitation after global ischemia such as cardiac arrest. Hypothermia and resuscitation during interventional neuroradiology are areas wide open for future research with immediate impact, while secondary injury after ischemia is at the cutting edge of neurosciences. The specialty of anesthesiology should be a much larger part of the revolution in modeling ischemia and in the development of computational neurosciences. Even those who are not a part of cutting edge advances can make valuable contributions and should follow gains in modeling and predicting ischemia and anesthetic action on consciousness.

RECOMMENDED FURTHER READING

Excellent reviews of a traditional view of neuroprotection as is commonly understood in routine neuroanesthesia in the United States can be found in the following articles:

- Excellent, comprehensive review of available animal and human trials' data; summarizes the few anesthetic, physiologic, or pharmacologic strategies with any documented benefit after ischemic-hypoxic insult to the CNS [5]

- A 2009 review of recent research that investigates cerebral protection including the use of anesthetic agents, as well as therapies targeted specifically at the complex cascades following brain injury [4]

- Concise summary of known pathways of secondary injury with illustrative figures [32]

- Recent review of pharmacology, neuroprotectants, and promising combined strategies in understanding the pathophysiology of brain ischemia and the role of clinical trials [31]

- Historical review of early approaches to brain protection, current methods of optimizing brain physiology, and a section on "new mechanisms of cerebral protection" and the role for old and new drugs in the future for brain protection [7]

- Chapter 1 by Kass, Cottrell, and Lei is a recent review of current state of neurophysiology and neurochemistry in the textbook by Cottrell and Young [35]

- Meta-analysis from 2011 SNACC Meeting that evaluated over 5900 clinical trials to conclude that only magnesium, lidocaine, erythropoietin, statins, piracetam, and remacemide showed any neuroprotective effects in the "perioperative" period [84]

For research topics with likely impact in the future, these key references are recommended:

- Description of spectral fingerprints of neuronal interactions [81]

- DeGracia's bistable network-based framework for state analysis of stress responses and cell death damage mechanisms [76–80]

- Postischemia immunology [55]

- Successful resuscitation after 15 minutes of complete global ischemia by controlled reperfusion [50–52]

- Coordinated multipathway approach for analyzing endogenous neuroprotection [38]

- Preoperative stress conditioning [39]

- Transient ischemic preconditioning [40, 43]

- Pharmacologic preconditioning [41]

These authors are at the forefront of *modeling states of consciousness*:

- Brown examines different arousal states with different intravenous anesthetics using a systems analysis [63–66].

- Mashour describes specifics of preferential inhibition of frontal parietal feedback connectivity underlying understanding anesthetic interference of consciousness [67, 68].

- Tononi proposes an integrated information theory of consciousness and applies this to pathologic cognitive function [69–71].

REFERENCES

1. Perdrizet GA. *Heat Shock Response and Organ Preservation: Models of Organ Conditioning*. Austin, TX: RG Landes; 1997.
2. Perdrizet GA. Hans Selye and beyond: responses to stress. *Cell Stress Chaperones*. 1997;2:214–219.
3. Roach GW, Newman MF, Murkin JM, et al. Ineffectiveness of burst suppression therapy in mitigating perioperative cerebrovascular dysfunction. *Anesthesiology*. 1999;90:1255–1264.
4. Sturgess J and Matta B. Brain protection: Current and future options. *Best Pract Res Clin Anesthesiol*. 2009;22:167–176.
5. Fukuda S, Warner DS. Cerebral protection. *Br J Anaesth*. 2007;99:10–17.
6. Warner DS, Takaoka S, Wu B, et al. Electroencephalographic burst suppression is not required to elicit maximal neuroprotection from pentobarbital in a rat model of focal cerebral ischemia. *Anesthesiology*. 1996;84:1475–1484.
7. Baughman VL. Brain protection during neurosurgery. *Anesthesiol Clin N Am*. 2002;20:315–327.
8. Vavilala MS, Lee LA, Lam AM. Cerebral blood flow and vascular physiology. *Anesthesiol Clin N Am*. 2002;20:247–264.
9. Dagal A, Lam A. Cerebral blood flow and the injured brain: how should we monitor and manipulate it? *Curr Opin Anaesthiol*. 2011;24:131–137.
10. Dagal A, Lam A. Cerebral autoregulation and anesthesia. *Curr Opin Anaesthiol*. 2009;22:547–552.
11. WIlson MH, Edsell MEG, Davagnanam I, et al. Cerebral artery dilatation maintains cerebral oxygenation at extreme altitude and in acute hypoxia—an ultrasound and MRI study. *J Cereb Blood Flow Metab*. 2011;31:2019–2029.
12. Apfel CC, Philip BK, Cakmakkaya OS, et al. Who is at risk for postdischarge nausea nd vomiting after ambulatory surgery? *Anesthesiology*. 2012;117:475–486.
13. Sloan TB. Anesthetics and the brain. *Anesthesiol Clin N Am*. 2002;20:265–292.
14. Oh HS, Jeon HS, Seo WS. Non-infectious hyperthermia in acute brain injury patients: relationships to mortality, blood pressure, intracranial pressure and cerebral perfusion pressure. *Int J Nurs Pract*. 2012;18:295–302.
15. Blanco M, Campos F, Rodriquez-Yanez M, et al. Neuroprotection or increased brain damage mediated by temperature in stroke is time dependent. *PLoS One*. 2012;7:e30700.
16. Nakagawa K, Hills NK, Kamel H, et al. The effect of decompressive hemicraniectomy on brain temperature after severe brain injury. *Neurocrit Care*. 2011;15:101.

17. Henker RA, Brown SD, Marion DW. Comparison of brain temperature with bladder and rectal temperatures in adults with severe head injury. *Neurosurgery*. 1998;42:1071–1075.

18. Mcilvoy L. Comparison of brain temperature to core literature: a review of the literature. *J Neurosci Nurs*. 2004;36:23–31.

19. Rumana CS, Gopinath SP, Uzura M, et al. Brain temperature exceeds systemic temperature in head-injured patients. *Crit Care Med*. 1998;26:562–567.

20. Roach GW, Mewman MF, Murkin JM, et al. Ineffectiveness of burst suppression therapy in mitigating perioperative cerebrovascular dysfunction. Multicenter Study of Perioperative Ischemia (McSPI) Research Group. *Anesthesiology*. 1999;90:1255–1264.

21. Kobayashi M, Takeda Y, Taninishi H, et al. Quantitative evaluation of the neuroprotective effects of thiopental sodium, propofol, and halothane on brain ischemia in the gerbil: effects of the anesthetics on ischemic depolarization and extracellular glutamate concentration. *J Neurosurg Anesthesiol*. 2007;19:171–178.

22. Mortier E, Struys M, Herregods L. Therapeutic coma or neuroprotection by anaesthetics. *Acta Neurol Belg*. 2000;100:225–228.

23. Kawaguchi M, Furuya H, Patel PM. Neuroprotective effects of anesthetic agents. *J Anesthesiol*. 2005;19:150–156.

24. Moller JT, Cluitmans P, Rasmussen LS, et al; ISPOCD Investigators. Long-term postoperative cognitive dysfunction in the elderly ISPOCD1 study. International Study of Post-Operative Cognitive Dysfunction. *Lancet*. 1998;351:857–861.

25. Jevtovic-Todorovic V, Hartman RE, Izumi Y, et al. Early exposure to common anesthetic agents causes widespread neurodegeneration in the developing rat brain and persistent learning deficits. *J Neurosci*. 2003;23:876–882.

26. Kudo M, Aono M, Lee Y, et al. Effects of volatile anesthetics on N-methyl-D-aspartate excitotoxicity in primary rat neuronal-glial cultures. *Anesthesiology*. 2001;95:756–765.

27. Homi HM, Mixco JM, Sheng H, et al. Severe hypotension is not essential for isoflurane neuroprotection against forebrain ischemia in mice. *Anesthesiology*. 2003;99:1145–1151.

28. Sanders RD, Ma D, Maze M. Anaesthesia induced neuroprotection. *Best Pract Res Clin Anaesthesiol* 2005;:19(3):461–474.

29. Urbano LA, Oddo M. Therapeutic hypothermia for traumatic brain injury. *Curr Neurol Neurosci Rep*. 2012;Epub:Jul 27.

30. Kaneko T, Kibayashi K. Mild hypothermia facilitates the expression of cold-inducible RNA-binding protein and heat shock protein 70.1 in mouse brain. *Brain Res*. 2012;1466:128–136.

31. Mantz J, Degos V, Laigle C. Recent advances in pharmacologic neuroprotection. *Eur J Anaesthesiol*. 2010;27:6–10.

32. Menon DK, Wheeler DW. Neuronal injury and neuroprotection. *Anaesth Intensive Care Med Neurosurg*. 2009;6:184–188.

33. Dumas TC, Sapolsky RM. Gene therapy against neurological insults: sparing neurons versus sparing function. *Trends Neurosci*. 2001;24:695–700.

34. Molina PE. Neurobiology of the stress response: contribution of the sympathetic nervous system to the neuroimmune axis in traumatic injury. *Shock*. 2005;24:3–10.

35. Kass IS, Cottrell JE, Lei B. Chapter 1. Brain metabolism, the pathophysiology of brain injury, and potential beneficial agents and techniques. In Cottrell JE, Young WL, eds. *Neuroanesthesia*. Philadelphia: Mosby Elsevier; 2011:1–16.

36. Loane DJ, Faden AI. Neuroprotection for traumatic brain injury: translational challenges and emerging therapeutic strategies. *Trends Pharmacol Sci*. 2010;31:596–604.

37. Yu Y, Crumiller M, Knight B, et al. Estimating the amount of information carried by a neuronal population. *Front Comput Neurosci*. 2010;4:1–10.

38. Iadecola C, Anrather J. Stroke research at a crossroad: asking the brain for directions. *Nature Neurosci*. 2011;14:1363–1368.

39. Perdrizet GA, Lena CJ, Shapiro DS, et al. Preoperative stress conditioning prevents paralysis after experimental aortic surgery: increased heat shock protein content is associated with ischemic tolerance of the spinal cord. *J Thorac Cardiovasc Surg*. 2002;124:162–170.

40. Gidday JM. Cerebral preconditioning and ischaemic tolerance. *Nat Rev Neurosci*. 2006;7:437–448.

41. Gidday JM. Pharmacologic preconditioning: translating the promise. *Transl Stroke Res*. 2010;1:19–30.

42. McGrath LB, Locke M, Cane M, et al. Heat shock protein (HSP 72) expression in patients undergoing cardiac operations. *J Thorac Cardiovasc Surg*. 1995;109:370–376.

43. Stenzel-Poore MP, Stevens SL, Xiong Z, et al. Effect of ischaemic preconditioning on genomic response to cerebral ischemia: similarity to neuroprotective strategies in hibernation and hypoxia-tolerant states. *Lancet*. 2003;362:1028–1037.

44. Sinclair HL, Andrews PJD. Bench-to-bedside review: hypothermia in traumatic brain injury. *Crit Care*. 2010;14:204:1–10.

45. Gow WG, Campbell K, Meade AJ, et al. Lack of neuroprotection of inhibitory peptides targeting Jun/JNK after transient focal cerebral ischemia in spontaneously hypertensive rats. *J Cereb Blood Flow Metab*. 2011;31:e1–e8.

46. Wu J, Hecker JG, Chiamvimonvat N. Antioxidant enzyme gene transfer for ischemic diseases. In Maeda H, ed. *Advanced Drug Delivery Reviews*. Philadelphia: Elsevier; 2009:351–363.

47. Anderson DM, Hall LL, Ayyalapu AR, et al. Stability of mRNA/cationic lipid lipoplexes in human and rat cerebrospinal fluid: methods and evidence for nonviral mRNA gene delivery to the central nervous system. *Hum Gene Ther*. 2003;14:191–202.

48. Nantz MH, Dicus CW, Hilliard B, et al. Unsymmetrical hydrophobic domains improve in vivo transfection efficiency. *Mol Pharmaceut*. 2010;7:786–794.

49. Hecker JG, Hall LL, Irion VR. Non-viral gene delivery to the lateral ventricles in rat brain: initial evidence for widespread distribution and expression in the central nervous system. *Mol Ther*. 2001;3:375–384.

50. Trummer G, Foerster KBG, Benk C, et al. Successful resuscitation after prolonged periods of cardiac arrest: a new field in cardiac surgery. *J Thorac Cardiovasc Surg*. 2010;139:1325–1332.

51. Brucken A, Kaab AB, Kottmann K, et al. Reducing the duration of 100% oxygen ventilation in the early reperfusion period after cardiopulmonary resuscitation decreases striatal brain damage. *Resuscitation*. 2010;81:1698–1703.

52. Buckberg GD. Controlled reperfusion after ischemia may be the unifying recovery denominator. *J Thorac Cardiovasc Surg*. 2010;140:12–18.

53. Allen BS, Buckberg GD. Studies of isolated global brain ischaemia: I. Overview of irreversible brain injury and evolution of a new concept- redefining the time of brain death. *Eur J Cardiothorac Surg*. 2012;41:1132–1137.

54. Meng L, Cannesson M, Alexander BS, et al. Effect of phenylephrine and ephedrine bolus treatment on cerebral oxygenation in anaesthetized patients. *Br J Anaesth*. 2011. doi:10.1093:1-9

55. Iadecola C, Anrather J. The immunology of stroke. *Nat Med*. 2011;17:796–808.

56. Highton DT, Ghosh A, Kolyva C, et al. Low frequency oscillations of NIRS in brain injury: relation to flow, intracranial pressure and blood pressure. *J Neurosurg Anesthesiol*. 2011;23:A4.

57. Lee JK, Brady KM, Mytar JO, et al. Cerebral blood flow and cerebrovascular autoregulation in a swine model of pediatric cardiac arrest and hypothermia. *Crit Care Med*. 2011;39:2337–2345.

58. Brady K, Joshi B, Zweifel C, et al. Real-time continuous monitoring of cerebral blood flow autoregulation using near-infrared spectroscopy in patients undergoing cardiopulmonary bypass. *Stroke*. 2010;41:1951–1956.

59. Klein KU, Fului K, Schramm P, et al. Human cerebral microcirculation and oxygen saturation during propofol-induced reduction of bispectral index. *Br J Anaesth*. 2011;107:735–741.

60. Klein KU, Stadie A, Fukui K, et al. Measurement of cortical microcirculation during intracranial aneurysm surgery by combined laser-Doppler flowmetry and photospectrometry. *Neurosurgery*. 2011;69:391–398.

61. Kircheiner J, Seeringer A, Godoy AL, et al. CYP2D6 in the brain: genotype effects on resting brain perfusion. *Mol Psychiatry*. 2011;16:333–341.

62. Navlakha S, Bar-Joseph Z. Algorithms in nature: the convergence of systems biology and computational thinking. *Mol Syst Biol.* 2011;7:1–11.

63. Ching S, Cimenser A, Purdon PL, et al. Thalamocortical model for a propofol-induced alpha-rhythm associated with loss of consciousness. *PNAS.* 2011;28:22665–22670.

64. Brown EN, Purdon PL, Van Dort CJ. General anesthesia and altered states of arousal: a systems neuroscience analysis. *Annu Rev Neurosci.* 2011;34:601–628.

65. Truccolo W, Donoghue JA, Hochberg LR, et al. Single-neuron dynamics in human focal epilepsy. *Nat Neurosci.* 2011;14:635–641.

66. Humphries C. The mystery behind anesthesia. MIT *Technol Rev.* Dec 2011; p. 5..

67. Ku SW, Lee U, Noh GJ, et al. Preferential inhibition of frontal-to-parietal feedback connectivity is a neurophysiologic correlate of general anesthesia in surgical patients. *PLoS One.* 2011;6:e25155.

68. Mashour G. Consciousness versus responsiveness: insights from general anesthetics. *Brain Cogn.* 2011;77:325–326.

69. Cheung BL, Riedner B, Tononi G, et al. Steady-state multivariate autoregressive models for estimation of cortical connectivity from EEG. *Conf Proc IEEE Engr Med Biol Soc.* 2011;2009:61–64.

70. Cirelli C, Pfister-Genskow M, McCarthy D, et al. Proteomic profiling of the rat cerebral cortex in sleep and waking. *Arch Ital Biol.* 2009;147:59–68.

71. Tononi G. Information integration: its relevance to brain function and consciousness. *Arch Ital Biol.* 2010;148:299–322.

72. Tymianski M. Emerging mechanisms of disrupted cellular signaling in brain ischemia. *Nat Neurosci.* 2011;14:1369–1373.

73. Lauritzen M, Dreier JP, Fabricus M, et al. Clinical relevance of cortical spreading depression in neurological disorders: migraine, malignant stroke, subarachnoid and intracranial hemorrhage, and traumatic brain injury. *J Cereb Blood Flow Metab.* 2011;31:17–35.

74. DeGracia DJ, Kumar R, Owen CR, et al. Molecular pathways of protein synthesis inhibition during brain reperfusion: implications for neuronal survival or death. *J Cereb Blood Flow Metab.* 2002;22:127–141.

75. DeGracia DJ, Kreipke CW, Kayali FM, et al. Brain endothelial HSP70 stress response coincides with endothelial and pericyte death after brain trauma. *Neurol Res.* 2007;29:356–361.

76. Hossmann K-A. The bistable network model of brain ischemia. *J Exp Stroke Transl Med.* 2010;3(1):56–58.

77. DeGracia DJ. Towards a dynamical network view of brain ischemia and reperfusion. Part I: background and preliminaries. *J Exp Stroke Transl Med.* 2010;3:Epub.

78. DeGracia DJ. Towards a dynamical network view of brain ischemia and reperfusion. Part II: a post-ischemic neuronal state space. *J Exp Stroke Transl Med.* 2010;3:72–89.

79. DeGracia DJ. Towards a dynamical view of brain ischemia and reperfusion. Part III: therapeutic implications. *J Exp Stroke Transl Med.* 2010;3:90–103.

80. DeGracia DJ. Towards a dynamical view of brain ischemia and reperfusion. Part IV; additional considerations. *J Exp Stroke Transl Med.* 2010;3:104–114.

81. Siegel M, Donner TH, Engel AK. Spectral fingerprints of large-scale neuronal interactions. *Nat Rev Neurosci.* 2012;13:121–134.

82. Waldrop MM. Brain in a box. *Nature.* 2012;482:457.

83. Brooks R, Hassabis D, Bray D, et al. Turing centenary: is the brain a good model for machine intelligence? *Nature.* 2012;482:462–463.

84. Doronzio A, Stasi E, Titi L, et al. Pharmacologic perioperative brain neuroprotection: a systemic review and meta-analysis of randomized clinical trials. *J Neurosurg Anesthesiol.* 2011;23:A121.

6.

NEUROIMAGING TECHNIQUES

Ramachandran Ramani

INTRODUCTION

Starting from a modest beginning with plain radiographs of the skull, neuroimaging techniques have reached a stage where precise localization of tumors as small as 2 to 3 mm can be achieved. During the past 5 to 10 years, neuroimaging techniques have become available in the operating room, allowing surgeons to perform precise biopsies and resections guided by high-quality images and accurate neuronavigation. In many cases, the quality of images is comparable to illustrations in a neuroanatomy text. The Brainlab Navigation system (Brainlab Inc., Westchester, IL) reconstructs magnetic resonance (MR) images so that the surgeon can view the reconstructed image of the lesion, as it would be seen in the surgical approach to the lesion. The navigation system creates a mathematical space (same as the physical space) within which the surgeon can work. This chapter discusses neuroimaging techniques currently in clinical use, including cerebral angiogram (a four-vessel, transfemoral, biplane digital subtraction angiogram), computed tomography (CT), and MR imaging (MRI). MRI includes a variety of imaging techniques such as MR angiography (MRA), diffusion-weighted MRI, perfusion-weighted MRI, diffusion tensor imaging, functional MRI (fMRI), and MR spectroscopy (MRS).

Although several neuroimaging techniques exist, the three most commonly used techniques are cerebral angiography, CT, and MRI. Each technique has its own specific pros and cons, and imaging modalities are often combined to provide adequate visualization. CT scans are rapid and can be obtained within minutes, making CT the technique of choice in an emergency (e.g., head trauma or acute neurologic deterioration). CT scan can image an intracerebral or extracerebral blood clot, a skull fracture, brain edema, or ventricular dilatation, which allows treatment to begin quickly. The CT angiogram was developed as an alternative to the conventional transfemoral angiogram that is less invasive and has fewer complications. Because of these advantages, the CT angiogram has gradually replaced the transfemoral angiogram for diagnostic vascular imaging. Transfemoral angiograms are now used primarily for endovascular interventional neurovascular procedures such as coiling or embolization. As per a recent review, more than 50% of neurovascular lesions are being treated through an endovascular approach with a GDC coil (Guglielmi Detachable Coil – Boston Scientific, Natick, MA) or embolization [1]. MRI offers high-resolution images that cannot be matched by other imaging techniques. It is most often used to diagnose structural lesions in the brain, and stereotactic neurosurgical systems allow the surgeon to view images that have been oriented to the surgical approach. Over the past several years, intraoperative MRI (iMRI) systems have become available. This technology offers brain imaging during surgery, which then allows the surgeons to gauge the extent of tumor resection and achieve maximal tumor excision while minimizing damage to normal tissue. MRI has some limitations: It cannot image vascular lesions, blood clots, calcifications, or bony lesions. MRA can image vascular lesions and can identify aneurysms as small as 2 mm. But CT angiogram (discussed later) images are far superior to MRA. This chapter discusses neuroradiology as it applies to the anesthesiologist, including CT scans, cerebral angiograms, and a comprehensive description of MRI, MR safety issues, American Society of Anesthesiologists (ASA) guidelines, and anesthetic considerations.

CEREBRAL ANGIOGRAPHY

Cerebral angiography is the technique of choice for diagnosing and treating neurovascular lesions such as intracranial aneurysms and arteriovenous malformations. All modern systems use digital subtraction angiograms (DSAs) to remove the static bone images from the display and improve the clarity of the image. The basic technique involves cannulation of carotid and vertebral arteries and injection of contrast dye. As alluded to earlier, the technique is highly refined to make it less invasive (compared with the direct puncture techniques) and at the same time improve the image quality. The transfemoral approach has become the technique of choice. Guidewires of various shapes are used to guide small catheters through the aorta and into distal branches in the vascular tree. The use of biplane angiography (i.e., two X-ray sources and detectors oriented in perpendicular planes) permits a simultaneous view of two planes, giving a three-dimensional view of the lesion. Serial images can be obtained after a bolus injection of contrast dye to get a dynamic view of the vascular anatomy.

CT SCANNING

CT is based on the principle of *differential X-ray beam attenuation* [2]. Collimated X-rays pass through the tissues (i.e., the brain) and are detected on the opposite side of the body. The signal sensed by the detector is proportional to the differential absorption of the photons by the tissues along the narrow X-ray beam. The beam is rotated, while calculating the differential absorption pattern of a slice of tissue. The differential absorption of the X-ray by the tissues is presented on a gray scale. Via a process referred to as projection reconstruction, modern CTs offer shorter imaging time, thinner slices, better quality of image, and less radiation exposure. Wider beams and multiple detectors have improved accuracy and sensitivity. Improved computational ability enables continuous imaging while the table is moving. This allows the entire brain to be imaged in less than 1 minute. The absorption within each pixel (a very small three-dimensional volume) within a slice of tissue is then reconstructed. This then allows structural images to be created from the differential absorption of various tissues. The spatial resolution of the image varies inversely with the size of the pixel, which currently can be as small as 1 mm × 0.3 mm × 0.3 mm. The relative density of the tissues is expressed in Hounsfield units (HU), which range between −1000 and +1000 (0 HU is equivalent to the density of water). Bone density is close to 1000 HU and air has a density of −1000 HU. The radio density of a given tissue depends on its protein content. In the brain, white and gray matter density varies between 30 and 50 HU, while a blood clot has a density of 50 to 80 HU and a calcified lesion might have a density of 150 HU.

The clinical indications for a CT scan include head trauma (e.g., bone injuries, blood clot, contusion), diagnosis and evaluation of patients with suspected subarachnoid hemorrhage, and imaging calcified lesions in the brain (e.g., oligodendroglioma, craniopharyngioma, retinoblastoma, meningioma, etc.). CT is also the preferred imaging technique for bony lesions in the cranium or spine, or for the evaluation of patients with spinal hardware. CT is the imaging technique of choice in patients for whom MRI is contraindicated.

In CT perfusion technique, a combination of O_2 and ^{133}Xe is inhaled to map the regional brain perfusion. Brain Xe concentration is determined by the concentration of Xe in the blood, cerebral blood flow, and duration of exposure. Iodinated contrast can also be used for CT semiquantitative perfusion studies. After rapid injection, the brain is continuously scanned and the contrast wash-in and wash-out times are analyzed. The mean transit time (MTT), cerebral blood volume (CBV), and cerebral blood flow (CBF) can be measured using the formula

$$\textbf{CBF} = \textbf{CBV/MTT}$$

MRI

Block and Purcell first described the phenomenon of nuclear MR (NMR) in 1945, and Paul Lauterbaur first described the technique of biological imaging using NMR in 1973. As this technology was introduced into clinical practice, its name was changed to *magnetic resonance imaging* (MRI). The term "nuclear" was removed because it falsely implied to patients and staff that that ionizing radiation was being used. *Magnetic resonance spectroscopy* (MRS) refers to the use of NMR technology for in situ biochemical imaging or measurement.

BASIC PRINCIPLES

Anesthesiologists must be familiar with the fundamentals of MRI to understand how this technology impacts patient care and to minimize the unique hazards of working in this environment [3, 4]. An MRI scanner uses three types of magnetic fields to create images: a static magnetic field, a time-varying magnetic field gradient, and radiofrequency (RF) energy. The static field is rated in *Tesla* (T). One Tesla is equivalent to 10,000 Gauss. The typical MRI scanner uses a static magnetic field between 1.5 and 3 T (15,000–30,000 Gauss). Research scanners may employ a field strength up to 7 T or even 14 T. By comparison, a refrigerator magnet has a strength of 50 G and the Earth's magnetic field is approximately 0.3 G. The iMRI scanners use lower field strength (0.05–0.12 T) as well as high field strength (0.5–3 T). Image quality improves with higher field strengths, although some centers prefer open MRI scanners because they require less stringent magnet safety requirements and access to the patient is better. Higher-strength magnets (>1.5 T) use superconductive coils that are cryogenically cooled with liquid nitrogen and liquid helium.

Elements with an odd number of electrons (^{1}H, ^{13}C, ^{19}F, ^{23}Na, ^{31}P) are *paramagnetic*; they act as a dipole in a magnetic field. Between 55% and 60% of the human body consists of water, and MR scanning is primarily a technique of proton (^{1}H) imaging. When protons are exposed to a magnetic field, they align themselves parallel and antiparallel to the field.

There are slightly more protons in the antiparallel alignment and these have a higher energy state, which increases with the strength of the external magnetic field. During MRI, a second magnetic field is applied perpendicular to the static magnetic field using a pulsed RF current. This second magnetic field changes the alignment of the protons, and when this magnetic field is interrupted, the protons flip back to their original alignment in the static magnetic field, emitting a low-amplitude RF signal. There is a RF coil which captures this signal, which is then converted to a structural image and plotted on a gray scale. The extremely low amplitude of the signal makes it prone to interference from external sources of RF energy. All equipments used in the entire MR environment must therefore be shielded and the scanner room itself is also shielded against external sources of RF energy.

The decay of the RF signal is called *relaxation* and has several characteristics that can be exploited to identify structures. The amount of time required for protons to recover to 63% of their original magnetic vector (longitudinal magnetization) is called T1, while T2 refers to the time required for protons to dissipate the energy acquired (transverse magnetization) during the RF pulse sequence (decay to 37% of the original value) [5]. Proton density and the T1 and T2 relaxation time are tissue specific. This allows white and gray matter, cerebrospinal fluid (CSF), blood, and pathological tissues to be visualized using the appropriate MR imaging parameters. The same principles can be applied to obtain biochemical images of hydrogen (glutamate, γ-aminobutyric acid [GABA]) or carbon (for glucose), fluorine (fluorinated compounds) and phosphorus (for ATP) with MRS [6].

FUNCTIONAL IMAGING

Most neuroimaging techniques (e.g., CT scan and MRI) create structural images that demonstrate anatomic features. *Functional imaging* is a technique by which the activity in specific areas of the brain can be imaged and linked to anatomic images. The spectrum of functional activity that can currently be imaged by MRI includes speech, visual, auditory, sensory activation, motor activation, and memory. The activation techniques might include asking a patient to speak (language), to view a moving image (visual), or to tap his or her fingers (motor). This powerful tool has applications in both research and clinical care. fMRI is used while planning a surgical approach to brain tumors that are located in proximity to eloquent areas of the brain, for example, a brain tumor that is located near a language center. Functional imaging can locate these critical areas and demonstrate their anatomic relationship to the brain tumor. A patient with a frontal lobe tumor near speech and motor areas might undergo functional imaging with speech activation and motor activation of the face. This allows the surgeons to identify the regions that control speech. This

image is then transposed on the anatomic image, delineating the relationship of the tumor to the functional regions. Functional imaging is also of use in neuropsychiatric disorders such attention-deficit disorder and speech and language disorders. fMRI enhances treatment planning and facilitates tracking of patients' progress. Functional imaging has applications in research, providing new insights into the basic functioning of the brain.

FUNCTIONAL IMAGING TECHNIQUES

MRI and positron emission tomography (PET) scanning are the two techniques most commonly used for functional imaging [7, 8]. The PET scan is similar to the autoradiographic technique for measuring cerebral metabolic rate oxygen consumption ($CMRo_2$) and CBF and is the gold standard for the measurement of CBF. PET uses ^{15}O-labeled water to measure CBF and ^{18}F-labeled glucose (^{18}FDG) to measure cerebral metabolism. Other compounds can be tagged with isotopes to image drug or neurotransmitter receptors, sites of action of chemotherapeutic agents, or other biochemical compounds in the brain. One major limitation of this technique is that while ^{15}O has a half-life of 2 minutes, the half-life of ^{18}F is 110 minutes. Measurements of CBF measurements can therefore be repeated every 15 minutes, but measurements of cerebral metabolism cannot be repeated because it takes 30 to 45 minutes for the ^{18}FDG to be trapped in the neurons.

As discussed earlier, structural MRI captures signals emanating from protons to create images. In fMRI the signal imaged is referred to as BOLD (blood oxygen level dependent contrast) that was first described by Ogawa and colleagues in 1990 [9], and it relies on the changes in oxyhemoglobin-deoxyhemoglobin ratio at the tissue level. Any neuronal activity in the brain increases the $CMRO_2$, causing a proportional increase in CBF. For a brief period, the increase in the regional blood flow is greater than the increase in metabolism. This disproportionate rise in regional CBF increases the oxyhemoglobin concentration and decreases the deoxyhemoglobin concentration. Deoxyhemoglobin has an affinity to a magnetic field (i.e., it is paramagnetic), while oxyhemoglobin is diamagnetic (has a poor affinity for a magnetic field). This alteration in the deoxyhemoglobin-oxyhemoglobin ratio creates the BOLD signal, which is directly proportional to the neuronal activity. BOLD is a qualitative signal; it is a dimensionless number, and the relative change is more important than an absolute value. BOLD images are therefore obtained before and after functional activation. The alteration in BOLD signal induced by neuronal activity is approximately 5% higher than the baseline BOLD signal. To amplify the signal and minimize the extraneous sources of signal interference unrelated to neuronal activity, multiple images are acquired and the data are averaged. A three-dimensional high-resolution structural image of the brain is also acquired during this process. The functional images are then overlaid on the anatomic (structural) image to identify the anatomic location of the functional activity.

MRS is a technique of imaging specific biochemical compounds [6]. Although the basic principles of MRS are similar to those of fMRI, molecules such as phosphorus, nitrogen, carbon, or fluorine (depending on the structure of the target compound) are the targeted sources of signal in MRS. MRS takes advantage of the differing proton density and the relaxation time that are determined by the chemical structure of the compound. Neurotransmitters glutamate and GABA can be imaged by using ^{1}H MRS. ATP can be demonstrated using phosphorus MRS. ^{13}C-labeled glucose can be infused to trace the dynamic distribution of the carbon atom in glucose between the neurons and glial cells. It can be used to track the synthesis and recycling of glutamate and GABA from the glucose in the citric acid cycle between the neurons and astroglia. Because of the low concentration of the neurotransmitters in the brain (compared with H$^+$ ions in H$_2$O), stronger magnetic fields are necessary to obtain high-resolution images. For ^{1}H MRS, a 3-T, 4-T, or 7-T MRI unit is used, which limits the use of this technique to research laboratories and specialized centers.

Origin of iMRI

After bipolar cautery and the operating microscope, iMRI is considered the third biggest advancement in neurosurgery [10, 11]. Although specialized neuronavigation tools have been developed over the past 20 years, MRI-based systems offer a significant improvement in image navigation technology. Successful resection of a lesion in the brain depends on the surgeon's ability to delineate its margins and to remove it without damaging the surrounding tissue. In patients undergoing surgical resection of an epileptic focus, the target area must be co-registered with an fMRI to ensure that eloquent areas of the brain are not damaged, and accuracy in registration is critical for a successful surgery. Some brain tumors (e.g., glioma) do not have a well-defined capsule. Hence, delineating the margin between the tumor and the normal brain within the surgical field can be challenging in such cases.

Stereotactic neurosurgical navigation systems use high-resolution MR images to precisely locate the surgical lesion within the brain. Systems either use a stereotaxic frame that is fixed to the patient's skull or merge a preoperative MR image with the patient's surface anatomy during a "registration" process (frameless system). Frame-based systems are generally more accurate and precise and can localize a target to within 1 to 2 mm. The frame must be attached to the patient before images are obtained, and the frame itself may limit access to the surgical field. This generally limits the use of frame-based technique to procedures that can be done through a burr hole (e.g., deep brain stimulator lead implantation, brain biopsy).

Frameless neuronavigation systems do not encroach on the surgical field and can be used for a wide variety of neurosurgical procedures. The navigation system creates a reconstructed image from the MR image and merges it with the patient's surface anatomy. These systems rely on an electromagnetic or optical sensor to track movement of the surgical instruments within the operating field and can project the position of the surgical instrument in the brain relative to the lesion. Images are generally acquired before surgery and are reconstructed in such a way that the pathologic lesion can be viewed in all three planes—sagittal, axial, and coronal. Frameless neuronavigation is, however, susceptible to several kinds of errors, since the reconstructed image is not a real time image of the brain. The brain may shift after the dura is opened. In addition to this, CSF drainage, brain retraction, and initial resection of the brain tumor all change the relative neuroanatomy. The reconstructed image therefore no longer precisely reflects the anatomy of the surgical field. The brain can move as much as 10 mm within 1 hour of opening of the dura and before the excision of the lesion, and perhaps even more if there is a preexisting loss of brain parenchyma or hydrocephalus [12, 13] (Figure 6.1). Acquisition of new images during surgery, after the brain has shifted, can improve the accuracy of the reconstructed images. MR images obtained intraoperatively can be used to identify the extent of resection of the tumor, alterations in neuroanatomy, and the presence of blood in the parenchyma. The potential of these applications to improve patient care has led to the

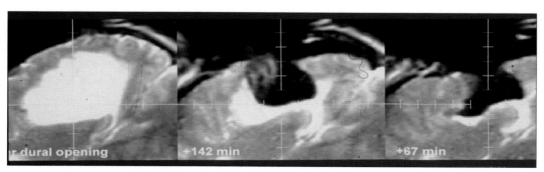

Figure 6.1   Shift in the brain position and size with time.

development of iMRI systems that can be used to image the patient during surgery.

iMRI

Over the past 15 years, three types of iMRI have been developed for use in the surgical suite [11]. The first system designed for clinical use incorporated a 0.5-T magnet in a "double donut" open configuration designed at Brigham and Women's Hospital in Boston, Massachusetts (Figure 6.2). A 70-cm space between the two magnets provided limited surgical access to the head. The introduction of this prototype raised concerns about magnet safety in the operating room. All surgical instruments, including the electrocautery, drill, and suction, had to be manufactured with non-ferrous material. The entire operating room was shielded against RF energy, which required extensive redesigning in the operating room. "Low-field" iMR imagers that used a smaller, portable magnet were then introduced. These systems could be stored within a lead shield in a separate location and brought into the operating when imaging is required. Low-field iMRI systems use a magnetic field strength between 0.12 and 0.15 T. Subsequently, a 0.5-T portable MRI was also introduced. These systems eliminated the need to redesign the entire operating room, and ferromagnetic surgical instruments could be moved away from the operting field during the imaging. In this model the size (and therefore the strength) of the magnet is limited by the requirement for portability, which decreases the available image resolution.

The current generation of iMRI systems use a closed bore magnet and are designed to be stored in a dedicated room adjacent to the operating room when not in use. The scanner moves on rails and is brought out when imaging is required, which allows a single system to be shared between two operating rooms. The operating rooms are custom-designed to incorporate RF shielding, and the 50-G and 5-G lines are marked on the floor. These "high-field" systems use a stronger magnetic field (1.5–3 T), which substantially improves image quality over the low-field systems. Most neurosurgeons use the system intermittently to obtain images during surgery, as they are needed. When the system is brought into the operating room, the operating field is draped, all surgical

instruments are moved outside the 5-G line, and the magnet is brought out for imaging. Anticipated future applications for high-field iMRI include precisely targeted instillation of chemotherapy and immune therapy and the use of MRS to track tumor resection. iMRI-guided laser-induced interstitial thermal treatment (LITT) is another application under development. A robotic arm that is currently under development will allow the surgeons to manipulate the targeted area during imaging.

MRI Hazards and Safety Considerations

The presence of the MRI scanner in the operating room presents unique problems of its own because of the constant presence of the powerful magnetic field [14, 15]. The RF energy also creates hazards that impact the management of patients undergoing surgery in the iMRI operating room. The RF signal of the iMRI can cause equipment to malfunction (anesthesia physiologic monitors and infusion pumps), while extraneous sources of RF signal (e.g., from unshielded anesthesia physiologic monitors) can interfere with the MRI signal and degrade image quality. MRI-related hazards result from:

1. Hazards related to the high-power magnetic field—biophysical or physical

2. Hazards related to the RF energy

3. Interference with the RF signal of MRI by the electrical noise in the room

4. Imaging problems: prolonged imaging time, noise, heating

5. Hazards related to the contrast agent

Magnetic Field

A 3-T magnet in an MRI scanner has a field strength 30,000 to 60,000 times stronger than that of the magnetic field of the earth (0.5–1 G). Ferromagnetic objects such as scissors, sitting stools, and oxygen tanks can be pulled along the gradient of the magnetic field at a very high velocity. This

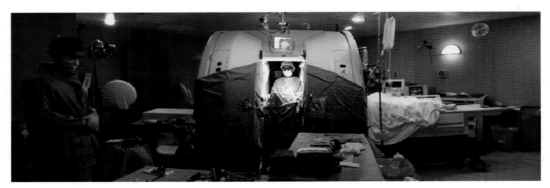

Figure 6.2   Double donut intraoperative MRI.

"missile effect" can cause extensive damage, and at least one death has been reported due to an oxygen tank being pulled into the scanner and crushing a patient. All ferromagnetic objects must be moved beyond the 5-G line to ensure that they will not be attracted by the magnetic field. Most studies have shown no evidence that strong magnetic fields have biological adverse effects, and even pregnant women have safely undergone MRI. One recent study suggests that the stray magnetic field from a 7-T research MRI scanner may have transient effects on memory and the ability to perform spatial tasks [16].

Medical devices such as permanent pacemakers (PPMs), implantable cardioverter-defibrillators (ICDs), or other implanted devices can be dislodged by the powerful magnetic field, potentially causing injury or death. To date there is only one case of fatality related to MR-unsafe aneurysm clip (MRI safety.com). Nonferromagnetic aneurysm clips made of titanium or cobalt-chromium (Phynox) are replacing the ferromagnetic clips. Before 1985, aneurysm clips were made of stainless steel and were ferromagnetic. Nonferromagnetic aneurysm clips (titanium and cobalt chromium clips) have been extensively checked and certified by the manufacturer for their MRI safety. Patients who have a history of neurovascular surgery should be carefully evaluated before they are allowed to enter the magnet room. Patient with titanium clips and cobalt chromium clips can be safely imaged in a 3-T magnet.

Most PPMs are affected by any magnetic field over 5 G, although some newer models are unaffected by magnetic field up to 1.5 T (discussed later). The chief hazard is that the programming of pacemakers, ICDs, neurostimulators, and infusion pumps may be altered during exposure to the magnetic field. Deaths due to pacemaker malfunction during MRI have been reported [17]. It has been estimated that there are 2 million patients with implanted pacemakers in Europe and that there is a 50% to 75% chance that they may need MRI in their lifetime. MRI is becoming safer in these patients as long as the manufacturers' recommendations are followed. Some MRI-conditional pacemakers are now available in the United States as well as in Europe [18]. A U.S. Food and Drug Administration (FDA)-approved MRI-conditional pacemaker is the Revo MRI Sure scan pacing system (Medtronics Inc., Minnesota, MN). The other MRI-conditional pacemakers available are the Biotronik system (Berlin, Germany) and the St. Jude system (St. Paul, MN). Although these MRI-conditional pacemakers are available, it is important to be aware that certain preconditions have to be fulfilled before imaging patients with an MRI-conditional pacemaker. These preconditions are [19]:

- MRI-conditional pacemaker is approved for a cylindrical bore 1.5-T magnet only.
- MRI device as well as lead should be MR compatible.

- The device should be implanted over the right or left pectoral region and should have been in place for more than 6 weeks.
- The transmitter and the receiving coil should not be placed over the pacing system.
- Patient should not be positioned on one side.
- The pacemaker device should be in asynchronous mode during the imaging.
- Hemodynamic monitoring should be carried out during the imaging, a cardiologist should be in attendance, and there should be a defibrillator device available.
- The pacemaker device should be interrogated after MRI to ensure that the pacemaker settings have not been altered.

A study by Raj and colleagues [19] reported that more than 400 patients with an MRI-conditional pacemaker have been imaged without any problems (average imaging time of 40 minutes).

RF Energy

RF energy is used to create a time-varying magnetic field that can induce an electrical current in any conductor. The RF energy creates a magnetic field that can induce electrical voltage and this voltage can be dissipated into the human body, creating heat. However, the overall rise in temperature during a standard FDA-approved MRI sequence is no more than 1°C. Electrical voltage can develop in any coil of wire within the magnetic field. And if this coil of wire is in contact with any part of the patient's body, at the point of contact electrical current can be dissipated, causing release of thermal energy and resulting in a burn. At the point of contact with the pulse oximeter probe or electrocardiographic (ECG) electrodes, burns can develop. This can be prevented by carefully avoiding any coil of wire (ECG, pulse oximeter wires) and by ensuring that there is no direct contact between these wires and skin. And periodically these wires should be inspected to ensure that their insulation is intact. Even tattoos and eyeliners have ferric oxide in them, which absorbs electrical energy releasing heat. However, this is a very rare occurrence. Subjects with a possible metallic foreign body should be carefully evaluated by a radiologist and the MRI technician prior to an MRI study.

Interference With the RF Signal

External sources of RF energy can interfere with the RF signal that is generated by the protons during relaxation (the tissue-specific primary signal in MRI). Anesthesia monitors, infusion pumps, and other electronic devices emit RF energy in the megahertz to gigahertz range. The MRI room is shielded to prevent any interference from extraneous sources of RF energy, and MRI-compatible anesthesia monitors and infusion pumps are also shielded. Unshielded equipment such as computers should be powered off during imaging. Portable MRI scanners are protected from RF interference by a Faraday cage that encloses the scanner and the patient while the images are obtained.

Problems Related to Imaging

For a physician, access to the patient is limited during the scan, and the length of time that the patient will be inaccessible depends on the number of images being acquired and the specific imaging sequences that will be used. Patients who are awake may find the noisy environment and confined space stressful and may require sedation. This is especially true for patients who are claustrophobic or who cannot lie flat for extended periods of time.

During image acquisition, the gradient coils are pulsed with RF energy, which causes them to vibrate. The sound pressure level increases with the strength of the static field and can exceed 100 dB. This is significantly louder than the 90-dB noise level permitted by the U.S. Occupational Safety and Health Administration (OSHA). Prolonged exposure to the scanner without hearing protection can cause irreversible hearing loss. Hearing protection is required for employees working in an environment with the sound pressure level above 85 dB. Sound protection should be provided for patients as well. Prolonged exposure to sounds that exceed 70 dB may also cause injury.

Contrast-Induced Toxicity

Gadolinium (Gd) is the most commonly used intravenous MRI contrast agent and is currently the only agent that is approved by the FDA [20]. It is administered to enhance blood vessels. MRI contrast agents are paramagnetic compounds, and they influence the T1-weighted image. Gd has a high therapeutic ratio and has a better safety profile than that of iodine-based contrast agents. However, headache, itching, burning, facial swelling, and thrombophlebitis have been reported with Gd administration. Nephrogenic systemic fibrosis (NSF) is a rare but potentially life-threatening side effect of Gd. NSF causes fibrosis of the joints, skin, eyes, and internal organs and has been reported to occur in patients with renal disease. Patients with a glomerular filtration rate (GFR) less than 30 mL/1.73 m²/min are at risk for developing NSF after administration of Gd. Renal function should be evaluated before subjecting a patient to an MRI study that requires contrast. If the patient has a low GFR, the need for Gd injection should be carefully evaluated with the risks involved. The lowest possible dose of Gd should be used, and contrast should not be readministered within 7 days. Gd-based contrast media has been classified into high-risk (gadopentolic acid), medium risk (gadobenic acid), and low risk (gadoteridol). Administration of high-risk Gd-based contrast agents to neonates or in patients who have recently undergone liver transplantation is not safe. Administration of any Gd contrast agent is not recommended during pregnancy.

MRI Safety Measures

The American College of Radiologists and the ASA have jointly published detailed guidelines for the care of patients in the MRI suite [21, 22]. These guidelines form the basis of policies and procedure that are developed by individual institutions to ensure safe practice in this unique environment. Safety protocols have been developed for each of four *zones* that are defined by their proximity to the magnetic field [22].

Zone I is open to general public, and includes areas such as a lobby or check-in area.

Zone II is the interface between zone I and potentially hazardous areas. Patients, visitors, and staff who might come into contact with the magnetic field are interviewed to ensure that there are no contraindications to being exposed to a strong magnetic field. Any item that will be brought into the scanner is inspected to ensure that no ferromagnetic objects are brought into the scanner.

Zone III is potentially hazardous and includes the MRI console room. A closed locked door that can be opened only by MRI personnel restricts entry.

Zone IV is the MRI magnet room. Ferromagnetic objects brought into this location may fly into the magnet, causing extensive property damage or severe injury to personnel. Access to zone IV is through a locked door that is directly supervised by an MRI technologist, either through direct line of sight or by a video monitor. A lighted warning sign is required.

Any equipment that is brought into zone III or IV should be clearly marked as *MRI Safe, MRI Conditional,* or *Unsafe*. The term *MRI Compatible* is no longer used. MRI-safe items are not ferromagnetic and are not affected by the magnetic field. MRI-conditional items are safe under specified conditions (e.g., they will tolerate exposure to a magnetic field of limited strength). For MRI-conditional items, the conditions under which the items are MRI safe should be clearly specified. The zoning refers to diagnostic MRI rooms only—not to the MRI operating room. For the iMRI room, the only working rule is the 50-G and 5-G line rule—all items are moved beyond the 5-G line except the anesthesia machine, monitor, and infusion pump, which remain beyond the 50-G line (because they are MRI conditional).

Anesthesia for Patients Undergoing MRI

Every day, thousands of patients undergo MRI in outpatient facilities with no sedation or monitoring. If, however, a patient is unable to tolerate a confined, loud environment or to hold still, or if the patient will undergo an MRI-guided invasive procedure, an anesthesiologist is likely to be present. A patient for MRI can be managed with any of the following:

- Monitoring alone
- Monitoring with sedation
- General anesthesia

The requirement for sedation or general anesthesia is decided based on the procedure:

- The anticipated level of discomfort
- The patient's age
- Comorbidities

For example, if the patient is very young or has impaired cognitive function, deep sedation or general anesthesia may be required for even a brief scan. On the other hand, a patient undergoing an MRI-guided neurosurgical procedure might require general anesthesia for the procedure. For patients who require routine imaging, the ASA has published practice guidelines for sedation and analgesia by nonanesthesiologists (Table 6.1) [23]. A patient who requires mild or moderate sedation (conscious sedation—the patient responds to verbal and tactile stimuli and does not require support of the airway, ventilation, or circulation) may be monitored by a trained nurse or physician. Patients who require deep sedation (i.e., the patient is unresponsive or requires support of the airway, ventilation, or circulation) must be cared for by trained anesthesia providers. ASA guidelines for nonoperating room anesthesia require that facilities be available for monitoring ventilation, circulation, and oxygenation during the procedure.

ASA PRACTICE ADVISORY ON ANESTHETIC CARE FOR MRI

The ASA practice advisory is a comprehensive, updated set of guidelines for the anesthetic management of patients in an MRI facility [22]. This advisory was published in 2009 and is based on scientific literature published between 1974 and 2008 and expert opinion. Part I of the advisory describes the various MRI facilities, which can be grouped under three categories depending on the type of monitoring and medical care that is available.

Level I MRI facilities do not offer any type of medical care during imaging. These facilities are not required to have any equipment for monitoring physiologic parameters or the ability to provide therapeutic intervention such as airway support.

Level II MRI facilities accept patients who may need physiologic monitoring or critical care services such as controlled ventilation or hemodynamic support.

Level III Operating rooms with iMRI capabilities.

Level II and III MRI facilities are required to have physiologic monitors and qualified medical personnel immediately available. Patients who are imaged in Level II and III facilities may require sedation, anesthesia, or critical care services such as airway management, mechanical ventilation, and hemodynamic support. Level III facilities that offer intraoperative imaging are likely to be equipped with surgical instruments as well. Health care providers in these areas include personnel who are not primarily associated with the MRI and include anesthesiologists, surgeons, and operating room nurses. This combination of ferromagnetic objects in a hybrid environment and staff members who may be unaware of the implications of working around a strong magnetic field therefore requires a high level of vigilance.

Table 6.1 **CONTINUUM OF DEPTH OF SEDATION: DEFINITION OF GENERAL ANESTHESIA AND LEVELS OF SEDATION-ANALGESIA**

CONSIDERATION	MINIMAL SEDATION (ANXIOLYSIS)	MODERATE SEDATION-ANALGESIA (CONSCIOUS SEDATION)	DEEP SEDATION-ANALGESIA	GENERAL ANESTHESIA
Responsiveness	Normal response to verbal stimulation	Purposeful response to verbal or tactile stimulation	Purposeful response after repeated or painful stimulation	Unarousable, even with painful stimulus
Airway	Unaffected	No intervention required	Intervention may be required	Intervention often
Spontaneous ventilation	Unaffected	Adequate	May be inadequate	Frequently inadequate
Cardiovascular function	Unaffected	Usually maintained	Usually maintained	May be impaired

Working in a Level II or III MRI facility requires a multifaceted approach that encompasses MRI safety and management of patients with multiple comorbidities who require invasive monitoring, airway management, and hemodynamic support. Part 2 of the ASA advisory covers the various aspects related to management in an MRI facility. Broadly these are:

- Education of the personnel
- Screening of the personnel
- Screening of the patients
- Preparations for anesthesia
- Patient management
- Emergency care
- Postanesthesia management

i. *Education:* All anesthesia personnel involved in anesthesia care should be educated about MRI safety, hazards related to MRI and how they can be prevented, dangers related to ferromagnetic substances and implanted medical devices, etc.

ii. *Screening of personnel likely to work in the MRI facility:* Screening requirements are the same for both patients as well as personnel working in an MRI facility (*Yale University, MRI safety questionnaire*) (see Figure 6.3) All personnel working in the MRI facility should be asked to fill out an MRI safety form and the MRI director should review this safety form to decide on the eligibility of the personnel to work in the MRI facility. Screening is primarily for implanted medical devices, prosthesis, valves, vascular stents, etc.

iii. *Screening the patients:* Screening a patient for MRI should cover the following:

a) Screening for medical illness. This should cover optimizing his medical status, need for monitoring during the imaging, continued critical care like ventilation, vasopressor support to stabilize the blood pressure etc. Management of the medical illnesses should be carried out in consultation with the physician caring for the patient. In patients with renal failure, administration of gadolinium (MRI contrast) is contraindicated.

b) Screening for any implanted medical devices like PPM, automatic implanted cardioverter-defibrillator (AICD), neurostimulators like vagus nerve stimulator (VNS), deep brain stimulator, etc. In patients with PPM or AICD, MRI is contraindicated, while patients with VNS or thermodilution catheter can have a limited MRI.

c) Screening for implanted ferromagnetic substances like prosthetic joints, aneurysm clips, prosthetic cardiac valves, etc.

d) Screening for ferromagnetic substances embedded in the body like metallic fragments.

iv. *Preparation for MRI:* Points to be considered during the preparation of a patient for MRI are

a) Duration of the MRI
b) Position of the patient during MRI
c) Position of the coil
d) Use of contrast agent (gadolinium)
e) Positioning of the anesthetic equipment and monitors in zone IV—MR-compatible anesthesia machines, monitors, infusion pumps should be placed outside the 50-G line.
f) Position of the anesthesiologist for monitoring the patient—in a conventional MRI, the anesthesiologist monitors the patient from the MRI console (zone III).
g) Plan for any emergency

v. *Patient management during MRI*

Monitoring:

a) As per the ASA basic monitoring standard ventilation, circulation, oxygenation, and temperature should be monitored during the procedure.
b) Only MRI-safe monitors should be used in zone 4 with additional display in zone 3.
c) ECG monitor has some limitations—because of superimposed voltage from the magnetic field—ST-segment and T-wave voltage will be altered even when it is filtered.
d) When ECG and pulse oximeter cables are connected, coiling of the cable should be avoided and the cables should not be in contact with the skin.

Anesthetic Management: Equipment for MRI anesthesia should be comparable to the equipment in any other anesthesia care facility. Because of the limited access to the airway and possible airway compromise with sedation, more proactive airway management consistent with the standard practice in the institution should be considered. Movement of the head can distort MR images, requiring repeat imaging, thus extending the imaging time. For any MRI, the region to be imaged has to be positioned at the center of the magnet. Because of this reason, the head (and the airway) cannot be accessed during the MRI. For the same reason, airway management should be planned in advance, and if airway devices like fiberoptic scope is required, this should be done outside in zone III. There should be a lower threshold for airway intervention in an MRI facility because of limited access to the patient.

MRI Safety Questionnaire

Name: _____   **Date of birth:** _____

Today's date: _____

Please read the following questions carefully. It is very important for us to know if you have any **metal devices** or **metal parts** anywhere in your body. If you do not understand a question, please ask us to explain! If you answer yes to any question, please contact the principal investigator.

1. Yes ☐ No ☐   Do you have a heart pacemaker? (if you have a pacemaker, **you cannot have an MRI**)
2. Yes ☐ No ☐   Did you ever have a device implanted somewhere in your body like a heart defibrillator?
3. Yes ☐ No ☐   Did you ever have an aneurysm clip implanted during brain surgery?
4. Yes ☐ No ☐   Do you have a Carotid Artery Vascular clamp?
5. Yes ☐ No ☐   Do you have nerve stimulators (neuron-stimulators also called TENS or wires)?
6. Yes ☐ No ☐   Do you have any devices to make bones grow (like bone growth or bone fusion stimulators)?
7. Yes ☐ No ☐   Do you have implants in your ear (like cochlear implants)?
8. Yes ☐ No ☐   Do you have a Vagus nerve stimulator to help you with convulsions or with epilepsy?
9. Yes ☐ No ☐   Do you have a filter for blood clots (Umbrella, Greenfield, bird's nest)?
10. Yes ☐ No ☐   Do you have embolization coils (Gianturco) in your brain?
11. Yes ☐ No ☐   Do you have implants in your eyes? Have you ever had cataract surgery?
12. Yes ☐ No ☐   Do you have any stents (small metal tubes used to keep blood vessels open)?
13. Yes ☐ No ☐   Do you have an implanted pump to deliver medication?
14. Yes ☐ No ☐   Do you have an artificial arm or leg?
15. Yes ☐ No ☐   Do you wear colored contact lenses?
16. Yes ☐ No ☐   Do you wear a patch to deliver medicines through the skin?
17. Yes ☐ No ☐   Do you have shrapnel or metal in your head, eyes or skin?
18. Yes ☐ No ☐   Have you ever worked with metal? (For example in a machine shop)? If yes, we need to obtain orbit x-rays.
19. Yes ☐ No ☐   Have you ever had metal removed from your eyes by a doctor?
20. Yes ☐ No ☐   Have you ever had a gunshot wound? Or a B-B gun injury?
21. Yes ☐ No ☐   Do you have body-piercing or jewelry on your body?
22. Yes ☐ No ☐   Do you have permanent eye liner? (We need to make sure it does not heat up during the MRI)
23. Yes ☐ No ☐   Do you use a hearing aid?
24. Yes ☐ No ☐   Do you wear braces on your teeth or have a permanent retainer?
25. Yes ☐ No ☐   Do you have a "shunt" (a tube to drain fluid) in your brain, spine or heart?
26. Yes ☐ No ☐   Do you have metal joints, rods, plates, pins, screws, nails, or clips in any part of your body?
27. Yes ☐ No ☐   Do you have a tattoo? (We need to make sure it does not heat up during the MRI)
28. Yes ☐ No ☐   Do you get upset or anxious in small spaces?
29. Yes ☐ No ☐   Do you have kidney disease, need dialysis or have diabetes?
30. Yes ☐ No ☐   Do you have asthma? Have you ever had an allergic reaction? If yes, to what? _____
31. Yes ☐ No ☐   Have you ever had any surgery? Please list all _____
32. Yes ☐ No ☐   Do you have hair extensions?

FOR WOMEN

33. Yes ☐ No ☐   Are you breastfeeding?
34. Yes ☐ No ☐   Do you use a diaphragm, IUD, or cervical pessary? If IUD, what brand? _____
35. Yes ☐ No ☐   Do you think there is any possibility that you might be pregnant? Date of last menstrual period _____

FOR MEN

36. Yes ☐ No ☐   Do you have a penile implant?

Weight _____   Height _____

Signature: _____   **Date:** _____

Figure 6.3   Yale University MRI safety questionnaire.

vi. Management of Emergencies: Every institution should develop its own protocol for managing any emergency in an MRI facility and personnel working in MRI facility should be familiar with this protocol. Some of the possible emergencies are—

a) Medical emergency (like cardiorespiratory arrest): In case of a cardiac arrest imaging should be immediately discontinued and the patient moved out of zone IV while doing a CPR (if indicated) and calling for help. Patient should be moved to a predetermined location from zone IV for resuscitation—this location should be close to zone IV and should have all the equipment for resuscitation.

b) Fire—In case of a fire, the team members should follow their pre assigned tasks, which includes moving the patient to a safe location, measures to put out the fire, resuscitation, etc.

c) Projectile emergency: In case of a projectile accident remove the patient from zone IV, controlled quench may be required to move the patient out and attend to the medical emergency if the patient is hurt.

d) Quench: Quenching refers to the sudden boiling of the coolant (liquid helium) in the superconductive MRI magnet. This results in venting of the helium into MRI room, which could cause a hypoxic environment—affecting the patient as well as the personnel in the MRI suite. Quenching occurs because of the sudden loss of super conductivity in the MRI magnet with rise in electrical resistance causing generation of heat. If a quench occurs remove the patient from zone IV and administer oxygen. Powerful static magnetic field still persists in zone IV—hence the routine MRI precautions should be followed during a quench.

As a general rule in case of an emergency, the emergency response team of the hospital should not enter zone IV.

vii. Postprocedure care: Postprocedure care of the patient following MRI should be consistent with the practice anywhere else in the hospital where sedation/anesthesia is being administered.

ANESTHETIC MANAGEMENT

As per the ASA practice guidelines for sedation and anesthesia by nonanesthesiologists, the various levels of sedation/anesthesia are [22, 23]:

- *Mild Sedation:* Patient has a normal response to verbal command and physiologic functions like airway, ventilation, and circulation are not affected.

- *Moderate Sedation:* Patient has a purposeful response to verbal and tactile stimulation and physiologic functions are not affected.

- *Deep Sedation:* Purposeful response to noxious stimuli. Airway and ventilation may be affected but circulation is not affected.

- *General Anesthesia:* As it implies, patient is not arousable and is likely to need airway, ventilation, and/or circulatory support.

ASA recommends that anything beyond moderate sedation should be managed only in the presence of trained anesthesia personnel.

For anesthetic management the important considerations are:

i) MRI safety standards

ii) Monitoring the patient

iii) Anesthetic management

1) *MRI safety:* MRI safety precautions discussed above should be strictly implemented in the MRI suite and iMRI operating room. MRI-unsafe equipment should not be permitted in the zone IV of an MRI suite. iMRI has the unique situation of a blending between zones 3 and 4 and should be treated as such. For safety purposes the regulations that should be followed are:

- The 50-G line and 5-G line should be clearly marked in the room.
- As far as possible, MRI-unsafe equipment should not be permitted in the room.
- Equipment/items that are MRI unsafe should be beyond the 5-G line during the imaging period.
- MRI-safe equipment (anesthesia machine, physiologic monitor, and infusion device) should be beyond the 50-G line.
- Every institution should develop its own checklist to ensure that the proper MRI safety regulations are followed.

2) *Monitoring:* As per the ASA Practice Guidelines, the patient monitoring standards in an MRI suite should be the same as in an operating room. Oxygenation, ventilation, circulation, and temperature should be monitored during the procedure. MRI-safe anesthesia equipment has been designed for use in an MRI room. The MRI magnet and the gradient coil interfere with the functioning of anesthesia monitors and other equipment and, conversely, the equipment in the operating room can interfere with the MRI signals. ECG tracing is most commonly affected. For monitoring design purposes, conductors, which carry electrical signals for monitoring physiological parameters, should be eliminated. In place of conductors either wireless technology or fiberoptic cables should be used. The gradient coil emits signals at 100-Hz frequency, which disturbs the ECG tracing (Figure 6.4). Monitors are equipped with high-frequency filters to eliminate this noise.

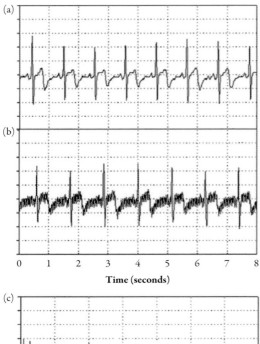

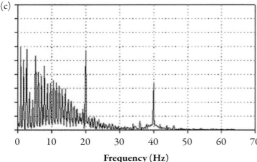

Figure 6.4 ECG disturbance with 0.15-T MRI.

- Hydromagnetic effect refers to the behavior of a fluid in the presence of a magnetic field. Blood flow in the aorta generates a low-amplitude signal, which can distort the ECG trace—T-wave voltage is altered. Distortion is proportional to the velocity and volume of blood flow and orientation of the vessel in relation to the magnetic field. To prevent/minimize the hydromagnetic effect, it is recommended that the electrodes be placed close together on the left side below the axilla.

The recommendations for ECG monitoring in an MRI room are:

- MRI-safe electrode should be used.

- ECG leads should be short, close together in order to minimize the hydromagnetic effect.

- Standard lead placement should be followed.

- ECG is distorted during MRI and is not reliable.

- If MRI time is more than 13 minutes, adjust the filter to minimize the electrical interference.

- If a cardiac event is suspected, remove the patient from the MRI console and institute standard ECG monitoring.

Pulse oximeter should be wireless and length of the wire should be short. Coiling of the wire and contact of the pulse oximeter wire with patient's skin should be avoided. Standard blood pressure cuff and end-tidal CO_2 monitor can be used. For temperature monitoring, only MRI-compatible temperature probe (fiberoptic cable) should be used. For invasive pressures, standard cable and transducer are used. The transducer should be clamped to a pole or operating room table.

3) Anesthetic management [24]

   i) Anesthesia set-up should be extremely meticulous and well planned because once the imaging commences, it is difficult to make any changes, alterations in the set-up.

   ii) Intravenous lines should have sufficiently long extension tubing to permit access to the injection port when the patient is in the scanner.

   iii) Similarly, tubing for oxygen supplementation, ventilator tubing, etc. should be long enough to be able to reach the patient.

   iv) All tubing should be clearly labeled.

   v) Faraday cage used for enclosing low-field magnets has an opening for tubing to exit.

   vi) MRI-compatible anesthesia machine should be used. Desflurane vaporizer is not MRI compatible because of the internal heating element. Isoflurane and sevoflurane vaporize are MRI compatible.

   vii) MRI-compatible infusion pump should be used.

   viii) Fluid warmer and patient warming device (Bear hugger) are not MRI compatible—hence, they should be disconnected and moved beyond the 5-G line during MRI.

Anesthetic Technique: No specific anesthetic technique has been recommended for MRI. ASA Practice Guideline also does not recommended any specific anesthetic agent for MRI. For diagnostic imaging, short-acting agents like propofol, remifentanil, and sevoflurane are preferred. With these agents, adequate depth of anesthesia can be achieved during the MRI, and at the end of the procedure it is possible to wake up the patient with minimal residual effect of anesthesia or sedation. It is important to ensure that the patient does not move during the imaging—movement can distort the image, and with excessive unanticipated movement, the patient can get injured in the restricted space of the MRI console. Airway emergencies are difficult to manage with the patient's head positioned for imaging with the sensing coil secured over the head. Hence, there should be a lower threshold for using airway support devices like nasal trumpet, laryngeal mask airway, or endotracheal tube. During an iMRI, the entire face and operating area are draped. Hence the endotracheal tubing should be secured properly, and ventilator hose should be well supported to prevent any drag on the endotracheal tube because of the length of the hose.

REFERENCES

1. Smith GA, Dagostino P, Maltenfort MG, et al. Geographic variation and regional trends in adoption of endovascular techniques for cerebral aneurysms. *J Neurosurg.* 2011;114:1768–1777.

2. Grossman RI, Yousem DM. *Neuroradiology.* 2nd edition. Philadelphia: Mosby; 2003.

3. Menon DK, Peden CJ, Hall AS, et al. Magnetic resonance for the anaesthetist. Part I: Physical principles, applications, safety aspects. *Anaesthesia.* 1992;47:240–255.

4. Huettel SA, McCarthy G. *Functional magnetic resonance imaging.* 2nd edition. Sunderland, MA: Sinauer Associates; 2009.

5. Smith RC, Lange RC. *Understanding magnetic resonance imaging.* New York: CRC Press; 1997.

6. Ross B, Bluml S. Magnetic resonance spectroscopy of the human brain. *Anat Rec.* 2001;265:54–84.

7. Heinke W, Schwarzbauer C. In vivo imaging of anaesthetic action in humans: approaches with positron emission tomography (PET) and functional magnetic resonance imaging (fMRI). *Br J Anaesth.* 2002;89:112–122.

8. Ramani R, Wardhan R. Understanding anesthesia through functional imaging. *Curr Opin Anaesthesiol.* 2008;21:530–536.

9. Ogawa S, Lee TM, Kay AR, et al. Brain magnetic resonance imaging with contrast dependent on blood oxygenation. *Proc Natl Acad Sci U S A.* 1990;87:9868–9872.

10. Mislow JM, Golby AJ, Black PM. Origins of intraoperative MRI. *Neurosurg Clin N Am.* 2009;20:137–146.

11. Foroglou N, Zamani A, Black P. Intra-operative MRI (iop-MR) for brain tumour surgery. *Br J Neurosurg.* 2009;23:14–22.

12. Nabavi A, Black PM, Gering DT, et al. Serial intraoperative magnetic resonance imaging of brain shift. *Neurosurgery.* 2001;48:787–797; discussion 797–788.

13. Hartkens T, Hill DL, Castellano-Smith AD, et al. Measurement and analysis of brain deformation during neurosurgery. *IEEE Trans Med Imaging.* 2003;22:82–92.

14. Farling PA, Flynn PA, Darwent G, et al. Safety in magnetic resonance units: an update. *Anaesthesia.* 2010;65:766–770.

15. Johnston T, Moser R, Moeller K, et al. Intraoperative MRI: safety. *Neurosurg Clin N Am.* 2009;20:147–153.

16. van Nierop, L. E., P. Slottje, et al. Effects of magnetic stray fields from a 7 tesla MRI scanner on neurocognition: a double-blind randomised crossover study. *Occup Environ Med.* 2012;69:759–766.

17. Ferris NJ, Kavnoudias H, Thiel C, et al. The 2005 Australian MRI safety survey. *AJR Am J Roentgenol.* 2007;188:1388–1394.

18. Shinbane JS, Colletti PM, Shellock FG. Magnetic resonance imaging in patients with cardiac pacemakers: era of "MR conditional" designs. *J Cardiovasc Magn Reson.* 2011;13:63.

19. Raj V, O'Dwyer R, Pathmanathan R, Vaidhyanath R. MRI and cardiac pacing devices—beware the rules are changing. *Br J Radiol.* 2011;84:857–859.

20. Shellock FG, Spinazzi A. MRI safety update 2008: part 1, MRI contrast agents and nephrogenic systemic fibrosis. *AJR Am J Roentgenol.* 2008;191:1129–1139.

21. Kanal E, Borgstede JP, Barkovich AJ, et al. American College of Radiology White Paper on MR safety. *AJR Am J Roentgenol.* 2002;178:1335–1347.

22. Practice advisory on anesthetic care for magnetic resonance imaging: a report by the Society of Anesthesiologists Task Force on Anesthetic Care for Magnetic Resonance Imaging. *Anesthesiology.* 2009;110:459–479.

23. Practice guidelines for sedation and analgesia by non-anesthesiologists. *Anesthesiology.* 2002;96:1004–1017.

24. Bergese SD, Puente EG. Anesthesia in the intraoperative MRI environment. *Neurosurg Clin N Am.* 2009;20:155–162.

7.
PHARMACOLOGY OF INTRAVENOUS SEDATIVE—HYPNOTIC AGENTS

Joshua H. Atkins and Jessica Dworet

INTRODUCTION

Intravenous anesthetic agents have always played a central role in neuroanesthetic management. The increasing role of intraoperative neurophysiologic monitoring, extensive clinical experience with easy to use drugs such as propofol and remifentanil, and the availability of sophisticated pharmacologic models to guide dosing has greatly expanded the use of total intravenous anesthesia. Investigations into cellular physiology offer insight into the molecular underpinnings of drug action and direct the development of even better agents. Clinical investigations have also revisited the benefits of older drugs such as ketamine. Only two new intravenous anesthetic agents—fospropofol and dexmedetomidine (DEX)—have been introduced to the clinic in the past decade. This chapter reviews the fundamental properties of intravenous anesthetic agents and how they affect central nervous system physiology. Key differences between agents are highlighted, as are recent research findings in controversial areas. A practical approach to the use of opioid and intravenous agents in the specific settings of awake craniotomy and spinal fusion with monitoring are included.

ANESTHETIC AGENTS AND CEREBRAL PHYSIOLOGY

Anesthetic agents produce significant changes in cerebral energy dynamics and blood flow, and a basic understanding of these effects is critical to anesthetic management in neurosurgery. Intravenous anesthetic agents as a group offer several advantages for neuroanesthesia over inhaled agents but subtle differences between drugs should be appreciated. Intravenous agents (with the exception of ketamine) reduce cerebral metabolic rate (CMR) and cerebral blood flow (CBF) while preserving autoregulation and flow–metabolism coupling. Intravenous agents also preserve responsiveness of CBF to changes in dissolved CO_2.

Volatile anesthetic agents disrupt CBF-CMR coupling in a dose-dependent fashion thereby increasing CBF out of proportion to metabolic needs although the magnitude of this effect varies by agent. The resulting increase in brain blood volume may increase intracranial pressure (ICP) and make surgical access more difficult. Barbiturates, etomidate, and propofol may therefore be preferable to high concentrations of an inhaled anesthetic in the neurosurgical patient.

Total intravenous anesthesia with propofol, etomidate, or barbiturates in conjunction with opioids can reduce ICP and cerebral blood volume (CBV), improving surgical access for craniotomy in patients with space occupying lesions. In several prospective, randomized clinical trials, patients receiving TIVA had decreased ICP and increased cerebral perfusion pressure (CPP) compared with patients receiving volatile anesthetics for elective craniotomies. Barbiturates and propofol produce a dose-dependent reduction in EEG activity and CMR [1]. The effect of propofol on ICP and CBF is similar to that of barbiturates, but propofol has a rapid onset and short half-life compared with barbiturates. In contrast to volatile anesthetic agents, which impair cerebral autoregulation in a dose-dependent fashion, propofol preserves autoregulation at a wide range of doses in healthy patients. In patients with brain injury, however, high doses of propofol (plasma concentration 4.3 µg/mL, dose >180 µg/kg/min) can impair autoregulation [2]. When used at doses that produce equivalent anesthetic depth, propofol and volatile agents reduce metabolic rate but only propofol reduces CBF and brain blood volume [1]. Propofol produced greater reductions in CMR for oxygen than did thiopental [3]. A prospective, randomized trial demonstrated that at levels of anesthesia corresponding to a bispectral index (BIS) of 35, TIVA with propofol and remifentanil preserved autoregulation and blood flow–metabolism coupling, while sevoflurane decoupled blood flow and metabolism. High CO_2 concentrations impaired cerebral autoregulation in the sevoflurane group but not in the TIVA group [4]. Together, remifentanil and propofol dose dependently reduced CBF but preserved cerebrovascular autoregulation [5].

The reduction in CBF induced by propofol has been associated with a decrease in cerebral oxygen saturation in specific circumstances. For example, if a patient receiving propofol is hyperventilated, regional hypoperfusion may occur in areas of hypoxic brain tissue [6]. Positron emission tomography (PET) studies in humans demonstrated that propofol-mediated metabolic suppression might exhibit regional differences. Regional CBF (rCBF) PET in healthy human volunteers demonstrated that propofol caused global dose-related decreases in CBF that were exaggerated in the thalamus, basal forebrain, posterior cingulate, and occipital cortices [7]. Indeed, functional imaging suggests that alterations in regional blood to the thalamus may be central to propofol-mediated unconsciousness [8]. In theory, regional alterations in CBF–metabolism coupling could cause susceptible areas of the brain to become hypoxic. These findings are likely of clinical relevance only in small subgroups of patients with susceptibility due to underlying neuropathology. In most circumstances, the numerous clinical benefits of propofol will outweigh this theoretical risk.

Etomidate has similar effects on ICP and CBF, has minimal effects on hemodynamics, and is not a significant respiratory depressant. A dose of 0.2 mg/kg significantly decreases ICP [9]. In dogs, etomidate reduced EEG activity and CMR in a dose-dependent fashion. The CMR reaches a minimum when the EEG becomes isoelectric, indicating that cellular homeostasis is the only energy-requiring process. The minimum CBF was achieved before the minimum metabolic rate for oxygen, and the proposed mechanism is cerebral vasoconstriction. Despite this characteristic, however, there were no signs of cerebral ischemia after etomidate administration [10].

The choice of a sedative-hypnotic in a particular patient for a neurosurgical procedure is determined by the clinical situation. Current understanding of pharmacodynamic differences between individual agents suggests that for many patients the use of a specific agent is unlikely to have a profound clinical impact except in very unique circumstances. Primary considerations in the selection of suitable intravenous agent are highlighted in Table 7.1.

Table 7.1 **CRITICAL ASPECTS OF PRE-OPERATIVE ASSESSMENT FOR CRANIOTOMY**

1. Surgical plan regarding neurologic intraoperative monitoring (NIOM)

2. Need for rapid emergence versus continued postoperative sedation

3. Intracranial compliance and intracranial pressure

4. Presence of traumatic brain injury

5. Seizure risk

6. Coexisting metabolic derangements (e.g., acidosis)

7. Cardiovascular/hemodynamic condition

8. Perceived risk of intraoperative cerebral ischemia

In most circumstances, these individual factors will help to guide the selection of a particular agent or combination of agents. Properties of the individual drugs that inform this selection are discussed in depth in the following sections.

INDIVIDUAL AGENTS: OVERVIEW AND PRACTICAL CONSIDERATIONS IN NEUROANESTHESIA

PROPOFOL (2,6-DIISOPROPYLPHENOL)

Propofol's current formulation uses an emulsion of soybean oil, egg phospholipid, glycerol, and propofol in water. Its introduction eliminated most of the disadvantages of prior intravenous anesthetics because its short duration of action and side effect profile allowed a rapid emergence with little "hangover." Propofol provides all of the components of general anesthesia except analgesia, but very high effect-site concentrations are needed to achieve surgical immobility if it is used as the sole anesthetic agent. Propofol is therefore most commonly used in combination with opioids, volatile agents, or other adjunctive anesthetics.

Propofol is a GABAergic drug that increases channel conductance, prolonging inhibitory postsynaptic currents mediated by γ-aminobutyric acid A (GABA$_A$) [11]. Propofol also blocks the N-methyl-D-aspartate (NMDA) receptor and calcium influx through slow calcium ion channels and modulates nitric oxide metabolism [12]. Unlike other hypnotic agents, it reduces postoperative nausea and vomiting (1) and also has some immunomodulatory activity that results in decreased inflammation [13]. A standard three-compartment model is used to describe the pharmacokinetics of propofol, although it does not account for all of the observed behavior. After a single IV bolus, propofol rapidly equilibrates with the effect site and reaches peak effect-site concentration within 2 minutes. It is extensively bound to plasma proteins and may undergo first-pass extraction in the lungs. Redistribution to inactive tissues (e.g., muscle and fat) produces a rapid fall in plasma concentration and prompt return of consciousness. Propofol also has a high metabolic clearance. It is metabolized by hepatic conjugation to inactive glucuronide metabolites, which are excreted through the kidneys. Multiple cytochrome enzymes are involved in propofol metabolism, including cytochrome P450 CYP2B6, CYP2C9, CYP2A6, CYP3C8, CYP2C18, CYP2C19, and CYP1A2. Thus, there are few drug interactions and limited interindividual variability in propofol metabolism between patients.

Because it accumulates in peripheral compartments, the context-sensitive half-time of propofol increases during prolonged infusion. For example, after a 10-day infusion, the half-time of propofol is 1 to 3 days, but for procedures of modest duration (less than 12 hours), the half-time rarely exceeds 1 hour. The time required for return to consciousness depends not only on the context-sensitive half-time but also on the effect-site concentration relative to the level at which return of consciousness will occur. If this ratio is high (i.e., the effect-site concentration needs to drop by greater than 30% for wake-up) dose reductions should be considered during protracted (hours to days) infusions of propofol [13]. After shorter infusions, the context sensitive half-time of propofol increases only slightly because of the large volume of distribution and rapid clearance. Adding an opioid permits the use of lower steady-state propofol concentrations and decreases the impact of the increasing context-sensitive half-time. Age also affects the ideal propofol dose. A smaller induction dose is needed in elderly patients and the drug should be administered slowly to account for a smaller plasma volume and potentially greater patient sensitivity. In contrast, children have a larger plasma volume and increased propofol metabolism and need a higher ideal induction dose [14].

There are growing examples of differences in propofol dose-responsiveness between genetically diverse patient populations [15]. Increasing doses of propofol produce a continuum of EEG changes starting with an increase in high frequency activity and then transitioning to mid- and then low-frequency activity. The process through which these effects occur is slowly being revealed. Propofol changes the topology and efficiency of networked interactions between frontal and parietal brain regions with a more profound effect on parietal EEG signals compared with frontal EEG. Intriguingly, the effects of propofol on EEG network connections, particularly during emergence, displayed a significant difference between two groups within the study population. The difference contributed to a longer time to return of consciousness in one group [16].

Burst suppression is seen during very deep anesthesia [17, 18]. Propofol has a significant depressant dose-dependent effect on bispectral analysis (BIS). The BIS nears 0 with propofol concentrations above 10 mg/L, which is associated with burst suppression [14]. Recent investigations using novel analytical methods (cortical electrorhythmogenesis), have attempted to discriminate the analgesic and hypnotic effects of propofol-remifentanil combinations on the EEG. In brief, remifentanil (opioids) suppresses input to the thalamus, while propofol (hypnotic) suppresses cortical responsiveness to thalamic input. As discussed in the opioid chapter, EEG mainly detects activity in the cortex, so a synergistic effect between propofol and remifentanil may be underestimated by current processed EEG algorithms (i.e., a higher reading despite deep anesthesia); but newer techniques hold promise in this regard [19].

Fospropofol is a new prodrug analog of propofol that was recently approved in the United States [20]. Phosphorylation of the hydroxyl group of propofol results in an ionized compound that is highly water soluble. This eliminates the need for a complex lipid emulsion used in commercial preparations of propofol. It is the lipid emulsion that is believed to be the cause of a number of side effects including anaphylaxis, pain on injection, and bacterial contamination. However, the phosphoryl group must be hydrolyzed for pharmacologic activity. This increases the amount of time between administration of the drug and its observed effect. There does not currently appear to be any strong clinical reason to use fospropofol in neurosurgical patients except perhaps in pediatric patients who may be less tolerant of pain.

Applications in Neuroanesthesia

Propofol has many characteristics that make it a useful anesthetic for neurosurgical patients. It generally reduces CBV leading to improved surgical exposure in the "tight brain" and reduced ICP in patients with reduced intracranial compliance. Rapid clearance with few residual effects enhances the likelihood of obtaining a rapid postoperative neurologic assessment. Propofol also reduces the risk of postoperative nausea and vomiting, which is undesirable in neurosurgical patients in part because it can be a symptom of neurologic deterioration and can increase ICP.

Propofol is not known to induce seizures and is generally considered to be an anticonvulsant. Although some studies suggest that propofol may have antiepileptic and proconvulsive properties, propofol generally acts as an anticonvulsant [21–23]. However, TIVA with propofol has, on rare occasions, been associated with seizure activity. Seizure-like activity observed with propofol may include convulsions or myoclonus and often occurs during times when propofol concentrations are changing such as induction or emergence. Such changes in propofol concentration may result in an imbalance in cerebral neurotransmitters such that excitatory pathways predominate. The clinical significance of these effects is unclear [6].

Brain "relaxation" limits surgical compression and focal brain ischemia. In a prospective, randomized trial of patients with brain tumors undergoing craniotomy, propofol administration resulted in lower ICP, less cerebral edema, and higher mean arterial pressure (MAP) and CPP compared with patients anesthetized with sevoflurane or isoflurane. Operating conditions were also improved with propofol compared with the volatile anesthetics [24]. Propofol similarly reduces CMR and regional CBF. Thus, it does not interfere with the metabolic–blood flow coupling as do volatile agents. However, propofol combined with hyperventilation may induce ischemia due to low CBF and pressure. Thus, hyperventilation should be used with caution for the adjuvant treatment of refractory ICP elevations when combined with propofol [25]. The use of propofol for sedation of spontaneously ventilating patients with intracranial tumors did not increase ICP compared with nonsedated patients [26]. Changes in CBV may cause the brain to shift, making stereotactic-guided craniotomies less accurate. Intraoperative imaging may be used to circumvent this problem.

Propofol may confer additional benefits in the management of patients with evolving neurologic injury and brain tissue at risk. In patients having a stroke, free radical production occurs during reperfusion after the initial ischemic event. Propofol is a free radical scavenger that may promote mitochondrial membrane stability during oxidative stress. In an animal model of traumatic brain injury, propofol decreased markers of oxidative stress [27]. Propofol also decreases lipid peroxidation, reduces the rate of oxygen consumption, and inhibits cellular oxidative damage [28]. Propofol exerts a complex modulation of nitric oxide pathways by increasing constitutive production and reducing inducible nitric oxide [29]. The downstream clinical effects will be dependent on the relative importance of each in a given physiologic state.

Propofol is highly compatible with neurophysiologic monitoring. Propofol has less of an effect on electrophysiologic monitoring than do volatile anesthetic agents [6]. Propofol is also synergistic with opioids, allowing a dramatic reduction in the doses needed to blunt the responses to painful stimuli. Moreover, propofol-opioid TIVA techniques preserve cerebral autoregulation at a wide range of doses [30]. Propofol has also been used successfully for provocative testing (Wada test) of patients for planned resection or embolization of AVM near eloquent brain areas [31, 32]. This is another area in which propofol has largely supplanted the previous use of barbiturates.

Concerns in Neuroanesthesia

Side effects of propofol include hypotension, decreased CPP, respiratory depression, propofol infusion syndrome, and delayed emergence after prolonged use.

Hypotension

Maintaining cardiovascular stability and an adequate CPP (between 60 and 70 mm Hg in most patients) is important for adequate oxygen delivery in most patients. Propofol is a myocardial depressant and commonly induces hypotension, especially in hypovolemic patients or those with intrinsic severe cardiac dysfunction. Hypotension due to propofol may be due to decreased sympathetic tone and impaired baroreflexes. Reduced calcium influx into cells induces arterial vasodilation. Reduced cytosolic calcium concentration in myocardial cells decreases inotropy. This effect may become especially clinically significant in elderly patients [14].

Propofol decreases CPP by approximately 10% [6]. Propofol sedation (0.5 mg/kg bolus followed by 50 μg/kg/min) resulted in a 14.3–mm Hg reduction in MAP compared with sedation with remifentanil [26]. Other groups have reported a similar 13% reduction in MAP with propofol sedation [33, 34]. This reduction in MAP resulted in a lower CPP in the propofol group. Administering a vasopressor such as phenylephrine can in most cases prevent propofol-induced hypotension [35, 36].

TIVA with propofol-remifentanil produces a low blood flow state but preserves cerebral autoregulation. Several studies have described a reduction in both cerebral metabolism and regional CBF with propofol [4, 37]. Other studies suggest that propofol decreases CBF more than it suppresses cerebral metabolism. In patients with a brain tumor undergoing a craniotomy, propofol decreased jugular bulb saturation more than that of nitrous oxide and isoflurane [38]. Similarly, propofol, but not isoflurane or sevoflurane, decreased jugular bulb saturation 1 hour after cardiopulmonary bypass [39]. Thus, hypotension induced by propofol may induce cerebral hypoxia. However, another study showed that propofol did not affect jugular venous bulb oxygen saturation in normothermic or hypothermic neurosurgical patients [40]. The effect of this low blood flow state on neurologic outcome, if any, is unclear.

Propofol Infusion Syndrome

Propofol infusion syndrome is primarily observed in patients who are young or those on long infusions in the critical care setting. Components include severe lactic acidosis, rhabdomyolysis, renal failure, cardiac dysrhythmias, and potential cardiovascular collapse. Patients with preexisting mitochondrial metabolic disorders are thought to be at higher risk for propofol infusion syndrome [41]. Additional risk factors for the development of propofol infusion syndrome include the accumulation of very large doses, critical illness, acute neurologic injury, low carbohydrate intake, high fat intake, and the use of vasopressors or steroids [42].

Although propofol infusion syndrome is rare, its development is unpredictable and potentially fatal. Propofol infusion syndrome is more common after prolonged infusion [43–45]. Although it has occurred after infusions of short duration, it is extremely uncommon during the relatively short durations of propofol administered in the operating room. In a retrospective study of 227 head-injured patients, 67 patients were diagnosed with propofol infusion syndrome and 7 patients died as a result (odds ratio 1.93 per unit increase in dose) [46]. The syndrome occurred more frequently in patients who received high cumulative propofol doses (greater than 80 μg/kg/min) for longer than 58 hours.

Delayed Emergence

An anesthetic plan that allows rapid emergence is critical to detect and care for surgical complications. Propofol has a longer context-sensitive half-life compared with other anesthetics such as desflurane, sevoflurane, and remifentanil. However, combining propofol with remifentanil allows lower propofol doses to be used and thus converts propofol to a nearly context-insensitive drug. Studies comparing the emergence time with propofol compared with sevoflurane or isoflurane have mostly failed to detect a clinically significant difference.

Differences in the emergence time between sevoflurane and propofol are generally not large (e.g., 9 versus 11 minutes) [47]. In a study of 103 patients undergoing short neuroradiology procedures, the use of sevoflurane resulted in a more rapid emergence compared with propofol, but the difference was not more than 4 minutes [48]. In one study of neurosurgical patients, there was no difference in emergence time in 50 intracranial surgical patients receiving sevoflurane or propofol [49]. There was no change in recovery and cognitive function in another study that compared propofol-remifentanil and sevoflurane-fentanyl in neurosurgical patients [50]. Propofol, isoflurane, and sevoflurane also produced no difference in emergence time in elderly patients [51]. There was also no difference in recovery times or psychomotor test performance between isoflurane, propofol, or mixed isoflurane-propofol anesthetics in patients undergoing craniotomy for brain tumor [52]. In one prospective randomized controlled study of 121 adult patients undergoing craniotomy for intracranial tumors, propofol-fentanyl resulted in a longer emergence from anesthesia than nitrous oxide-fentanyl [53]. In contrast, other studies have demonstrated a more rapid recovery after TIVA compared with sevoflurane anesthesia. Differences in the recovery times between these studies could be due to protocol design, delayed discontinuation of the anesthetic agent, concomitant opioid administration, or baseline neurologic impairment. The potential prolonged emergence time seen with high-dose propofol infusions can be diminished if the propofol infusion is discontinued and volatile agent is begun after the removal of the intracranial mass, at which time a moderate increase in CBV will have less significance. Alternatively, the infusion rate can be guided in part by processed EEG monitoring. Time of emergence must also be balanced with hemodynamics (e.g., avoidance of hypertension) and bucking (e.g., avoidance of ICP increases).

ETOMIDATE [ETHYL 3-(1-PHENYLETHYL) IMIDAZOLE-4-CARBOXYLATE]

Etomidate is an imidazole-derived short-acting sedative-hypnotic that was introduced in Europe in 1972 and in the United States in 1983. Etomidate produces hypnosis by stimulating $GABA_A$ receptors. Etomidate produces changes in the EEG that are similar to other GABAergic drugs. Processed EEG signals appear to correlate with etomidate plasma levels [54]. Etomidate pharmacology is best described by a two-compartment model and demonstrates rapid effect-site equilibration. Distribution away from the central compartment allows a rapid induction and emergence.

Etomidate is particularly useful due to its low incidence of cardiovascular or respiratory depression. It has been frequently administered to facilitate endotracheal intubation in patients requiring rapid sequence intubation due to the need for a predictable hemodynamic response given the inability to titrate to clinical effect under emergency conditions. Side effects, which include reduced seizure threshold and adrenal suppression, limit its routine use in neuroanesthesia to specific applications involving neurophysiologic monitoring or to single-bolus doses for induction of general anesthesia.

Applications in Neuroanesthesia

Etomidate decreases ICP, CBF, and CMR for oxygen. CPP and the ratio of oxygen delivery to metabolic demand are increased [55]. Cerebrovascular reactivity to carbon dioxide is maintained. The cardiovascular system is much more stable at doses of etomidate used for deep anesthesia and potential brain protection (burst suppression) compared with propofol or barbiturates. Under circumstances where CPP is already marginal etomidate may be an appropriate choice for maintenance of anesthesia when a total intravenous technique is necessary for indications such as transcranial motor evoked potential (TcMEP) monitoring. A typical regimen consists of a continuous infusion in the range of 10 to 25 µg/kg/min after induction with 0.1 to 0.3 mg/kg.

Etomidate does not significantly affect evoked potentials and can be used during electrocorticography for epilepsy surgery to activate seizure foci. It is particularly useful for monitoring of cortical somatosensory evoked potentials (SSEPs) and TcMEPs because it augments the signals. Thus, high doses of etomidate (greater than 20 µg/kg/min) could be used for induced burst suppression while still allowing reproducible neuromonitoring [56]. Both ketamine and etomidate evoke hyperactivity of the motor central nervous system. Evidence of motor hyperactivity induced by etomidate includes brief twitches, mild tremors, and generalized myoclonic-like activity. This could be problematic in the absence of neuromuscular blockade or may contribute to artifactual elevation of the processed EEG value. Due to the significant side effect profile the duration of etomidate infusion should be as short as possible. During intracranial procedures requiring TcMEPs, it is advisable to use etomidate to the critical periods from the raising of the dural flap to completion of the critical resection and to use an alternative regimen during opening and closing. Processed EEG may be useful to monitor depth of anesthesia as well as to detect seizure activity. The long duration of monitoring required for procedures on the spine and the challenge of spine surgery with increased muscle tone as might occur with etomidate limit the use of etomidate infusions to those patients with significant underlying cardiovascular compromise or those in which muscle relaxant is compatible.

Concerns in Neuroanesthesia

Etomidate had a high incidence of side effects when it was used along with fentanyl in 20 patients for outpatient cystoscopy. Venous pain occurred after injection in 68% of patients, 50% had pain or swelling at the injection site, 50% exhibited skeletal movements, 40% exhibited nausea and vomiting, and 25% had emergence psychoses [57]. Myoclonic movements occur in 10% to 70% of the time with etomidate and are reduced by premedication with benzodiazepines or opioids [55]. There is some evidence that etomidate may decrease the seizure threshold, and in some cases, seizure activity has been associated with etomidate infusion [58]. Its use has been suggested to reduce the seizure threshold and increase seizure duration in patients undergoing electroconvulsive (ECT) therapy for depression or schizophrenia [59]. Despite the evidence that etomidate may lower the seizure threshold in some patients, the overall reported incidence of seizures is low. Etomidate also has anticonvulsant activity and has been used to treat refractory status epilepticus. Etomidate should, however, be used with caution in most patients with refractory epilepsy and in patients who have had recent seizures [60].

Etomidate may also inhibit nitric oxide production. In a rodent model of ischemia produced by temporary middle cerebral artery occlusion, ischemic damage was worse in rats under etomidate-induced burst suppression compared with deep halothane anesthesia. This difference was erased by pretreatment with a nitric oxide synthase inhibitor and overcome by treatment with the nitric oxide synthase precursor and substrate L-arginine [61]. This may be of particular relevance in patients with existing cerebral vasospasm from acute injury. A single case report of inadvertent injection of etomidate into the brain parenchyma was associated with worsening vasospasm, and a number of mechanisms, including decreased nitric oxide production and vasoactive effects of the diluent could be involved [62].

Emergence Phenomena

Emergence delirium is characterized by agitation, restlessness, and hyperactivity and may interfere with extubation and postanesthetic neurologic evaluation. Emergence delirium does not fluctuate and lasts for a short amount of time. The incidence of emergence delirium ranges from 3% to 6% after routine general anesthesia [63]. A prospective observational study analyzed the risk factors for inadequate emergence after anesthesia in 1868 adult patients. Of the 1868 patients enrolled in the study, 93 patients exhibited emergence delirium. Induction of anesthesia with etomidate was a significant risk factor for emergence delirium; 12.6% of patients who received etomidate exhibited emergence delirium compared with 3.8% of patients who received propofol and 5.3% of those who received thiopental [64]. The transient postoperative cognitive impairment observed with etomidate may result from the activation of localized GABA receptors by subanesthetic concentrations of the drug. In a mouse study, emergence after deep etomidate anesthesia resulted in a long lasting decrease in theta-peak frequency on the EEG, signifying persistent etomidate activity [65].

It is possible that the ongoing activity of etomidate at these receptor subtypes could also contribute to emergence phenomena [64]. For these reasons, routine use of etomidate for intracranial procedures is not recommended.

Adrenocortical Suppression

As etomidate infusions first started to be used, mortality appeared to increase in critically ill trauma patients [57, 66, 67]. This was thought to be caused by etomidate-induced adrenocortical suppression. Etomidate reversibly inhibits 11β-hydroxylase, which catalyzes the conversion of deoxycortisol to cortisol. Cortisol and aldosterone levels are decreased 30 minutes after a single dose of etomidate, and this effect can persist for up to 24 hours. Adrenocortical suppression is pronounced during prolonged etomidate infusions and is of particular concern in the patient with traumatic brain injury who may require prolonged sedation in the ICU [68].

The effect of etomidate after a single induction dose has been studied in several trials. Healthy patients induced with etomidate for elective surgery exhibited transient adrenocortical suppression, but it is not known if this suppression is clinically significant. The administration of a single dose of etomidate has been linked to a transient adrenal suppression in elective surgery, emergency department, and critically ill patients [69, 70]. Trauma patients who received etomidate for intubation had lower cortisol levels and a decreased response to a cortisol stimulation test than did patients who received midazolam and fentanyl. Patients who received etomidate required a longer ICU stay, had more ventilator-dependent days, had a longer total hospital admission, and required more intravenous fluids/blood products in the first 24 hours than did patients who had received midazolam and fentanyl, despite a similar degree of injury in both groups. Thus, a single etomidate dose in trauma patients resulted in adrenocortical insufficiency that affected clinical outcome [71].

Etomidate blood concentrations after an IV bolus or continuous infusion greatly exceed that needed to inhibit adrenal steroidogenesis. The blood cortisol decrease in response to etomidate was dose dependent. Aldosterone levels are either unchanged or reduced after etomidate. After an etomidate infusion, blood cortisol levels are reduced and an inhibited response to ACTH persists for 8 to 22 hours. After an etomidate infusion of 25.5 µg/kg/min, serum cortisol response to ACTH was completely blocked for 24 hours after the infusion. Cortisol and aldosterone levels were reduced for up to 4 days after the infusion was stopped [72]. Coadministration of steroids with etomidate may decrease the mortality associated with the use of etomidate [72]. However, smaller trials failed to show the same mortality benefit of steroids in patients in septic shock. Steroid administration could be considered in patients who received etomidate and who remain hypotensive after adequate fluid resuscitation and vasopressor administration

[70, 73]. Particular attention should be given to patients at elevated risk for adrenocortical insufficiency, especially if etomidate is given as a continuous infusion.

Propylene Glycol Toxicity

Etomidate is manufactured with a propylene glycol solvent in the United States. This preparation is more likely to cause pain on injection. Venous complications, including phlebitis, thrombosis, and thrombophlebitis, occur frequently (up to 43% of patients) after intravenous etomidate administration [74]. Propylene glycol is generally considered to be nontoxic, but there are reports of propylene glycol toxicity consisting of an increased anion gap metabolic acidosis due to lactic acidosis, hemolysis, hyperosmolality, and acute renal injury resulting in renal failure. A sepsis-like syndrome may also occur. Large intravenous doses of propylene glycol administered over a short time period can be toxic, and this risk is increased by renal and hepatic disease. The liver metabolizes propylene glycol to lactate, acetate, and pyruvate, while 12% to 45% of propylene glycol is excreted in the urine. Propylene glycol has also been associated with renal insufficiency. The mechanism for acute kidney injury includes proximal tubular necrosis. Saturation of proximal tubular secretion of propylene glycol causes renal clearance to decrease at high doses. Chronic alcohol abuse decreases the metabolism of propylene glycol and increases the risk of toxicity [75]. There have been reports of propylene glycol toxicity during prolonged etomidate infusions in a patient with intracerebral hemorrhage [76] and for cerebral protection during resection of a large intracranial AVM [77]. In both of these cases, acidosis resolved on discontinuation of etomidate infusion. Treatment of propylene glycol toxicity may necessitate intermittent dialysis. Prevention includes avoiding large doses of propylene glycol. Appropriate limits to propylene glycol doses include 290 to 2900 mg/h or 6.9 to 69 g/d. In patients with risk factors, the dose should be reduced by 50% [75]. Propylene glycol is easily cleared by dialysis.

KETAMINE [(±)-2-(2-CHLOROPHENYL)-2-(METHYLAMINO)CYCLOHEXANONE]

Ketamine is a dissociative anesthetic that is used primarily in hemodynamically unstable patients. The drug is also used to provide brief periods of sedation and analgesia for procedures (e.g., dressing changes in burn patients) and as an adjunctive analgesic in patients with chronic pain. Ketamine provides hemodynamic stability and minimal respiratory depression while preserving airway reflexes. CO_2 responsiveness of the cerebral vasculature is generally maintained with ketamine. In the neurosurgical population, these pharmacologic features are often overshadowed by concern regarding the side effects of ketamine.

Ketamine interacts with multiple receptors. Its primary anesthetic action is mediated by noncompetitive antagonism of the excitatory, glutaminergic NMDA receptor. Ketamine binds at a site independent of glutamate such that antagonism cannot be overcome by increased neurotransmitter concentrations. Ketamine also binds to the nicotinic cholinergic receptor, opioid receptors, and monoamine receptors such as dopamine D2 and serotonin (5-HT) receptors. Ketamine exists as an enantiomeric mixture of stereoisomers (R, S). Extensive clinical investigation has revealed significant differences in the pharmacologic profile of the individual isomers and the particular clinical utility of the S isomer [78, 79]. (S)-Ketamine is more than twice as potent as the R-enantiomer and exhibits similar pharmacokinetics at onset but with more rapid recovery. The side effect profile may be more limited with (S)-ketamine and several nonhuman studies hint that the neurologic profile, particularly with regard to potential for neuroprotection at the cellular level, may be improved. Enantiomerically pure ketamine is not available for clinical use in the United States

Ketamine can produce hallucinations and altered mental status. Risk factors and dose–response curves for these effects are not well established, nor are there good data to define the dose of GABAergic drugs to mitigate these effects. As a primary agent, ketamine likely increases CMR and CBV as a result of increased synaptic activation. This is of particular concern in a brain-injured patient experiencing neuronal ischemia and in patients with elevated ICP. In awake, healthy patients, low- to moderate-dose ketamine infusion increases heart rate and MAP. A direct, dose-dependent increase in CBF averages approximately 30% at the highest target concentrations (300 ng/mL) but is very modest at lower concentrations (30 ng/mL) [80]. Ketamine is reported to increase ICP in humans [81], but this is based on observational data in a small number of trials in spontaneously breathing patients anesthetized with ketamine who may have become simultaneously hypercarbic. There may be significant regional differences in the effect of ketamine on both cerebral consumption of glucose and local blood flow. As some studies suggest, this may even vary at the microvascular level with disease pathophysiology [82].Given these many variables- it is particularly difficult to extrapolate in vitro animal data to a specific patient population with significant confidence.

More recently, human studies in clinically relevant populations suggest that combining ketamine with other sedative-hypnotic agents and controlled ventilation improves the physiologic profile of ketamine in the neurosurgical population. Alabanese and colleagues have investigated ketamine sedation in the brain-injured patient [83]. In a prospective trial comparing ketamine-midazolam to sufentanil-midazolam for sedation of patients with severe traumatic injury, patients sedated with ketamine demonstrated decreased need for interventions to treat hypotension. There was no statistically significant difference in mean ICP, ICP elevations, or need for additional ICP-lowering therapy between the groups. Arterial carbon dioxide tension in these patients was controlled by mechanical ventilation. Additional studies fail to demonstrate an increase in middle cerebral artery velocity when ketamine is administered in conjunction with midazolam or propofol [84]. There is also data indicating that ketamine (up to 30 μg/kg/min) reduces ICP when added to a methohexital or propofol infusion for ICU sedation in adults and children [85, 86]. Finally, DEX may play a role in limiting the side effect profile of ketamine such that the combination of these drugs is gaining clinical use [87, 88].

A reasonable conclusion from the existing data is that ketamine is not strictly contraindicated in the brain injured or neurosurgical patient if it is not used as the primary agent. The addition of supplemental ketamine to a propofol, benzodiazepine, or DEX infusion, provided appropriate monitoring is in place, may be reasonable in patients with refractory elevations in ICP, complex analgesic needs, concomitant hypotension, or low amplitude evoked potentials. The analgesic effect of the ketamine may also help to reduce hemodynamic instability associated with pain.

NMDA antagonists have been associated with neurologic injury in multiple in vitro studies. The effects may be different on the developing brain (fetus, neonate, pediatrics) versus the adult brain and in the presence or absence of ischemia–reperfusion conditions. However, under certain conditions, ketamine may be neuroprotective. This is discussed in the section on neuroprotection later in this chapter.

Ketamine amplifies evoked potentials and can be an excellent adjunct during TcMEP monitoring for spine surgery [89, 90]. A loading dose of 0.5 to 1.0 mg/kg followed by an infusion of 0.3 mg/kg/h has been recommended for spine surgeries. Ketamine increases high-frequency EEG activity, and in some patients this is reflected as an increase in the processed EEG (qEEG) value despite increased depth of anesthesia [91]. This may complicate interpretation of qEEG during ketamine-based anesthesia.

Ketamine has recently regained popularity for analgesia in patients with acute and chronic pain [92–95]. Studies in a wide variety of settings are equivocal with regard to the efficacy of low-dose ketamine boluses (less than 0.5 mg/kg) or infusions in reducing perioperative pain. The use of ketamine infusions on the floor for analgesia requires careful coordination and adoption of systemwide protocols coordinated by an acute pain service. Many view the risk–benefit ratio of a trial of perioperative ketamine to favor its use in patients with chronic pain or those undergoing invasive spinal surgery but favor avoidance in intracranial procedures. Further studies are necessary to clarify the role of ketamine for the treatment of postcraniotomy pain [96].

BARBITURATES (THIOPENTAL AND PENTOBARBITAL)

Barbiturates are $GABA_A$ agonists that produce hypnosis and amnesia while reducing CMR, CBF, and CBV. Thiopental and pentobarbital are barbiturates with a long established history as effective sedative-hypnotic agents. However, propofol has now largely supplanted barbiturates for use in general anesthesia for neuroanesthesia. Moreover, as of this printing, thiopental is no longer available in the United States.

Barbiturates, especially thiopental, have a significantly increased context-sensitive half-time after a prolonged infusion. Pentobarbital is an active metabolite of thiopental and is partially responsible for increasing its context-sensitive half-time. Residual barbiturates make it difficult to obtain a rapid neurologic examination. For these reasons, barbiturates are no longer routinely used in neuroanesthesia. Their use is currently reserved for three indications: (1) elevated ICP or status epilepticus that is refractory to alternative strategies, (2) induction of deep general anesthesia with burst suppression or isoelectric EEG as part of a brain protection strategy in anticipation of or immediately following cerebral ischemia, and (3) provocative Wada testing.

Several animal studies with thiopental revealed that it provided neuroprotection from ischemia and hypotension, and the use of thiopental has been linked to a reduction in morbidity and mortality in animal studies of ischemia. Barbiturates cause a dose-dependent reduction in CMR along with an associated progressive slowing of the EEG, a reduction in ATP consumption and protection from incomplete cerebral ischemia [97]. The effect on CMR and CBF is coupled and the reduction in metabolic rate is associated with a parallel decrease in CPP and ICP [1]. Pentobarbital depresses the central nervous system as well as cortical and subcortical structures and suppresses EEG responses [11]. The decrease in ICP induced by thiopental is dependent on normal cerebral vasoreactivity [98]. Patients with preserved cerebral vasoreactivity had a decrease in CMR of 28%, accompanied by a decrease in CBF of 29% when treated with a thiopental bolus followed by an infusion. Patients with impaired cerebral vasoreactivity did not exhibit changes in CMR for oxygen, CBF, or ICP. In large doses, however, thiopental may decrease arterial blood pressure, stroke volume, and cardiac output. Its use was associated with the need for increased inotropic and chronotropic support [99].

DEXMEDETOMIDINE [(S)-4-[1-(2,3-DIMETHYLPHENYL) ETHYL]-3H-IMIDAZOLE]

DEX is a novel intravenous adrenoreceptor agonist with a relatively unique clinical profile that has several applications in neuroanesthesia. DEX is similar to clonidine but displays enhanced selectivity (1200:1) for the α_2-receptor subtype of which there are several subtypes [100]. Clinical effects of DEX include sympatholysis (decreased blood pressure, bradycardia), anxiolysis, and "sleep" as opposed to typical hypnosis. The drug also acts as an analgesic and mild antisialogogue. Importantly, when used as a sole agent, DEX produces amnesia in some, but not all, patients [101]. DEX is produces sedation in both intubated and unintubated patients that more closely mimics sleep than any typical sedative-hypnotic or benzodiazepine. DEX is not a complete anesthetic but can be used as an adjunctive agent to reduce the dose of other sedative-hypnotic agents during the maintenance of general anesthesia, to amplify the analgesic effects of opiates or ketamine, to reduce sympathetic activation and smooth emergence, or to provide sedation in the ICU.

The mechanism of action of DEX is widely believed to involve suppression of noradrenergic output, although there is evidence that alternative pathways, such as non-adrenergic alpha receptors, may be important [102]. The locus ceruleus (LC) in the pons is the primary source of noradrenergic projections in the brain. These projections are diverse, and the LC is centrally involved in the modulation of sleep, consciousness, and the transition between the two [103]. Of all sedative-hypnotic agents used in anesthesia, DEX produces a state closest to physiologic sleep in both behavior and neurophysiologic (EEG) phenotype [104]. The advantage of this is that "sleeping" patients can generally be readily aroused for clinical assessment with appropriate stimulation. However, patients sedated with DEX for procedural sedation may be startled by sudden stimulation or ambient noise.

Due primarily to a decrease in plasma concentrations of norepinephrine modest drops in MAP and heart rate (20% to 25%) can be anticipated during DEX infusion. The lower blood pressure and heart rate may persist for 1 to 2 hours after the cessation of the infusion. In the majority of patients, these hemodynamic effects are self-limited. Rare reports document severe bradycardia when a loading dose of DEX is given or with infusion rates greater than 0.7 μg/kg/h. There has been no formal study of the role of prophylactic anticholinergics; however, atropine (0.4 to 1 mg) is reported to be effective in the treatment of hemodynamically significant bradycardia [105]. Chronic β-blockade does not appear to exacerbate this effect and may blunt the chronotropic response to DEX administration [106]. The decrease in sympathetic tone may be used to clinical advantage to reduce tachycardia, hypertension, and responsiveness to the endotracheal tube during emergence. This was specifically studied in patients undergoing elective craniotomy with a balanced opioid/potent agent general anesthetic titrated to BIS scores. Similar to propofol and thiopental, the α_2-agonist clonidine and DEX cause slowing of EEG waveforms and a decrease in the quantitative EEG. Addition of DEX (1 μg/kg load; 0.5 μg/kg/h) resulted in fewer episodes of treatable hypertension, decreased postoperative opioid consumption, and no clinically significant postoperative hypotension [107]. Similar findings regarding emergence hemodynamic stability and utility of DEX to abolish stimulation from Mayfield pin application were reported in separate studies [108, 109].

Although rare, refractory cardiogenic shock after DEX administration in patients with limited cardiac reserve has been reported [110]. DEX can certainly be used safely in the average patient with cardiac disease, but alternative approaches should be considered in the patient with severe reduction in cardiac output related to cardiomyopathy.

DEX is remarkable for its lack of significant respiratory depression. Unlike opioid associated respiratory depression, DEX does not depress the ventilatory response to CO_2 or predispose to central apnea [111, 112]. At clinically useful doses, DEX may produce a small increase in respiratory rate and minute ventilation. In patients receiving DEX for sedation with a natural airway, dynamic airway obstruction can occur in susceptible patients while in healthy patients airway caliber is minimally affected [113]. DEX is most closely associated with stage 2 sleep, while apnea from OSA typically manifests during REM sleep. Therefore, obstruction is primarily associated with the concomitant use of other sedative agents such as benzodiazepines, which may be used to increase the likelihood of amnesia during DEX sedation.

α_2-Adrenoreceptor agonists are reported to inhibit insulin secretion, but the magnitude of this effect and its clinical relevance is not well defined. However, the neuroendocrine stress response during surgery or brain injury and the common concomitant use of perioperative steroids predispose the neurosurgical patient to dysregulation of glucose control. Because hyperglycemia has been associated with worsened neurologic outcome in numerous clinical studies, this should be kept in mind when using DEX in certain subsets (i.e., traumatic brain injury, subarachnoid hemorrhage) of neurosurgical patients.

Applications in Neuroanesthesia:

DEX is ideally suited to procedures simultaneously requiring sedation and cooperation in which inadvertent respiratory depression would present a significant management issue. The "awake" craniotomy and carotid endarterectomy are typical procedures for which the unique pharmacologic profile of DEX is of benefit. DEX is also useful for procedures during which there is limited access to the airway (e.g., prone vertebroplasty). DEX is also useful for sedation of intubated patients in the neuro ICU in whom reliable, serial neurologic examination are planned despite the ongoing need for sedation to tolerate ventilation or to treat refractory elevations in ICP. Finally, DEX has a role as an adjunctive anesthetic agent to reduce the dose of other drugs (e.g., inhaled potent agents or propofol) that may alter evoked potential signals during neurophysiologic monitoring.

DEX can provide analgesia via modulation of pain signaling by receptors in the dorsal horn of the spinal cord, but the effect is not sufficient to use this agent as a primary analgesic. DEX appears to enhance the analgesia derived from opioid analgesics. DEX may be an excellent choice to supplement analgesia in patients on chronic opioid therapy undergoing complex spine procedures using neurophysiologic monitoring. The utility of agents such as DEX to diminish the risk of hyperalgesia that may occur with high-dose infusions of ultrapotent opioids is unknown but may be an area for active future investigation.

DEX is not a "magic bullet." but is a versatile agent [87, 114]. However, significant advantages of DEX include compatibility with evoked potential monitoring, modulation of sympathetic activation during emergence and extubation, adjuvant analgesia without respiratory depression, and MAC-sparing qualities. DEX should be used with caution in patients with significant cardiac dysfunction or intrinsic cardiac conduction pathology or patients who are fundamentally dependent on high sympathetic tone to maintain cardiac output. If a loading dose of DEX is administered, transient hypertension is possible in some patients due to peripheral vasoconstriction mediated by α_{2B}-receptors on the vasculature that is observed at higher plasma levels [115]. Infusions of DEX longer than 1 hour result in an increase in the context-sensitive half-time. The clinical relevance of this is only significant when at least a 50% drop in plasma concentration is intended in close proximity to the end of surgery [116]. Otherwise, plasma concentrations can remain at clinically relevant levels for hours after an infusion, and this may be beneficial for analgesia and sympatholysis [117]. This should be considered when monitoring patients in the postoperative period. Thus, routine sedation with DEX for cases such as neurointerventional diagnostics (angiogram, etc.) may not be optimal in a high throughput clinical setting as PACU discharge may be delayed while awaiting patient recovery to baseline values.

Studies of cerebral physiology under DEX infusion to three clinically relevant target plasma levels (0.6, 1.2, and 1.6 ng/mL) in normal human subjects demonstrate the safety of DEX. The data exhibit (1) preservation of CBF/CMR ratio (i.e., proportional decrease in both with DEX sedation, (2) an appropriate increase in CBF during arousal from DEX-induced sleep, and (3) a decrease in the middle cerebral blood velocity responsiveness to CO_2 challenge [118]. A limited, retrospective analysis of patients with cerebrovascular injury receiving DEX infusion showed no evidence of DEX-mediated cerebral vasoconstriction. Patients in this study had stable brain oxygen levels in proximity to the compromised tissue [119]. The effect of DEX on cerebral autoregulation is not clear and needs further study, although it seems to have no effect on static (slow component) cerebral autoregulation in healthy volunteers. However, it may impair dynamic (fast component) autoregulation by delaying the restoration of CBF velocity to normal with a reduction in blood pressure [120].

A typical dosing regimen for DEX involves a loading dose followed by steady state infusion. The recommended loading dose varies from 0.5 to 1 μg/kg over 5 to 10 minutes, with more rapid administration causing hypertension. The loading dose can be avoided unless rapid effect-site levels must be obtained such as for immediate sedation for airway management or block placement for awake craniotomy. Avoidance of the loading dose may reduce the delayed and potentially significant hypotension seen with the higher concentrations of drug achieved with rapid loading. When used for sedation, the slow bolus infusion can be titrated to the pharmacodynamic end point of maintained eye closure and then stopped and a continuous infusion initiated. In the experience of the authors, a typical infusion rate of 0.3 to 0.5 μg/kg/h is adequate when used as an adjunct to general anesthesia and the typical range is 0.3 to 0.8 μg/kg/h when used for sedation.

INTRAVENOUS AGENTS AND EVOKED POTENTIAL MONITORING

All anesthetic agents affect evoked potentials. The type of monitoring, the baseline neurologic and physiologic status of the patient, and the effects of a given anesthetic technique on evoked potentials guide the selection of a specific agent. In general, intravenous agents are more compatible with monitoring modalities than inhaled potent agents. This is particularly true in patients with marginal presurgical baseline signals.

In general, longer neurologic pathways with multiple synapses are more affected by anesthetic agents due to depression of neural synaptic activity. Thus, cortical SSEPs or TcMEPs that depend on multiple synapses are more sensitive to anesthetic agents. Anesthetics have a strong inhibitory effect on the synapse of motor neurons in the anterior horn of the spinal cord, but most agents, except for neuromuscular blocking agents, have a minimal effect on motor signals at the neuromuscular junction (i.e., EMG). Anesthetic agents have a significant impact on visual evoked potentials but little effect on brainstem auditory evoked potentials [121].

SOMATOSENSORY EVOKED POTENTIALS (SSEPS)

Barbiturates increase the latency and decrease the amplitude of cortical SSEPs. An induction dose of thiopental (5 mg/kg) increases latency by 10% to 20% and decreases amplitude by 20% to 30% for less than 10 minutes [121]. Propofol has a similar effect on SSEPs. Propofol decreases the amplitude of cortical SSEPs, but there is a rapid recovery after the infusion is terminated. Propofol interferes with SSEP signals less than does isoflurane [122]. In addition, the combination of propofol with opioids interferes less with SSEP amplitude than does nitrous oxide or midazolam [123]. The combination of propofol and remifentanil allows consistent SSEP monitoring and is therefore a favored anesthetic choice. Ketamine also increases cortical SSEP amplitude but has no effect on cortical latency or subcortical signals. DEX affects SSEP amplitude minimally and blunts isoflurane's effect on SSEP amplitude [124]. Opioids produce a small decrease in amplitude and increase in latency in cortical signals that are not typically of clinical significance. Remifentanil has a minimal effect on SSEP amplitude and thus it is an excellent opioid choice for SSEP monitoring.

Etomidate increases cortical SSEP amplitude but does not affect subcortical SSEPs; this effect is related to myoclonus and increased cortical excitability. Etomidate infusion enhances SSEP signals and is especially useful in patients with preexisting neurologic deficits and weak SSEPs. Administration of an etomidate bolus of 0.1 to 0.3 mg/kg followed by an infusion of 10 to 30 µg/kg/min can be used to augment SSEP signals. There may be concern that etomidate could interfere with the detection of early warning signs of CNS hypoxia, which causes the amplitude of the SSEPs to transiently increase. However, etomidate has not been shown to mask spinal cord injury when used during SSEP monitoring [124].

Etomidate boluses or continuous infusions augment the amplitude of early cortical SSEPs and can be helpful particularly when the cortical signals are small. Etomidate allows reliable monitoring of SSEPs and auditory evoked potentials and has little or no effect on cervical and subcortical potentials [125]. The aforementioned side effects and limitations of etomidate infusions should be considered.

MOTOR EVOKED POTENTIALS

TcMEP monitoring is performed during spine and intracranial procedures to decrease the risk injury to the descending motor pathways. TcMEPs monitor the integrity of the spinal cord supplied by the anterior spinal artery (mainly the corticospinal tract) as well as the subcortical motor pathways through the internal capsule and cerebral peduncle. Ligation of this artery would not affect the dorsal columns; SSEPs could, therefore, miss potential injury caused by damage to the anterior spinal artery. TcMEPS are very sensitive to anesthetic agents [126].

Opioids, propofol, and thiopental all suppress myogenic but not neurogenic MEPs in a dose-dependent fashion. Neurogenic MEPs (e.g., D-waves) are difficult to monitor as they require placement of epidural electrodes and so are not commonly used except in intramedullary spinal cord surgery when other potentials may be reduced by the nature of the surgery and disease process. Propofol, methohexital, and thiopental were all shown to impair magnetic TcMEP monitoring, but intraoperative monitoring used needle electrodes less vulnerable to anesthetic-induced depression. Thiopental transiently depresses the amplitude and increases the latency of TcMEPs [121]. Increasing doses of propofol progressively depress TcMEP amplitude but have no effect on MEP latency. DEX acts as an adjunct to other anesthetic agents, and its use may decrease the amount of

propofol required to maintain general anesthesia, potentially improving MEP monitoring. Successful TcMEP monitoring is dependent on a consistent baseline and is easiest to interpret when the anesthetic doses are not altered rapidly during monitoring through bolusing [126]. All changes in anesthetic regimen should be promptly communication to the monitoring team.

Monitoring MEPs in patients with abnormal preoperative motor function is more difficult due to a reduction in amplitude [113]. However, the majority of patients with abnormal preoperative motor function due to spinal cord injury successfully underwent TcMEP monitoring in one study with propofol as the only anesthetic [127]. Compared with volatile anesthetics, propofol has less of an effect on motor evoked potentials, median nerve SSEPs, and mid-latency auditory evoked potentials [6]. Propofol combined with opioids (especially remifentanil) has been used successfully for monitoring cortical SSEPs and epidural MEPs. Poor baseline potentials or the need for high current to generate adequate potentials during surgery should provoke consideration to reduced propofol dose, conversion to etomidate infusion, or addition of other adjuncts such as ketamine.

Opioids have little effect on TcMEP monitoring. Opioids produce only a minimal decrease in amplitude or increase in latency of myogenic MEPs. An anesthetic technique that includes high-dose opioids is therefore often preferred when monitoring myogenic TcMEPs. Fentanyl may improve muscle recordings by decreasing the background interference created by spontaneous muscle contractions. Remifentanil exerted the least suppressive effects and, when added to propofol, improves the quality of evoked potentials [128].

Ketamine enhances cortical MEP and SSEP signals. A ketamine loading dose of 0.5 to 1.0 mg/kg followed by an infusion of 0.3 mg/kg/h is recommended [90]; the effects of ketamine on subcortical and peripheral SSEPs and myogenic MEPs are minimal. Thus, ketamine may be useful when monitoring responses that are susceptible to other anesthetic agents. However, it is generally avoided in patients with cranial pathology due to the potential for increase in ICP and psychological effects such as hallucinations that could interfere with the postoperative neurologic examination.

Mahmoud et al. [129] studied the effect of target-controlled DEX and propofol infusion on the amplitude of motor evoked potentials (TcMEPs) in 40 pediatric patients undergoing posterior spinal fusion. DEX produced a dose-dependent reduction in MEP amplitude that was most pronounced (greater than 50% reduction) at plasma levels of 0.6 ng/mL or greater. The effect of DEX on these potentials was independent of propofol (high/low) dose. SSEP signals were unaffected by the DEX infusion. They concluded that low doses of DEX (plasma levels of 0.4 ng/mL) should have minimal effect on TcMEP amplitude. If amplitude is decreased, the signals generally return to at least 70% of baseline within 1 hour after cessation of the DEX infusion. Other studies have consistently demonstrated that DEX does not impair SSEP potentials. Results from those studies are equivocal regarding the effect on TcMEP. Studies of TcMEP under different anesthetic regimens can be profoundly influenced by (1) stimulation protocol, (2) baseline patient clinical variables including neurologic impairment, and (3) intrinsic trial-to-trial variability in MEP signals.

In the authors' clinical practice, propofol with remifentanil and low-dose DEX infusion (0.4 µg/kg/h with no load) reliably produces adequate anesthesia for monitoring of TcMEP in patients with relatively normal baseline function. An alternative approach uses an etomidate infusion for patients undergoing craniotomy with TcMEP monitoring. A ketamine infusion is preferable for spinal procedures. When etomidate is used, anesthesia is induced and maintained with propofol and opioid until incision. Propofol is discontinued and etomidate is started at the onset of bone drilling. An etomidate bolus of 0.2 mg/kg is followed by an infusion of 20 µg/kg/min, titrated to a minimum of 10 µg/kg/min depending on indicators of anesthetic depth (qEEG, blood pressure, heart rate). Etomidate is discontinued when motor mapping is finished. At this point, less than 0.5 MAC of a potent volatile anesthetic is started along with a neuromuscular blocking agent to allow for a rapid emergence.

BRAINSTEM AUDITORY EVOKED POTENTIALS

Intravenous anesthetics have little effect on brainstem auditory evoked potentials (BAEPs). Opioids, barbiturates, etomidate, and ketamine do not affect BAEPs and propofol has a minimal effect. Induction doses of barbiturates, propofol, and etomidate cause complete suppression of mid-latency auditory evoked potential (MLAEP) potentials. Maintenance with propofol at 3 to 5 mg/kg/h caused MLAEP latency prolongation and amplitude reduction. Midazolam and ketamine do not affect MLAEP waveforms. Opioids produce only partial suppression of MLAEP.

NEUROPROTECTION: AN ONGOING CONTROVERSY

The role of pharmacologic suppression of brain metabolic activity as a mode of brain protection during ischemia remains highly controversial despite an appealing theoretical explanation and a body of literature derived from experiments in the laboratory. Most recently, attention has focused on complementary mechanisms such as antioxidant activity, modulation of other signaling pathways including adenosine, NMDA, and calcium signaling. The

broader topic of anesthetic agent mediated neuroprotection and the specific issue of barbiturate for the control of ICP have recently been reviewed [130]. Many agents may provide some degree of neuroprotection in different studies (mostly in rodents or in vitro) under varying conditions, but there is a paucity of human clinical data to guide anesthetic selection in neurologically vulnerable patients. This puts the practitioner in the position of selecting agents that are most compatible with the clinical situation and the patient's comorbidities.

Intravenous anesthetic agents like propofol and barbiturates enhance $GABA_A$-mediated inhibitory pathways, which reduce excitotoxicity [6]. A vast amount of research has been done on the neuroprotective properties of barbiturates [131]. The mechanism by which barbiturates provide neuroprotection has been thought to be due to reduced cerebral metabolism, but barbiturates also reduce brain temperature (due to decreased CMR and CBF) and thus could induce hypothermia-related neuroprotection [41]. In general, the clinical use of barbiturates is in rapid decline, there are confounders such as inadequate control for temperature, and these data are in many ways no longer applicable to present clinical practice. Limited data from comparative studies in humans exist but suggest that when using barbiturates to treat refractory ICP, thiopental is preferred to pentobarbital [132]. There is less work done on the potential neuroprotective effects of propofol. There are several animal studies but only a few human clinical studies that demonstrate a neuroprotective effect of propofol [41, 133]. The effect of propofol on CBF, CMR, ICP, EEG, and free radical scavenging activity is similar to barbiturates and thus it is thought that propofol may have neuroprotective potential. Propofol is also desirable because of its shorter context-sensitive half-life compared with that of barbiturates. Propofol also has some beneficial effect in focal and global ischemia in animal models [134, 135]. When propofol was initiated within 2 hours of an induced infarction and infused for an additional 3 hours, it initially reduced infarct volume and lead to functional improvement after 14 to 21 days in treated animals. However, the infarct size was unchanged when analyzed at 21 days [136]. The benefits of propofol as an anesthetic for its neuroprotective effects are theoretical at best. High propofol doses, such as those used to achieve burst suppression, may cause potential side effects such as hypotension and reduced CPP. Although it is occasionally used to induce burst suppression (i.e., minimal synaptic brain activity) during temporary intracerebral artery occlusion, the clinical benefit of this approach is unsubstantiated. In humans, there are no data on the optimal dose of propofol to achieve neuroprotection or to guide potential clinical use [137]. Animal studies of cerebral ischemia with propofol titrated to burst suppression are inconclusive, and there are some reports in which it fails to protect. In human studies of the effects of propofol infusion titrated to burst suppression, there was no effect on neurologic function in patients undergoing cardiac valve surgery [138, 139]. Propofol may be effective in mild ischemic insults, but this effect is not sustained in more severe insults [13].

Although ketamine was once believed to be entirely neurotoxic, it may have some neuroprotective effects that are now under active investigation [140–143]. Indeed, a number of animal studies hint at the possibility of a neuroprotective effect of ketamine by reduction of excitotoxic glutaminergic injury after ischemia, anti-inflammatory actions, or other ill-defined mechanisms. Preliminary data in humans suggest that ketamine may reduce post coronary surgery neurologic deficits [141].

There is some theoretical evidence from animal studies that DEX may be neuroprotective [144]. Some laboratory results suggest that the risk of neuronal death after global ischemia or subarachnoid hemorrhage in brain regions such as the hippocampus is decreased if the ischemic brain is treated with DEX immediately following injury [145, 146]. Finally, a preconditioning effect of DEX on injury related to hypoxemia and decreased glucose supply in rodents has also been demonstrated [147, 148]. In some cases, DEX may be associated with hyperglycemia associated with decreased pancreatic insulin secretion, but this is not typically pronounced. Clinical evidence in humans does not support the routine use of DEX infusion for the specific purpose of neuroprotection. However, use could be considered in specific cases in which intraoperative cerebral ischemia is expected or confirmed as there are few alternative therapies.

In summary, the selection of a particular intravenous anesthetic agent for the purpose of neuroprotection cannot at present be guided by consistent experimental data and therefore use for this purpose should be guided by careful consideration of the relative risk–benefit profile of the intended dosing regimen.

Case I **AWAKE CRANIOTOMY**

A 26-year-old woman presents for removal of an astrocytoma located in Broca's area that presented with seizure. Past medical history is notable for anxiety, morbid obesity, and sleep apnea with no other medical problems. Medications include levetiracetam, dexamethasone, sertraline, and lorazepam. She uses CPAP 10 cm H_2O at night. Polysomnography revealed an AHI index of 25. She is 62 inches tall and weighs 118 kg (body mass index 47.5). The preoperative neurologic examination was normal without any focal neurologic deficits. Functional MRI revealed the location of the lesion was impinging on eloquent cortex involved in the motor production of speech. Preoperative vital signs are heart rate 64 bpm, blood pressure 120/80 mm Hg, and oxygen saturation on room air 100%. Airway examination reveals a short neck, Mallampati class II, with normal mouth opening, subluxation, and

mento-hyoid distance. No other abnormalities are noted on physical examination.

The surgical plan is for awake craniotomy and intraoperative speech mapping. After arrival in the operating room and placement of standard monitors, ondansetron 4 mg was administered intravenously and a remifentanil infusion was begun at 0.05 μg/kg/min after a 0.25 μg/kg bolus. A DEX bolus of 1 μg/kg over 8 minutes was started followed by an infusion of 0.5 μg/kg/hr using an adjusted body weight of 77 kg (dose adjustment is optional). An additional 16 g peripheral IV and a radial arterial line were then placed. The nares were then topicalized with 2% lidocaine-soaked pledgets with added oxymetazoline and then lubricated nasal trumpets (32F) were inserted into each naris. The nasal trumpets were then connected to the anesthesia machine circuit via a double-lumen ETT connector that was subsequently attached to ventilator circuit. Pressure support ventilation of 10 cm H_2O was initiated. Scalp blocks were performed using 0.5% ropivacaine with epinephrine (1:200,000). Remifentanil was adjusted to 0.08 μg/kg/min for supplemental analgesia during scalp blocks. After the scalp blocks were performed, propofol was started at 40 μg/kg/min and local anesthetic injected at the pinning sites by the surgeon. At this point, Mayfield pinning was performed. During pinning, the patient experienced some pain, which was treated with a small propofol bolus (20 mg), the propofol was adjusted to 50 μg/kg/min and the remifentanil infusion was adjusted to 0.1 μg/kg/min. The patient was positioned such that visual access was maintained with the patient's face. Prior to incision the patient had a small amount of obstruction, which required an increase in the pressure support to 15 cm H_2O. Once the bone flap was off, all agents were discontinued until the patient was responsive. Once responsive, DEX was restarted at 0.3 μg/kg/hr. Remifentanil 0.06 μg/kg/min was restarted for supplemental analgesia and titrated up to 0.1 μg/kg/min until the patient was comfortable. Once the tumor was excised, propofol was restarted. When the pins were removed, all agents were discontinued and fentanyl titrated for pain management. This protocol allowed adequate motor and speech mapping and the tumor was successfully removed without any postoperative neurologic deficits.

DISCUSSION

The patient's cooperation may be necessary during neurosurgery when lesions are located close to functional areas of the brain, including vision, language, and motor areas. These cases require a sufficient anesthesia depth during opening and closure and full consciousness during functional testing. They also require a smooth transition between unconsciousness and consciousness, adequate ventilation, immobility, and comfort throughout the procedure. When propofol infusion is combined with remifentanil and DEX, patients usually wake up within 5 to 15 minutes after stopping the propofol infusion. Propofol is a good agent for awake craniotomy because it is easily titratable, allows rapid recovery without confusion and has antiemetic properties [149].

Types of surgeries in which patient cooperation and responsiveness may be beneficial include craniotomies for electrode implantation, deep brain stimulation for the treatment of Parkinson's disease, and surgical management of epilepsy, tumors, or vascular lesions located close to functional eloquent areas of the brain important for motor, vision, or language. Surgeries involving Broca's and Wernicke's speech areas necessitate verbal contact to be maintained with the patient.

Different techniques have been used during these cases, ranging from alternating asleep-awake-asleep techniques with the use of an LMA or ETT to manage the airway during the asleep portions of the case to continuous sedation with rapidly acting agents in which the patient breaths spontaneously. Nasopharyngeal airways have been used in some centers in these cases. Total intravenous anesthesia is favored due to rapid titration, faster awakening, less interference with monitoring, and decreased tendency for coughing and other deleterious emergence effects. Sedation with propofol and narcotics leads to a high incidence of respiratory depression, which frequently results in the need for placement of a supraglottic airway. Without topicalization, the intraoperative placement of airway devices can precipitate coughing that is dangerous while the head is fixed in Mayfield pins and the cranium is open. The use of propofol-remifentanil had demonstrated fewer respiratory issues compared with the use of propofol-fentanyl [150]. Remifentanil is the most appropriate narcotic used during awake craniotomy because its levels can be rapidly changed. Significant respiratory depression can occur but this is much less likely when remifentanil levels are titrated slowly [151]. However, hypercarbia and brain swelling will always be of concern when opioids are used. DEX is a highly specific α_2-receptor agonist that produces sedation, anxiolysis, and analgesia without respiratory depression. It has an anesthetic-sparing effect and allows patients to be awakened easily by verbal stimulation. BIS decreases during DEX infusion but returns to baseline values when patients are simulated. It produces a dose-dependent bradycardia and hypotension [150]. Typically, a loading dose is given (0.5 to 1.0 μg/kg) slowly to avoid significant hypertension. A continuous infusion of 0.5 to 1.0 μg/kg/h usually results in adequate anxiolysis. DEX produces unreliable amnesia.

The preemptive placement of bilateral nasal airways will in most cases prevent substantial obstruction, thereby preserving a conduit for ventilation, oxygenation, and continuous capnometry. In the case of patients with significant obstructive sleep apnea in whom tongue base rather than soft palate obstruction may occur, the trumpets allow a means for delivery of noninvasive positive pressure airway support. Positive inspiratory and expiratory pressure has been applied through bilateral cannulation of the nares during the asleep phases of the craniotomy and can successfully improve ventilation in patients with obstructive sleep apnea [122]. Nerve blocks of the scalp are performed and include six nerves on each side [152]. Generally, 2 to 3 mL of local anesthetic (ropivacaine or bupivacaine 0.5% with epinephrine) is deposited at each of the auriculotemporal, zygomaticotemporal, supraorbital, supratrochlear, and lesser occipital and greater occipital nerves. Long-acting local anesthetics are preferred. Because the scalp is highly vascular, ropivacaine and levobupivacaine are preferred over bupivacaine due to their lower cardio/neurotoxicity. Epinephrine is added to minimize acute rises in plasma concentration and maximize the block duration [153]. In some patients, intravenous esmolol or metoprolol may be considered to blunt a significant chronotropic response to the catecholamines. Potential complications of awake craniotomies include upper airway obstruction, respiratory depression, cerebral edema, nausea and vomiting, seizures, decreased consciousness, neurologic deficit, and loss of patient's cooperation. One study of 178 patients found a 16% overall complication rate [149]. The challenges are increased in the patient with sleep apnea, obesity, and a difficult airway. DEX is an excellent option in such patients as the risk of significant respiratory depression is minimal and cooperative sedation is reliable. In the clinical experience of the authors, DEX use allows the dose of remifentanil to be substantially reduced, thereby lessening the risk of respiratory depression that results in both hypoxia and hypercarbia with deleterious brain swelling. Airway obstruction can still occur, especially when DEX is combined with propofol or midazolam.

Case II SPINAL FUSION, NEUROMONITORING, TIVA

The patient is a 60-year-old man with a history of severe spinal stenosis who presents for C8-T2 spinal fusion in the prone position. The surgical team plans to use SSEP and TcMEP monitoring throughout the case. The patient has a history of hypertension well controlled on a calcium channel blocking agent and diabetes mellitus on oral medications. He takes oral Percocet intermittently and gabapentin daily for chronic leg pain. His baseline visual analog pain score on analgesic medications is 5/10. He has no known drug allergies and underwent uneventful general anesthesia for cholecystectomy 3 years earlier. Physical examination reveals a well-nourished, nonsmoking man (American Society of Anesthesiologists [ASA] II, 5 ft 6 in, 275 lb, body mass index 44.4, blood pressure 140/85, heart rate 82, respirations 14, oxygen saturation 99% on room air) with a Mallampati II airway, a Maryland bridge at tooth 8, a normal cardiopulmonary examination, and intact neurologic examination except for significant bilateral leg weakness (3/5). ECG reveals normal sinus rhythm and a stress-echocardiogram

3 months prior demonstrated normal ventricular function, no ischemia, and no hemodynamically significant valvular disease. Labs show hemoglobin 11 g/dL and creatinine 1.2 ml/dL and are otherwise within normal limits.

The patient is consented for general anesthesia with invasive arterial monitoring. In addition, the risks of perioperative vision loss and dislodgement of the Maryland bridge are explicitly discussed. Two milligrams of midazolam are administered, availability of an active type and screen is confirmed, and the patient is brought to the operating suite. ASA standard monitors and a processed EEG monitor are placed, and 60 mg of intravenous lidocaine administered, the lungs are denitrogenated and the patient induced with propofol (1000 μg/kg) followed by infusion at 330 μg/kg/min and sufentanil (100 μg) followed by infusion at 0.2 μg/kg/h. Mask ventilation is accomplished with the ventilator set to pressure-cycled ventilation (driving pressure 20 cm H_2O), rate 10, inspiratory:expiratory ratio 1:1) Eight minutes after the start of induction laryngoscopy is performed with a Glidescope (to minimize risk of bridge damage), 4 mL of 4% lidocaine is sprayed on the cords and in the trachea via an atomizer and a unstyletted 8.0 ETT is introduced into the trachea atraumatically. The Maryland bridge is confirmed to be intact. The tube is secured with silk and clear tape, the eyes are lubricated and taped, and a bite-block is placed between the left molar teeth. Propofol infusion is reduced to 80 μg/kg/min. Phenylephrine infusion is initiated to maintain blood pressure within 10% of baseline. Intravenous ketamine (0.5 mg/kg followed by infusion at 0.25 mg/kg/h) is administered with no measureable effect on the processed EEG reading. Two large-bore intravenous catheters are placed along with a left-radial arterial line in-line with a pressurized extension tubing to accommodate proning. A bolus of 10 μg of sufentanil is administered 5 minutes before the head is secured in Mayfield pins, and after an additional bolus of 500 μg/kg of propofol, the patient is positioned prone on a prepadded Jackson table with careful attention to avoidance of pressure on the eyes, nose, and face. The arms are secured at the sides with the palms facing the hips with sheets and towel clips. Rectal acetaminophen suppository (1 g) is placed. Baseline SSEP potentials are intact and show adequate amplitude. TcMEPs are intact but show generally low amplitude in the lower extremities and higher amplitude in the arms. Surgery proceeds uneventfully with 850 mL of blood loss (250 mL of which is returned as cell-saver) and no change in baseline potentials. Propofol infusion during the case is titrated in the range of 70 to 110 μg/kg/min to hemodynamics, response to surgical stimulation, and processed EEG reading (to maintained an average reading of 50. Sufentanil (15 μg) is bolused in response to any patient movement, significant increase in blood pressure and heart rate, or attempted spontaneous ventilation, and after 4 hours the infusion is reduced to 0.1 μg/kg/h with no increase in blood pressure or processed EEG value. After 5 hours, an intraoperative CT scan reveals adequate alignment of the fused spine. Approximately 30 minutes before the end of the case, the ketamine and sufentanil infusions are stopped, propofol titrated to a processed EEG reading at the upper range of adequate depth, and ondanestron administered. The patient is returned to the spine position, propofol infusion stopped, the patient thoroughly suctioned, and the trachea extubated upon resumption of a regular respiratory pattern without damage to the Maryland bridge. Neurologic examination is performed in the postanesthesia recovery unit and reveals no new deficits.

DISCUSSION

Preexisting diabetes, hypertension, and neurologic deficit predispose to difficulty in obtaining adequate TcMEPs. A propofol-opioid technique without ketamine may be adequate in patients without these risk factors. Avoidance of inhaled potent agents during planned monitoring of TcMEPs is consistent with the demonstrated significant reduction of amplitude and latency found with the agents. Remifentanil would be an alternative opioid. However, in this patient with chronic pain aggressive titration of an intermediate- or long-active opioid may provide for better analgesia at emergence and during transition to the recovery area. Remifentanil has in some studies been linked to hyperalgesia, although this remains controversial and is not a widespread observation. Fentanyl can also be used as a perioperative infusion and can be titrated preinduction to appropriate effect-site concentrations to achieve analgesia in a patient with chronic pain. Fentanyl, however, does have a significant increase in context sensitive half-time in longer cases, may be subject to delayed peak due to enterohepatic recirculation, and in an effort to reduce total dose cannot be used as aggressively to blunt intraoperative changes to transient increases in levels of surgical stimulus as sufentanil or remifentanil. Substantial clinical experience suggests that deep propofol-opioid anesthesia with adjuvant topical lidocaine provides excellent intubating conditions and obviates the need for muscle relaxation [154, 155]. Succinylcholine is associated with significant risk of perioperative myalgia [156, 157]. Nondepolarizing muscle relaxants can be of variable duration and their use for intubation often necessitates intraoperative dosing of reversal agents that can decrease the depth of anesthesia, increase heart rate, increase the risk of nausea and vomiting, and complicate subsequent dosing of neuromuscular blocking agents should that be desired at a later point in the surgery [158].

REFERENCES

1. Cole CD, Gottfried ON, Gupta DK, et al. Total intravenous anesthesia: advantages for intracranial surgery. *Neurosurgery*. 2007;61(5 Suppl 2):369, 377; discussion 377–378.
2. Steiner LA, Johnston AJ, Chatfield DA, et al. The effects of large-dose propofol on cerebrovascular pressure autoregulation in head-injured patients. *Anesth Analg*. 2003;97:572–576.

3. Newman MF, Murkin JM, Roach G, et al. Cerebral physiologic effects of burst suppression doses of propofol during nonpulsatile cardiopulmonary bypass. CNS subgroup of McSPI. *Anesth Analg.* 1995;81:452–457.

4. Conti A, Iacopino DG, Fodale V, et al. Cerebral haemodynamic changes during propofol-remifentanil or sevoflurane anaesthesia: transcranial Doppler study under bispectral index monitoring. *Br J Anaesth.* 2006;97:333–339.

5. Dagal A, Lam AM. Cerebral autoregulation and anesthesia. *Curr Opin Anaesthesiol.* 2009;22:547–552.

6. Engelhard K, Werner C. Inhalational or intravenous anesthetics for craniotomies? pro inhalational. *Curr Opin Anaesthesiol.* 2006;19:504–508.

7. Gyulai FE. Anesthetics and cerebral metabolism. *Curr Opin Anaesthesiol.* 2004;17:397–402.

8. Xie G, Deschamps A, Backman SB, et al. Critical involvement of the thalamus and precuneus during restoration of consciousness with physostigmine in humans during propofol anaesthesia: a positron emission tomography study. *Br J Anaesth.* 2011;4:548–557.

9. Moss E, Powell D, Gibson RM, et al. Effect of etomidate on intracranial pressure and cerebral perfusion pressure. *Br J Anaesth.* 1979;51:347–352.

10. Milde LN, Milde JH, Michenfelder JD. Cerebral functional, metabolic, and hemodynamic effects of etomidate in dogs. *Anesthesiology.* 1985;63:371–377.

11. Franceschini MA, Radhakrishnan H, Thakur K, et al. The effect of different anesthetics on neurovascular coupling. *Neuroimage.* 2010;51:1367–1377.

12. Miyawaki I, Nakamura K, Terasako K, Toda H, Kakuyama M, Mori K. Modification of endothelium-dependent relaxation by propofol, ketamine, and midazolam. 1995;81:474–479.

13. Kotani Y, Shimazawa M, Yoshimura S, et al. The experimental and clinical pharmacology of propofol, an anesthetic agent with neuroprotective properties. *CNS Neurosci Ther.* 2008;14:95–106.

14. Lichtenbelt BJ, Mertens M, Vuyk J. Strategies to optimise propofol-opioid anaesthesia. *Clin Pharmacokinet.* 2004;43:577–593.

15. Dahaba AA, Zhong T, Lu HS, et al. Geographic differences in the target-controlled infusion estimated concentration of propofol: bispectral index response curves. *Can J Anaesth.* 2011;58(4):364–370.

16. Lee U, Müller M, Noh GJ, Choi B, Mashour GA. Dissociable network properties of anesthetic state transitions. *Anesthesiology.* 2011;114:872–881.

17. Kortelainen J, Koskinen M, Mustola S, et al. EEG spectral changes and onset of burst suppression pattern in propofol/remifentanil anesthesia. *Conf Proc IEEE Eng Med Biol Soc.* 2008;2008:4980–4983.

18. Kortelainen J, Koskinen M, Mustola S, et al. Effects of remifentanil on the spectrum and quantitative parameters of electroencephalogram in propofol anesthesia. *Anesthesiology.* 2009;111:574–583.

19. Liley DT, Sinclair NC, Lipping T, Heyse B, Vereecke HE, Struys MM. Propofol and remifentanil differentially modulate frontal electroencephalographic activity. *Anesthesiology.* 2010;113:292–304.

20. Garnock-Jones KP, Scott LJ. Fospropofol. *Drugs.* 2010;70:469–477.

21. De Riu PL, Petruzzi V, Testa C, et al. Propofol anticonvulsant activity in experimental epileptic status. *Br J Anaesth.* 1992;69:177–181.

22. Makela JP, Iivanainen M, Pieninkeroinen IP, et al. Seizures associated with propofol anesthesia. *Epilepsia.* 1993;34:832–835.

23. Holtkamp M. Treatment strategies for refractory status epilepticus. *Curr Opin Crit Care.* 2010 Dec 21.

24. Petersen KD, Landsfeldt U, Cold GE, et al. Intracranial pressure and cerebral hemodynamic in patients with cerebral tumors: a randomized prospective study of patients subjected to craniotomy in propofol-fentanyl, isoflurane-fentanyl, or sevoflurane-fentanyl anesthesia. *Anesthesiology.* 2003;98:329–336.

25. Hans P, Bonhomme V. Why we still use intravenous drugs as the basic regimen for neurosurgical anaesthesia. *Curr Opin Anaesthesiol.* 2006;19:498–503.

26. Girard F, Moumdjian R, Boudreault D, et al. The effect of sedation on intracranial pressure in patients with an intracranial space-occupying lesion: remifentanil versus propofol. *Anesth Analg.* 2009;109:194–198.

27. Ozturk E, Demirbilek S, Kadir But A, et al. Antioxidant properties of propofol and erythropoietin after closed head injury in rats. *Prog Neuropsychopharmacol Biol Psychiatry.* 2005;29:922–927.

28. Vasileiou I, Xanthos T, Koudouna E, et al. Propofol: a review of its non-anaesthetic effects. *Eur J Pharmacol.* 2009:605:1–8.

29. Gonzalez-Correa JA, Cruz-Andreotti E, Arrebola MM, et al. Effects of propofol on the leukocyte nitric oxide pathway: in vitro and ex vivo studies in surgical patients. *Naunyn Schmiedebergs Arch Pharmacol.* 2008;376:331–339.

30. Dagal A, Lam AM. Cerebral autoregulation and anesthesia. *Curr Opin Anaesthesiol.* 2009;22:547–552.

31. Feliciano CE, de Leon-Berra R, Hernandez-Gaitan MS, et al. Provocative test with propofol: experience in patients with cerebral arteriovenous malformations who underwent neuroendovascular procedures. *AJNR Am J Neuroradiol.* 2010;31:470–475.

32. Kim JH, Joo EY, Han SJ, et al. Can pentobarbital replace amobarbital in the Wada test? *Epilepsy Behav.* 2007;11:378–383.

33. Roekaerts PM, Huygen FJ, de Lange S. Infusion of propofol versus midazolam for sedation in the intensive care unit following coronary artery surgery. *J Cardiothorac Vasc Anesth.* 1993;7:142–147.

34. Chamorro C, de Latorre FJ, Montero A, et al. Comparative study of propofol versus midazolam in the sedation of critically ill patients: results of a prospective, randomized, multicenter trial. *Crit Care Med.* 1996;24:932–939.

35. Imran M, Khan FH, Khan MA. Attenuation of hypotension using phenylephrine during induction of anaesthesia with propofol. *J Pak Med Assoc.* 2007;57:543–547.

36. El-Tahan MR. Preoperative ephedrine counters hypotension with propofol anesthesia during valve surgery: a dose dependent study. *Ann Card Anaesth.* 2011;14:30–40.

37. Nakamura K, Hatano Y, Hirakata H, et al. Direct vasoconstrictor and vasodilator effects of propofol in isolated dog arteries. *Br J Anaesth.* 1992;68:193–197.

38. Jansen GF, van Praagh BH, Kedaria MB, et al. Jugular bulb oxygen saturation during propofol and isoflurane/nitrous oxide anesthesia in patients undergoing brain tumor surgery. *Anesth Analg.* 1999;89:358–363.

39. Nandate K, Vuylsteke A, Ratsep I, et al. Effects of isoflurane, sevoflurane and propofol anaesthesia on jugular venous oxygen saturation in patients undergoing coronary artery bypass surgery. *Br J Anaesth.* 2000;84:631–633.

40. Iwata M, Kawaguchi M, Inoue S, et al. Effects of increasing concentrations of propofol on jugular venous bulb oxygen saturation in neurosurgical patients under normothermic and mildly hypothermic conditions. *Anesthesiology.* 2006;104:33–38.

41. Pasternak JJ, Lanier WL. Neuroanesthesiology update. *J Neurosurg Anesthesiol.* 2010;22:86–109.

42. Meyer MJ, Megyesi J, Meythaler J, et al. Acute management of acquired brain injury, part II: an evidence-based review of pharmacological interventions. *Brain Inj.* 2010;24:706–721.

43. Bonhomme V, Demoitie J, Schaub I, et al. Acid-base status and hemodynamic stability during propofol and sevoflurane-based anesthesia in patients undergoing uncomplicated intracranial surgery. *J Neurosurg Anesthesiol.* 2009;21:112–119.

44. Rozet I, Tontisirin N, Vavilala MS, et al. Prolonged propofol anesthesia is not associated with an increase in blood lactate. *Anesth Analg.* 2009;109:1105–1110.

45. Liolios A, Guerit JM, Scholtes JL, et al. Propofol infusion syndrome associated with short-term large-dose infusion during surgical anesthesia in an adult. *Anesth Analg.* 2005;100:1804–1806.

46. Cremer OL, Moons KG, Bouman EA, et al. Long-term propofol infusion and cardiac failure in adult head-injured patients. *Lancet.* 2001;357:117–118.

47. Nishikawa K, Nakayama M, Omote K, et al. Recovery characteristics and post-operative delirium after long-duration laparoscope-assisted surgery in elderly patients: propofol-based vs. sevoflurane-based anesthesia. *Acta Anaesthesiol Scand.* 2004;48:162–168.

48. Castagnini HE, van Eijs F, Salevsky FC, et al. Sevoflurane for interventional neuroradiology procedures is associated with more rapid early recovery than propofol. *Can J Anaesth.* 2004;51:486–491.

49. Sneyd JR. Bispectral index and propofol induction: beware of inappropriate conclusions. *Anesth Analg.* 2005;100:904-5; author reply 905.

50. Magni G, Baisi F, La Rosa I, et al. No difference in emergence time and early cognitive function between sevoflurane-fentanyl and propofol-remifentanil in patients undergoing craniotomy for supratentorial intracranial surgery. *J Neurosurg Anesthesiol.* 2005;17:134–138.

51. Arar C, Kaya G, Karamanlioglu B, et al. Effects of sevoflurane, isoflurane and propofol infusions on post-operative recovery criteria in geriatric patients. *J Int Med Res.* 2005;33:55–60.

52. Talke P, Caldwell JE, Brown R, et al. A comparison of three anesthetic techniques in patients undergoing craniotomy for supratentorial intracranial surgery. *Anesth Analg.* 2002;95:430, 435, table of contents.

53. Todd MM, Warner DS, Sokoll MD, et al. A prospective, comparative trial of three anesthetics for elective supratentorial craniotomy. Propofol/fentanyl, isoflurane/nitrous oxide, and fentanyl/nitrous oxide. *Anesthesiology.* 1993;78:1005–1020.

54. Kaneda K, Yamashita S, Woo S, et al. Population pharmacokinetics pharmacodynamics of brief etomidate infusion in healthy volunteers. *J Clin Pharmacol.* 2011: 51(4):.482–491.

55. Griffeth BT, Mehra A. Etomidate and unpredicted seizures during electroconvulsive therapy. *J ECT.* 2007;23:177–178.

56. Ghaly RF, Lee JJ, Ham JH, et al. Etomidate dose-response on somatosensory and transcranial magnetic induced spinal motor evoked potentials in primates. *Neurol Res.* 1999;21:714–720.

57. Yelavich PM, Holmes CM. Etomidate: a foreshortened clinical trial. *Anaesth Intensive Care.* 1980;8:479–483.

58. Sen H, Algul A, Senol MG, et al. Epileptic seizure during anaesthesia induction with etomidate. *Middle East J Anesthesiol.* 2010;20:723–725.

59. Avramov MN, Husain MM, White PF. The comparative effects of methohexital, propofol, and etomidate for electroconvulsive therapy. *Anesth Analg.* 1995;81:596–602.

60. Khalid N, Atkins M, Kirov G. The effects of etomidate on seizure duration and electrical stimulus dose in seizure-resistant patients during electroconvulsive therapy. *J ECT.* 2006;22:184–188.

61. Drummond JC, McKay LD, Cole DJ, et al. The role of nitric oxide synthase inhibition in the adverse effects of etomidate in the setting of focal cerebral ischemia in rats. *Anesth Analg.* 2005;100:841, 846.

62.. Etomidate, nitric oxide, and cerebral vasospasm. *Anesth Analg.* 2008; 107:343.

63. Lepousé C, Lautner CA, Liu L, Gomis P, Leon A. Emergence delirium in adults in the post-anaesthesia care unit. 2006;96:747–753.

64. Radtke FM, Franck M, Hagemann L, et al. Risk factors for inadequate emergence after anesthesia: emergence delirium and hypoactive emergence. *Minerva Anestesiol.* 2010;76:394–403.

65. Butovas S, Rudolph U, Jurd R, et al. Activity patterns in the prefrontal cortex and hippocampus during and after awakening from etomidate anesthesia. *Anesthesiology.* 2010;113:48–57.

66. Ledingham IM, Watt I. Influence of sedation on mortality in critically ill multiple trauma patients *Lancet* 1983;1:1270.

67. Watt I, Ledingham IM. Mortality amongst multiple trauma patients admitted to an intensive therapy unit. *Anaesthesia.* 1984;39:973–981.

68. Chan CM, Mitchell AL, Shorr AF. Etomidate is associated with mortality and adrenal insufficiency in sepsis: a meta-analysis. *Crit Care Med.* 2012;40:2945–2953.

69. Schenarts CL, Burton JH, Riker RR. Adrenocortical dysfunction following etomidate induction in emergency department patients. *Acad Emerg Med.* 2001;8:1–7.

70. Zed PJ, Mabasa VH, Slavik RS, et al. Etomidate for rapid sequence intubation in the emergency department: is adrenal suppression a concern? *CJEM.* 2006;8:347–350.

71. Hildreth AN, Mejia VA, Maxwell RA, et al. Adrenal suppression following a single dose of etomidate for rapid sequence induction: a prospective randomized study. *J Trauma.* 2008;65:573–579.

72. Preziosi P, Vacca M. Adrenocortical suppression and other endocrine effects of etomidate. *Life Sci.* 1988;42:477–489.

73. Annane D, Sebille V, Charpentier C, et al. Effect of treatment with low doses of hydrocortisone and fludrocortisone on mortality in patients with septic shock. *JAMA.* 2002;288:862–871.

74. Korttila K, Aromaa U. Venous complications after intravenous injection of diazepam, flunitrazepam, thiopentone and etomidate. *Acta Anaesthesiol Scand.* 1980;24:227–230.

75. Zar T, Graeber C, Perazella MA. Recognition, treatment, and prevention of propylene glycol toxicity. *Semin Dial.* 2007;20:217–219.

76. Bedichek E, Kirschbaum B. A case of propylene glycol toxic reaction associated with etomidate infusion. *Arch Intern Med.* 1991;151:2297–2298.

77. Van de Wiele B, Rubinstein E, Peacock W, et al. Propylene glycol toxicity caused by prolonged infusion of etomidate. *J Neurosurg Anesthesiol.* 1995;7:259–262.

78. Adams HA, Werner C. From the racemate to the eutomer: (S)-ketamine. renaissance of a substance? *Anaesthesist.* 1997;46:1026–1042.

79. Aroni F, Iacovidou N, Dontas I, et al. Pharmacological aspects and potential new clinical applications of ketamine: reevaluation of an old drug. *J Clin Pharmacol.* 2009;49:957–964.

80. Langsjo JW, Kaisti KK, Aalto S, et al. Effects of subanesthetic doses of ketamine on regional cerebral blood flow, oxygen consumption, and blood volume in humans. *Anesthesiology.* 2003;99:614–623.

81. Gardner AE, Dannemiller FJ, Dean D. Intracranial cerebrospinal fluid pressure in man during ketamine anesthesia. *Anesth Analg.* 1972;51:741–745.

82. Chi OZ, Wei HM, Klein SL, et al. Effect of ketamine on heterogeneity of cerebral microregional venous O2 saturation in the rat. *Anesth Analg.* 1994;79:860–866.

83. Albanese J, Arnaud S, Rey M, et al. Ketamine decreases intracranial pressure and electroencephalographic activity in traumatic brain injury patients during propofol sedation. *Anesthesiology.* 1997;87:1328–1334.

84. Sakai K, Cho S, Fukusaki M, et al. The effects of propofol with and without ketamine on human cerebral blood flow velocity and CO response. *Anesth Analg.* 2000;90:377–382.

85. Schmittner MD, Vajkoczy SL, Horn P, et al. Effects of fentanyl and S(+)-ketamine on cerebral hemodynamics, gastrointestinal motility, and need of vasopressors in patients with intracranial pathologies: a pilot study. *J Neurosurg Anesthesiol.* 2007;19:257–262.

86. Bar-Joseph G, Guilburd Y, Tamir A, et al. Effectiveness of ketamine in decreasing intracranial pressure in children with intracranial hypertension. *J Neurosurg Pediatr.* 2009;4:40–46.

87. Mahmoud M, Tyler T, Sadhasivam S. Dexmedetomidine and ketamine for large anterior mediastinal mass biopsy. *Paediatr Anaesth.* 2008;18:1011–1013.

88. Iravani M, Wald SH. Dexmedetomidine and ketamine for fiberoptic intubation in a child with severe mandibular hypoplasia. *J Clin Anesth.* 2008;20:455–457.

89. Erb TO, Ryhult SE, Duitmann E, et al. Improvement of motor-evoked potentials by ketamine and spatial facilitation during spinal surgery in a young child. *Anesth Analg.* 2005;100:1634–1636.

90. Pajewski TN, Arlet V, Phillips LH. Current approach on spinal cord monitoring: the point of view of the neurologist, the anesthesiologist and the spine surgeon *Eur Spine J* 2007;16(Suppl 2):S115–S129.

91. Bennett C, Voss LJ, Barnard JP, et al. Practical use of the raw electroencephalogram waveform during general anesthesia: the art and science. *Anesth Analg.* 2009;109:539–550.

92. Angst MS, Clark JD. Ketamine for managing perioperative pain in opioid-dependent patients with chronic pain: a unique indication? *Anesthesiology.* 2010;113:514–515.

93. Domino EF. Taming the ketamine tiger. *Anesthesiology.* 2010;113:678–684.

94. Minville V, Fourcade O, Girolami JP, et al. Opioid-induced hyperalgesia in a mice model of orthopaedic pain: preventive effect of ketamine. *Br J Anaesth.* 2010;104:231–238.

95. Loftus RW, Yeager MP, Clark JA, et al. Intraoperative ketamine reduces perioperative opiate consumption in opiate-dependent patients with chronic back pain undergoing back surgery. *Anesthesiology*. 2010;113:639–646.

96. Flexman AM, Ng JL, Gelb AW. Acute and chronic pain following craniotomy. *Curr Opin Anaesthesiol*. 2010;23:551–557.

97. Franceschini MA, Radhakrishnan H, Thakur K, et al. The effect of different anesthetics on neurovascular coupling. *Neuroimage*. 2010;51:1367–1377.

98. Nordstrom CH, Messeter K, Sundbarg G, et al. Cerebral blood flow, vasoreactivity, and oxygen consumption during barbiturate therapy in severe traumatic brain lesions *J Neurosurg*. 1988;68:424–431.

99. Turner BK, Wakim JH, Secrest J, et al. Neuroprotective effects of thiopental, propofol, and etomidate. *AANA J*. 2005;73:297–302.

100. Fairbanks CA, Stone LS, Wilcox GL. Pharmacological profiles of alpha 2 adrenergic receptor agonists identified using genetically altered mice and isobolographic analysis. *Pharmacol Ther*. 2009;123(2):224–238.

101. Hall JE, Uhrich TD, Barney JA, et al. Sedative, amnestic, and analgesic properties of small-dose dexmedetomidine infusions. *Anesth Analg*. 2000;90:699–705.

102. Gilsbach R, Roser C, Beetz N, et al. Genetic dissection of alpha2-adrenoceptor functions in adrenergic versus nonadrenergic cells. *Mol Pharmacol*. 2009;75:1160–1170.

103 Sara SJ. The locus coeruleus and noradrenergic modulation of cognition. *Nat Rev Neurosci*. 2009;10:211–223.

104. Huupponen E, Maksimow A, Lapinlampi P, et al. Electroencephalogram spindle activity during dexmedetomidine sedation and physiological sleep. *Acta Anaesthesiol Scand*. 2008;52:289–294.

105. Gerlach AT, Murphy CV. Dexmedetomidine-associated bradycardia progressing to pulseless electrical activity: case report and review of the literature. *Pharmacotherapy*. 2009;29:1492.

106. Ebert TJ, Hall JE, Barney JA, Uhrich TD, Colinco MD. The effects of increasing plasma concentrations of dexmedetomidine in humans. The effects of increasing plasma concentrations of dexmedetomidine in humans. *Anesthesiology*. 2000;93:382–394.

107. Bekker A, Sturaitis M, Bloom M, et al. The effect of dexmedetomidine on perioperative hemodynamics in patients undergoing craniotomy. *Anesth Analg*. 2008;107:1340–1347.

108. Tanskanen PE, Kytta JV, Randell TT, et al. Dexmedetomidine as an anaesthetic adjuvant in patients undergoing intracranial tumour surgery: a double-blind, randomized and placebo-controlled study. *Br J Anaesth*. 2006;97:658–665.

109. Uyar AS, Yagmurdur H, Fidan Y, et al. Dexmedetomidine attenuates the hemodynamic and neuroendocrine responses to skull-pin head-holder application during craniotomy *J Neurosurg Anesthesiol*. 2008;20:174–179.

110. Fischer GW, Silverstein JH. Dexmedetomidine and refractory cardiogenic shock. *Anesth Analg*. 2009;108:380.

111. Hsu YW, Cortinez LI, Robertson KM, et al. Dexmedetomidine pharmacodynamics: part I: crossover comparison of the respiratory effects of dexmedetomidine and remifentanil in healthy volunteers. *Anesthesiology*. 2004;101:1066–1076.

112. Belleville JP, Ward DS, Bloor BC, et al. Effects of intravenous dexmedetomidine in humans. I. Sedation, ventilation, and metabolic rate. *Anesthesiology*. 1992;77:1125–1133.

113. Mahmoud M, Radhakrishnan R, Gunter J, et al. Effect of increasing depth of dexmedetomidine anesthesia on upper airway morphology in children. *Paediatr Anaesth*. 2010:20:506–515.

114. Ebert T, Maze M. Dexmedetomidine: another arrow for the clinician's quiver. *Anesthesiology*. 2004;101:568–570.

115. Talke P, Stapelfeldt C, Lobo E, et al. Alpha-2B adrenoceptor polymorphism and peripheral vasoconstriction. *Pharmacogenet Genom*. 2005;15:357–363.

116. Dyck JB, Maze M, Haack C, Azarnoff DL, Vuorilehto L, Shafer SL. Computer-controlled infusion of intravenous dexmedetomidine hydrochloride in adult human volunteers. *Anesthesiology*. 1993;78:821–828.

117. Petroz GC, Sikich N, James M, et al. A phase I, two-center study of the pharmacokinetics and pharmacodynamics of dexmedetomidine in children. *Anesthesiology*. 2006;105:1098–1110.

118. Drummond JC, Dao AV, Roth DM, et al. Effect of dexmedetomidine on cerebral blood flow velocity, cerebral metabolic rate, and carbon dioxide response in normal humans. *Anesthesiology*. 2008;108:225–232.

119. Drummond JC, Sturaitis MK. Brain tissue oxygenation during dexmedetomidine administration in surgical patients with neurovascular injuries. *J Neurosurg Anesthesiol*. 2010;22:336–341.

120. Dagal A, Lam AM. Cerebral autoregulation and anesthesia. *Curr Opin Anaesthesiol*. 2009;22:547–552.

121. Sloan TB, Heyer EJ. Anesthesia for intraoperative neurophysiologic monitoring of the spinal cord. *J Clin Neurophysiol*. 2002;19:430–443.

122. Hans P, Bonhomme V. Anesthetic management for neurosurgery in awake patients. *Minerva Anestesiol*. 2007;73:507–512.

123. Franceschini MA, Radhakrishnan H, Thakur K, Wu W, Ruvinskaya S, Carp S, Boas DA. The effect of different anesthetics on neurovascular coupling. *Neuroimage*. 201015;51:1367–1377.

124. Banoub M, Tetzlaff JE, Schubert A. Pharmacologic and physiologic influences affecting sensory evoked potentials: implications for perioperative monitoring. *Anesthesiology*. 2003;99:716–737.

125. Ghaly RF, Stone JL, Levy WJ, et al. The effect of etomidate on motor evoked potentials induced by transcranial magnetic stimulation in the monkey. *Neurosurgery*. 1990;27:936–942.

126. Wang AC, Than KD, Etame AB, et al. Impact of anesthesia on transcranial electric motor evoked potential monitoring during spine surgery: a review of the literature. *Neurosurg Focus*. 2009;27:E7.

127. Jellinek D, Jewkes D, Symon L. Noninvasive intraoperative monitoring of motor evoked potentials under propofol anesthesia: effects of spinal surgery on the amplitude and latency of motor evoked potentials. *Neurosurgery*. 1991;29:551–557.

128. Fodale V, Schifilliti D, Pratico C, et al. Remifentanil and the brain. *Acta Anaesthesiol Scand*. 2008;52:319–326.

129. Mahmoud M, Sadhasivam S, Salisbury S, et al. Susceptibility of transcranial electric motor-evoked potentials to varying targeted blood levels of dexmedetomidine during spine surgery. *Anesthesiology*. 2010;112:1364–1373.

130. Schifilliti D, Grasso G, Conti A, et al. Anaesthetic-related neuroprotection: intravenous or inhalational agents? *CNS Drugs*. 2010;24:893–907.

131. Pittman JE, Sheng H, Pearlstein R, et al. Comparison of the effects of propofol and pentobarbital on neurologic outcome and cerebral infarct size after temporary focal ischemia in the rat. *Anesthesiology*. 1997;87:1139–1144.

132. Perez-Barcena J, Llompart-Pou JA, Homar J, et al. Pentobarbital versus thiopental in the treatment of refractory intracranial hypertension in patients with traumatic brain injury: a randomized controlled trial. *Crit Care*. 2008;12:R112.

133. Hollrigel GS, Toth K, Soltesz I. Neuroprotection by propofol in acute mechanical injury: role of GABAergic inhibition. *J Neurophysiol*. 1996;76:2412–2422.

134. Adembri C, Venturi L, Pellegrini-Giampietro DE. Neuroprotective effects of propofol in acute cerebral injury. *CNS Drug Rev*. 2007;13:333–351.

135. Adembri C, Venturi L, Tani A, et al. Neuroprotective effects of propofol in models of cerebral ischemia: inhibition of mitochondrial swelling as a possible mechanism. *Anesthesiology*. 2006;104:80–89.

136. Bayona NA, Gelb AW, Jiang Z, et al. Propofol neuroprotection in cerebral ischemia and its effects on low-molecular-weight antioxidants and skilled motor tasks. *Anesthesiology*. 2004;100:1151–1159.

137. Warner DS, Takaoka S, Wu B, et al. Electroencephalographic burst suppression is not required to elicit maximal neuroprotection from pentobarbital in a rat model of focal cerebral ischemia. *Anesthesiology*. 1996;84:1475–1484.

138. Roach GW, Newman MF, Murkin JM, et al. Ineffectiveness of burst suppression therapy in mitigating perioperative cerebrovascular dysfunction. Multicenter study of perioperative ischemia (McSPI) research group. *Anesthesiology*. 1999;90:1255–1264.

139. Fukuda S, Warner DS. Cerebral protection. *Br J Anaesth*. 2007;99:10–17.

140. Hudetz JA, Pagel PS. Neuroprotection by ketamine: a review of the experimental and clinical evidence. *J Cardiothorac Vasc Anesth*. 2010;24:131–142.

141. Hudetz JA, Iqbal Z, Gandhi SD, et al. Ketamine attenuates post-operative cognitive dysfunction after cardiac surgery. *Acta Anaesthesiol Scand*. 2009;53:864–872.

142. Reeker W, Werner C, Mollenberg O, et al. High-dose S(+)-ketamine improves neurological outcome following incomplete cerebral ischemia in rats. *Can J Anaesth*. 2000;47:572–578.

143. Shibuta S, Varathan S, Mashimo T. Ketamine and thiopental sodium: individual and combined neuroprotective effects on cortical cultures exposed to NMDA or nitric oxide. *Br J Anaesth*. 2006;97:517–524.

144. Sanders RD, Xu J, Shu Y, et al. Dexmedetomidine attenuates isoflurane-induced neurocognitive impairment in neonatal rats. *Anesthesiology*. 2009;110:1077–1085.

145. Eser O, Fidan H, Sahin O, et al. The influence of dexmedetomidine on ischemic rat hippocampus. *Brain Res*. 2008;1218:250–256.

146. Cosar M, Eser O, Fidan H, et al. The neuroprotective effect of dexmedetomidine in the hippocampus of rabbits after subarachnoid hemorrhage. *Surg Neurol*. 2009;71:54,9; discussion 59.

147. Dahmani S, Rouelle D, Gressens P, et al. Characterization of the postconditioning effect of dexmedetomidine in mouse organotypic hippocampal slice cultures exposed to oxygen and glucose deprivation. *Anesthesiology*. 2010;112:373–383.

148. Mantz J, Josserand J, Hamada S. Dexmedetomidine: new insights. *Eur J Anaesthesiol*. 2011;28:3–6.

149. Bonhomme V, Franssen C, Hans P. Awake craniotomy. *Eur J Anaesthesiol*. 2009;26:906–912.

150. Frost EA, Booij LH. Anesthesia in the patient for awake craniotomy. *Curr Opin Anaesthesiol*. 2007;20:331–335.

151. Olofsen E, Boom M, Nieuwenhuijs D, et al. Modeling the non-steady state respiratory effects of remifentanil in awake and propofol-sedated healthy volunteers. *Anesthesiology*. 2010;112:1382–1395.

152. Osborn I, Sebeo J. "Scalp block" during craniotomy: a classic technique revisited. *J Neurosurg Anesthesiol*. 2010;22:187–194.

153. Costello TG, Cormack JR. Anaesthesia for awake craniotomy: a modern approach. *J Clin Neurosci*. 2004;11:16–19.

154. Alexander R, Olufolabi AJ, Booth J, et al. Dosing study of remifentanil and propofol for tracheal intubation without the use of muscle relaxants. *Anaesthesia*. 1999;54:1037–1040.

155. Baillard C, Adnet F, Borron SW, et al. Tracheal intubation in routine practice with and without muscular relaxation: an observational study. *Eur J Anaesthesiol*. 2005;22:672–677.

156. Tejirian T, Lewis CE, Conner J, et al. Succinylcholine: a drug to avoid in bariatric surgery. *Obes Surg*. 2009;19:534–536.

157. Allen TK, Habib AS, Dear GL, et al. How much are patients willing to pay to avoid postoperative muscle pain associated with succinylcholine? *J Clin Anesth*. 2007;19:601–608.

158. Vasella FC, Frascarolo P, Spahn DR, et al. Antagonism of neuromuscular blockade but not muscle relaxation affects depth of anaesthesia. *Br J Anaesth*. 2005;94:742–747.

8.

PHARMACOLOGY OF OPIOIDS

Joshua H. Atkins and Jessica Dworet

INTRODUCTION/OVERVIEW

Opioids are a fundamental component of most neurosurgical anesthetics. They provide for post-operative analgesia, intraoperative blunting of hemodynamic responses to surgical stimulus and laryngoscopy, and immobility for procedures that require avoidance of neuromuscular blockade. Moreover pharmacodynamic synergy of opioids with intravenous hypnotics such as propofol provides for significant reductions in the effect-site concentrations required to achieve the desired clinical endpoint. Herein is reviewed basic pharmacology of opioids, properties of individual agents, and the pharmacologic principles underlying interactions with intravenous sedative-hypnotics.

PHARMACODYNAMICS OF OPIOIDS

Opioids produce analgesia by binding to G protein–coupled receptors located throughout the central and peripheral nervous system. The agonists most commonly used as adjuncts in balanced anesthesia and for perioperative analgesia are morphine, hydromorphone, fentanyl, remifentanil, and sufentanil. Methadone is a very long-acting narcotic and *N*-methyl-D-aspartate (NMDA) antagonist that may be useful in patients with chronic pain syndromes or who are resistant to other opioids. Opioids produce undesirable side effects that include respiratory depression, muscle rigidity, nausea, vomiting, and pruritis [1].

The discovery of opioid receptors in 1973 led to the identification of endogenous peptides with opioid activity. Study of these substances revealed a series of opioid receptor subtypes that were subsequently shown to be members of the G protein–receptor superfamily [2]. Activation of the opioid receptor triggers a range of physiologic responses mediated by downstream phosphorylation. Opioids also activate presynaptic receptors on γ-aminobutyric acid (GABA) neurons, which inhibit the release of GABA. This

allows dopaminergic neurons to fire more vigorously, resulting in extra dopamine in the nucleus accumbens, which is intensely pleasurable [3].

The three classic opioid receptors are μ, δ and γ. A fourth related, nonclassic receptor (ORL-1 or KOR-3) for nociceptin/orphanin was recently identified. The structure of this receptor and the signal transduction pathways activated by its stimulation reveal that it likely evolved from the opioid receptor family. Neither opioid drugs nor nonselective antagonists have affinity for this receptor [4]. Endogenous ligands (i.e., dynorphins, endorphins, and enkephalins) exist for these receptors, although they are not yet used clinically [5]. Genes encoding the three families of opioid peptides and their receptors have been cloned and characterized. This information continues to drive the development of novel opioids with targeted effects and a more narrow side effect profile [6, 7].

Opioid action in the brain is concentrated in discrete regions and the clinical profile of a given agent may be a function of subtle, still-undefined differences in localized receptor activity. The thalamus, caudate, putamen, amygdala, periaqueductal gray, and anterior cingulate have the highest opioid receptor binding potential [8]. There is also a dense concentration of opioid receptors in the locus ceruleus, the substantia gelatinosa of the spinal cord, the brain stem, and vagal nuclei such as the nucleus ambiguous and nucleus solitarius [9]. Opioid receptors are also found as genetically distinct subtypes and are distributed differently throughout the central nervous system (CNS); μ1, δ1, and κ3 are supraspinal, while μ2 is spinal and δ2, κ1, and μ3 are located within the spine and are also supraspinal [10].

μ-OPIOID RECEPTORS

Opioid analgesic activity is predominantly mediated by the μ-opioid receptor (MORs) [6]. This receptor also mediates respiratory depression, euphoria, sedation, decreased gastrointestinal motility, and physical dependence. When activated, the μ1-opioid receptor produces analgesia, while μ2 receptor subtypes produce respiratory depression, pruritis, and sedation [3]. The MOR agonists produce the most effective antinociception but also have the highest abuse potential. Most of the clinically used opioids demonstrate highest affinity for the MOR with variable affinity for other opioid receptor types.

Patients on chronic opioid therapy frequently demonstrate tolerance and the need for dose escalation. This is largely due to opioid receptor desensitization. A mechanistic understanding of the desensitization process at the protein level is evolving and suggests that desensitization may begin as early as a few minutes after drug exposure [11]. Some clinicians choose to minimize intraoperative opioid therapy for this reason, although the clinical significance of acute desensitization is questionable in the majority of patients.

δ-OPIOID RECEPTORS

The δ-opioid receptors (DORs) are located in the periphery, dorsal root ganglion, spinal cord, and supraspinal regions associated with pain control through inhibition of CNS pathways including those in the medulla and periaqueductal gray matter [12]. The DOR agonists may play a role in reversing or preventing hyperalgesia, inflammatory pain, and chronic pain after injury. The DOR agonists have minimal effects on respiration and the gastrointestinal system. Seizures may occur due to the chemical structure of some of the opioid-specific agonists [12]. DOR knock-out mice have unaffected analgesia but have reduced opioid tolerance [4]. The δ-specific opioid agonists have reduced abuse potential in animal studies compared with μ opioids and are under clinical development [7, 13]. Because of these effects, there may be an increased interest in drugs that act on the secondary opioid receptors in coming decades.

Recent data suggest that blocking DORs while activating MORs produces analgesia without the development of tolerance. Simultaneous targeting of these receptors can be accomplished by coadministration of two selective drugs, administering one nonselective drug or designing a single drug that contains two active sites separated by a spacer. For example, linking the MOR agonist oxymorphone to the DOR antagonist naltrindole produces a bivalent ligand that produced analgesia with reduced tolerance, decreased physical dependence, reduced respiratory depression, and decreased gastrointestinal inhibition in animal studies [4]. Selective synthetic ligands for the DOR have been identified but remain confined to laboratory use.

κ-OPIOID RECEPTORS

The κ-opioid receptors (KORs) are found in the limbic and other diencephalic areas, the brain stem, and spinal cord and are responsible for spinal analgesia, sedation, dyspnea, dependence, dysphoria, and respiratory depression. Kappa receptors seem to be important in the regulation of analgesia during inflammation [4]. Peripherally restricted KOR agonists target KORs located on visceral and somatic afferent nerves and produce inflammatory, visceral, and neuropathic chronic pain relief. The use of κ agonists in analgesia is limited, however, due to dysphoric side effects. In one clinical study, the κ agonist enadoline (25 μg) produced analgesia equivalent to 10 mg of morphine, but dysphoria was dose limiting. KOR agonists that target receptors on visceral and somatic afferent nerves without crossing the blood–brain barrier have also been investigated. These agonists were effective for chronic visceral pain such as that due to chronic pancreatitis [12].

GENETICS AND OPIOID ACTION

Genetic factors affect opioid efficacy, metabolism, and side effects and influence pain management strategies [14]. A single nucleotide polymorphism (SNP) is a point mutation for which alternative nucleotide pairings occur at the same chromosomal position in different individuals. One common SNP may be present in 22% of patients and is associated with reduced endogenous opioid binding, altered opioid requirements, and decreased opioid associated side effects [15]. Carriers of this variant had reduced analgesic requirements for intravenous morphine in one study [16]. In one study of Chinese patients, fentanyl consumption was increased in patients with this SNP and similar findings have been reported elsewhere [17]. The *OPRM1* genotype may also be an important factor in pharmacodynamic interactions between two classes of agents such as that found in patients administered a benzodiazepine-methadone combination [18].

Variation in the *COMT* gene on chromosome 22 may contribute to variability in analgesic response to opioids as well as variations in opioid dependence and addiction. The COMT enzyme metabolizes catecholamines such as dopamine and norepinephrine, which are secondarily involved in the modulation of pain. An SNP in the *COMT* gene causes decreased COMT enzyme activity. Patients with the most frequent COMT haplotype required lower daily morphine doses than the other COMT haplotypes. There is an association between morphine side effects of drowsiness, confusion, hallucinations, and nightmares with variations in the *COMT* gene [16]. The effect of opioids on the brain may be impacted by genotypic variation in genes with no direct relationship to the opioid system. For example, the effect of remifentanil infusion on cerebral blood flow (CBF) is related to an apolipoprotein E polymorphism [19].

Genetic profiling of individual patients for receptor and metabolic enzyme genotype has yet to reach clinical practice but may become a part of routine testing in the future. Genetic profiling will help future physicians select and dose opioids to achieve both postoperative analgesia and adequate depth of total intravenous anesthesia.

OPIOID RECEPTOR ANTAGONISTS

In clinical practice, opioid receptor antagonism is an important aspect of opioid therapy and used primarily to rescue patients from opioid-related side effects. Naloxone and naltrexone are commonly used nonselective MOR antagonists.

Naloxone is a MOR, DOR, and KOR antagonist and is used to treat opioid-induced respiratory depression. It has the greatest affinity for the μ-opioid site [20] and has a rapid onset and short duration of action after intravenous administration. When administered in low doses (0.25 or 1 μg/kg/h), naloxone reduces the incidence of pruritis, nausea, and vomiting without affecting analgesia. Interestingly, the lower-dose naloxone infusion resulted in less morphine consumption during patient controlled analgesia. [21].

Opioid reversal with naloxone may cause acute pain, nausea, vomiting, acute withdrawal, sweating, anxiety, restlessness, hypertension, tremor, seizures, ventricular tachycardia, and pulmonary edema. These side effects are more likely to occur in a patient who is receiving chronic opioid therapy. Naloxone is typically administered in 40- to 80-μg increments to reverse respiratory depression in patients emerging from general anesthesia. This dose may be repeated every 3 minutes until the desired clinical effect is obtained. The duration of action of naloxone is shorter than that of some opioids, so respiratory depression may recur. Naloxone may produce seizure activity and hypertension, so it should be used judiciously in neurosurgical patients. Despite its intrinsic epileptogenic potential, naloxone has exhibited some efficacy in the treatment of tramadol-induced seizure activity [22].

Naltrexone is a long-acting MOR antagonist and is rarely used in the acute setting. Methylnaltrexone is a charged derivative that does not cross the blood–brain barrier and is used to treat opioid-associated ileus. Nalbuphine is an MOR antagonist and a KOR agonist and has been shown to be as potent an analgesic as morphine. Nalbuphine has analgesic synergy and reduced pruritis when combined 1:1 with morphine and could be considered in exceptional cases of patients with severe pruritis [4].

OPIOID SIDE EFFECTS

The two most common side effects are constipation (to which tolerance does not develop) and nausea [23]. Sedation, nausea, vomiting, constipation, physical dependence, tolerance, and respiratory depression are also common. Additional side effects include delayed gastric emptying, hyperalgesia, immunologic and hormonal dysfunction, muscle rigidity, and myoclonus. Rapid administration of large doses of high-potency opioids such as remifentanil and fentanyl causes muscle rigidity and may impair ventilation. Several regions of

the brain are thought to be involved in opioid-induced muscle rigidity, including the basal ganglia, nucleus raphe pontis, periaqueductal gray, and locus ceruleus [24, 25]. These effects are probably specific to receptor subtypes.

Selective KOR or GOR agonists have their own array of side effects, including diuresis, sedation, and dysphoria.

Opioid-induced nausea and vomiting can have special consequences for the neurosurgical patient because vomiting increases intracranial pressure (ICP). Postoperative nausea and vomiting occur in 30% of postoperative patients, and craniotomy causes a relatively high incidence of postoperative nausea vomiting. Opioids stimulate the chemoreceptor trigger zone in the brain stem, which activates the emetic center in the brain through the release of dopamine and serotonin. Opioids increase the sensitivity of the middle ear to movement, which activates the medullary vomiting center through the release of histamine and acetylcholine from vestibular fibers [26].

TOLERANCE AND HYPERALGESIA

Tolerance is defined as a loss of analgesic potency that causes increasing dose requirements and decreased effectiveness over time. *Physical dependence* is the development of an altered state including autonomic and somatic hyperactivity that is revealed by opioid withdrawal. Opioid-induced hyperalgesia is a phenomenon in which intraoperative opioids may increase the baseline pain perception acutely and is probably distinct from tolerance. Remifentanil, particularly at high doses, has been associated with postoperative hyperalgesia in both healthy human volunteers and animal studies [27]. Patients with opioid-induced hyperalgesia become more sensitive to painful stimuli. Hyperalgesia is probably caused by sensitization of pronociceptive pathways [28, 29] and inhibition of descending inhibitory pathways in the peripheral and central nervous systems. Clinical studies remain inconclusive, but it is probably a rare occurrence.

Treatment of opioid-induced hyperalgesia consists of rotating between different opioids. Propofol may modulate opioid-induced hyperalgesia possibly through interactions GABAA receptors at the supraspinal level. Propofol had analgesic effects at subhypnotic doses and delays the onset of antianalgesia after remifentanil infusion. Clonidine (an α$_2$-agonist) attenuated opioid-induced postinfusion secondary hyperalgesia in one study [30, 31]. NMDA antagonists (e.g., ketamine and preoperative gabapentin) have also been shown to block this effect, and methadone is particularly effective due to its NMDA receptor–blocking effects. These drugs may be considered in patients who are at high risk for postoperative pain [29, 32].

RESPIRATORY DEPRESSION

Respiratory depression is a significant risk when opioids are used for postoperative pain. Respiratory depression in the neurosurgical patient produces an acute increase in arterial carbon dioxide tension. The resultant increase in CBF may produce intracranial hypertension in a patient with decreased intracranial compliance.

Opioids decrease respiratory rate, tidal volume, or both, impair the response to hypoxia, shift the CO_2–response curve down and to the right, and act directly on brainstem respiratory pattern generating nuclei. Opioids may also depress respiration indirectly through inhibition of pain. Breathing may become irregular and periodic. Respiration is controlled through medullary respiratory centers and modulated by input from peripheral and central chemoreceptors, the vagus nerve, and supraspinal sources [33]. Opioids exert their primary action at the pre-Bötzinger nucleus in the brain stem [34, 35]. Paired peripheral chemoreceptors in the carotid bodies are stimulated by hypoxia, decreased pH, and, to a lesser extent, elevated CO_2. Afferent signals travel through the glossopharyngeal nerve to respiratory centers in the medulla. Central chemoreceptors are responsible for 80% of the response to CO_2 (through changes in CSF pH) but are not responsive to hypoxia. Central respiratory depression occurs when the respiratory centers in the medulla fail to respond appropriately to hypoxia or hypercapnea. Opioids raise the level of blood CO_2 necessary to stimulate breathing (apneic threshold) by producing respiratory inhibition at the chemoreceptors via MORs and in the medulla via MORs and DORs. Tolerance to respiratory depression may be slower than tolerance to euphoric or analgesic effects, but it is usually possible to titrate opioids to the combined goal of adequate respiratory drive and patient comfort. Because of its high potency and rapid effect-site equilibration, remifentanil produces profound respiratory depression when it is given as a bolus or its infusion rate is increased rapidly. All agents may have a lower therapeutic window in patients with baseline neurologic impairment, obstructive sleep apnea, and morbid obesity [34, 35].

SEIZURES

Opioids may be proconvulsant when given in extremely high doses. The resulting seizures increase cerebral metabolic rate and CBF. Remifentanil produces dose related limbic system activation in humans and brain damage in rats and supports electroconvulsive therapy–induced seizures in humans, but the clinical significance of these effects is unclear [36]. Morphine can induce seizure-like activity when applied directly to the mouse hippocampus. The effect was mediated by MORs and KORs only [37]. Opioids are thought to produce seizures by blocking inhibitory neurons, which causes disinhibition of glutamatergic excitatory neurons [38]. The doses of opioids used in common anesthesia practice are much lower than those used in the animal studies that produced seizures and neurotoxicity and are unlikely to cause seizure activity. Moreover, opioids are typically used in conjunction with anticonvulsant sedative-hypnotic agents in the neurosurgical setting, which raise the seizure threshold. Opioid-induced seizures are therefore very rare in humans and do not represent a significant clinical risk.

Patients who receive large doses of morphine or hydromorphone have exhibited neuroexcitatory side effects that include allodynia, myoclonus, and seizures. More than half of a dose of morphine or hydromorphone is metabolized by the liver to morphine-3-glucuronide (M3G) and hydromorphone-3-glucuronide (H3G), respectively. The M3G and H3G compounds lack analgesic activity and evoke a range of dose dependent excitatory behaviors. M3G crosses the blood–brain barrier, allowing an accumulation of its concentration in the CSF. Smith and colleagues have suggested that when the M3G or H3G concentration in the CSF exceeds the neuroexcitatory threshold, excitatory behaviors may occur [39, 40]. Accumulation of these metabolites is of particular concern in the patient with clinically significant renal dysfunction [41]. Large bolus doses or continuous infusions of hydromorphone and morphine should therefore be used with caution in the neurosurgical patient with significant kidney failure. Fentanyl, sufentanil, and remifentanil do not produce metabolites with significant clinical effects in patients with renal failure. The parent compounds are not removed by dialysis thereby rendering stable therapeutic levels throughout the acute period where analgesia is needed throughout regular dialysis therapy.

Finally, two opioids used uncommonly in neurosurgical patients that have independently demonstrated seizure potential in certain subsets of patients are tramadol and meperidine.

OPIOIDS, SYNERGY, AND CONTEXT-SENSITIVE HALF-TIME

Opioids exhibit pharmacodynamic synergy with most sedative-hypnotics [44]. Opioids and inhaled anesthetics generally also act synergistically for hypnosis and the suppression of movement. The opioid effect is not limited to propofol as sevoflurane and remifentanil are also strongly synergistic for sedation [44, 52]. This property can be used to great benefit during neurosurgical procedures to minimize the probability of movement in response to noxious stimulus while decreasing the dose of hypnotic agent required to maintain general anesthesia. The key to this technique is to maintain the propofol effect-site concentration at a low enough level that less than a 50% decrease in effect-site concentration is required to cross the awake threshold. One should choose an opioid for which context-sensitive half-time does not increase during prolonged use. This permits the anesthesiologist to use techniques that provide rapid emergence for immediate postoperative neurologic assessment [45–47].

Pharmacokinetic-pharmacodynamic computer simulation predicts the optimal propofol concentration in the context of the duration of the infusion and the choice of opioid [48–51]. As the decay in the opioid concentration relative to the decay in the propofol concentration becomes more rapid, the optimal ratio shifts to a lower propofol and a higher opioid concentration, unless spontaneous respiration is desired [46]. Thus, the optimal propofol concentration is much lower when it is combined with remifentanil compared with fentanyl, sufentanil in part because much higher doses can be used without concern for post-operative over sedation.

Total intravenous anesthesia introduces significant intra-individual and interindividual dose–response differences due to the combination of pharmacokinetic and phamacodynamic variability. Using a higher dose of remifentanil may allow the dose of propofol to be decreased, shortening the time required for emergence. Infusions of fentanyl that last more than several hours dramatically increase its context-sensitive half-time, while sufentanil exhibits a more modest increase. Longer-acting opioids (e.g., morphine and hydromorphone) are not well suited to continuous perioperative infusion for the maintenance of general anesthesia. Potential interventions to ensure appropriate dosing include the avoidance of muscle relaxation, the use of processed EEG monitoring, and the addition of low concentrations of potent volatile anesthetics or the addition of adjuvant agents such as dexmedetomidine.

CEREBRAL PHYSIOLOGY AND OPIOIDS

FLOW–METABOLISM COUPLING/ UNCOUPLING

Cerebral autoregulation ensures that a constant supply of nutrients and oxygen is delivered to the brain by the cerebral circulation despite variations in cerebral perfusion pressure (CPP) [53]. Autoregulation maintains adequate cerebral perfusion between the limits of autoregulation, approximately 50 to 150 mm Hg in normal patients. There is, however, a wide range of individual variation, especially in patients with chronic hypertension. Cerebral autoregulation may also be impaired in severe traumatic brain injury. Because they do not impair autoregulation, opioids are especially well suited to the neurosurgical setting. In general, opioids at doses used for clinical neuroanesthesia have little *intrinsic* effect on cerebral metabolism and CBF but may reduce CBF at very high doses (e.g., remifentanil infused at 3 μg/kg/min, which is significantly higher than the highest recommended dose) [54]. Opioid administration may, however, reduce blood pressure, leading to an autoregulatory cerebral vasodilation to compensate for decreased blood flow. Opioid-induced respiratory depression in a spontaneously breathing patient, such as during an awake craniotomy or ICU sedation, will increase $PaCO_2$ and increase CBF [55].

Opioids produce modest decreases in cerebral metabolic rate and ICP, but these changes are influenced by the use of other drugs [56]. Remifentanil, alfentanil, and fentanyl produce regional changes in CBF in both humans and animals [28, 57]. In one study, moderate doses of fentanyl (25 μg/kg) or sufentanil (3 μg/kg) did not change CBF velocity, heart rate, end-tidal CO_2, or $PaCO_2$, in patients undergoing elective coronary artery bypass graft surgery, but infusion of high-dose sufentanil (6 μg/kg) was associated with a 27% to 30% decrease in CBF velocity. Sufentanil may produce a dose-dependent cerebral vasoconstriction if $PaCO_2$ is held constant [58], while fentanyl decreases both CBF and cerebral metabolic rate of oxygen [59]. In general, opioids cause relatively little change in cerebral metabolism or CBF at standard doses and are used routinely in almost all neuroanesthesia cases.

EFFECTS ON CO_2 REGULATION, CBF, AND ICP

Anesthetic agents may significantly influence CBF and ICP through their effects on $PaCO_2$. It is, however, difficult to isolate the effect of a single pharmacologic agent on a physiologic parameter like ICP that is determined by so many factors. The effects of opioids on ICP are determined by a variety of factors, including level of consciousness, whether the patient is being ventilated or is breathing spontaneously, and whether a single or multiple agents are used. The most clinically relevant studies are those in patients receiving a combination of opioids and another sedative-hypnotic. In patients with acquired brain injury, five studies reported increases in ICP, two found no increase, and one reported a decrease in ICP after opioid administration. Infusion of remifentanil usually decreases ICP with minimal CPP changes.

Rates of CSF production and reabsorption are not affected by remifentanil. The increase in cerebral perfusion caused by remifentanil is most likely due to hypercapnia-induced vasodilation [8]. One prospective, randomized study compared the effects on ICP and CPP of remifentanil versus propofol titrated for equal sedation in spontaneously ventilating patients having stereotactic intracranial tumor biopsy. Patients who received remifentanil had a lower respiratory rate (11 versus 15 breaths/min), a higher arterial PCO_2 (48 versus 43 mm Hg), and a higher MAP, but there was no difference in ICP. This is clinically important for patients who may be receiving sedation during evaluation of neuropathology (i.e., angiogram for intracranial bleed, magnetic resonance imaging to evaluate intracranial mass) because increasing CBF in patients with decreased intracranial compliance may increase ICP and precipitate neurologic deterioration. The higher MAP in the remifentanil group resulted in a higher CPP. Thus, CPP was well preserved with remifentanil [60, 61]. Sedation with remifentanil, fentanyl, or morphine in addition to propofol or midazolam did not alter mean ICP or CPP in mechanically ventilated ICU patients with acute brain injury or postoperative neurosurgical patients.

In general, opioids do not independently increase CBF or ICP when used for general anesthesia or sedation with controlled mechanical ventilation. Their effects on ICP and CPP should not be a primary concern with the use of opioids as part of a balanced anesthetic for neurosurgery but should be kept in mind when using opioid-benzodiazepine or opioid-propofol combinations for procedural sedation. Very high opioid doses can increase cerebral metabolic rate and ICP due to seizure activity and/or decreased MAP.

EFFECTS ON EEG/PROCESSED EEG

EEG and processed EEG (pEEG) are commonly used for procedures including cerebrovascular surgery, spine surgery, or as an indicator of anesthetic depth. Opioids have variable, mostly dose-dependent effects on the EEG. MOR agonists including remifentanil tend to decrease frequency and increase EEG amplitude, eventually producing delta waves (0.5–4 Hz) at the drug's maximal effect. As the opioid dose increases, the EEG changes from low-amplitude, high-frequency signal to a high-amplitude, low-frequency signal [46].

Opioid have variable effects on the bispectral index (BIS). High doses of opioids can paradoxically increase the pEEG scores because muscle rigidity produces a strong EMG component. Several studies suggest that the BIS monitor is insensitive to opioids, but others detected a sedation effect of opioids similar to other hypnotics with pEEG.[28].

Addition of opioids to other anesthetics reduces the dose of anesthetic required to prevent recall and movement. Adding opioids to the anesthetic will either decrease the BIS or reduce the likelihood of movement or awakening at a given BIS score. In one study, high-frequency (>14 Hz) activity during light anesthesia was decreased in patients who received a combination of remifentanil and propofol, while extended α (7–14 Hz) activity increased and γ activity decreased during deep anesthesia. Remifentanil suppressed some of the changes propofol induced in the EEG (i.e., β activity during light anesthesia and delta activity during deep anesthesia) [65]. Loss of consciousness after administration of propofol occurs at higher BIS values when opioids are preadministered compared with when propofol is given alone.

Processed EEG should be considered in any neurosurgical procedure that relies primarily on intravenous agents to provide the major component of a general anesthestic, but it should not be considered as a primary monitor of depth of anesthesia. The information provided is more useful when data collection begins before induction of anesthesia, allowing the response to induction drugs, laryngoscopy, positioning, and subsequent bolus drug administration can be measured. Raw EEG (e.g., burst suppression), EMG, and signal quality scores can be correlated to changes in the pEEG. pEEG is particularly effective in distinguishing between conscious and unconscious states, but pEEG scores

may not correlate with effect-site concentration of intravenous hypnotics, particularly when they are used in combination with high-dose opioid infusions [66, 67].

PRACTICAL CONSIDERATIONS: IS THERE AN "IDEAL" OPIOID FOR NEUROANESTHESIA?

A neurosurgical anesthetic is designed to provide analgesia, amnesia, immobility, and hemodynamic stability while optimizing surgical exposure and neurophysiologic monitoring. At the end of the procedure, the patient should be awake and able to cooperate with a neurologic examination.. Patients undergoing neurosurgical procedures may have a variety of comorbidities that make them and may be more vulnerable to opioid-related side effects. Physicians tend to underestimate postoperative pain, particularly in neurosurgical patients [68]. An infusion of a short- to intermediate-acting opioid will maintain relative steady-state concentrations during total intravenous anesthesia or neurophysiologic monitoring. The choice of a specific drug and dosing regimen depends on experience and specific patient issues.

REMIFENTANIL

Remifentanil is the newest intravenous opioid to be introduced to the market. Remifentanil offers several advantages, including very rapid (1 minute) effect-site equilibration; ultra short half-life (3 to 4 minutes) that is independent of hepatic metabolism, renal excretion, or duration of infusion; and high potency. Remifentanil is an ester that is readily hydrolyzed by nonspecific plasma esterases to remifentanil acid, a metabolite with very low potency. Its metabolism is unaffected by pseudocholinesterase deficiency. Remifentanil can be used in doses sufficient to blunt the response to rapidly varying levels of surgical stimulation without delaying emergence or impairing the postoperative neurologic examination.

Remifentanil is synergistic with propofol. Surface-response models and isobolograms for propofol-remifentanil are well developed and readily available, allowing a specific dose to be chosen (Figure 8.1). These properties make remifentanil an optimal choice for neurosurgical cases that may require significant amounts of opioid to achieve balanced anesthesia.

Remifentanil can also be used as part of a balanced total intravenous anesthetic when neurophysiologic monitoring precludes the use of neuromuscular blocking agents. The combination is also particularly effective for intubation and may eliminate the need for the use of muscle relaxant on induction [69]. A bolus of remifentanil (1 μg/kg) blunts the autonomic response to transient stimuli such as laryngoscopy, Mayfield pinning, or surgical positioning. Last, remifentanil acts synergistically with propofol, whose

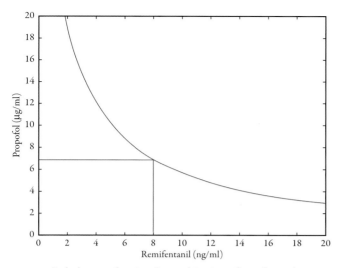

Figure 8.1   Isobologram showing the combination of remifentanil and propofol effect-site concentrations predicted to produce a 99% probability of no response to endotracheal intubation.

context-sensitive halftime becomes longer during an infusion, and allows a lower dose of propofol to be used.

The primary disadvantages of remifentanil include cost, rapid awakening if the infusion is interrupted, a theoretical risk of hyperalgesia, and the need for immediate transition to longer-acting opioids by the end of surgery to prevent postoperative pain. Because of its high potency, remifentanil may be associated with significant bradycardia as well as muscle and glottic rigidity, particularly during induction of anesthesia. The drug is typically administered as an infusion dosed at a rate of 0.1 to 0.4 µg/kg/min. Infusions are usually continued until the procedure is completed and the dressing is applied. In morbidly obese patients, the dose of remifentanil should be adjusted to ideal body weight or lean body mass, particularly when the effects of opioid-propofol combinations on blood pressure are of concern [70].

SUFENTANIL

Sufentanil is an ultrapotent opioid with an extensive history of clinical use as a perioperative infusion. It has a relatively long terminal elimination half-life (average 769 minutes), but the average time for plasma concentration to drop 50% after a continuous infusion is 33 minutes compared with 262 minutes for fentanyl [71]. Sufentanil is principally cleared by hepatic extraction, and dose adjustments are not necessary in patients with renal failure but interpatient variability may be enhanced [72]. Sufentanil has a relatively slow effect-site equilibration, with its peak occurring 7 to 8 minutes after a bolus dose. As a result, sufentanil must be administered well before a stimulus in order to provide an adequate level of analgesia or reflex suppression. Despite these limitations, sufentanil is an effective narcotic for patients undergoing craniotomy [73]. Emergence from

anesthesia is slightly prolonged in patients who have received sufentanil (as opposed to remifentanil), but patients who have received sufentanil have decreased opioid requirements in the immediate postoperative period [74, 75]. and an intraoperative conversion to a longer acting opioid is generally not necessary. Sufentanil commonly produces an post-operative analgesic "window" of 30 to 60 minutes in duration that is ideal for transporting and assessing the patient after surgery. Pharmacokinetic and pharmacodynamic models for sufentanil are available but are not as well characterized as those for remifentanil [76–78]. As long as moderate plasma concentrations are targeted (4–8 ng/mL), plasma concentrations of sufentanil fall more rapidly than fentanyl [78]. Patients who receive propofol and sufentanil infusions do take longer to emerge than those who have received remifentanil. This may be caused by a longer context-sensitive half-time and the use of higher doses of propofol to maintain a similar depth of anesthesia. In one small study of propofol and sufentanil infusions in obese patients, the results supported choosing the dose based on total body weight [79]. The average induction dose of sufentanil is 0.5 to 2.0 µg/kg followed by an infusion maintained at 0.1 to 0.3 µg/kg/h. The higher induction doses are necessary for intubation without muscle relaxants. In general, sufentanil infusions can be decreased by approximately 50% after 2 to 3 hours in order to accommodate for the modest increase in context-sensitive half-time [76]. This dose should be adjusted to accommodate individual patient factors and patient responsiveness (e.g., a sympathetic response to surgical stimulation) to a dose reduction may help guide dosing.

Sufentanil can also be administered in bolus doses (10–20 µg) if the patient responds to a painful stimulus, but the peak effect-site concentration will not be obtained until 7 to 8 minutes after the bolus. Large bolus doses of sufentanil in an awake patient may trigger coughing and a feeling of chest tightness. In most cases, the infusion is discontinued 30 minutes before the end of surgery.

FENTANYL

Fentanyl is a highly potent synthetic opioid drug with a well-established clinical profile [80]. Fentanyl equilibrates with the effect site within 3 to 5 minutes and has limited cardiovascular effects. It has no active metabolites. Fentanyl, like other opioids, is used commonly to blunt the autonomic response to painful stimuli (e.g., laryngoscopy and intubation, application of the headholder, and incision). Tachyphylaxis, a significant increase in context-sensitive half-time, and a delay in peak plasma concentration may occur when fentanyl is used at higher doses or continuous infusions.

Fentanyl is initially distributed out of the plasma to other compartments within the first hour after administration. This may, however, result in a slower overall decrease in plasma (and effect-site) concentration after longer infusions and high doses.

Fentanyl can be administered by as a bolus or as a continuous infusion. Fentanyl offers an excellent balance between titration, duration of action, analgesic potency, and side effect profile. One proposed approach to fentanyl titration, particularly in the opioid-dependent patient, is to determine a dose–response curve by titrating fentanyl to respiratory depression during induction of anesthesia [81]. The infusion rate can then be guided by the measured response curve. Such an approach should be used with caution in neurosurgical patients who may have decreased intracranial compliance. This technique may, however, be considered in patients undergoing complex spine surgery on chronic opioid therapy. In patients undergoing intracranial procedures, 3 to 5 μg/kg may be administered as a bolus at induction, followed by 2 μg/kg when the headholder is applied and 2 μg/kg at the time of incision. In this approach the majority of the opioid is administered at the beginning of the procedure and only small boluses (50 μg) or used for the remainder of the surgery.

MORPHINE

Morphine has been used as part of a balanced general anesthetic and is commonly used for longer-acting postoperative analgesia. Because of its longer half-life, delayed emergence may occur if morphine is used as the primary opioid as part of a balanced anesthetic technique. Morphine also has an active metabolite. M6G is a potent analgesic with a unique MOR profile. M6G may have a better therapeutic ratio (analgesia to respiratory depression) than morphine, but equilibration with the central nervous system is exceptionally slow [82].

Morphine has a variety of side effects. Bolus administration of morphine may cause transient vasodilation and hypotension, likely related to histamine release [83]. Some studies suggest that morphine may be more sedating than fentanyl and is also more likely to cause nausea and vomiting [84].

HYDROMORPHONE

Hydromorphone is a long-acting opioid that is 3 to 7 times more potent then morphine [85]. Clinical experience suggests that hydromorphone and morphine are clinically similar. Hydromorphone has no active metabolites and is therefore safer than morphine in renal failure. The administration of large doses or prolonged infusions of hydromorphone may result in accumulation of the neuroexcitatory compound H3G. Hydromorphone equilibration with the effect site may be slightly faster than morphine and the duration of action is similar (3–4 hours). A routine starting dose for postoperative analgesia is 0.01 to 0.2 mg (10 to 20 μg/kg). There are virtually no published data on the pharmacodynamic interaction profile of hydromorphone and intravenous agents such as propofol.

METHADONE

Methadone is a long-acting opioid that is not routinely used in neuroanesthesia. It has a long clinical history for the treatment of heroin dependence as well as management of chronic pain. Methadone is an NMDA receptor antagonist and there is a resurgence in its use for patients with chronic pain. Methadone has analgesic properties similar to a combination of opioid and ketamine and is used in the perioperative period as a potent analgesic. The effect-site equilibration time is similar to hydromorphone (7–10 minutes), but the duration of action is up to 36 hours. Thus, a single dose (0.1–0.2 mg/kg) can be given at the time of induction, and no further "guesswork" is typically necessary to determine the need for additional opioids. Intravenous methadone for acute perioperative analgesia may have a role in complex spine surgery and in patients with a history of tolerance to high-dose opioids [86, 87]. Management of these patients in the postoperative period, particularly if methadone will be continued, requires a multidisciplinary approach involving pain specialists. Methadone must be used with caution, especially if repeat doses are given, to avoid accumulation and the sudden onset of respiratory depression.

THE GRAY ZONE

Are opioids neuroprotective or neurotoxic?

Several animal studies have shown a neuroprotective effect of opioids but the clinical evidence in humans is scant. Opioid preconditioning is a phenomenon by which exposure of neurons to opioid before ischemia induces ischemic tolerance. Morphine pretreatment 24 hours before middle cerebral artery occlusion in rats reduced brain infarct volume and improved neurologic functional outcome [88]. KOR agonists are neuroprotective in animal models of global and focal cerebral ischemia. A KOR agonist administered to Wistar rats subjected to middle cerebral artery occlusion (focal ischemia) for 2 hours followed by reperfusion decreased the size of the infarct volume and mortality when administered at the onset of reperfusion [89].

Opioid preconditioning may induce opioid receptor–dependent neuroprotection against focal cerebral ischemia. Pretreatment with fentanyl in rats subjected to unilateral middle cerebral artery occlusion exhibited an improvement in regional CBF compared with control. Thus, pretreatment with fentanyl could possibly be beneficial in improving regional CBF after focal cerebral ischemia [90]. The neuroprotective activity of opioids can have important clinical implications. Opioid treatment in newborns improved neurologic outcome and decreased intracranial hemorrhage. Newborns with perinatal asphyxia treated with opioids in their first week of life had less brain structure injury on magnetic resonance imaging and better neurologic function assessed by a neurologist [88]. Morphine infusion for up to 7 days decreased the occurrence of periventricular and intraventricular hemorrhage in newborns ventilated in the neonatal intensive care unit [91].

In addition to the studies that demonstrate a neuroprotective effect of opioids, there are several animal studies that suggest that opioids can be neurotoxic. Opioid administration can induce apoptosis in animal models. Knockout of MORs enhances the survival of hippocampal granule cells. Morphine has an anticancer effect mediated through apoptosis [92]. Chronic morphine use induces apoptosis in parietal, frontal, temporal, occipital, entorhinal, piriform, and hippocampal CA1, CA2, and CA3 regions of rat brains and the spinal cord [93].

Opioids, when used alone and in large doses, may produce brain damage, especially in the limbic system. Alfentanil, sufentanil, and fentanyl all induce limbic system (hippocampus, amygdale, septal nuecleus, cingulated and entorhinal cortices, dentate gyrus) hypermetabolism, seizures, and histologic lesions in rat brains when administered in large doses. The relationship between opioid dose and severity of brain damage was analyzed in rats. Fentanyl doses from 50 to 3200 μg/kg induced a dose-dependent effect on the development of histologic evidence of brain damage in the limbic system of rats. Fentanyl administration was associated with activation of EEG in rats. Fentanyl induced evidence of brain damage when administered over a range of doses, including that corresponding to the doses used clinically in humans [37]. In contrast, another study revealed no effect (protective or toxic) of fentanyl on focal ischemia related brain damage in rats anesthetized with isoflurane [94].

In light of the conflicting evidence, opioid selection cannot be based solely on a goal of neuroprotection. Similarly, the evidence does not support a neurotoxic effect of opioids when used as a component of balanced anesthesia or for postoperative analgesia neurosurgical patients.

REFERENCES

1. Servin FS, Billard V. Remifentanil and other opioids. *Handb Exp Pharmacol.* 2008;**182**:283–311.
2. Standifer KM, Pasternak GW. G proteins and opioid receptor-mediated signalling. *Cell Signal.* 1997;**9**(3–4):237–248.
3. Trescot AM, Datta S, Lee M, et al. Opioid pharmacology. *Pain Physician.* 2008;**11**(2 Suppl):S133–S153.
4. Dietis N, Guerrini R, Calo G, et al. Simultaneous targeting of multiple opioid receptors: a strategy to improve side-effect profile. *Br J Anaesth.* 2009;**103**:38–49.
5. Sauriyal DS, Jaggi AS, Singh N. Extending pharmacological spectrum of opioids beyond analgesia: multifunctional aspects in different pathophysiological states. *Neuropeptides.* 2011 45(3): 175–188
6. Kieffer BL. Opioids: First lessons from knockout mice. *Trends Pharmacol Sci.* 1999;**20**:19–26.
7. Lee YS, Kulkarani V, Cowell SM, et al. Development of potent mu and delta opioid agonists with high lipophilicity. *J Med Chem.* 2011 Jan 13;54(1):382–386
8. MacIntosh BJ, Pattinson KT, Gallichan D, et al. Measuring the effects of remifentanil on cerebral blood flow and arterial arrival time using 3D GRASE MRI with pulsed arterial spin labelling. *J Cereb Blood Flow Metab.* 2008;**28**:1514–1522.
9. Snyder SH, Pasternak GW. Historical review: opioid receptors. *Trends Pharmacol Sci.* 2003;**24**:198–205.
10. Holden JE, Jeong Y, Forrest JM. The endogenous opioid system and clinical pain management. *AACN Clin Issues.* 2005;**16**:291–301.
11. Berger AC, Whistler JL. How to design an opioid drug that causes reduced tolerance and dependence. *Ann Neurol.* 2010;**67**:559–569.
12. Vanderah TW. Delta and kappa opioid receptors as suitable drug targets for pain. *Clin J Pain.* 2010;**26**(Suppl 10):S10–S15.
13. Janecka A, Perlikowska R, Gach K, et al. Development of opioid peptide analogs for pain relief. *Curr Pharm Des.* 2010;**16**:1126–1135.
14. Lloret Linares C, Hajj A, Poitou C, et al. Pilot study examining the frequency of several gene polymorphisms involved in morphine pharmacodynamics and pharmacokinetics in a morbidly obese population. *Obes Surg.* 21(8):1257–1264.
15. Mura E, Govoni S, Racchi M, Carossa V, Ranzani GN, Allegri M, van Schaik RH. Consequences of the 118A>G polymorphism in the OPRM1 gene: translation from bench to bedside? *J Pain Res.* 2013;6:331–353.
16. Kosarac B, Fox AA, Collard CD. Effect of genetic factors on opioid action. *Curr Opin Anaesthesiol.* 2009;**22**:476–482.
17. Zhang W, Yuan JJ, Kan QC, et al. Study of the OPRM1 A118G genetic polymorphism associated with postoperative nausea and vomiting induced by fentanyl intravenous analgesia. *Minerva Anestesiol.* 2011;77(1):33–9.
18. Bunten H, Liang WJ, Pounder D, et al. CYP2B6 and OPRM1 gene variations predict methadone-related deaths. *Addict Biol.* 2011;**16**:142–144.
19. Kofke WA, Blissitt PA, Rao H, et al. Remifentanil-induced cerebral blood flow effects in normal humans: Dose and ApoE genotype. *Anesth Analg.* 2007;**105**:167–175.
20. Orman JS, Keating GM. Buprenorphine/naloxone: a review of its use in the treatment of opioid dependence. *Drugs.* 2009;**69**:577–607.
21. Gan TJ, Ginsberg B, Glass PS, et al. Opioid-sparing effects of a low-dose infusion of naloxone in patient-administered morphine sulfate. *Anesthesiology.* 1997;**87**:1075–1081.
22. Saidi H, Ghadiri M, Abbasi S, et al. Efficacy and safety of naloxone in the management of postseizure complaints of tramadol intoxicated patients: A self-controlled study. *Emerg Med J.* 2010;**27**:928–930.
23. Benyamin R, Trescot AM, Datta S, et al. Opioid complications and side effects. *Pain Physician.* 2008;**11**(2 Suppl):S105–S120.
24. Vankova ME, Weinger MB, Chen DY, et al. Role of central mu, delta-1, and kappa-1 opioid receptors in opioid-induced muscle rigidity in the rat. *Anesthesiology.* 1996;**85**:574–583.
25. Drummond GB. The abdominal muscles in anaesthesia and after surgery. *Br J Anaesth.* 2003;**91**:73–80.
26. Miaskowski C. A review of the incidence, causes, consequences, and management of gastrointestinal effects associated with postoperative opioid administration. *J Perianesth Nurs.* 2009;**24**:222–228.
27. Fodale V, Schifilliti D, Pratico C, et al. Remifentanil and the brain. *Acta Anaesthesiol Scand.* 2008;**52**:319–326.
28. Colvin LA, Fallon MT. Opioid-induced hyperalgesia: A clinical challenge. *Br J Anaesth.* 2010;**104**:125–127.
29. Gottschalk A, Yaster M. The perioperative management of pain from intracranial surgery. *Neurocrit Care.* 2009;**10**:387–402.
30. Chu LF, Angst MS, Clark D. Opioid-induced hyperalgesia in humans: molecular mechanisms and clinical considerations. *Clin J Pain.* 2008 Jul-Aug;**24**:479–496.
31. Chu LF, Clark DJ, Angst MS. Opioid tolerance and hyperalgesia in chronic pain patients after one month of oral morphine therapy: a preliminary prospective study. *J Pain.* 2006;7:43–48.
32. Minville V, Fourcade O, Girolami JP, et al. Opioid-induced hyperalgesia in a mice model of orthopaedic pain: preventive effect of ketamine. *Br J Anaesth.* 2010;**104**:231–238.
33. Dahan A, Teppema LJ. Influence of anaesthesia and analgesia on the control of breathing. *Br J Anaesth.* 2003;**91**:40–49.
34. Pattinson KT, Mitsis GD, Harvey AK, et al. Determination of the human brainstem respiratory control network and its

cortical connections in vivo using functional and structural imaging. *Neuroimage*. 2009;**44**:295–305.

35. Feldman JL, Del Negro CA. Looking for inspiration: new perspectives on respiratory rhythm. *Nat Rev Neurosci*. 2006;**7**:232–242.

36. Kofke WA. Anesthetic management of the patient with epilepsy or prior seizures. *Curr Opin Anaesthesiol*. 2010;**23**:391–399.

37. Brull R, McCartney CJ, Chan VW, et al. Neurological complications after regional anesthesia: contemporary estimates of risk. *Anesth Analg*. 2007;**104**:965–974.

38. Kofke WA, Garman RH, Stiller RL, et al. Opioid neurotoxicity: fentanyl dose-response effects in rats. *Anesth Analg*. 1996;**83**:1298–1306.

39. Smith MT. Neuroexcitatory effects of morphine and hydromorphone: evidence implicating the 3-glucuronide metabolites. *Clin Exp Pharmacol Physiol*. 2000;**27**:524–528.

40. Wright AW, Mather LE, Smith MT. Hydromorphone-3-glucuronide: A more potent neuro-excitant than its structural analogue, morphine-3-glucuronide. *Life Sci*. 2001;**69**:409–420.

41. Niscola P, Scaramucci L, Vischini G, et al. The use of major analgesics in patients with renal dysfunction. *Curr Drug Targets*. 2010;**11**:752–758.

42. Voss LJ, Sleigh JW, Barnard JP, et al. The howling cortex: Seizures and general anesthetic drugs. *Anesth Analg*. 2008;**107**:1689–1703.

43. McGuire G, El-Beheiry H, Manninen P, et al. Activation of electrocorticographic activity with remifentanil and alfentanil during neurosurgical excision of epileptogenic focus. *Br J Anaesth*. 2003;**91**:651–655.

44. Hendrickx JF, Eger EI 2nd, Sonner JM, et al. Is synergy the rule? A review of anesthetic interactions producing hypnosis and immobility. *Anesth Analg*. 2008;**107**:494–506.

45. Short TG. Using response surfaces to expand the utility of MAC. *Anesth Analg*. 2010;**111**:249–251.

46. Lichtenbelt BJ, Mertens M, Vuyk J. Strategies to optimise propofol-opioid anaesthesia. *Clin Pharmacokinet*. 2004;**43**:577–593.

47. Shafer SL, Varvel JR. Pharmacokinetics, pharmacodynamics, and rational opioid selection. *Anesthesiology*. 1991;**74**:53–63.

48. Tallarida RJ. An overview of drug combination analysis with isobolograms. *J Pharmacol Exp Ther*. 2006;**319**:1–7.

49. Kern SE, Xie G, White JL, et al. A response surface analysis of propofol-remifentanil pharmacodynamic interaction in volunteers. *Anesthesiology*. 2004;**100**:1373–1381.

50. Minto C, Vuyk J. Response surface modelling of drug interactions. *Adv Exp Med Biol*. 2003;**523**:35–43.

51. Bouillon TW, Bruhn J, Radulescu L, et al. Pharmacodynamic interaction between propofol and remifentanil regarding hypnosis, tolerance of laryngoscopy, bispectral index, and electroencephalographic approximate entropy. *Anesthesiology*. 2004;**100**:1353–1372.

52. Schifilliti D, Grasso G, Conti A, et al. Anaesthetic-related neuroprotection: intravenous or inhalational agents? *CNS Drugs*. 2010 Nov 1;**24**:893–907.

53. Dagal A, Lam AM. Cerebral autoregulation and anesthesia. *Curr Opin Anaesthesiol*. 2009;**22**:547–552.

54. Paris A, Scholz J, von Knobelsdorff G, et al. The effect of remifentanil on cerebral blood flow velocity. *Anesth Analg*. 1998;**87**:569–573.

55. Lam AM, Mayberg TS. Opioids and cerebral blood flow velocity. *Anesthesiology*. 1993;**79**:616–617.

56. Cole CD, Gottfried ON, Gupta DK, et al. Total intravenous anesthesia: advantages for intracranial surgery. *Neurosurgery*. 2007;**61**(5 Suppl 2):369,77; discussion 377–378.

57. Gyulai FE. Anesthetics and cerebral metabolism. *Curr Opin Anaesthesiol*. 2004;**17**:397–402.

58. Hanel F, Werner C, von Knobelsdorff G, et al. The effects of fentanyl and sufentanil on cerebral hemodynamics. *J Neurosurg Anesthesiol*. 1997;**9**:223–227.

59. Franceschini MA, Radhakrishnan H, Thakur K, et al. The effect of different anesthetics on neurovascular coupling. *Neuroimage*. 2010 Jul 15;**51**:1367–1377.

60. Girard F, Moumdjian R, Boudreault D, et al. The effect of sedation on intracranial pressure in patients with an intracranial

61. Pasternak JJ, Lanier WL. Neuroanesthesiology update. *J Neurosurg Anesthesiol*. 2010;**22**:86–109.

62. Sperry RJ, Bailey PL, Reichman MV, et al. Fentanyl and sufentanil increase intracranial pressure in head trauma patients. *Anesthesiology*. 1992;**77**:416–420.

63. Kofke WA, Tempelhoff R. Increased intracranial pressure in head trauma patients given fentanyl or sufentanil. *Anesthesiology*. 1993;**78**:620–621.

64. Scholz J, Bause H, Schulz M, et al. Pharmacokinetics and effects on intracranial pressure of sufentanil in head trauma patients. *Br J Clin Pharmacol*. 1994;**38**:369–372.

65. Kortelainen J, Koskinen M, Mustola S, et al. Effects of remifentanil on the spectrum and quantitative parameters of electroencephalogram in propofol anesthesia. *Anesthesiology*. 2009;**111**:574–583.

66. Hoymork SC, Hval K, Jensen EW, et al. Can the cerebral state monitor replace the bispectral index in monitoring hypnotic effect during propofol/remifentanil anaesthesia? *Acta Anaesthesiol Scand*. 2007;**51**:210–216.

67. Hoymork SC, Raeder J, Grimsmo B, et al. Bispectral index, serum drug concentrations and emergence associated with individually adjusted target-controlled infusions of remifentanil and propofol for laparoscopic surgery. *Br J Anaesth*. 2003;**91**:773–780.

68. Gottschalk A. Craniotomy pain: trying to do better. *Anesth Analg*. 2009;**109**:1379–1381.

69. Alexander R, Olufolabi AJ, Booth J, et al. Dosing study of remifentanil and propofol for tracheal intubation without the use of muscle relaxants. *Anaesthesia*. 1999;**54**:1037–1040.

70. Egan TD, Huizinga B, Gupta SK, et al. Remifentanil pharmacokinetics in obese versus lean patients. *Anesthesiology*. 1998;**89**:562–573.

71. Westmoreland CL, Hoke JF, Sebel PS, et al. Pharmacokinetics of remifentanil (GI87084B) and its major metabolite (GI90291) in patients undergoing elective inpatient surgery. *Anesthesiology*. 1993;**79**:893–903.

72. Davis PJ, Stiller RL, Cook DR, et al. Pharmacokinetics of sufentanil in adolescent patients with chronic renal failure. *Anesth Analg*. 1988;**67**:268–271.

73. Gerlach K, Uhlig T, Huppe M, et al. Remifentanil-propofol versus sufentanil-propofol anaesthesia for supratentorial craniotomy: a randomized trial. *Eur J Anaesthesiol*. 2003;**20**:813–820.

74. Bilotta F, Caramia R, Paoloni FP, et al. Early postoperative cognitive recovery after remifentanil-propofol or sufentanil-propofol anaesthesia for supratentorial craniotomy: a randomized trial. *Eur J Anaesthesiol*. 2007;**24**:122–127.

75. Derrode N, Lebrun F, Levron JC, et al. Influence of peroperative opioid on postoperative pain after major abdominal surgery: Sufentanil TCI versus remifentanil TCI. A randomized, controlled study. *Br J Anaesth*. 2003;**91**:842–849.

76. Gepts E, Shafer SL, Camu F, et al. Linearity of pharmacokinetics and model estimation of sufentanil. *Anesthesiology*. 1995;**83**:1194–1204.

77. Hudson RJ, Bergstrom RG, Thomson IR, et al. Pharmacokinetics of sufentanil in patients undergoing abdominal aortic surgery. *Anesthesiology*. 1989;**70**:426–431.

78. Zhao Y, Zhang LP, Wu XM, et al. Clinical evaluation of target controlled infusion system for sufentanil administration. *Chin Med J (Engl)*. 2009 Oct 20;**122**:2503–2508.

79. Slepchenko G, Simon N, Goubaux B, et al. Performance of target-controlled sufentanil infusion in obese patients. *Anesthesiology*. 2003;**98**:65–73.

80. Peng PW, Sandler AN. A review of the use of fentanyl analgesia in the management of acute pain in adults. *Anesthesiology*. 1999;**90**:576–599.

81. Davis JJ, Swenson JD, Hall RH, et al. Preoperative "fentanyl challenge" as a tool to estimate postoperative opioid dosing in chronic opioid-consuming patients. *Anesth Analg*. 2005;**101**:389,95, table of contents.

82. Hammoud HA, Aymard G, Lechat P, et al. Relationships between plasma concentrations of morphine, morphine-3-glucuronide, morphine-6-glucuronide, and intravenous morphine titration outcomes in the postoperative period. *Fundam Clin Pharmacol.* 2011;25(4):518–527.

83. Rosow CE, Moss J, Philbin DM, et al. Histamine release during morphine and fentanyl anesthesia. *Anesthesiology.* 1982;**56**:93–96.

84. Claxton AR, McGuire G, Chung F, et al. Evaluation of morphine versus fentanyl for postoperative analgesia after ambulatory surgical procedures. *Anesth Analg.* 1997;**84**:509–514.

85. Dunbar PJ, Chapman CR, Buckley FP, Gavrin JR. Clinical analgesic equivalence for morphine and hydromorphone with prolonged PCA. *Pain.* 1996;68(2–3):265–270.

86. Gottschalk A, Durieux ME, Nemergut EC. Intraoperative methadone improves postoperative pain control in patients undergoing complex spine surgery. *Anesth Analg.* 2011 Jan;112(1): 218–223.

87. Kharasch ED. Intraoperative methadone: rediscovery, reappraisal, and reinvigoration? *Anesth Analg.* 2011;**112**:13–16.

88. Zhao P, Huang Y, Zuo Z. Opioid preconditioning induces opioid receptor-dependent delayed neuroprotection against ischemia in rats. *J Neuropathol Exp Neurol.* 2006;**65**:945–952.

89. Zhang Z, Chen TY, Kirsch JR, et al. Kappa-opioid receptor selectivity for ischemic neuroprotection with BRL 52537 in rats. *Anesth Analg.* 2003;**97**:1776–1783.

90. Chi OZ, Hunter C, Liu X, et al. Effects of fentanyl pretreatment on regional cerebral blood flow in focal cerebral ischemia in rats. *Pharmacology.* 2010;**85**:153–157.

91. Simons SH, van Dijk M, van Lingen RA, et al. Routine morphine infusion in preterm newborns who received ventilatory support: a randomized controlled trial. *JAMA.* 2003 Nov 12;**290**:2419–2427.

92. Cui J, Chen Q, Yu LC, et al. Chronic morphine application is protective against cell death in primary human neurons. *Neuroreport.* 2008;**19**:1745–1749.

93. Zhang Y, Chen Q, Yu LC. Morphine: A protective or destructive role in neurons? *Neuroscientist.* 2008;**14**:561–570.

94. Soonthon-Brant V, Patel PM, Drummond JC, et al. Fentanyl does not increase brain injury after focal cerebral ischemia in rats. *Anesth Analg.* 1999;**88**:49–55.

9.

INHALED ANESTHETICS

Ariane Rossi and Luzius A. Steiner

During neurosurgery the brain is particularly vulnerable to insults due to the surgical procedure itself as well as systemic insults and consequences of insufficient control of physiologic variables. The aim of intraoperative anesthetic management is to protect the brain as much as possible with the means available to the anesthesiologist. The goals of intraoperative management for neurosurgical patients are shown in Table 9.1.

Hemodynamic stability and adequate cerebral perfusion must be maintained. Arterial hypotension may decrease cerebral perfusion pressure (CPP), leading to cerebral ischemia. Arterial hypertension and excessive cerebral perfusion increase the risk of intracerebral hemorrhage and vasogenic cerebral edema. While cerebral blood flow (CBF) in patients without intracranial pathology is assumed to remain more or less constant over a wide range of arterial pressures, this may not be the case in neurosurgical patients. Autoregulatory dysfunction increases the brain's vulnerability to changes in systemic hemodynamics. Brain edema and intracranial hypertension not only may be detrimental because they will reduce CPP but also may make dissection difficult. Cerebral vasodilatation and increases in cerebral blood volume (CBV) will increase intracranial pressure (ICP), particularly when the brain's ability to compensate is impaired. Furthermore, changes in secretion and reabsorption of cerebrospinal fluid (CSF) or increases in the permeability of the blood–brain barrier (BBB) induced by anesthetics could theoretically also increase ICP. During some neurosurgical procedures, such as when temporary vascular clips are used, cerebral protection (i.e., pronounced suppression of the brain's electrical activity to a burst suppression pattern in the EEG) may be required. Rapid recovery at the end of the procedure is critical to allow neurologic assessment in the immediate postoperative period. Accordingly, the characteristics of the ideal anesthetic agent for neuroanesthesia include providing stability of systemic hemodynamics and cerebral perfusion, preventing rises in ICP and providing a slack brain for the surgeon, providing neuroprotection when required, and facilitating rapid recovery.

At a first glance, many of the characteristics of inhaled anesthetics seem to be incompatible with several of these criteria. Under clinical conditions, all inhaled anesthetic agents can increase CBV, CBF, and ICP due to their intrinsic vasodilating effects. There are, however, differences in potency regarding these effects, and in many cases inhaled anesthetics can be safely used for neuroanesthesia.

We will first consider the commonly used drugs halothane, isoflurane, sevoflurane, and desflurane as far as their characteristics as "ideal" agents for neurosurgical procedures are concerned and then address some of the particularities of nitrous oxide (N_2O) and xenon.

SYSTEMIC HEMODYNAMIC STABILITY

All inhaled anesthetics have similar effects on the cardiovascular system. Cardiac index declines most with halothane and less so with isoflurane, sevoflurane, or desflurane. Heart rate increases with all inhaled anesthetics. The increase is dose-dependent with isoflurane; desflurane and sevoflurane have a similar effect but only at high doses [1]. Halothane causes the most pronounced decrease in arterial blood pressure predominantly through myocardial depression. Isoflurane, sevoflurane and desflurane cause significant decreases in systemic vascular resistance. While these properties may seem to be less than optimal for neuroanesthesia, it is important to realize that intravenous anesthetics such as propofol also produce decreases in systemic vascular resistance and myocardial depression. Sevoflurane preserves myocardial function better than propofol and in patients without cardiovascular disease sevoflurane is superior to propofol in preserving left ventricular relaxation and maintaining estimated CPP [2].

CEREBROVASCULAR EFFECTS OF INHALED ANESTHETICS

Inhaled anesthetics produce a dose-related suppression of cerebral electrical activity and hence cerebral metabolism (see

Table 9.1 GOALS OF INTRAOPERATIVE MANAGEMENT IN NEUROSURGERY AND CHARACTERISTICS OF THE IDEAL ANESTHETIC FOR NEUROSURGICAL PROCEDURES

GOALS OF INTRAOPERATIVE MANAGEMENT IN NEUROANESTHESIA	IMPLICATION FOR THE IDEAL ANESTHETIC FOR NEUROSURGICAL PROCEDURES
Hemodynamic stability	Not negative inotrope, no decrease of systemic vascular resistance
Adequate cerebral perfusion	Does not disturb cerebrovascular autoregulation, CO_2 reactivity, or flow metabolism coupling
Low ICP	No cerebral vasodilatation, no increase in CBV, no increase in CSF secretion or decrease in CSF resorption, does not increase BBB permeability.
Cerebral protection	Burst suppression achievable at non-toxic concentrations
Rapid recovery	Low blood:gas partition coefficient for inhaled anesthetics or short half-life for intravenous anesthetics

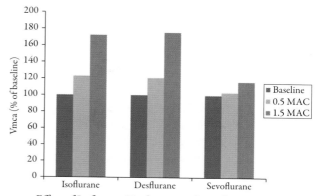

Figure 9.1 Effect of Isoflurane, Desflurane, and Sevoflurane on CBF. Vmca, flow velocity in the middle cerebral artery. The effect of sevoflurane on CBF (estimated by transcranial Doppler) even at 1.5 MAC is considerably lower than that of isoflurane or desflurane. (Based on Matta et al. [5, 6].)

later), which leads to a reduction in CBF as a result of the preserved flow–metabolism coupling [1–3]. However, all inhaled anesthetics also have a dose-dependent direct vasodilator effect on the cerebral vessels that increases CBV and CBF. The net effect results from the balance between these two mechanisms, entailing a decrease in CBF at low concentrations and an increase in CBV and CBF at high concentrations [3]. The changes in CBF induced by inhaled anesthetics are variable depending on the brain region [1, 4]. The vasoactive potency and consequently the end-tidal concentration above which CBF will increase differs from one anesthetic agent to the other. The vasodilatatory properties of halothane are much more pronounced than those of enflurane, which are in turn greater than those of desflurane and isoflurane. Sevoflurane is the inhaled anesthetic with the least vasodilator properties [3, 5]. At concentrations below 1 minimal alveolar concentration (MAC), sevoflurane has almost no effect on CBV and CBF [2] (Figure 9.1). In clinical practice, enflurane and halothane are no longer used in many countries.

The clinical question is whether the change in CBV or CBF increases ICP. Changes in CBF do not necessarily directly reflect changes in CBV. CBF and CBV are correlated, but the magnitude of variations in CBF is considerably greater than those in CBV. Halothane and enflurane are known to increase ICP at doses above 0.5 MAC and 1.5 MAC, respectively [3]. In contrast, isoflurane and desflurane increase CBF at concentrations of 1 MAC, but no change in ICP has been found in normocapnic patients undergoing removal of supratentorial brain tumors [7]. Sevoflurane does not increase ICP either [8], but these studies have mostly been performed in patients with preserved intracranial compensatory reserve (i.e., normal compliance). In patients with decreased intracranial compliance, the effects of inhaled anesthetics on ICP may be different.

Cerebral autoregulation is the homeostatic mechanism that keeps CBF relatively constant, despite changes in mean arterial pressure (MAP) or CPP, by changing the resistance of the precapillary arterial cerebral vasculature. The physiologic limits of this protective mechanism in healthy volunteers are assumed to be 60 to 160 mm Hg (MAP) or 50 to 150 mm Hg (CPP). Above or below these thresholds CBF varies directly with changes in pressure. Loss of cerebral autoregulation increases the risk of cerebral hypoperfusion in the setting of arterial hypotension or increases in CBV and ICP with rising MAP.

Cerebral vasodilators such as inhaled anesthetics impair the effectiveness of autoregulation. Inhaled anesthetics have a dose-dependent depressive effect on cerebral autoregulation; the agents that produce the most vasodilation have the greatest impact. At 1 MAC of desflurane, autoregulation is impaired, and it is nearly abolished at 1.5 MAC [9]. This effect is less pronounced with similar concentrations of isoflurane [10]. Low-dose isoflurane (0.5 MAC) delays but does not reduce the autoregulatory response. Higher concentrations (1.5 MAC) significantly impair cerebral autoregulation [10]. Sevoflurane seems to have a minimal impact on cerebral autoregulation at concentrations less than 1.5 MAC [11, 12], although some studies show a deterioration of dynamic autoregulation already at lower concentrations [2].

CO_2 reactivity (i.e., the ability to change the vascular diameter in response to changes in the arterial partial pressure of CO_2) is another important regulatory mechanism. Control of $PaCO_2$ is a very important means to control CBV and ICP in neurosurgical patients. CO_2 reactivity is a relatively robust mechanism compared with autoregulation. CO_2 reactivity seems to be preserved with all inhaled anesthetics in normal brain and at clinically used concentrations [3].

INHALED ANESTHETICS AND CEREBRAL METABOLISM

All volatile anesthetics suppress cerebral electrical activity and hence cerebral metabolism in a dose-related but not linear manner [13, 14]. The maximal reduction is reached when the EEG is completely suppressed (i.e., "flat"). At this point, cerebral metabolism is reduced to approximately 40% of the awake state. The remaining energy consumption is required for membrane and cell homeostasis, which is not affected by inhaled anesthetics. The metabolic rates for oxygen ($CMRo_2$) and glucose ($CMR_{glucose}$) are reduced variably depending on the brain region [4, 15]. Several studies [4, 15–18] have quantified the decrease in $CMRo_2$ and $CMR_{glucose}$ caused by inhaled anesthetics, but the results are quite variable. In summary, at 1 MAC, sevoflurane reduces $CMRo_2$ by 47% to 74% and $CMR_{glucose}$ by about 40%, isoflurane reduces $CMRo_2$ by 40% to 60% and $CMR_{glucose}$ by 43%, and desflurane reduces $CMRo_2$ by approximately 50% and $CMR_{glucose}$ in the order of 35%.

INHALED ANESTHETICS AND THE EEG

Volatile anesthetic agents influence the EEG activity in a dose-related manner; the changes are specific to each given agent [13, 14]. Sevoflurane, desflurane, and isoflurane cause similar changes in the EEG [13, 19], and MAC equivalent administration of these three inhaled anesthetics is associated with equipotent EEG suppression [14, 19, 20]. With increasing concentrations, the signal evolves from a low-voltage, fast-wave to a high-voltage, slow-wave pattern, to burst suppression [19] (Figure 9.2).

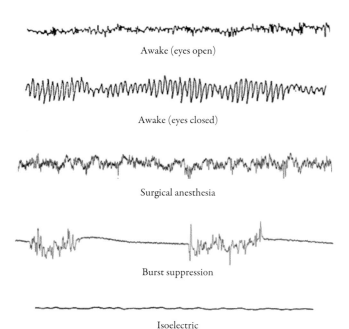

Figure 9.2   EEG Patterns Induced by Inhaled Anesthetics. With increasing concentrations of isoflurane, desflurane, or sevoflurane, an increase in the slow delta and theta range and a decrease in the fast beta and alpha domain are seen on the EEG. At higher concentrations burst suppression and finally an isoelectric EEG is observed.   (Based on EEG tracings from Kroeger [21], Metrowestneurofeedback [22], and Ferron [23].)

All three agents increase the slow delta and theta waves and decrease the fast beta and alpha waves [13], and all produce burst suppression patterns. In contrast, halothane does not produce burst suppression at clinically relevant concentrations. Neither desflurane nor isoflurane causes epileptic activity at any concentration [14]; sevoflurane can produce epileptiform waves, especially in children and at high concentrations [24]. However, although sevoflurane may be associated with cortical epileptiform EEG patterns, these are usually not clinically significant under most circumstances and do not limit the usefulness of sevoflurane in neuroanesthesia [24]. In contrast, enflurane, which is not commonly used in clinical practice, should be avoided in neurosurgical patients because of its potentially proconvulsant effects. Below 0.7 MAC, enflurane produces slowing and increasing amplitude of the EEG, as is seen with the other inhaled anesthetic agents as a result of cortical depression [25]. At higher concentrations, however, enflurane induces paroxysmal epileptiform discharges that may occasionally progress to generalized seizure activity [26].

The reproducible EEG changes induced by inhaled anesthetics allow monitoring of anesthetic depth. While a recent study shows that anesthesiologists may indeed be able to judge anesthetic depth on a frontal EEG [27], it is often assumed that the standard EEG is too complex for real-time intraoperative monitoring of anesthetic depth. Therefore, several devices have been developed that estimate anesthetic depth using processed EEG: the bispectral index (BIS), entropy, the Patient State Index (PSI™), and the Narcotrend™. The topographic distribution of cerebral electrical activity changes between the awake state and anesthesia [28] and the BIS was designed to detect anesthetic-induced frontal alterations in EEG, and it has recently been shown that BIS values obtained from occipitally positioned electrodes cannot be used interchangeably with values obtained from frontal electrodes [29].

EFFECTS OF INHALED ANESTHETICS ON CEREBROSPINAL FLUID AND THE BBB

Numerous studies have been conducted in animals to explore the effects of the various inhaled anesthetics on secretion and reabsorption of CSF, which are summarized in Table 9.2.

The balance between CSF secretion and reabsorption may affect ICP. In theory, in a patient with poor intracranial compliance, enflurane and perhaps desflurane should be avoided, but there are no clinical data to support this hypothesis. Even if sevoflurane does not seem to influence the secretion and reabsorption of CSF in rabbits [36], it has been suspected to increase CSF pressure in humans [37, 38], as do desflurane and isoflurane [39]. However, this effect was interpreted to be secondary to the changes in

Table 9.2 EFFECTS OF INHALED ANESTHETICS ON SECRETION AND REABSORPTION OF CSF

ANESTHETIC AGENT	CSF SECRETION	CSF REABSORPTION
Halothane	↓	↓
Enflurane	↑	↓
Isoflurane	No effect	↑
Desflurane	↑	No effect
Sevoflurane	No effect	No effect

Based on References 30 to 36.

CBV discussed earlier rather than changes in CSF secretion and reabsorption.

Investigations regarding the effects of volatile anesthetics on the BBB have been performed in animals [40–42] and in in vitro models [43]. To the best of our knowledge, no studies have been performed in humans, not all inhaled agents have been tested in vivo, and the available data are conflicting. Under normotensive conditions, one study has concluded that isoflurane increases the permeability of the BBB at high concentrations [40], but another study had opposite findings [41]. An older study has suggested that in contrast to thiopental, halothane enhances the extravasation of plasma proteins into the normal brain during acute extreme hypertension in rabbits [42]. Fischer and colleagues [43] have tested the effect of halothane, enflurane, isoflurane, desflurane, and sevoflurane at very high concentrations (4 MAC) on cultures of porcine brain microvascular endothelial cells without finding any effect on the permeability of the BBB. In summary, there is no certain evidence that volatile anesthetics posses intrinsic properties that affect the BBB.

MECHANISMS OF ACTION AND NEUROPROTECTIVE AND NEUROTOXIC EFFECTS

The specific mechanism of action of inhaled anesthetics remains unclear and is the focus of numerous research studies. It is known that inhaled anesthetics have agonist effects on GABA and glycine receptors, both of which are inhibitory neurotransmitters. Inhaled anesthetics also exert antagonist effects on neuronal nicotinic acetylcholine receptors, glutamate receptors, and voltage-activated potassium, sodium, and calcium channels. The anesthetic effect is most likely due to the effects of these drugs on one or more of these receptors [44].

The volatile anesthetics seem to have both protective and toxic effects on the central nervous system. These effects are mediated by different mechanisms, depending on the exposure time and concentration that is delivered. Almost all data are based on in vitro or animal models, which are often difficult to compare because of the multitude of models, methods, and outcomes that are used.

NEUROPROTECTION

It has long been assumed that because volatile anesthetics suppress cerebral metabolic demand, they should improve neuronal survival during periods of cerebral ischemia. The rationale for this effect is that reducing cerebral electrical activity conserves energy that may then be used for basal neuronal metabolism [45]. Even though current clinical practice is based on this concept, the mechanisms involved in neuroprotection are far more complex. There are several theories about whether and how neuroprotection occurs, all of which are based on the pathophysiology of cerebral ischemia [45]. They include blocking the release of excitatory neurotransmitters such as glutamate and aspartate by presynaptic neurons, enhancing the release of inhibitory neurotransmitters such as GABA, inhibiting the postsynaptic neurons activated by glutamate and aspartate, blocking of calcium influx into neurons, up-regulation of antiapoptotic factors such as MAP kinases, inhibition of lipid peroxidation, reduction of inflammatory cytokines, decreasing free radicals, and augmentation of peri-ischemic CBF [46].

Ischemic neuronal injury is characterized by early cell death mediated by excitotoxicity (i.e., excessive stimulation of postsynaptic glutamate NMDA and AMPA receptors and by delayed death caused by apoptosis). Halothane [47], desflurane [48], sevoflurane [47], and isoflurane [49] may protect neurons against excitotoxicity early during an ischemic episode. It has been shown that halothane antagonizes NMDA mediated excitotoxicity [50] and that isoflurane reduces excitotoxicity mediated by NMDA [51] and AMPA [52] receptors. Isoflurane mediated neuroprotection seems to also involve GABA$_A$ receptors [53]. The neuroprotective effect of desflurane in rat models seems to be greater than that conferred by halothane [48, 54]. In contrast, some data suggest that neuroprotection produced by isoflurane and desflurane could be related to a reduction in sympathetic activity rather than a decrease in the cerebral metabolic rate or modulation of glutamate metabolism [55].

There are conflicting explanations for the effects of inhaled anesthetics on apoptosis. In in vitro models, desflurane and sevoflurane lead to a significant reduction of neuronal cell death caused by oxygen-glucose deprivation, regardless of the concentrations to which the neurons are exposed [54, 56], suggesting that these drugs may also offer protection from neuronal apoptosis. Other studies suggest that neuroprotection may be sustained if the ischemic insult is relatively mild but that in the setting of moderate to severe insults, neuronal protection is not sustained, which suggests that volatile agents do not reduce delayed neuronal death caused by apoptosis [57]. A recent study concluded that sevoflurane may offer long-term neuroprotection [58], but this seems not to be the case for isoflurane [59, 60].

Enflurane has been observed to have limited effects in vitro, and no animal studies have been performed evaluating its neuroprotective potential [61].

The benefits of preconditioning with inhaled anesthetics may extend to the brain [62]. Prior exposure to halothane, desflurane, isoflurane, and sevoflurane seems to induce neuroprotection in a concentration-dependent manner [54], possibly by modification of glutamate transporter activity [63].

At the present time, there are no studies that offer a direct comparison of cerebral protection between the various volatile anesthetics [46]. It is, therefore, impossible to recommend a specific inhaled anesthetic as the best neuroprotective agent in neurosurgical patients.

NEUROTOXICITY

Multiple in vitro and in vivo animal studies have been performed to evaluate potential neurotoxic effects of inhaled anesthetics [64, 65], but there are few human studies and it is difficult to extrapolate the data that do exist to humans.

Eckenhoff and colleagues [66] have found that halothane and isoflurane enhanced in vitro amyloid beta peptide oligomerization and cytotoxicity, a process that is also implicated in the pathogenesis of Alzheimer's disease. In a further in vitro study, sevoflurane induced apoptosis and increased beta-amyloid protein levels [67]. The same was shown for clinically relevant concentrations of desflurane [68]. In vivo studies in animals have shown the importance of the stage of brain development on potential neurotoxicity. Immature and senescent brains seem to be more vulnerable. For example, blockade of NMDA receptors caused excessive neuronal apoptosis in neonate rats [69]. Potentiation of $GABA_A$ receptors had the same neurodegenerative effects in the developing brain. Depolarization and excitation were observed instead of inhibition of neurons [70]. In contrast, sevoflurane did not seem to generate apoptotic neurodegeneration in the developing animal brain [71, 72]. These studies triggered a debate in pediatric anesthesia [73] because such neurodegenerative changes have been associated with learning disability and delayed behavioral development in animals [65, 74]. In contrast,

the relationship between the density of amyloid plaques and cognitive impairment is less clear. An in vivo study [75] exposing mice to halothane and isoflurane anesthesia could not confirm a relationship between the density of amyloid plaques and cognitive impairment. A study investigating a large cohort of monozygotic twins aged 3 to 12 who were exposed to anesthesia, not necessarily to inhaled anesthetics, found no evidence for a causal relationship between anesthesia and later learning-related outcomes [76]. At the present time, there is no proven relationship in humans between general anesthesia, particularly inhaled anesthetics, and postoperative cognitive dysfunction or Alzheimer's disease [77–79].

Several studies have shown that inhaled anesthetics induce modulations in gene expression in animal brains [64, 80, 81], which has direct effects on the synthesized proteins coded by these genes [82]. These changes have not only been seen during or immediately following anesthesia but also seem to persist after the anesthetics should have been completely eliminated [83]. However, it remains unclear if these considerations are applicable to humans, whether the effect would be neuroprotective or neurotoxic, or if this effect has any clinical significance.

In summary, there is ample evidence that inhaled anesthetics may cause long-lasting changes in the brain, but intravenous anesthetics may also have similar effects. Currently, there is insufficient evidence that would justify changing clinical practice [84].

RECOVERY FROM ANESTHESIA

Rapid recovery from anesthesia is essential in neuroanesthesia because it is important to obtain a neurologic assessment soon after surgery and also because a depressed level of consciousness is the most consistent clinical presentation of postoperative intracranial hematoma [85]. The blood:gas partition coefficient is an important factor in the speed of onset and recovery from inhaled anesthetics: the lower this coefficient, the faster is recovery (Table 9.3). A systematic review comparing the recovery profiles of isoflurane, sevoflurane, and desflurane after ambulatory surgery

Table 9.3 **BLOOD:GAS PARTITION COEFFICIENTS, EMERGENCE AND RECOVERY TIMES OF SOME VOLATILE ANESTHETICS**

ANESTHETIC AGENT	BLOOD:GAS PARTITION COEFFICIENT	EMERGENCE (MIN)	EARLY RECOVERY (MIN)
Halothane	2.3	10 ± 4	21 ± 8
Isoflurane	1.4	9 ± 3	11 ± 3
Desflurane	0.42	5 ± 3	9 ± 5
Sevoflurane	0.65	7 ± 3	11 ± 5

Emergence: time to extubation, early recovery: eye opening and obeying simple commands.

Based on data from References 1, 87, and 88. Data are not available for all inhaled anesthetics.

[86] concluded that emergence (i.e., time to extubation), and early recovery characterized by eye opening and obeying simple commands are more rapidly achieved after desflurane than after sevoflurane, which in turn allows faster emergence than isoflurane.

There were also small differences in late recovery (defined as "home readiness") between the drugs, but these were most likely of minimal clinical significance. A limitation of many studies on this topic is that volatile anesthetics are rarely used alone in daily clinical practice. The use of concomitant medication, especially opioids and benzodiazepines, has a significant effect on emergence and recovery times [89]. Several studies have compared the characteristics of recovery between inhaled anesthetics mainly sevoflurane in the more recent publications and propofol, with conflicting results [2, 86]. However, even if some of the reported the differences are statistically significant, they are probably clinically irrelevant. Some studies have suggested that monitoring of anesthetic depth may accelerate early recovery [90–92] because this allows more precise titration of anesthetic agents, but this remains controversial.

CLINICAL CONSIDERATIONS

Modern inhalational agents can be used safely for most neurosurgical procedures, including craniotomies, but some specific aspects need to be considered. Arterial $PaCO_2$ should be kept in the normal to moderately low range throughout the procedure in patients with space occupying lesions. In most of these patients, inhalation induction or maintenance of spontaneous ventilation during the procedure should be avoided, with the possible exception of those pediatric patients, in whom insertion of an intravenous catheter is impossible while awake. Furthermore, the excitation that may occur during inhalational induction is undesirable as it may increase ICP. Anesthesia in patients undergoing craniotomy is typically induced with a rapid-acting intravenous agent.

High concentrations of the volatile anesthetics may cause cerebral vasodilatation and loss of autoregulation, so a combination of a volatile agent and an opioid is typically used during the maintenance phase to avoid inhaled concentrations above 1 MAC. Sevoflurane at a concentration below 1 MAC should have only a minimal impact on intracranial hemodynamics. Should a period of burst suppression be required during the procedure (e.g., during placement of a temporary vascular clip), it would theoretically be possible to increase the concentration of the inhaled anesthetic. In dogs, 2.17 and 2.14 MAC of isoflurane and sevoflurane, respectively, are required to achieve burst suppression [93]. Because of the cerebral vasodilation that occurs at such concentrations, however, an intravenous anesthetic such as propofol is typically used for this purpose.

During emergence from volatile anesthetics, a phase of excitation, which may include coughing and fighting the ventilator, should be avoided as it will always increase ICP. One potential solution is to remove the endotracheal tube very early during emergence, but this is contraindicated in many patients because of concerns regarding airway patency and protection and also because control of arterial CO_2 is lost. Alternatively, using a short-acting opioid such as remifentanil at a relatively high dose until the end of the procedure will greatly improve the patient's ability to tolerate the endotracheal tube and allow extubation of a patient who is awake but not coughing. Alternatively, reversal of opioid effects with naloxone is an option if longer acting opioids are used. If coughing does occur during emergence and immediate extubation is not possible, intravenous lidocaine (1 mg/kg) may be used to treat coughing.

The physiology of the spinal cord is similar to that of the brain in terms of CO_2 reactivity, autoregulation, and a high metabolic rate and blood flow have been documented. The gray matter of the spinal cord is particularly vulnerable to ischemia. There is also a mechanism similar to that of the BBB. However, measures to reduce spinal cord swelling are rarely used. During surgery of the spinal cord, evoked potentials are often monitored, and the choice of anesthetic agent can have significant effects on the ability to record responses to stimulation. Most often, somatosensory evoked potentials (SSEPs) are monitored. SSEPs are recorded after electric stimulation of a peripheral mixed nerve—typically, the median nerve and the posterior tibial nerve. Despite the fact that SSEPs primarily monitor the integrity of the sensory components of the spinal cord, the very low incidence of postoperative paraplegia on awakening without any intraoperative changes in SSEPs suggests that to some extent motor pathways are also monitored. If specific monitoring of motor pathways is desired, motor evoked potentials (MEPs) evoked by transcranial electric or magnetic stimulation are typically used. Sevoflurane and isoflurane increase the latency of SSEPs and depress MEPs in a dose-dependent manner and should therefore be avoided in these patients [2]. During MEP monitoring, neuromuscular blockers cannot be used. If no electrophysiologic monitoring is planned, inhaled anesthetics can be safely used in spinal surgery. As in intracranial surgery, the important point is to be aware of the general goals of neuroanesthesia (Table 9.1) rather than to focus on the question of inhalational versus intravenous anesthesia.

NITROUS OXIDE

N_2O has played an important role in the history of anesthesia since the 19th century, when its anesthetic, analgesic, and amnesic properties were first recognized [94] N_2O does not seem to be carcinogenic, but it is possibly teratogenic. Although exposure to higher doses for less than 6 hours is generally considered to be harmless, prolonged exposure to N_2O has known toxic effects: it oxidizes vitamin B12 and inactivates methionine synthase. Both ultimately lead to a clinical syndrome including megaloblastic anemia and neurotoxicity. N_2O may also be involved in the development of hyperhomocysteinemia [95].

N_2O has negligible effects on $GABA_A$ receptors but significantly inhibits postsynaptic glutaminergic transmission via NMDA glutamate receptor blockade [96]. It also produces sympathomimetic effects [96, 97]. N_2O has a very low potency (MAC 104%). It is not suitable for use as a sole anesthetic but is typically used in combination with other inhalational or intravenous agents [98].

N_2O increases CBF partly as a consequence of its sympathoadrenergic stimulating effect, without significant changes in CBV [99]. Inhalation of 50% to 70% N_2O will increase CBF by about 20% [100], but considerable variations in the magnitude of this effect are seen, depending on the presence or absence of other anesthetic drugs. The administration of N_2O alone can cause substantial significant increase in CBF and ICP, while using N_2O in combination with an inhaled anesthetic produces a moderate increase in CBF and cerebral metabolism [4]. The N_2O-induced vasodilatation seems to be correlated with the concentration of the other inhaled drug [101]. Conversely, the cerebral vasodilating effect of N_2O is attenuated or even completely inhibited when it is administered in combination with intravenous drugs, including barbiturates, benzodiazepines, opioids, and propofol, although not all anesthetics have been evaluated and the dose–response relationships are not well defined. There are conflicting data on the effects of N_2O on cerebrovascular autoregulation and CO_2 reactivity [98], but the CBF response to CO_2 seems to be preserved [102]. Although some of the data are contradictory [103, 104], N_2O also seems to increase CMR, especially $CMRo_2$ [4] without a strict correlation with the variation of CBF.

Administration of N_2O initially leads to decreases in frequency and amplitude of alpha activity and, in a second phase with the occurrence of analgesia and depressed consciousness, to increases in beta range activity [96]. Administration of N_2O alone or adding it to a fentanyl-midazolam anesthetic [105] or a propofol-remifentanil anesthetic did not change the BIS in one study [106]. In another study, increases in BIS were observed when N_2O was added to isoflurane [107]. Another small study found that the BIS decreased when N_2O was used in combination with volatile aesthetics [108]. As the data are contradictory, it is probably prudent not to rely on BIS monitoring when N_2O is used.

Some older animal studies suggest that N_2O might exacerbate ischemic brain injury or attenuate the neuroprotective effects of other anesthetics [109, 110]. Moreover, prolonged anesthesia with N_2O seems to induce inflammation of the cerebral microcirculation and the brain [111]. In contrast, some recent research suggests that N_2O might

have neuroprotective properties, when used at concentrations up to 75% [112]. A recent study in humans [113] has shown that N_2O does not have any detrimental or beneficial effect on neurologic or neuropsychological outcomes in a population of patients at risk for ischemic brain damage.

Many anesthesiologists consider N_2O to be unsuitable for neuroanesthesia primarily because of its effects on cerebral hemodynamics. The cerebral vasodilatation caused by N_2O can be significant in neurosurgical patients with reduced intracranial compliance. N_2O quickly enters a closed gas space and may potentially produce a pneumocranium in the presence of a closed intracranial gas space. It has also been proposed that using N_2O during procedures involving breach of the dura mater could facilitate the occurrence of a tension pneumocephalus after dural closure [98], but one randomized study has disproved this theory [114]. In contrast, N_2O facilitates rapid emergence and recovery from anesthesia, allowing early neurologic assessment after surgery [98]. N_2O seems to cause more postoperative nausea and vomiting (PONV) than other volatile anesthetics, but primarily in patients who are already at a high risk for PONV [115]. In neurosurgical patients vomiting may increase intracranial pressure (ICP) transiently and N_2O-associated PONV could be mistaken for nausea and vomiting due to neurogenic causes [98]. Even if the neurotoxic or neuroprotective potential of N_2O is controversial, and avoidance of N_2O in specific circumstances is warranted, it has been widely used in neurosurgery, and according to the accumulated experience, there is no reason to completely avoid it in neurosurgical patients.

XENON

Xenon is a noble gas and is the only inert gas that has anesthetic and analgesic properties under normobaric conditions. Several animal studies have shown that xenon has no mutagenic, carcinogenic, embryotoxic, or teratogenic properties. It is not allergenic and it does not trigger malignant hyperthermia [116, 117].

Although its mechanism of action has not been fully elucidated, it has been shown that the anesthetic effects of xenon are primarily mediated by noncompetitive inhibition of postsynaptic NMDA receptors, with a minor effect on $GABA_A$ receptors or non-NMDA glutamatergic receptors [118]. Other studies have established that xenon has noncompetitive and voltage-independent inhibitory actions at the nicotinic acetylcholine receptors and competitively blocks the $5\text{-}HT_{3A}$ receptor [116]. Xenon has little or no presynaptic effect. The MAC of xenon was first estimated to be 71%, but more recent investigations have established it to be 63% in humans [119]. Its MAC seems to be sex- and age-dependent, a value of 51% having been determined in elderly women [120].

Effects of xenon on CBF are controversial. Some studies suggest that xenon increases CBF in the first 5 minutes of exposure, but this effect appears to decrease after the initial effect [117]. Other animal studies report no changes in CBF at all [121]. Yet, a recent study in humans showed increases and decreases in CBF depending on the cerebral region [122]. Despite changes in CBF, CO_2 reactivity is maintained and hyperventilation can reverse the changes in CBF [117]. Cerebrovascular autoregulation remains unaffected [123, 124]. Animal data have shown that ICP is not increased by xenon administration at 0.3 and 0.7 MAC regardless of whether intracranial hypertension is present [117, 125]. Other investigations have shown clinically significant increases in ICP and reduction in CPP, albeit without an increase in cerebral arteriovenous oxygen content differences, which would be indicative of cerebral oligemia or ischemia [117, 126]. Further research is required to define the effect of xenon on cerebral metabolism. Some studies do not show any significant changes in metabolism [127], whereas others suggest that xenon reduces $CMR_{glucose}$ and fluctuations in cerebral arteriovenous oxygen content difference [116, 126].

Xenon induces EEG changes that are similar to those of N_2O [117]. At lower concentrations alpha waves are attenuated. At higher concentrations, slow and synchronized waveforms in the delta and theta range without burst suppression are observed [116, 128]. The effect of xenon anesthesia on BIS monitoring has not yet been clarified. Initially, it was thought, that the anesthetic effect of xenon was not reflected by the BIS because of the NMDA antagonism, which is known to have the opposite effect on EEG and BIS than GABAergic anesthetics [117]. However, a recent study has shown the contrary [129].

Xenon has putative dose-dependent neuroprotective effects [130, 131] because of its inhibition of the excitatory NMDA pathway, but there is currently only limited data in adult subjects. The neuronal and glial cell damage in cerebral cortex of mice after NMDA or glutamate application or after oxygen deprivation is reduced by xenon [131]. Xenon can reduce both functional and histologic ischemic cerebral injury [116, 132]. Moreover, xenon preconditioning seems to decrease the vulnerability of the brain to ischemic injury and significantly reduces infarction size [133]. However, a possible neurotoxic effect of xenon at higher concentrations cannot be excluded [116].

Although the use of xenon in neurosurgical patients has not been evaluated, many of its characteristics could make xenon an attractive substance for neuroanesthesia. Because of its low blood:gas partition coefficient of 0.12 (sevoflurane 0.65), xenon allows extremely short induction and emergence times, 2 to 3 times faster than any other inhalational anesthetic or propofol [134, 135]. Furthermore, prolonged xenon anesthesia does not lengthen the emergence time [117]. Although recovery from xenon anesthesia is more rapid, no significant differences in postoperative cognitive function have been found in patients exposed to xenon compared with desflurane [136]. Xenon can diffuse into air-containing spaces such as the bowel, although this occurs to less of an extent than with N_2O [137]. Nevertheless, in patients with intracranial air, xenon should be used with caution. Characteristics that have a negative impact on a widespread use of xenon are its high price (1 L currently costs approximately US$10) and the limited number of ventilators able to deliver this gas as closed circuits and recycling systems are required.

CONCLUSION

In neuroanesthesia, the choice of anesthetic agents is most likely less important than a very carefully conducted anesthetic. Neuroanesthesia can be safely performed with modern inhaled anesthetics, provided agent-specific dose ranges are not exceeded. Isoflurane and sevoflurane are less prone to increase CBV and to disturb cerebrovascular autoregulation than is desflurane. Sevoflurane allows faster emergence than does isoflurane and is, in our opinion, the agent of choice if inhaled anesthetics are to be used. For spinal surgery, inhaled anesthetics can also be used safely as long as they do not interfere with electrophysiologic spinal cord monitoring.

REFERENCES

1. Preckel B, Bolten J. Pharmacology of modern volatile anaesthetics. *Best Pract Res Clin Anaesthesiol*. 2005;19:331–348.
2. Engelhard K, Werner C. Inhalational or intravenous anesthetics for craniotomies? Pro inhalational. *Curr Opin Anaesthesiol*. 2006;19:504–508.
3. Sloan TB. Anesthetics and the brain. *Anesthesiol Clin North America*. 2002;20:265–292.
4. Kaisti KK, Langsjo JW, Aalto S, et al. Effects of sevoflurane, propofol, and adjunct nitrous oxide on regional cerebral blood flow, oxygen consumption, and blood volume in humans. *Anesthesiology*. 2003;99:603–613.
5. Matta BF, Heath KJ, Tipping K, et al. Direct cerebral vasodilatory effects of sevoflurane and isoflurane. *Anesthesiology*. 1999;91:677–680.
6. Matta BF, Mayberg TS, Lam AM. Direct cerebrovasodilatory effects of halothane, isoflurane, and desflurane during propofol-induced isoelectric electroencephalogram in humans. *Anesthesiology*. 1995;83:980–985; discussion 927A.
7. Fraga M, Rama-Maceiras P, Rodino S, et al. The effects of isoflurane and desflurane on intracranial pressure, cerebral perfusion pressure, and cerebral arteriovenous oxygen content difference in normocapnic patients with supratentorial brain tumors. *Anesthesiology*. 2003;98:1085–1090.
8. Bundgaard H, von Oettingen G, Larsen KM, et al. Effects of sevoflurane on intracranial pressure, cerebral blood flow and cerebral metabolism. A dose-response study in patients subjected to craniotomy for cerebral tumours. *Acta Anaesthesiol Scand*. 1998;42:621–627.
9. Bedforth NM, Girling KJ, Skinner HJ, et al. Effects of desflurane on cerebral autoregulation. *Br J Anaesth*. 2001;87:193–197.
10. Strebel S, Lam AM, Matta B, et al. Dynamic and static cerebral autoregulation during isoflurane, desflurane, and propofol anesthesia. *Anesthesiology*. 1995;83:66–76.

11. Duffy CM, Matta BF. Sevoflurane and anesthesia for neurosurgery: a review. *J Neurosurg Anesthesiol*. 2000;12:128–140.
12. Gupta S, Heath K, Matta BF. Effect of incremental doses of sevoflurane on cerebral pressure autoregulation in humans. *Br J Anaesth*. 1997;79:469–472.
13. Freye E, Bruckner J, Latasch L. No difference in electroencephalographic power spectra or sensory-evoked potentials in patients anaesthetized with desflurane or sevoflurane. *Eur J Anaesthesiol*. 2004;21:373–378.
14. Rampil IJ, Lockhart SH, Eger EI 2nd, et al. The electroencephalographic effects of desflurane in humans. *Anesthesiology*. 1991;74:434–439.
15. Lenz C, Rebel A, van Ackern K, et al. Local cerebral blood flow, local cerebral glucose utilization, and flow-metabolism coupling during sevoflurane versus isoflurane anesthesia in rats. *Anesthesiology*. 1998;89:1480–1488.
16. Mielck F, Stephan H, Weyland A, et al. Effects of one minimum alveolar anesthetic concentration sevoflurane on cerebral metabolism, blood flow, and CO_2 reactivity in cardiac patients. *Anesth Analg*. 1999;89:364–369.
17. Mielck F, Stephan H, Buhre W, et al. Effects of 1 MAC desflurane on cerebral metabolism, blood flow and carbon dioxide reactivity in humans. *Br J Anaesth*. 1998;81:155–160.
18. Alkire MT, Haier RJ, Shah NK, et al. Positron emission tomography study of regional cerebral metabolism in humans during isoflurane anesthesia. *Anesthesiology*. 1997;86:549–557.
19. Schwender D, Daunderer M, Klasing S, et al. Power spectral analysis of the electroencephalogram during increasing end-expiratory concentrations of isoflurane, desflurane and sevoflurane. *Anaesthesia*. 1998;53:335–342.
20. Rehberg B, Bouillon T, Zinserling J, et al. Comparative pharmacodynamic modeling of the electroencephalography-slowing effect of isoflurane, sevoflurane, and desflurane. *Anesthesiology*. 1999;91:397–405.
21. Kroeger D: http://archimede.bibl.ulaval.ca/archimede/fichiers/25863/ch05.html
22. Metrowestneurofeedback: http://www.metrowestneurofeedback.com/index.php?page=faq&PHPSESSID=d54732beed6cdaf5955a28feee0bdc17
23. Ferron JF:http://archimede.bibl.ulaval.ca/archimede/fichiers/25863/ch03.html
24. Constant I, Seeman R, Murat I. Sevoflurane and epileptiform EEG changes. *Paediatr Anaesth*. 2005;15:266–274.
25. Jameson LC, Sloan TB. Using EEG to monitor anesthesia drug effects during surgery. *J Clin Monit Comput*. 2006;20:445–472.
26. Sleigh JW, Vizuete JA, Voss L, et al. The electrocortical effects of enflurane: experiment and theory. *Anesth Analg*. 2009;109:1253–1262.
27. Bottros MM, Palanca BJ, Mashour GA, et al. Estimation of the bispectral index by anesthesiologists: an inverse turing test. *Anesthesiology*. 2011 May;114:1093–1101.
28. Scherer GB, Mihaljevic VG, Heinrichs MA, et al. Differences in the topographical distribution of EEG activity during surgical anaesthesia and on emergence from volatile anesthetics. *Int J Clin Monit Comput*. 1994;11:179–183.
29. Dahaba AA, Xue JX, Zhao GG, et al. BIS-vista occipital montage in patients undergoing neurosurgical procedures during propofol-remifentanil anesthesia. *Anesthesiology*. 2010;112:645–651.
30. Artru AA. Effects of halothane and fentanyl on the rate of CSF production in dogs. *Anesth Analg*. 1983;62:581–585.
31. Artru AA. Effects of enflurane and isoflurane on resistance to reabsorption of cerebrospinal fluid in dogs. *Anesthesiology*. 1984;61:529–533.
32. Artru AA. Isoflurane does not increase the rate of CSF production in the dog. *Anesthesiology*. 1984;60:193–197.
33. Artru AA. Effects of halothane and fentanyl anesthesia on resistance to reabsorption of CSF. *J Neurosurg*. 1984;60:252–256.
34. Artru AA. Concentration-related changes in the rate of CSF formation and resistance to reabsorption of CSF during enflurane and isoflurane anesthesia in dogs receiving nitrous oxide. *J Neurosurg Anesthesiol*. 1989;1:256–262.
35. Artru AA. Rate of cerebrospinal fluid formation, resistance to reabsorption of cerebrospinal fluid, brain tissue water content, and electroencephalogram during desflurane anesthesia in dogs. *J Neurosurg Anesthesiol*. 1993;5:178–186.
36. Artru AA, Momota T. Rate of CSF formation and resistance to reabsorption of CSF during sevoflurane or remifentanil in rabbits. *J Neurosurg Anesthesiol*. 2000;12:37–43.
37. Liao R, Li J, Liu J. Volatile induction/maintenance of anaesthesia with sevoflurane increases jugular venous oxygen saturation and lumbar cerebrospinal fluid pressure in patients undergoing craniotomy. *Eur J Anaesthesiol*. 2010;27:369–376.
38. Talke P, Caldwell JE, Richardson CA. Sevoflurane increases lumbar cerebrospinal fluid pressure in normocapnic patients undergoing transsphenoidal hypophysectomy. *Anesthesiology*. 1999;91:127–130.
39. Talke P, Caldwell J, Dodsont B, et al. Desflurane and isoflurane increase lumbar cerebrospinal fluid pressure in normocapnic patients undergoing transsphenoidal hypophysectomy. *Anesthesiology*. 1996;85:999–1004.
40. Tetrault S, Chever O, Sik A, et al. Opening of the blood-brain barrier during isoflurane anaesthesia. *Eur J Neurosci*. 2008;28:1330–1341.
41. Chi OZ, Anwar M, Sinha AK, et al. Effects of isoflurane on transport across the blood-brain barrier. *Anesthesiology*. 1992;76:426–431.
42. Forster A, Van Horn K, Marshall LF, et al. Anesthetic effects on blood-brain barrier function during acute arterial hypertension. *Anesthesiology*. 1978;49:26–30.
43. Fischer S, Renz D, Kleinstuck J, et al. [In vitro effects of anaesthetic agents on the blood-brain barrier]. *Anaesthesist*. 2004;53:1177–1184.
44. Stachnik J. Inhaled anesthetic agents. *Am J Health Syst Pharm*. 2006;63:623–634.
45. Baughman VL. Brain protection during neurosurgery. *Anesthesiol Clin North America*. 2002;20:315–327, vi.
46. Matchett GA, Allard MW, Martin RD, et al. Neuroprotective effect of volatile anesthetic agents: molecular mechanisms. *Neurol Res*. 2009;31:128–134.
47. Warner DS, McFarlane C, Todd MM, et al. Sevoflurane and halothane reduce focal ischemic brain damage in the rat. Possible influence on thermoregulation. *Anesthesiology*. 1993;79:985–992.
48. Haelewyn B, Yvon A, Hanouz JL, et al. Desflurane affords greater protection than halothane against focal cerebral ischaemia in the rat. *Br J Anaesth*. 2003;91:390–396.
49. Soonthon-Brant V, Patel PM, Drummond JC, et al. Fentanyl does not increase brain injury after focal cerebral ischemia in rats. *Anesth Analg*. 1999;88:49–55.
50. Beirne JP, Pearlstein RD, Massey GW, et al. Effect of halothane in cortical cell cultures exposed to N-methyl-D-aspartate. *Neurochem Res*. 1998;23:17–23.
51. Harada H, Kelly PJ, Cole DJ, et al. Isoflurane reduces N-methyl-D-aspartate toxicity in vivo in the rat cerebral cortex. *Anesth Analg*. 1999;89:1442–1447.
52. Kimbro JR, Kelly PJ, Drummond JC, et al. Isoflurane and pentobarbital reduce AMPA toxicity in vivo in the rat cerebral cortex. *Anesthesiology*. 2000;92:806–812.
53. Bickler PE, Warner DS, Stratmann G, et al. gamma-Aminobutyric acid-A receptors contribute to isoflurane neuroprotection in organotypic hippocampal cultures. *Anesth Analg*. 2003;97:564–571, table of contents.
54. Schifilliti D, Grasso G, Conti A, et al. Anaesthetic-related neuroprotection: intravenous or inhalational agents? *CNS Drugs*. 2010;24:893–907.
55. Engelhard K, Werner C, Reeker W, et al. Desflurane and isoflurane improve neurological outcome after incomplete cerebral ischaemia in rats. *Br J Anaesth*. 1999;83:415–421.
56. Wise-Faberowski L, Raizada MK, Sumners C. Desflurane and sevoflurane attenuate oxygen and glucose deprivation-induced neuronal cell death. *J Neurosurg Anesthesiol*. 2003;15:193–199.

57. Kawaguchi M, Furuya H, Patel PM. Neuroprotective effects of anesthetic agents. *J Anesth*. 2005;19:150–156.

58. Pape M, Engelhard K, Eberspacher E, et al. The long-term effect of sevoflurane on neuronal cell damage and expression of apoptotic factors after cerebral ischemia and reperfusion in rats. *Anesth Analg*. 2006;103:173–179, table of contents.

59. Elsersy H, Sheng H, Lynch JR, et al. Effects of isoflurane versus fentanyl-nitrous oxide anesthesia on long-term outcome from severe forebrain ischemia in the rat. *Anesthesiology*. 2004;100:1160–1166.

60. Kawaguchi M, Drummond JC, Cole DJ, et al. Effect of isoflurane on neuronal apoptosis in rats subjected to focal cerebral ischemia. *Anesth Analg*. 2004;98:798–805, table of contents.

61. Kitano H, Kirsch JR, Hurn PD, et al. Inhalational anesthetics as neuroprotectants or chemical preconditioning agents in ischemic brain. *J Cereb Blood Flow Metab*. 2007;27:1108–1128.

62. Xiong L, Zheng Y, Wu M, et al. Preconditioning with isoflurane produces dose-dependent neuroprotection via activation of adenosine triphosphate-regulated potassium channels after focal cerebral ischemia in rats. *Anesth Analg*. 2003;96:233–237, table of contents.

63. Wang C, Jin Lee J, Jung HH, et al. Pretreatment with volatile anesthetics, but not with the nonimmobilizer 1,2-dichlorohexafluorocyclobutane, reduced cell injury in rat cerebellar slices after an in vitro simulated ischemia. *Brain Res*. 2007;1152:201–208.

64. Perouansky M. Liaisons dangereuses? General anaesthetics and long-term toxicity in the CNS. *Eur J Anaesthesiol*. 2007;24:107–115.

65. Culley DJ, Xie Z, Crosby G. General anesthetic-induced neurotoxicity: an emerging problem for the young and old? *Curr Opin Anaesthesiol*. 2007;20:408–413.

66. Eckenhoff RG, Johansson JS, Wei H, et al. Inhaled anesthetic enhancement of amyloid-beta oligomerization and cytotoxicity. *Anesthesiology*. 2004;101:703–709.

67. Dong Y, Zhang G, Zhang B, et al. The common inhalational anesthetic sevoflurane induces apoptosis and increases beta-amyloid protein levels. *Arch Neurol*. 2009;66:620–631.

68. Mandal PK, Fodale V. Isoflurane and desflurane at clinically relevant concentrations induce amyloid beta-peptide oligomerization: an NMR study. *Biochem Biophys Res Commun*. 2009;379:716–720.

69. Ikonomidou C, Bosch F, Miksa M, et al. Blockade of NMDA receptors and apoptotic neurodegeneration in the developing brain. *Science*. 1999;283(5398):70–74.

70. Leinekugel X, Khalilov I, McLean H, et al. GABA is the principal fast-acting excitatory transmitter in the neonatal brain. *Adv Neurol*. 1999;79:189–201.

71. Bercker S, Bert B, Bittigau P, et al. Neurodegeneration in newborn rats following propofol and sevoflurane anesthesia. *Neurotox Res*. 2009;16:140–147.

72. Berns M, Zacharias R, Seeberg L, et al. Effects of sevoflurane on primary neuronal cultures of embryonic rats. *Eur J Anaesthesiol*. 2009;26:597–602.

73. Anand KJ, Soriano SG. Anesthetic agents and the immature brain: are these toxic or therapeutic? *Anesthesiology*. 2004;101:527–530.

74. Jevtovic-Todorovic V, Hartman RE, Izumi Y, et al. Early exposure to common anesthetic agents causes widespread neurodegeneration in the developing rat brain and persistent learning deficits. *J Neurosci*. 2003;23:876–882.

75. Bianchi SL, Tran T, Liu C, et al. Brain and behavior changes in 12-month-old Tg2576 and nontransgenic mice exposed to anesthetics. *Neurobiol Aging*. 2008;29:1002–1010.

76. Bartels M, Althoff RR, Boomsma DI. Anesthesia and cognitive performance in children: no evidence for a causal relationship. *Twin Res Hum Genet*. 2009;12:246–253.

77. Baranov D, Bickler PE, Crosby GJ, et al. Consensus statement: First International Workshop on Anesthetics and Alzheimer's disease. *Anesth Analg*. 2009;108:1627–1630.

78. Bohnen N, Warner MA, Kokmen E, et al. Early and midlife exposure to anesthesia and age of onset of Alzheimer's disease. *Int J Neurosci*. 1994;77(3-4):181–185.

79. Bohnen NI, Warner MA, Kokmen E, et al. Alzheimer's disease and cumulative exposure to anesthesia: a case-control study. *J Am Geriatr Soc*. 1994;42:198–201.

80. Hamaya Y, Takeda T, Dohi S, et al. The effects of pentobarbital, isoflurane, and propofol on immediate-early gene expression in the vital organs of the rat. *Anesth Analg*. 2000;90:1177–1183.

81. Takayama K, Suzuki T, Miura M. The comparison of effects of various anesthetics on expression of Fos protein in the rat brain. *Neurosci Lett*. 1994;176:59–62.

82. Futterer CD, Maurer MH, Schmitt A, et al. Alterations in rat brain proteins after desflurane anesthesia. *Anesthesiology*. 2004;100:302–308.

83. Culley DJ, Yukhananov RY, Xie Z, et al. Altered hippocampal gene expression 2 days after general anesthesia in rats. *Eur J Pharmacol*. 2006;549(1-3):71–78.

84. Perouansky M, Hemmings HC Jr. Neurotoxicity of general anesthetics: cause for concern? *Anesthesiology*. 2009;111:1365–1371.

85. Kalfas IH, Little JR. Postoperative hemorrhage: a survey of 4992 intracranial procedures. *Neurosurgery*. 1988;23:343–347.

86. Gupta A, Stierer T, Zuckerman R, et al. Comparison of recovery profile after ambulatory anesthesia with propofol, isoflurane, sevoflurane and desflurane: a systematic review. *Anesth Analg*. 2004;98:632–641, table of contents.

87. Nathanson MH, Fredman B, Smith I, et al. Sevoflurane versus desflurane for outpatient anesthesia: a comparison of maintenance and recovery profiles. *Anesth Analg*. 1995;81:1186–1190.

88. Welborn LG, Hannallah RS, Norden JM, et al. Comparison of emergence and recovery characteristics of sevoflurane, desflurane, and halothane in pediatric ambulatory patients. *Anesth Analg*. 1996;83:917–920.

89. Dexter F, Tinker JH. Comparisons between desflurane and isoflurane or propofol on time to following commands and time to discharge. A metaanalysis. *Anesthesiology*. 1995;83:77–82.

90. White PF. Use of cerebral monitoring during anaesthesia: effect on recovery profile. *Best Pract Res Clin Anaesthesiol*. 2006;20:181–189.

91. Recart A, Gasanova I, White PF, et al. The effect of cerebral monitoring on recovery after general anesthesia: a comparison of the auditory evoked potential and bispectral index devices with standard clinical practice. *Anesth Analg*. 2003;97:1667–1674.

92. Drover DR, Lemmens HJ, Pierce ET, et al. Patient State Index: titration of delivery and recovery from propofol, alfentanil, and nitrous oxide anesthesia. *Anesthesiology*. 2002;97:82–89.

93. Scheller MS, Nakakimura K, Fleischer JE, et al. Cerebral effects of sevoflurane in the dog: comparison with isoflurane and enflurane. *Br J Anaesth*. 1990;65:388–392.

94. Hopkins PM. Nitrous oxide: a unique drug of continuing importance for anaesthesia. *Best Pract Res Clin Anaesthesiol*. 2005;19:381–389.

95. Weimann J. Toxicity of nitrous oxide. *Best Pract Res Clin Anaesthesiol*. 2003;17:47–61.

96. Hirota K. Special cases: ketamine, nitrous oxide and xenon. *Best Pract Res Clin Anaesthesiol*. 2006;20:69–79.

97. Mennerick S, Jevtovic-Todorovic V, Todorovic SM, et al. Effect of nitrous oxide on excitatory and inhibitory synaptic transmission in hippocampal cultures. *J Neurosci*. 1998;18:9716–9726.

98. Pasternak JJ, Lanier WL. Is nitrous oxide use appropriate in neurosurgical and neurologically at-risk patients? *Curr Opin Anaesthesiol*. 2010;23:544–550.

99. Reinstrup P, Ryding E, Ohlsson T, et al. Cerebral blood volume (CBV) in humans during normo- and hypocapnia: influence of nitrous oxide (NO). *Anesthesiology*. 2001;95:1079–1082.

100. Reinstrup P, Ryding E, Algotsson L, et al. Effects of nitrous oxide on human regional cerebral blood flow and isolated pial arteries. *Anesthesiology*. 1994;81:396–402.

101. Strebel S, Kaufmann M, Anselmi L, et al. Nitrous oxide is a potent cerebrovasodilator in humans when added to isoflurane. A transcranial Doppler study. *Acta Anaesthesiol Scand*. 1995;39:653–658.

102. Hormann C, Schmidauer C, Haring HP, et al. Hyperventilation reverses the nitrous oxide-induced increase in cerebral blood flow velocity in human volunteers. *Br J Anaesth*. 1995;74:616–618.

103. Baughman VL, Hoffman WE, Miletich DJ, et al. Cerebrovascular and cerebral metabolic effects of N_2O in unrestrained rats. *Anesthesiology*. 1990;73:269–272.

104. Pelligrino DA, Miletich DJ, Hoffman WE, et al. Nitrous oxide markedly increases cerebral cortical metabolic rate and blood flow in the goat. *Anesthesiology*. 1984;60:405–412.

105. Barr G, Jakobsson JG, Owall A, et al. Nitrous oxide does not alter bispectral index: study with nitrous oxide as sole agent and as an adjunct to i.v. anaesthesia. *Br J Anaesth*. 1999;82:827–830.

106. Coste C, Guignard B, Menigaux C, et al. Nitrous oxide prevents movement during orotracheal intubation without affecting BIS value. *Anesth Analg*. 2000;91:130–135.

107. Puri GD. Paradoxical changes in bispectral index during nitrous oxide administration. *Br J Anaesth*. 2001;86:141–142.

108. Oda Y, Tanaka K, Matsuura T, et al. Nitrous oxide induces paradoxical electroencephalographic changes after tracheal intubation during isoflurane and sevoflurane anesthesia. *Anesth Analg*. 2006;102:1094–1102.

109. Baughman VL, Hoffman WE, Thomas C, et al. The interaction of nitrous oxide and isoflurane with incomplete cerebral ischemia in the rat. *Anesthesiology*. 1989;70:767–774.

110. Sakabe T, Kuramoto T, Inoue S, et al. Cerebral effects of nitrous oxide in the dog. *Anesthesiology*. 1978;48:195–200.

111. Lehmberg J, Waldner M, Baethmann A, et al. Inflammatory response to nitrous oxide in the central nervous system. *Brain Res*. 2008;1246:88–95.

112. Haelewyn B, David HN, Rouillon C, et al. Neuroprotection by nitrous oxide: facts and evidence. *Crit Care Med*. 2008;36:2651–2659.

113. McGregor DG, Lanier WL, Pasternak JJ, et al. Effect of nitrous oxide on neurologic and neuropsychological function after intracranial aneurysm surgery. *Anesthesiology*. 2008;108:568–579.

114. Domino KB, Hemstad JR, Lam AM, et al. Effect of nitrous oxide on intracranial pressure after cranial-dural closure in patients undergoing craniotomy. *Anesthesiology*. 1992;77:421–425.

115. Tramer M, Moore A, McQuay H. Omitting nitrous oxide in general anaesthesia: meta-analysis of intraoperative awareness and postoperative emesis in randomized controlled trials. *Br J Anaesth*. 1996;76:186–193.

116. Preckel B, Schlack W. Inert gases as the future inhalational anaesthetics? *Best Pract Res Clin Anaesthesiol*. 2005;19:365–379.

117. Sanders RD, Franks NP, Maze M. Xenon: no stranger to anaesthesia. *Br J Anaesth*. 2003;91:709–717.

118. Franks NP, Dickinson R, de Sousa SL, et al. How does xenon produce anaesthesia? *Nature*. 1998;396(6709):324.

119. Nakata Y, Goto T, Ishiguro Y, et al. Minimum alveolar concentration (MAC) of xenon with sevoflurane in humans. *Anesthesiology*. 2001;94:611–614.

120. Goto T, Nakata Y, Morita S. The minimum alveolar concentration of xenon in the elderly is sex-dependent. *Anesthesiology*. 2002;97:1129–1132.

121. Fink H, Blobner M, Bogdanski R, et al. Effects of xenon on cerebral blood flow and autoregulation: an experimental study in pigs. *Br J Anaesth*. 2000;84:221–225.

122. Laitio RM, Kaisti KK, Laangsjo JW, et al. Effects of xenon anesthesia on cerebral blood flow in humans: a positron emission tomography study. *Anesthesiology*. 2007;106:1128–1133.

123. Marx T, Schmidt M, Schirmer U, et al. Xenon anaesthesia. *J R Soc Med*. 2000;93:513–517.

124. Schmidt M, Marx T, Papp-Jambor C, et al. Effect of xenon on cerebral autoregulation in pigs. *Anaesthesia*. 2002;57:960–966.

125. Schmidt M, Marx T, Armbruster S, et al. Effect of xenon on elevated intracranial pressure as compared with nitrous oxide and total intravenous anesthesia in pigs. *Acta Anaesthesiol Scand*. 2005;49:494–501.

126. Plougmann J, Astrup J, Pedersen J, et al. Effect of stable xenon inhalation on intracranial pressure during measurement of cerebral blood flow in head injury. *J Neurosurg*. 1994;81:822–828.

127. Frietsch T, Bogdanski R, Blobner M, et al. Effects of xenon on cerebral blood flow and cerebral glucose utilization in rats. *Anesthesiology*. 2001;94:290–297.

128. Stuttmann R, Schultz A, Kneif T, et al. Assessing the depth of hypnosis of xenon anaesthesia with the EEG / Bestimmung der Hypnosetiefe bei Xenon-Narkosen mit dem EEG. *Biomed Tech (Berl)*. 2010;55:77–82.

129. Fahlenkamp AV, Peters D, Biener IA, et al. Evaluation of bispectral index and auditory evoked potentials for hypnotic depth monitoring during balanced xenon anaesthesia compared with sevoflurane. *Br J Anaesth*. 2010;105:334–341.

130. Ma D, Wilhelm S, Maze M, et al. Neuroprotective and neurotoxic properties of the "inert" gas, xenon. *Br J Anaesth*. 2002;89:739–746.

131. Wilhelm S, Ma D, Maze M, et al. Effects of xenon on in vitro and in vivo models of neuronal injury. *Anesthesiology*. 2002;96:1485–1491.

132. Homi HM, Yokoo N, Ma D, et al. The neuroprotective effect of xenon administration during transient middle cerebral artery occlusion in mice. *Anesthesiology*. 2003;99:876–881.

133. Ma D, Hossain M, Pettet GK, et al. Xenon preconditioning reduces brain damage from neonatal asphyxia in rats. *J Cereb Blood Flow Metab*. 2006;26:199–208.

134. Goto T, Saito H, Shinkai M, et al. Xenon provides faster emergence from anesthesia than does nitrous oxide-sevoflurane or nitrous oxide-isoflurane. *Anesthesiology*. 1997;86:1273–1278.

135. Nakata Y, Goto T, Morita S. Comparison of inhalation inductions with xenon and sevoflurane. *Acta Anaesthesiol Scand*. 1997;41:1157–1161.

136. Coburn M, Baumert JH, Roertgen D, et al. Emergence and early cognitive function in the elderly after xenon or desflurane anaesthesia: a double-blinded randomized controlled trial. *Br J Anaesth*. 2007;98:756–762.

137. Reinelt H, Schirmer U, Marx T, et al. Diffusion of xenon and nitrous oxide into the bowel. *Anesthesiology*. 2001;94:475–477.

10.

NEUROMUSCULAR BLOCKADE IN THE PATIENT WITH NEUROLOGIC DISEASE

Anup Pamnani and Vinod Malhotra

Neuromuscular blocking agents (NMBs) are frequently used in the anesthetic management of the patient undergoing neurosurgical procedures. The use of NMBs facilitates tracheal intubation and reduces the risk of inadvertent patient movement during critical portions of the surgical procedure. The skilled neuroanesthetist is able to adjust the level of neuromuscular blockade to ensure patient immobility without compromising the ability to obtain a rapid recovery and immediate neurologic assessment. Such precise titration requires a thorough knowledge of neuromuscular junction physiology and the pharmacology of NMBs.

PHYSIOLOGY OF THE NEUROMUSCULAR JUNCTION

The nicotinic acetylcholine receptor is a pentameric ion channel located in skeletal muscle and is the primary site of action of both depolarizing and nondepolarizing NMBs. It is closed in the resting state [1, 2]. There are currently three known isoforms of the nicotinic acetylcholine receptor: a junctional mature receptor, an extrajunctional immature receptor, and a neuronal $\alpha7$ receptor (Figure 10.1).

Acetylcholine is synthesized in motor neurons and stored in small packages termed vesicles. Stimulation of the neuron causes vesicles to migrate to the surface of the nerve and discharge acetylcholine into the cleft separating the nerve from muscle (Figure 10.2). When two acetylcholine molecules bind to the mature nicotinic receptor, the ion channel undergoes a conformational change to an open state that allows sodium ions to enter the muscle cell. This causes the cell to depolarize and which generate an action potential. The action potential then propagates via further activation of sodium channels along the length of a muscle fiber, initiating contraction [1, 2].

The acetylcholine is degraded in the neuromuscular cleft by the enzyme acetylcholinesterase. This terminates the action of the acetylcholine molecules [1–4].

Both immature and neuronal $\alpha7$ receptors are upregulated after denervation injury. Immature receptors are more sensitive to depolarizing blockade and have a longer mean channel open time than mature receptors. Potassium efflux from these receptors is therefore significantly greater (Figure 10.3). Neuronal $\alpha7$ receptors may also be implicated in the resistance to nondepolarizing NMBs seen in pathologic states such as cerebrovascular accident, denervation injuries, and spinal cord trauma [3, 5, 6].

DEPOLARIZING NEUROMUSCULAR BLOCKADE

Succinylcholine is the only depolarizing NMB that is used clinically in North America. It is composed of two acetylcholine molecules linked to each other at the methyl ends. Succinylcholine binds noncompetitively to the nicotinic acetylcholine receptor, opening the ion channel and depolarizing the muscle cell. Because succinylcholine is not degraded by acetylcholinesterase, it remains in the neuromuscular cleft. The resulting prolonged refractory period prevents further propagation of action potentials and produces neuromuscular blockade. Succinylcholine slowly diffuses out of the neuromuscular junction and into the circulation, where it is rapidly hydrolyzed to succinylmonocholine and choline by butyrylcholinesterase. Butyrylcholinesterase is particularly efficient at degrading succinylcholine, which accounts for its very short duration of action.

Succinylcholine has a rapid onset of action. When administered in doses 2 to 3 times its ED_{95}, effective muscle relaxation can be achieved in as little as 45 to 70 seconds [7–9]. Recovery of muscle function typically occurs in as little as 6 to 9 minutes [10]. Succinylcholine's rapid onset and short duration of action is of value when tracheal intubation must be accomplished rapidly or to allow the patient to regain spontaneous ventilation in a "can't intubate/can't ventilate" scenario. Several neurologic conditions, including

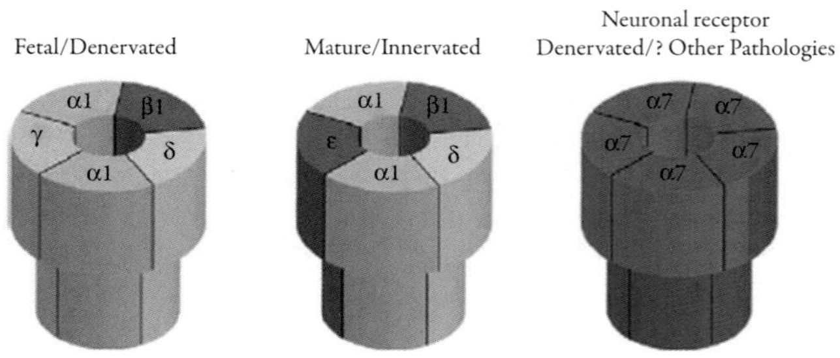

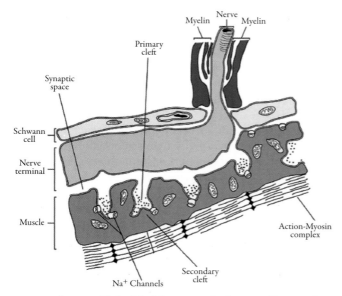

Figure 10.1 Isoforms of the nicotinic acetylcholine receptor. (Reprinted from Shear TD, Martyn JA. Physiology and biology of neuromuscular transmission in health and disease. J Crit Care. 2009;24:8, with permission from Elsevier).

acromegaly and cervical disc disease, may be associated with a difficult airway, making succinylcholine a valuable adjunct to the neuroanesthesiologist's armamentarium.

Depolarizing NMBs may also produce a second block component that is not the direct result of endplate depolarization. This phenomenon, called a *phase II block*, typically occurs after a large (7–10 mg/kg) dose, repeated administration, or an infusion of succinylcholine. It may even occur to some degree after single bolus administration [11]. The mechanisms underlying this change in pharmacologic action are not exactly clear, but a phase II block is similar to that produced by nondepolarizing agents. A phase II block will produce fade with train-of-four stimulation and posttetanic potentiation. Such a phase II block will also respond to reversal agents such as neostigmine. Once phase II block is clinically evident, the duration of action of succinylcholine becomes somewhat unpredictable. This property, along with undesirable side effects discussed later, render succinylcholine unsuitable for maintenance of neuromuscular blockade during neurosurgical procedures [7–9, 11, 12].

Figure 10.2 Synaptic Cleft of the Neuromuscular Junction (Reprinted from Shear TD, Martyn JA. Physiology and biology of neuromuscular transmission in health and disease. J Crit Care. 2009;24:7, with permission from Elsevier).

NONDEPOLARIZING NEUROMUSCULAR BLOCKADE

Nondepolarizing NMBs act by competitively inhibiting acetylcholine binding to the postjunctional nicotinic acetylcholine receptor. Nondepolarizing NMBs bind to the receptor without activating it and preventing acetylcholine from accessing the site. The two major classes of nondepolarizing blocker in current clinical use today include steroidal compounds (e.g., vecuronium, rocuronium, and pancuronium) and benzylisoquinolinium compounds (e.g., mivacurium and cisatracurium).

The onset of neuromuscular blockade after administration of a nondepolarizing NMB is slower than that of succinylcholine. Most drugs require 3 to 5 minutes to produce clinically observed relaxant effects. This reflects the time required for the drug concentration to build up in the neuromuscular junction and for a sufficient number of receptors to become occupied [2, 7, 13]. In general, the onset of neuromuscular blockade with nondepolarizing drugs is inversely correlated with potency. This is due to the fact that more drug molecules are available when a less potent agent is administered [14].

The duration of action of nondepolarizing neuromuscular block varies from short to long and is dependent on their mode of elimination. Mivacurium, a short-acting drug, has duration of minutes after bolus administration due to its rapid elimination by butyrylcholinesterase [15]. Intermediate-duration nondepolarizing agents, such as rocuronium and vecuronium, typically undergo significant hepatic elimination. Cisatracurium, an intermediate-duration nondepolarizing drug, is unique in that it is eliminated by an organ-independent mechanism. This process, termed Hoffman elimination, is purely chemical and results in the production of laudanosine, a byproduct with no known neuromuscular blocking properties [16]. In contrast, pancuronium, a long-acting drug, is eliminated primarily by the kidney.

This diversity in duration of action of nondepolarizing relaxants provides several options for reliable neuromuscular blockade during neurosurgical procedures. Moreover, nondepolarizing NMBs are eliminated by a variety of mechanisms. This allows a drug to be selected on the basis of medical conditions (e.g., hepatic or renal disease) and the coadministration of medications that may alter pharmacokinetics.

Rocuronium has a rapid onset of action and can produce intubating conditions similar to succinylcholine [17]. When 1.2 mg/kg is administered, excellent intubating conditions can be obtained in 60 to 90 seconds. This may be of benefit in the neurosurgical patient who might not tolerate the increase in intracranial pressure (ICP) or the fasciculations caused by depolarizing NMBs. The duration of action of rocuronium is, however, considerably longer than that of succinylcholine. Rocuronium may not be the best choice if difficult airway management is anticipated and spontaneous ventilation may need to be restored quickly.

Because of their prolonged duration of action, many clinicians administer an anticholinesterase agent at the end of

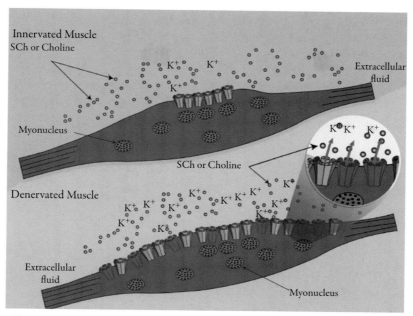

Figure 10.3   Succinylcholine (SCh)–induced potassium release in an innervated (top) and denervated muscle (bottom) (Reprinted from Martyn JA, Richtsfeld M. Succinylcholine-induced hyperkalemia in acquired pathologic states: etiologic factors and molecular mechanisms. Anesthesiology. 2006;104:164, with permission from Elsevier).

the surgical procedure to help speed recovery from neuromuscular block. These drugs also decrease the incidence of residual postoperative paralysis. The most commonly used anticholinesterase drugs are edrophonium and neostigmine. Although they are frequently referred to as *reversal agents*, these drugs work indirectly by inhibiting degradation of acetylcholine within the neuromuscular junction. This increases concentration of acetylcholine molecules in the synaptic cleft, leading to competitive antagonism of nondepolarizing block. Acetylcholinesterase inhibition is achieved by one of two mechanisms: Edrophonium produces a rapid but weak electrostatic bond to the anionic site, while neostigmine creates a stronger but slower covalent bond at the esteratic site.

The introduction of sugammadex, a new cyclodextrin NMB antagonist, will significantly change management of nondepolarizing neuromuscular block. Sugammadex can rapidly reverse moderate and deep neuromuscular blockade. Sugammadex binds the steroidal NMBs rocuronium, vecuronium, and pancuronium with varying affinity to form an inactive complex (Figure 10.4) that is then excreted through the kidney. Rapid reversal of nondepolarizing blockade would allow maintenance of profound muscle relaxation during delicate neurosurgical procedures with rapid recovery after the procedure, making it possible to obtain a neurologic examination [18–20].

SIDE EFFECTS OF NEUROMUSCULAR BLOCKADE

Both depolarizing and nondepolarizing NMBs have undesirable side effects. A thorough understanding of these

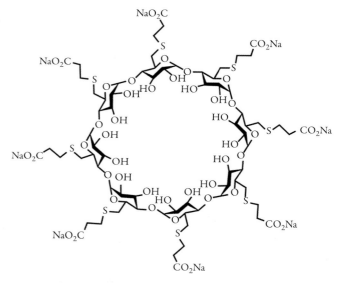

Figure 10.4   Structure of Sugammadex—a Υ cyclodextrin (Reprinted from Brydion® package insert).

effects and how they impact the neurosurgical procedure is essential to management of the neurosurgical patient.

ADVERSE EFFECTS OF DEPOLARIZING NMBS

Succinylcholine has numerous adverse effects including some with significant risk of morbidity and mortality. It may increase plasma potassium levels, potentially causing cardiac dysrhythmias. It may also increase ICP in patients with intracranial lesions. Last, it may also trigger an episode of malignant hyperthermia.

Table 10.1 CONDITIONS ASSOCIATED WITH SIGNIFICANT HYPERKALEMIA AFTER USE OF DEPOLARIZING BLOCKERS

Spinal cord transection

Stroke

Trauma

Significant burns

Prolonged immobility

Upper/lower motor neuron denervation

Prolonged chemical denervation by NMBs

Infection

Muscle tumor

Muscle inflammation

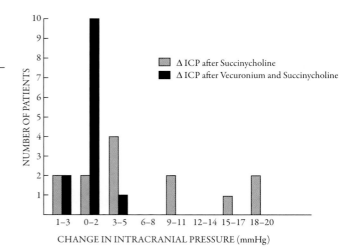

Figure 10.5 Peak increases in ICP after 1mg/kg Succinylcholine with and without prior depolarizing neuromuscular blockade with 0.14mg/kg vecuronium. (Reprinted from Minton MD, Grosslight K, Stirt JA, et al. Increases in intracranial pressure from succinylcholine: prevention by prior nondepolarzing blockade. Anesthesiology. 1986;65:167, with permission from Wolters Kluwer).

Administration of succinylcholine typically increases plasma potassium concentration by 0.5 to 1.0 mEq/L in a normal patient. Life-threatening hyperkalemia may occur in patients with recent burn injuries or neurologic conditions such as spinal cord injuries, stroke, or trauma (see Table 10.1). Hyperkalemia is thought to be caused by upregulation and spread of acetylcholine receptors outside the neuromuscular junction as discussed earlier. Activation of these receptors by succinylcholine leads to massive muscle depolarization. The resultant potassium efflux from the muscle cells can cause profound hyperkalemia [5, 6].

Muscle fasciculations, which commonly occur after administration of succinylcholine, may cause direct injury to the patient or exacerbate intracranial hypertension. Although fasciculations are generally thought to be benign, vigorous movement may cause injury to the patient or to health care providers. Muscle pains commonly occur in the postoperative period after succinylcholine administration, most frequently in young patients. The practice of "precurarization," or the administration of a small dose of nondepolarizing muscular blocker several minutes before the administration of succinylcholine, has been shown to reduce the incidence of myalgias and fasciculation [21, 22].

The ability of succinylcholine to increase ICP and the cause of this increase are the subject of some controversy. There is some evidence to suggest that succinylcholine elevates ICP in patients with cerebral tumors, and some animal studies suggest that neuromuscular blockade with succinylcholine may be contraindicated [23]. Conversely, in brain-injured patients, the use of succinylcholine does not appear to alter cerebral blood flow or ICP [24]. The mechanism by which succinylcholine administration increases ICP is incompletely understood but may be related to an increase in afferent neural traffic that originates in muscle spindle receptors. This hypothesis is supported by the observation that the rise in ICP is prevented by pretreatment with a nondepolarizing NMB (Figure 10.5)

[25, 26]. Because of this uncertainty, it is probably best avoided in patients known to have intracranial hypertension or who are otherwise at risk for cerebral herniation. If, however, emergent or complex airway management is anticipated, most clinicians agree that the admittedly theoretical concerns about increased ICP may not contraindicate succinylcholine use.

Sinus bradycardia, junctional rhythms, and ventricular escape beats have been reported after a bolus of succinylcholine. The cardiac effects seem to be more common after repeated administration. Patients with certain types of severe neurologic complications, such as subarachnoid hemorrhage or elevated ICP, may have preexisting dysrhythmias and may therefore be more susceptible to the effects of succinylcholine. This drug should therefore be used with caution in this patient population, and consideration should be given to whether airway management can be accomplished with nondepolarizing NMBs.

No discussion of depolarizing neuromuscular blockade would be complete without mention of malignant hyperthermia (MH): an inherited, potentially fatal disorder due to accelerated skeletal muscle metabolism associated with administration of succinylcholine and volatile anesthetics. Although not specifically associated with neurologic disease, it is seen in conjunction with rare myopathies such as central core disease, brody syndrome and others which the neuroanesthetist may occasionally encounter. MH susceptible patients should not receive volatile anesthetics or succinylcholine. Treatment of MH is outside the scope of this chapter and is extensively covered in publications by the Malignant Hyperthermia Association of the United States (MHAUS) which also maintains an MH hotline and a registry of MH susceptible individuals [27–30].

ADVERSE EFFECTS OF NONDEPOLARIZING NMBS

In general, nondepolarizing NMBs have fewer side effects than succinylcholine. The most common complication of nondepolarizing NMBs is prolonged or residual neuromuscular blockade that is caused by these drugs' longer duration of action.

Residual neuromuscular block due to the use of nondepolarizing NMBs is relatively common. In the patient with severe neurologic impairment, respiratory and swallowing function may already be dysfunctional and may become significantly impaired in the setting of residual neuromuscular blockade. Residual blockade may cause postoperative respiratory failure, upper airway collapse, and inhibition of swallowing and gag. Urgent reintubation of the trachea may be required, and aspiration of gastric contents, neurologic injury, and death have occurred as a result of this complication [31–34]. Residual neuromuscular blockade may also make it difficult or impossible to obtain a postoperative neurologic examination, potentially delaying the diagnosis of a life-threatening complication such as intracranial hemorrhage.

Residual neuromuscular blockade has many etiologies. Hypothermia, acidosis, use of a long-acting drug (e.g., pancuronium), and overdosage may be responsible for prolonged neuromuscular blockade. Failure to use neuromuscular monitoring, inadequate or inappropriate dosing of reversal agents, residual anesthesia, and synergistic effects of other medications, such as lidocaine, β-blockers, and calcium channel blockers, have also been implicated in potentiating residual neuromuscular blockade.

The choice of nondepolarizing agent should take into consideration the duration of the procedure and the physiology of drug elimination. Chronic antiepileptic therapy can lead to resistance to antiepileptic drugs by increasing the proportion of relaxant that is protein bound (thus reducing the free fraction), inducing hepatic cytochrome P450 isoforms, which break down nondepolarizing drugs (e.g., vecuronium or rocuronium) or decreasing hepatic production of plasma esterase (which break down drugs like mivacurium). The presence of liver or kidney disease should also influence which agent is chosen. A neuromuscular monitoring device should always be used whenever neuromuscular blockade is initiated.

Each nondepolarizing NMB has specific adverse effects that must be considered before use in the neurosurgical patient. Mivacurium and atracurium, for example, may cause histamine release, producing hypotension, tachycardia, and, in severe cases, bronchospasm and cardiovascular collapse [35, 36]. Atracurium and cisatracurium, which spontaneously degrade by Hoffman elimination, are converted to laudanosine. Laudanosine may cause seizures, hypotension, and bradycardia if it accumulates. Although laudanosine toxicity is unlikely to occur in the perioperative setting, it should be considered when using a prolonged high-dose infusion of these drugs in the intensive care unit (ICU), particularly in patients with renal insufficiency [37].

NEUROMUSCULAR BLOCK IN THE PATIENT WITH COEXISTING NEUROLOGIC AND NEUROMUSCULAR DISEASE

The management of neuromuscular blockade in the setting of neuromuscular disease requires a thorough understanding of the underlying pathology. A comprehensive review is outside the scope of this chapter, so a concise guide to the management of neuromuscular blockade in the setting of the major neuromuscular syndromes is presented next.

MYASTHENIC SYNDROMES

The myasthenic syndromes consist of a diverse group of neuromuscular junction diseases including myasthenia gravis (MG) and Lambert-Eaton syndrome (LES), as well as less common illnesses such as congenital myasthenic syndromes.

MG is caused by the production of antibodies against endplate acetylcholine receptors. This causes a decrease in the number of functional acetylcholine receptors, which in turn results in an abnormal response to NMBs. Patients with MG are abnormally sensitive to the effects of nondepolarizing NMBs. Variability in the severity of clinical presentation makes estimating nondepolarizing NMB requirements and management of these patients challenging [38–40]. Patients with MG also have a significant resistance to depolarizing NMBs. Dose requirements for succinylcholine may be more than doubled in these patients [41] due to the inability of succinylcholine to depolarize antibody-bound acetylcholine receptors. The duration of depolarizing block may also be prolonged due to anticholinesterase inhibition of pseudocholinesterase. These patients may also be at increased risk for development of a phase II block [38, 42].

The perioperative management of patients being treated for MG with anticholinesterase medications remains controversial. Although these medications may theoretically augment depolarizing blockade and inhibit nondepolarizing blockade, there appears to be little clinical evidence to suggest that clinical outcome and likelihood of postoperative mechanical ventilation are altered. Most clinicians, therefore, continue anticholinesterase medications throughout the perioperative period to maintain muscle strength. Plasmapheresis and intravenous immunoglobulin may also improve muscle strength in these patients [43, 44].

Because of the unpredictability of NMBs in the myasthenic patient, consideration should be given to avoiding these drugs when possible. Regional anesthesia should be considered if appropriate, and if general anesthesia is required, neuromuscular blockade should be avoided. If appropriate, the use of a laryngeal mask airway (if appropriate) may allow the airway to be managed without NMBs. It may also be possible to intubate the trachea without neuromuscular blockade under deep anesthesia to blunt tracheal and laryngeal reflexes. When rapid sequence intubation is indicated, these patients' potential resistance to succinylcholine and prolongation of its effects should be taken into account. Long-acting NMBs such as pancuronium are best avoided. If a nondepolarizing NMB is administered, neuromuscular function should be monitored with the use of a peripheral nerve stimulator. Respiratory function should be carefully assessed before extubation. Respiratory parameters such as negative inspiratory force may predict respiratory muscle strength.

The novel reversal agent sugammadex may also simplify the management of nondepolarizing NMBs in patients with MG. Recently published case reports describe the full recovery of respiratory muscle strength after nondepolarizing neuromuscular blockade in MG patients following reversal with sugammadex [45–47].

NMBs must also be used with caution in patients with LES, an acquired paraneoplastic disorder that causes decreased presynaptic acetylcholine release. Patients with LES are highly sensitive to the effects of both depolarizing and nondepolarizing NMBs. As in patients with MG, the use of NMBs should be avoided if possible. When neuromuscular blockade is necessary, these drugs should be used with caution, and the patient must demonstrate the full return of muscle strength before extubation of the trachea.

MYOTONIA

The myotonias are a diverse group of diseases characterized by delayed skeletal muscle relaxation. Myotonic dystrophy, an inherited autosomal defect of chromosome 19, is the most common of the myotonic syndromes.

Management of neuromuscular blockade in the myotonic patient is guided by the effects of the specific NMBs and the clinical situation. Succinylcholine can precipitate muscle spasm and should be avoided in these patients. Patients with myotonia often have exaggerated sensitivity to nondepolarizing blockade. As with the myasthenic patient, the need for neuromuscular blockade should be carefully considered and alternative options explored. When neuromuscular blockade must be used, NMBs should be titrated judiciously and postoperative respiratory muscle function should be carefully assessed before extubation of the trachea. Peripheral nerve stimulation may provoke localized muscle spasm, which can confound neuromuscular monitoring. Neuromuscular blockade may not reliably suppress myotonic contractions that occur in response to surgical stimulation and electrocautery. Additional pharmacologic therapy with membrane stabilizing medications such as procainamide and phenytoin may aid in producing muscle relaxation [48–50].

AMYOTROPHIC LATERAL SCLEROSIS

Amyotrophic lateral sclerosis (ALS) is a degenerative disease of anterior horn motor neurons that carries a poor prognosis. It is characterized by weakness of skeletal, pharyngeal, and respiratory muscles. Patients eventually develop respiratory failure and death. Succinylcholine should be avoided in patients with ALS because of the proliferation of extrajunctional acetylcholine receptors. Administration of succinylcholine may therefore cause a massive depolarization of skeletal muscle, causing life-threatening hyperkalemia. Patients with ALS may also be sensitive to the effects of nondepolarizing NMBs. This may be due to decreased presynaptic transmission of acetylcholine in these patients [51–53].

GUILLAIN-BARRE SYNDROME

Guillain-Barre syndrome (GBS) is an acute inflammatory demyelinating polyneuropathy characterized by generalized muscle weakness, areflexia, and ascending paralysis. Pharyngeal and respiratory muscle weakness may cause difficulty with ventilation and inability to protect the airway. Severe hyperkalemia may result if succinylcholine is administered due to the proliferation of extrajunctional immature acetylcholine receptors. Patients may also be sensitive to nondepolarizing NMBs. These drugs and administration should be administered judiciously and guided by monitoring with a nerve stimulator. Nondepolarizing NMBs that release histamine, such as mivacurium and atracurium, should be avoided because these patients frequently display significant autonomic dysfunction [54–56].

NEUROMUSCULAR BLOCKADE IN THE PATIENT WITH ELEVATED INTRACRANIAL PRESSURE

The patient with a space occupying lesion, cerebral edema, or traumatic brain injury is particularly vulnerable to cerebral injury. Management of the patient with intracranial hypertension is discussed elsewhere and may involve the use of multiple pharmacologic, physiologic, and surgical therapies.

Nondepolarizing neuromuscular blockade can be a valuable adjunct to the management of these patients. Although neuromuscular blockade does not directly impact intracranial compliance, it can be particularly useful in the ventilated patient with intracranial hypertension. Coughing caused by surgical or tracheal stimulation can lead to a significant increase in ICP in the patient with decreased intracranial compliance. Ensuring adequate neuromuscular blockade during airway management and surgery helps to avoid these deleterious increases in ICP [57–61].

As discussed earlier, the use of depolarizing blockade in the patient with intracranial hypertension is controversial.

The use of succinylcholine is, however, considered in these patients when it may facilitate complex airway management. The introduction of reversal agents that reliably terminate nondepolarizing neuromuscular blockade (e.g., sugammadex) may make complex airway management with rapid acting NMBs, such as rocuronium, an attractive alternative in this patient population.

NEUROMUSCULAR BLOCKADE AND NEUROPHYSIOLOGIC MONITORING

Intraoperative neurophysiologic monitoring is used during neurosurgical procedures to reduce the risk of nerve injury. Neurophysiologic monitoring is frequently used during neurosurgical procedures involving the spine but has a role in intracranial procedures as well.

The use of neuromuscular blockade in the perioperative period can significantly degrade the signals needed to perform neurophysiologic monitoring. It is therefore critical for the anesthesiologist to carefully discuss the anesthetic plan, including use of neuromuscular blockade, with the neurophysiologist and surgeon.

Somatosensory evoked potentials, visual evoked potentials, and brainstem evoked potentials test for afferent (sensory) impulses to the central nervous system. Although many anesthetic drugs have a significant effect on these measurements, they are unaffected by neuromuscular blockade. Conversely, motor evoked potentials (MEPs) (Figure 10.6) and electromyography (EMG) assess the integrity of the efferent (motor) impulses transmitted peripherally from the central nervous system. NMBs interfere with impulse transmission at the neuromuscular junction and can significantly diminish or eliminate the detected response.

When monitoring of motor pathways is planned, two distinct strategies can be used with regard to neuromuscular blockade. The first strategy involves avoidance of neuromuscular blockade during the maintenance phase of the anesthetic. Baseline signals are obtained before induction. Either a single dose of a relatively short-acting nondepolarizing agent or succinylcholine can facilitate endotracheal intubation. Monitoring is initiated after the patient has sufficiently recovered from blockade. The advantage of this technique is that motor signals to be recorded without being impeded by neuromuscular blockade. The disadvantage of this strategy is that the patient may move during motor testing or stimulating phases of the surgical procedure. Patient movement can be particularly problematic during spine surgery, when the patient is frequently in the prone position, possibly in head pins, undergoing manipulation of delicate neurologic structures under a microscope [62–64].

An alternative strategy of partial neuromuscular blockade may decrease the risk of patient movement when monitoring MEPs or using EMG. Neuromuscular blockade is carefully titrated to a level at which 20% to 50% of the receptors are blocked (as assessed by measuring two to four twitches remaining by train-of-four testing). This is typically achieved with drug infusion and avoiding boluses that may produce excessive blockade. Using these techniques, it is possible to produce a stable surgical field without significantly compromising adequate neurophysiologic monitoring. This should, however, be used with caution in patients with preoperative neurologic dysfunction who may have a significant baseline reduction in MEP amplitude. Avoiding neuromuscular blockade during neurophysiologic monitoring in these patients may be a better strategy [65, 66].

NEUROMUSCULAR BLOCKADE IN THE CRITICALLY ILL NEUROSURGICAL PATIENT

Long-term neuromuscular blockade is occasionally used in the postoperative period in neurosurgical patients. The most common reasons for this are to facilitate ventilation, control ICP, and reduce oxygen consumption in those patients who are critically ill. Prolonged neuromuscular blockade is a common complication of neuromuscular blockade in the ICU patient with multiple comorbidities. Failure to adequately monitor depth of blockade with neuromuscular monitoring devices can lead to significant accumulation of NMBs. Prolonged blockade may also be caused by renal insufficiency. Prolonged infusions of vecuronium, pancuronium, or other drugs that depend on renal elimination can lead to accumulation of active metabolites that

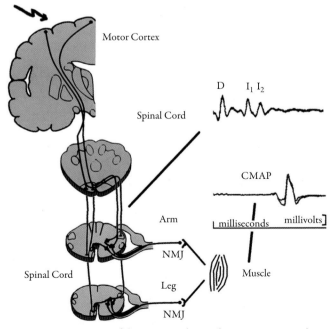

Figure 10.6   Monitoring of the motor pathways during neurosurgical procedures using Motor Evoked Potentials (MEPs). (Reprinted from Jameson LC, Sloan TB. Monitoring of the brain and spinal cord. Anesthesiol Clin. 2006;24:783, with permission from Elsevier).

may persist for several days after these drugs are discontinued. Use of a drug such as cisatracurium, which is metabolized by an organ-independent process, may be beneficial. Additional risk factors for prolonged blockade include metabolic acidosis, hypermagnesemia, nutritional deficiencies, administration of certain antibiotics, and hypothermia. Minimizing these risk factors can reduce the incidence of prolonged neuromuscular blockade in the ICU patient [67–70].

The use of NMBs in the critically ill patient has also been associated with the development of myopathy. Critical illness myopathy (CIM) is a diffuse myopathy, characterized by muscle fiber atrophy, fatty degeneration, and fibrosis, and has been associated with neuromuscular blockade. ICU patients concurrently receiving steroid medications are particularly vulnerable to this devastating complication. The mechanism of injury may be related to chemical denervation by NMBs causing proliferation of steroid receptors at the muscle membrane. This may in turn lead to increased susceptibility of muscle tissue to steroid toxicity. Sepsis is another major risk factor for the development of CIM. The inflammatory cytokines associated with the systemic inflammatory response syndrome (SIRS) may damage the muscle membrane allowing greater entry of NMBs and steroids into the sarcolemma. Hyperglycemia, prolonged ventilation and multiple organ dysfunction syndrome (MODS) are other associated risk factors [69–71].

The management of CIM is primarily supportive and includes nutritional support, physical therapy, daily attempts to wean ventilation, and glucose control. The most effective strategy in high-risk patients, however, is prevention. The need for prolonged neuromuscular blockade should be carefully assessed in critically ill patients, and feasible, alternative strategies, such as deep sedation, should be used whenever possible. If the use of NMBs is unavoidable, depth of blockade should be closely monitored and drugs should be titrated to minimize excessive blockade. Prevention of sepsis is another effective strategy. SIRS and MODS can significantly increase the risk of CIM in the patient receiving NMBs and steroids. Thus, prevention of nosocomial infection is a vital component of the management strategy against CIM [71, 72].

ADVANCES IN NEUROMUSCULAR BLOCKADE FOR THE NEUROSURGICAL PATIENT

There have been many advances in the field of neuromuscular blockade. These advances are particularly relevant to the neurosurgical patient and have the potential to significantly improve patient safety in the perioperative period. The new drug sugammadex, a selective binding reversal agent that terminates neuromuscular blockade, has been discussed in some detail earlier. Its ability to rapidly reverse even

profound levels of neuromuscular blockade could prove particularly advantageous in the neurosurgical patient. The incidence of postoperative residual neuromuscular blockade in patients arriving in the postanesthesia care unit, when using conventional reversal agents, may be as high as 50% [34]. Any residual paralysis in patients with neurological disease can be a particularly serious complication since these patients may frequently have impaired pharyngeal and respiratory function at baseline. Further, hypoventilation will lead to hypercapnia and hypercarbia with unwanted effects of increased ICP. The use of a reversal agent that rapidly and reliably terminates the effects of neuromuscular blockade has the potential to be of immense benefit in this patient population. At this time, sugammadex is unavailable in the United States.

Currently available acetylcholinesterase antagonists, such as neostigmine, have many adverse effects associated with their administration. These effects are typically attributed to the unintended stimulation of muscarinic cholinergic synapses prevalent throughout the autonomic nervous system. Bradycardia, copious secretions, increased gastrointestinal motility, bronchospasm, and nausea have all been reported as side effects of neostigmine administration [73]. As a result, acetylcholinesterase antagonists are frequently administered along with an antimuscarinic drug such as atropine and glycopyrrolate. Nevertheless, despite antimuscarinic coadministration, autonomic dysfunction frequently occurs with the administration of these reversal agents. The use of new drugs, such as sugammadex and others, could potentially avoid some of these adverse effects. However, their use may be associated with other side effects that are still under investigation. In the case of sugammadex, clinical trials have documented adverse effects such as anaphylaxis, anaphylactoid reactions, pyrexia, prolonged QT interval, constipation, and procedural blood pressure changes [18–20, 74].

Two new investigational NMBs, both of the fumarate class, are also particularly worthy of discussion in this section (Figure 10.7). The first of these, gantacurium (AV430A), is a new class of nondepolarizing NMB: asymmetric mixed-onium chlorofumarates. It has a pharmacodynamic profile similar to that of succinylcholine. In addition, it is degraded by rapid formation of an inactive adduction product with the amino acid cysteine by a chemical reaction. Administration of exogenous cysteine significantly speeds up this reaction, allowing for rapid antagonism of even deep neuromuscular block. Initial testing has shown transient cardiovascular side effects at high doses (presumed to be related to histamine release). Clinical trials of this drug are currently ongoing.

CW002 (AV002), a benzylisoquinolinium fumarate ester-based compound, is a second such novel investigational NMB. It is an intermediate-duration NMB. Like gantacurium, it is rapidly inactivated by the endogenous amino acid cysteine via an adduction mechanism.

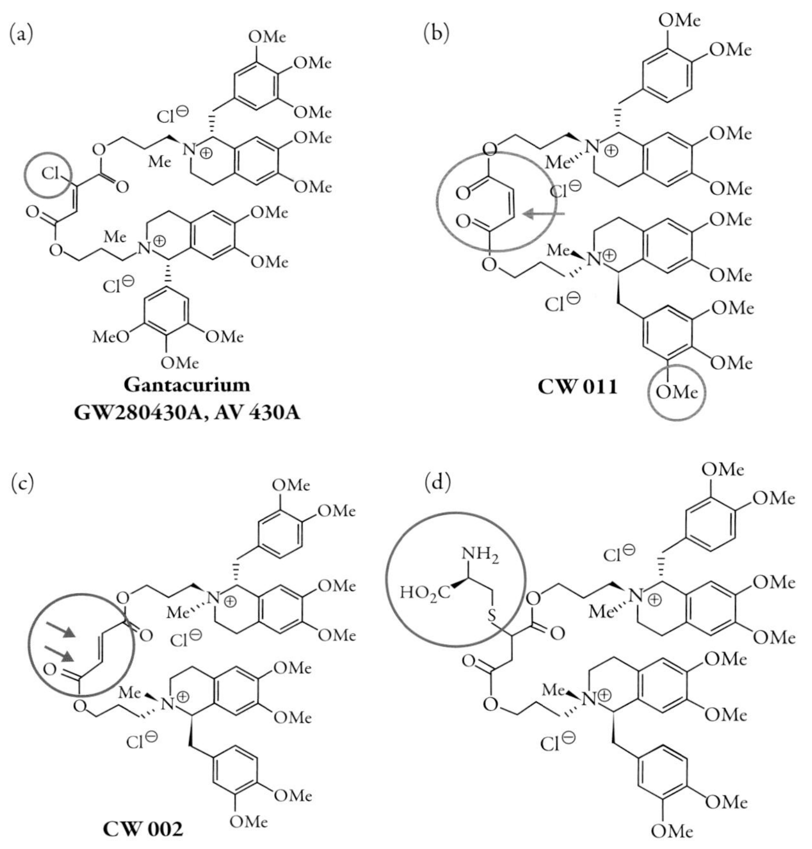

Figure 10.7   The chemical formulae of gantacurium (a), CW 011 (d), and CW 002 (c). The L-Cystein adduct of CW002 is shown in (d). (Reprinted from Savarese JJ, McGilvra JD, Sunaga H, et al. Rapid chemical antagonism of neuromuscular blockade by L-cysteine adduction to and inactivation of the olefinic (double-bonded) isoquinolinium diester compounds gantacurium (AV430A), CW 002, and CW 011. Anesthesiology. 2010;113:59).

Exogenous administration of cysteine also speeds up antagonism of neuromuscular blockade with this drug. Although high-dose cysteine administration has been reported to cause neurotoxicity in some animal species, this has not thus far been reported in humans. In addition, clinical testing thus far does not appear to display any organ toxicity associated with cysteine reversal of CW002 [75–78].

Current research in neuromuscular blockade is moving in a very exciting direction, with new drugs on the horizon that possess minimal adverse effects. In the future, these advances will undoubtedly further the safety of perioperative care delivered to the neurosurgical patient

REFERENCES

1. Grosman C, Zhou M, Auerbach A. Mapping the conformational wave of acetylcholine receptor channel gating. *Nature.* 2000;403:773–776.
2. Prior CB, Marshall IG. Neuromuscular junction physiology. In Hemmings HC, Hopkins PM, eds. *Foundations of Anesthesia.* 2nd edition. Philadelphia: Elsevier; 2006:435–460.
3. Shear TD, Martyn JA. Physiology and biology of neuromuscular transmission in health and disease. *J Crit Care.* 2009;24:5–10.
4. Bowman WC. Neuromuscular block. *Br J Pharmacol.* 2006;147: S277–S286.
5. Martyn JA, Richtsfeld M. Succinylcholine-induced hyperkalemia in acquired pathologic states: etiologic factors and molecular mechanisms. *Anesthesiology.* 2006;104:158–169.
6. Martyn JA, Fukushima Y, Chon JY, et al. Muscle relaxants in burns, trauma, and critical illness. *Int Anesthesiol Clin.* 2006;44:123–143.
7. Donati F, Bevan DR. Neuromuscular blocking agents. In Barash PG, Stoelting RK, Cahalan MK, Stock MC, eds. *Clinical Anesthesia.* 6th edition. Philadelphia: Lippincott Williams and Wilkins; 2009:498–530.
8. Martyn JA. Neuromuscular physiology and pharmacology. In Miller RD, Eriksson LI, Fleisher LA, Wiener-Kronish JP, Young WL, eds. *Miller's Anesthesia.* 7th edition. Philadelphia: Churchill Livingstone Elsevier; 2010:341–360.
9. Hemmerling TM, Schmidt J, Wolf T, et al. Surface vs. intramuscular laryngeal electromyography. *Can J Anaesth.* 2000;47:860–865.
10. Kopman AF, Zhaku B, Lai KS. The intubating dose of succinylcholine: the effect of decreasing doses on recovery time. *Anesthesiology.* 2003;99:1050–1054.
11. Naguib M, Lien CA, Aker J, et al. Posttetanic potentiation and fade in the response to tetanic and train-of-four stimulation during succinylcholine-induced block. *Anesth Analg.* 2004;98:1686–1691.
12. Ramsey FM, Lebowitz PW, Savarese JJ, et al. Clinical characteristics of long-term succinylcholine neuromuscular blockade during balanced anesthesia. *Anesth Analg.* 1980;59:110–116.

13. Bowman WC. Neuromuscular block. *Br J Pharm*. 2006;147:S277–S286.
14. Kopman AF, Klewicka MM, Kopman DJ, et al. Molar potency is predictive of the speed of onset of neuromuscular block for agents of intermediate, short and ultrashort duration. *Anesthesiology*. 1999;90:425.
15. Frampton JE, McTavish D. Mivacurium. A review of its pharmacology and therapeutic potential in general anaesthesia. *Drugs*. 1993;45:1066–1089.
16. Lien CA, Schmith VD, Belmont MR, et al. Pharmacokinetics of cisatracurium in patients receiving nitrous oxide/opioid/barbiturate anesthesia. *Anesthesiology*. 1996;84:300–308.
17. Perry JJ, Lee JS, Sillberg VA, et al. Rocuronium versus succinylcholine for rapid sequence induction intubation. *Cochrane Database Syst Rev*. 2008;2:CD002788.
18. Abrishami A, Ho J, Wong J, et al. Sugammadex, a selective reversal medication for preventing postoperative residual neuromuscular blockade. *Cochrane Database Syst Rev*. 2009;4:CD007362.
19. Rex C, Bergner UA, Pühringer FK. Sugammadex: a selective relaxant-binding agent providing rapid reversal. *Curr Opin Anaesthesiol*. 2010;23:461–465.
20. Kovac AL. Sugammadex: the first selective binding reversal agent for neuromuscular block. *J Clin Anesth*. 2009;21:444–453.
21. Wong SF, Chung F. Succinylcholine-associated postoperative myalgia. *Anaesthesia*. 2000;55:144–152.
22. Cannon JE. Precurarization. *Can J Anaesth*. 1994;41:177–183
23. Cottrell JE, Hartung J, Giffin JP, et al. Intracranial and hemodynamic changes after succinylcholine administration in cats. *Anesth Analg*. 1983;62:1006–1009.
24. Kovarik WD, Mayberg TS, Lam AM, et al. Succinylcholine does not change intracranial pressure, cerebral blood flow velocity, or the electroencephalogram in patients with neurologic injury. *Anesth Analg*. 1994;78:469–473.
25. Minton MD, Grosslight K, Stirt JA, et al. Increases in intracranial pressure from succinylcholine: prevention by prior nondepolarzing blockade. *Anesthesiology*. 1986;65:165–169.
26. Book JW, Mark A, Eisenkraft JB. Adverse effects of depolarizing neuromuscular blocking agents. *Drug Saf*. 1994;10: 331–349.
27. Strazis KP, Fox AW. Malignant hyperthermia: a review of published cases. *Anesth Analg*. 1993;77:297–304.
28. Larach MG, Gronert GA, Allen GC, et al. Clinical presentation, treatment, and complications of malignant hyperthermia in North America from. 1987 to. 2006. *Anesth Analg*. 2010;110:498–507.
29. Managing an MH crisis for health professionals. MHAUS website. http://www.mhaus.org/healthcare-professionals. Accessed on May 22, 2013.
30. The North American Malignant Hyperthermia Registry of MHAUS. MHAUS website. http://www.mhaus.org/registry. Accessed on May 22, 2013.
31. Debaene B, Plaud B, Dilly MP, et al. Residual paralysis in the PACU after a single intubating dose of nondepolarizing muscle relaxant with an intermediate duration of action. *Anesthesiology*. 2003;98:1042–1048.
32. Kopman AF, Yee PS, Neuman GG. Relationship of the train-of-four fade ratio to clinical signs and symptoms of residual paralysis in awake volunteers. *Anesthesiology*. 1997;86:765–771.
33. Murphy GS, Szokol JW, Marymont JH, et al. Residual neuromuscular block and critical respiratory events in the postanesthesia care unit. *Anesth Analg*. 2008;107:130–137.
34. Plaud B, Debaene B, Donati F, et al. Residual paralysis after emergence from anesthesia. *Anesthesiology*. 2010;112:1013–1022.
35. Bishop MJ, O'Donnell JT, Salemi JR. Mivacurium and bronchospasm. *Anesth Analg*. 2003;97:484.
36. Siler JN, Mager JG, Wyche MQ. Atracurium: hypotension, tachycardia and bronchospasm. *Anesthesiology*. 1985;62:645–646.
37. Fodale V, Santamaria LB. Laudanosine, an atracurium and cisatracurium metabolite. *Eur J Anaesthesiol*. 2002;19:466–473.
38. Baraka A. Anaesthesia and myasthenia gravis. *Can J Anesth*. 1992;39:476–486.
39. Abel M, Eisenkraft JB. Anesthetic implications of myasthenia gravis. *Mt Sinai J Med*. 2002;69:31–37.
40. Eisenkraft JB, Book WJ, Papatestas AE. Sensitivity to vecuronium in myasthenia gravis: a dose-response study. *Can J Anaesth*. 1990;37:301–306.
41. Eisenkraft. Resistance to succinylcholine in myasthenia gravis: a dose-response study. *Anesthesiology*. 1988;69:670–673.
42. Baraka A, Wakid N, Mansour R, et al. Effect of neostigmine and pyridostigmine on the plasma cholinesterase activity. *Br J Anesth*. 1981;53:849–851.
43. Dillon FX. Anesthesia issues in the perioperative management of myasthenia gravis. *Semin Neurol*. 2004;24:83–94.
44. Kernstine KH. Preoperative preparation of the patient with myasthenia gravis. *Thorac Surg Clin*. 2005;15:287–295.
45. de Boer HD, van Egmond J, Driessen JJ, et al. Sugammadex in patients with myasthenia gravis. *Anaesthesia*. 2010;65:653.
46. Petrun AM, Mekis D, Kamenik M. Successful use of rocuronium and sugammadex in a patient with myasthenia. *Eur J Anaesthesiol*. 2010;27:917–918.
47. Unterbuchner C, Fink H, Blobner M. The use of sugammadex in a patient with myasthenia gravis. *Anaesthesia*. 2010;65:302–305.
48. Russell SH, Hirsch NP. Anaesthesia and myotonia. *Br J Anaesth*. 1994;72:210–216.
49. Rosenbaum HK, Miller JD. Malignant hyperthermia and myotonic disorders. *Anesthesiol Clin N Am*. 2002;20:623–664.
50. Neuman GG, Kopman AF. Dyskalemic periodic paralysis and myotonia. *Anesth Analg*. 1993;76:426–428.
51. Rowland LP, Shneider NA. Amyotrophic lateral sclerosis. *N Engl J Med*. 2001;344:1688–1700.
52. Cooperman LH, Strobel GE Jr, Kennell EM. Massive hyperkalemia after administration of succinylcholine. *Anesthesiology*. 1970;32:161–164.
53. Rosenbaum KJ, Neigh JL, Strobel GE. Sensitivity to nondepolarizing muscle relaxants in amyotrophic lateral sclerosis: report of two cases. *Anesthesiology*. 1971;35: 638–641.
54. Pritchard J. Guillain-Barré syndrome. *Clin Med*. 2010;10: 399–401.
55. Dua K, Banerjee A. Guillain-Barré syndrome: a review. *Br J Hosp Med (Lond)*. 2010;71:495–498.
56. Kocabas S, Karaman S, Firat V, et al. Anesthetic management of Guillain-Barré syndrome in pregnancy. *J Clin Anesth*. 2007;19:299–302.
57. Pasternak JJ, Lanier WL. Diseases affecting the brain. In Hines RL, Marschall KE, eds. *Stoelting's Anesthesia and Coexisting Diseases*. 5th edition. Philadelphia: Churchill Livingstone; 2008:199–238.
58. Castillo LR, Shankar G, Robertson CS. Management of intracranial hypertension. *Neurol Clin*. 2008;26:521–541.
59. Lescot T, Abdennour L, Boch AL, et al. Treatment of intracranial hypertension. *Curr Opin Crit Care*. 2008;14:129–134.
60. Rangel-Castilla L, Gopinath S, Robertson CS. Management of intracranial hypertension. *Neurol Clin*. 2008;26:521–541.
61. Werba A, Weinstabl C, Petricek W, et al. Requisite muscle relaxation using vecuronium for tracheobronchial suction in neurosurgical intensive care patients. *Anaesthesist*. 1991;40:328–331.
62. Lotto ML, Banoub M, Schubert A. Effects of anesthetic agents and physiologic changes on intraoperative motor evoked potentials. *J Neurosurg Anesthesiol*. 2004;16:32–42.
63. Sloan TB, Heyer EJ. Anesthesia for intraoperative neurophysiologic monitoring of the spinal cord. *J Clin Neurophysiol*. 2002;19:430–443.
64. Jameson LC, Sloan TB. Monitoring of the brain and spinal cord. *Anesthesiol Clin*. 2006;24:777–791.
65. Lang EW, Beutler AS, Chesnut RM, et al. Myogenic motor-evoked potential monitoring using partial neuromuscular blockade in surgery of the spine. *Spine*. 1996;21:1676–1686.
66. Kalkman CJ, Drummond JC, Kennelly NA, et al. Intraoperative monitoring of tibialis anterior muscle motor evoked responses to

transcranial electrical stimulation during partial neuromuscular blockade. *Anesth Analg.* 1992;75:584–589.

67. Marshall IG, Gibb AJ, Durant NN. Neuromuscular and vagal blocking actions of pancuronium bromide, its metabolites, and vecuronium bromide (Org NC45) and its potential metabolites in the anaesthetized cat. *Br J Anaesth.* 1983;55:703–714.

68. Segredo V, Caldwell JE, Matthay MA, et al. Persistent paralysis in critically ill patients after long-term administration of vecuronium. *N Engl J Med.* 1992;327:524–528.

69. Pandit L, Agrawal A. Neuromuscular disorders in critical illness. *Clin Neurol Neurosurg.* 2006;108:621–627.

70. Murphy GS, Vender JS. Neuromuscular-blocking drugs. Use and misuse in the intensive care unit. *Crit Care Clin.* 2001;17:925–942.

71. Murray MJ, Brull SJ, Bolton CF. Brief review: Nondepolarizing neuromuscular blocking drugs and critical illness myopathy. *Can J Anaesth.* 2006;53:1148–1156.

72. Chawla J, Gruener G. Management of critical illness polyneuropathy and myopathy. *Neurol Clin.* 2010;28:961–977.

73. Caldwell JE. Clinical limitations of acetylcholinesterase antagonists. *J Crit Care.* 2009;24:21–28.

74. Caldwell JE, Miller RD. Clinical implications of sugammadex. *Anaesthesia.* 2009;64(Suppl 1):66–72.

75. Lien CA, Savard P, Belmont M, et al. Fumarates: unique nondepolarizing neuromuscular blocking agents that are antagonized by cysteine. *J Crit Care.* 2009;24:50–57.

76. Naguib M, Brull SJ. Update on neuromuscular pharmacology. *Curr Opin Anaesthesiol.* 2009;22:483–490.

77. Savarese JJ, McGilvra JD, Sunaga H, et al. Rapid chemical antagonism of neuromuscular blockade by L-cysteine adduction to and inactivation of the olefinic (double-bonded) isoquinolinium diester compounds gantacurium (AV430A), CW 002, and CW 011. *Anesthesiology.* 2010;113:58–73.

78. Sunaga H, Malhotra JK, Yoon E, et al. Cysteine reversal of the novel neuromuscular blocking drug CW002 in dogs: pharmacodynamics, acute cardiovascular effects, and preliminary toxicology. *Anesthesiology.* 2010;112:900–909.

11.

FLUID MANAGEMENT IN THE NEUROSURGICAL PATIENT

Markus Klimek and Thomas H. Ottens

INTRODUCTION

Good fluid management in neurosurgical patients can be summarized in one easy sentence: *Give the right amount of the right fluid to the right patient.* But something that sounds so easy can be quite challenging. Properly planned and calculated fluid management around neurosurgical procedures is more critical than for, say, an orthopedic day case surgery [1]. Edema may occur under a variety of neurologic conditions and can have disastrous effects. The brain is involved in regulating the fluid balance through hypothalamic antidiuretic hormone (ADH) production, and disturbances of ADH production and secretion are frequently seen in neurosurgical patients. Furthermore, fluid management also includes the therapeutic use of fluids like mannitol and hypertonic saline solutions, which are frequently used in neurosurgical patients. Finally, an adequate perioperative coagulation status is mandatory around neurosurgical procedures, because they can be complicated by major bleeding. This chapter will provide a physiologic and pharmacologic background, which is useful to find out how to give "the right amount of the right fluid to the right patient."

PHYSIOLOGIC ASPECTS

To maintain an adequate systemic blood pressure (and thus adequate cerebral perfusion pressure [CPP]), the cardiovascular system must be properly filled. One aspect of fluid management is that the volume required to keep the intravascular space filled must be replaced in proportion to ongoing losses in the surgical field. In hypovolemic and hypotensive patients, cerebral perfusion can become compromised, so normovolemia should be the goal in most neurosurgical patients. Although all fluids are administered into the extracellular, intravascular space, they invariably

affect the intracellular space as well. Osmotic and oncotic forces drive water from the intravascular (blood) to the extravascular space (tissue) and vice versa. Inside the rigid intracranial space, water moving into (swelling) and out of (shrinking) brain tissue will affect the intracranial pressure (ICP) and the cerebral blood flow (CBF). Both fluid volume and composition must therefore be carefully chosen to suit the clinical situation. Maintaining adequate perfusion while preventing intracranial hypertension will ultimately maintain adequate brain perfusion.

When choosing the right type of fluid, a rule of thumb is to use a fluid that is similar to the fluid that the patient lost. Sweat, gastric contents, insensible perspiration, urine, and cerebrospinal fluid can be replaced by crystalloids, while colloids, and/or blood products should be used to replace blood loss.

FLUID COMPARTMENTS

Water is the most important component of the human body, it accounts for 60% of the body weight. This so-called total body water (TBW) is divided into three important compartments (see Figure 11.1):

1. The intracellular space (two-thirds of TBW, approximately to 28 L in a 70-kg adult)

2. The extracellular space (one-third of TBW, approximately to 14 L in a 70-kg adult). The extracellular space is divided into:

    a. The interstitial space (80%), fluid in the space between the cells, but not contained within the blood vessels.
    b. The intravascular space (20%), consisting mostly of plasma.

Water-permeable membranes separate these compartments from each other. The cell membrane divides the intracellular

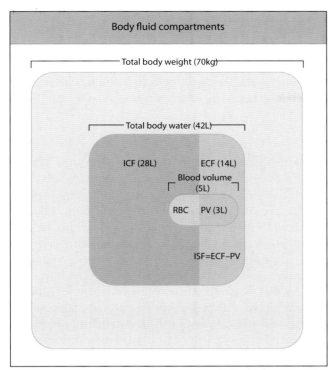

Figure 11.1   ICF, intracellular fluid; ECF, extracellular fluid; RBC, red blood cells; PV, plasma volume; ISF, interstitial fluid.

[From Hemmings, HC, Hopkins PM. *Foundations of anesthesia: basic sciences for clinical practice* (2nd ed.). Philadelphia: Elsevier; 2006.]

and the extracellular space, and the capillary membrane divides the intravascular and interstitial space. Fluid therefore moves across the membranes as the osmolarity in one compartment changes relative to another. As a result, fluid therapy may dramatically affect cellular function in the entire body.

Although the osmolarity in all compartments is normally equal, the compositions of the different fluids in each compartment are quite different: intracellular fluids are rich in potassium, whereas sodium is the most abundant ion in extracellular fluids.

INTRACRANIAL COMPARTMENTS

Many problems in neurosurgical anesthesia and neurocritical care are linked to the fact that a rigid skull encases our brain. Therefore, any increase in intracranial volume will cause an increase in ICP. Of the intracranial compartments, brain tissue occupies the most volume (1400 mL), followed by cerebrospinal fluid (150 mL), venous blood (120 mL), and arterial blood (30 mL). Within certain limits, fluids can easily move in and out of the skull to keep the ICP constant and the volume of an intracranial mass (e.g., tumor or hematoma) can grow without increasing the ICP, as long as this growth is matched by a decrease in volume of blood and/or cerebrospinal fluid. However, this compensation mechanism fails when the intracranial mass becomes too big or the

patient is positioned with his or her head down or if neck torsion obstructs venous drainage. In these cases, ICP will ultimately rise.

CPP is determined by the formula

$$\mathbf{CPP = MAP - ICP}$$

As a result, elevated ICP, especially in the presence of hypotension, may result in cerebral ischemia. Maintaining an adequate CPP while preventing an increase in ICP is part of the anesthetic (fluid) management in neuroanesthesia.

BLOOD–BRAIN BARRIER

The blood vessels in the brain have a unique endothelium, characterized by tight junctions between the endothelial cells, forming the blood–brain barrier (BBB) [2] The BBB restricts the movement of ions, molecules, and water between the brain and plasma. Only a few areas of the brain lack tight junctions and are permeable to drugs, hormones, and toxins. Examples of such areas are the choroid plexus, the pituitary gland, and the area postrema, the area of the brain that can trigger nausea and vomiting. Ischemia and trauma (including surgical manipulation) are the most important causes of disruption of the BBB. If the BBB becomes leaky, larger molecules can enter the interstitium of the brain, where they can attract water and produce "vasogenic" brain edema [3]

OSMOLALITY, TONICITY, AND ONCOTIC PRESSURE

The term *osmolarity* describes the number of osmotically active particles per liter of solution. Osmolarity is calculated by adding up all osmotically active particles in a liter of solution and is expressed as mOsm/L.

Osmolality describes the number of osmotically active particles relative to 1 kg of water. Because 1 L of water weighs 1 kg, the difference between the two only becomes interesting for fluids that do not consist solely of water (such as blood). The osmolality of plasma can be approximated by using the following formula (Na^+, glucose, and blood urea in mmol/L):

$$\mathbf{Osmolality\ (mOsm/kg\ H_2O)}$$
$$= (\mathbf{serum\ [Na^+] \times 2) + blood\ glucose + blood\ urea}$$

According to the principle of osmosis, water will cross a semipermeable membrane dividing two fluid compartments with different osmolarity until the osmolarity is equal in both compartments. In other words: osmolarity is the force that drives fluids to shift between compartments.

Both small molecules (e.g., sodium, glucose, urea) and larger molecules (e.g., proteins, sugars, and starch polymers) are capable of attracting water. The water attracting capacity of large molecules is called "oncotic pressure." The oncotic pressure counteracts the hydrostatic force that the arterial blood pressure exerts on tissues. Thus, when the concentration of large molecules falls, the oncotic pressure drops, allowing the hydrostatic force of the blood pressure to push fluid out of the blood vessels and into the tissue. This explains why patients with protein deficiencies tend to develop edema.

Fluid management in neuroanesthesia must aim to keep the osmotic and oncotic pressures of the patient within normal physiologic ranges to avoid edema formation. This requires that an appropriate amount of the correct fluids be administered, tailored to the volume and type of fluid lost by the patient [4].

PHARMACOLOGIC ASPECTS

CRYSTALLOIDS

Crystalloids contain electrolytes, sometimes mixed with sugars and other small molecules. They are commonly used to correct the extravascular volume and move freely between the intravascular and extravascular space along concentration gradients. Crystalloids come in many varieties, ranging from the simple, cheap, and widely used NaCl 0.9% to the more complex "balanced" solutions, designed to mimic the composition of blood. Hypertonic solutions, such as mannitol and hypertonic saline, are crystalloids designed for specialized uses, which may serve other purposes than correction of the extravascular volume. They are discussed in more detail next (see also Table 11.1).

NaCl 0.9%

Physiologic sodium chloride solution is commonly used to compensate for extravascular volume deficiency, such as dehydration. After infusion, NaCl 0.9% (normal saline [NS]) is distributed to the entire extracellular compartment.

Specific advantages of NS are its low cost and wide availability, applicability, and compatibility. It is, however, unbuffered and acidic, and the infusion of large volumes of NS may produce hyperchloremic acidosis. Physiologic saline is not actually physiologic: its sodium concentration is 154 mmol/L, making it a hyperosmolar solution.

Glucose 5%

This simple glucose solution, sometimes denoted "D5W," contains 50 g of glucose/L. Glucose solutions are cheap and widely available. They may be used to prevent hypoglycemia, especially in young children and infants. Glucose, sometimes called dextrose, is rapidly taken up into the cells, leaving free water to distribute across the other compartments. The infusion of large volumes of glucose-containing fluids may result in hyponatremia and hyperglycemia, both of which may worsen cerebral edema and neurologic injury. After the glucose has been taken up into cells, "glucose 5%" is just water and decreases plasma osmolarity. As plasma osmolarity falls, water diffuses into tissues, including the brain, increasing ICP and potentially reducing CBF.

In patients with liver failure or hypernatremia, glucose-containing solutions may be useful, but they should not be part of a standard fluid regimen in adult neurosurgical patients.

Ringer's Lactate

Ringer's lactate (RL) became popular when evidence accumulated about hyperchloremic acidosis caused by infusion of large volumes of NS. The substitution of the chloride anion for lactate, which is metabolized in the liver, reduces the risk of hyperchloremic acidosis. RL also contains 4 to 5 mmol/L potassium and should therefore be used with caution in patients with kidney failure. The liver metabolizes lactate to bicarbonate, which slightly increases oxygen consumption and $PaCO_2$. Like in case of glucose infusion, via this metabolism a part of the RL solution becomes

Table 11.1 **TYPICAL ANALYSIS OF HUMAN PLASMA AND THE CLASSIC CRYSTALLOIDS**

	PLASMA (HUMAN)	NS (NaCl 0.9%)	GLUCOSE 5% (D5W)	RL*
Na+, mmol/L	142	154		130
K+, mmol/L	4.5			4
Ca2+, mmol/L	2.5			1
Mg2+, mmol/L				1
Cl−, mmol/L	103	154		112
Lactate−, mmol/L				27
Glucose, g/L	$7–11 \times 10^{-3}$		50 (5%)	
Osmolarity, mOsmol/L	291	308	0†	276

* The composition of RL varies slightly between manufacturers.
† In vivo.

free water. Infusion of large volumes of RL may therefore decrease plasma osmolarity, increasing ICP and reducing CBF in the compromised patient. Note that the infusion of RL should be considered in the interpretation of elevated plasma lactate levels in the operating room and intensive care unit, especially in patients with limited liver function.

"Balanced" Solutions

Classic solutions such as NS and RL contain nonphysiologic concentrations of electrolytes and may alter plasma osmolality and acid-base balance. Balanced solutions are designed to mimic the composition of plasma as closely as possible (see also Table 11.2). Instead of just lactate, balanced crystalloids contain other metabolizable anions to buffer the solution, such as gluconate, acetate, and the divalent malate, which are also metabolized to bicarbonate but with reduced oxygen requirement compared with lactate. Balanced crystalloids may also contain glucose, potassium, magnesium, and calcium. There is no evidence that one of these anions is better than the other one, and most of these solutions seem to be interchangeable.

Hypertonic Saline

Hypertonic saline was first used for resuscitation of massive hemorrhage in the prehospital setting. The hypertonic (hyperosmolar) solution causes water to move from the intracellular and extracellular compartment to the bloodstream. Thus, in contrast to normotonic crystalloid solutions, hypertonic saline expands the intravascular volume, so that smaller volumes of crystalloid are required to restore the circulating volume: a concept known as *small volume resuscitation*. Hypertonic saline administration can reduce the ICP, as it will cause water from the brain to move into the bloodstream, thus reducing intracranial tissue volume [5, 6] Hypertonic saline solutions may also be used with caution to correct hyponatremia. Rapid correction of chronic hyponatremia may, however, result in (irreversible) central pontine myelinolysis. Hypertonic solutions may cause phlebitis when administered via peripheral veins. There is also an intrinsic risk of hypernatremia and/or hyperchloremic acidosis when hypertonic saline solutions are used, especially in large volumes.

Mannitol

Mannitol is a sugar solution that is not used to replace volume loss but rather as an osmotic diuretic [7–9]. Commercially available preparations typically contain 150 or 200 g of mannitol/L (15 or 20%), dissolved in water without added electrolytes. It is excreted by the kidneys and minimally reabsorbed. It thus increases the tonicity of the tubular fluid and attracts water from the bloodstream, producing a brisk diuresis of very dilute urine. This may result in hypovolemia and hypokalemia. Like hypertonic saline, mannitol causes water to move from the extravascular into the intravascular space. Compared with hypertonic saline, mannitol has additional properties that may contribute to its therapeutic potential: mannitol has been shown to inhibit apoptosis and has radical scavenging properties. Mannitol passes easily across damaged endothelium and may cause osmotic edema. This is of particular concern to patients with a damaged BBB, in whom mannitol may cause cerebral edema and raised ICP. Therefore, mannitol should be used quite carefully, especially in patients with longer-lasting pathologies (e.g., >24 hours after brain injury).

Mannitol is often used to protect the kidneys from the effects of contrast dye or chemotherapy, but recent evidence renders this practice obsolete.

COLLOIDS

Colloid solutions contain both electrolytes and large, heavy molecules, such as starch polymers or proteins. They can be used to replace intravascular volume loss. Many varieties

Table 11.2   TYPICAL ANALYSIS OF HUMAN PLASMA AND SOME BALANCED CRYSTALLOID SOLUTIONS

	PLASMA(HUMAN)	PLASMALYTEA (BAXTER)	PLASMALYTE146 (BAXTER)	STEROFUNDIN ISO (B. BRAUN)
Na^+, mmol/L	142	140	140	145
K^+, mmol/L	4.5	5	5	4
Ca^{2+}, mmol/L	2.5			2.5
Mg^{2+}, mmol/L	1.25	3	3	1
Cl^-, mmol/L	103	98	98	127
Acetate, mmol/L		27	27	24
$Malate^{2-}$, mmol/L				5
$Gluconate^-$, mmol/L		23	23	
Glucose, g/L	$7–11 \times 10^{-3}$		50 (5%)	
Osmolarity, mOsmol/L	291	294	547*	309

*Due to glucose, will be much lower in vivo after cellular uptake.

exist, ranging from simple enriched NS to "balanced colloids." The oncotic pressure exerted by the large molecules keep the infused volume inside the blood vessels and will even attract some additional fluid from the extravascular compartments. This is why they are also known as "plasma expanders": their effect on intravascular volume exceeds the infused volume. This is important in hypovolemic patients, in whom infusion of colloids might induce further intracellular volume depletion. It is therefore uncommon to use colloids as the first intravenous fluid to administer to a patient.

In patients with damaged endothelium, colloid molecules may leak out of the blood vessels, resulting in formation of interstitial edema. Colloids may also impair coagulation and cause allergic reactions. As a result, the safety and efficacy of colloids, their use in different conditions, and their relationship with cheaper crystalloids are the subjects of ongoing debate. The most important colloids are discussed next.

Hydroxyethyl Starch

Hydroxyethyl starch (HES) is the most commonly used artificial colloid worldwide. HES is a heavy, branched starch molecule, in which some glucose units have been substituted with hydroxyethyl groups. HES molecules come in three varieties. The first generation of very high molecular weight (>450 kDa) is known as hetastarch. The second generation, medium molecular weight (220 kDa), is known as pentastarch. The third generation has a lower molecular weight (130 kDa) and a molecular substitution grade of 0.4, which means 40% of the glucose units in the starch molecule are substituted with hydroxyethyl groups. This is denoted as HES 130/0.4.

After administration, small HES molecules are eliminated rapidly by the kidneys, and larger molecules undergo degradation by plasma α-amylase before excretion. In health, elimination half-life ($t_{1/2}\beta$) of 6% HES 130/0.4 is 12 hours. Terminal half-life is not affected in mild to moderate kidney failure [11]. The volume effect of HES-based colloid solutions lasts approximately 6 hours. HES is also available in a "balanced crystalloid" solution, marketed as Tetraspan or Volulyte in Europe.

HES, especially the older high molecular weight varieties, adversely affect coagulation by reducing the activity of factor VIII and von Willebrand factor. However, the effect of third generation HES products on coagulation seems to be clinically irrelevant within the recommended dosing limit (50 mL/kg/d). In case of volume resuscitation for major blood loss, these dose limits can be applied less strictly. High molecular weight HES also increases the risk of kidney failure in critically ill patients [10]. All HES-containing solutions may cause intense pruritus, but this risk seems to be smaller with third-generation formulations. Recently, several articles of one author supporting the use of HES in different states of critical illness and perioperative care have been retracted due to lack of ethical approval or scientific frauds. Furthermore, some recent studies have shown an increased incidence of renal failure in ICU-patients treated with HES-products. Nevertheless, several studies, as well as the personal experience of the authors support the use of 130/0.4 HES solution for compensation of perioperative blood loss.

Dextrans

Dextrans are solutions of polysaccharide molecules, numbered for their average molecular weight in kDa (40, 60, and 70). Dextran 40 reduces blood viscosity. As with the HES family, the dextrans interfere with coagulation by reducing the activity of factor VIII. This von Willebrand disease–like state may be partly remedied by administration of desmopressin (0.3 μg/kg). After administration, the smallest dextran variety (40) is eliminated by the kidneys, whereas the larger (60 and 70) dextrans are hydrolyzed after distribution into tissues. Unlike HES, dextrans do not cause pruritus, but they have a high risk of allergic reactions. The risk of allergic reactions can be reduced by administering a dextran monomer solution (marketed as Promit or Promiten) which inhibits hapten formation. In general, there is no indication for using dextrans in neurosurgical patients.

Gelatin

Gelatins are prepared from bovine collagen and have an average molecular weight of 35 kDa. The two most common varieties are essentially different: Haemaccel, which is urea-crosslinked, contains sodium (145 mmol/L), calcium (6.25 mmol/L), and potassium (5.1 mmol/L), whereas Gelofusin, the succinylated gelatin, is dissolved in normal saline and does not contain calcium or potassium. Gelatin does not seem to have any intrinsic effects on coagulation. Rapid infusion of gelatin-containing products may lead to histamine release, bronchospasm, and hypotension. Gelatin molecules will leak into tissues when the endothelial barrier is damaged. Gelatin solutions are not currently approved for use in the United States. Moreover, because gelatin is an animal product, the risk of transmission of prion diseases still is not completely excluded. Gelatins are rapidly eliminated by the kidneys and have a much shorter $t_{1/2}\beta$ compared with dextrans and HES.

Albumin

Commercial albumin preparations are prepared from donated human plasma and must therefore be considered a blood product. It is, therefore, more expensive than other colloid solutions. Albumin is available in 5% and 20% ("salt-free") solutions. The 20% solution is hypertonic and is capable of expanding plasma by 4 to 5 times the infused volume, similar to hypertonic saline. In otherwise healthy patients, the $t_{1/2}\beta$ of albumin is approximately 16 hours. In general, albumin should only be given in patients with reduced plasma albumin (<25 g/L). If albumin is given, one should be aware that it is not just an intravenous fluid but that it also has buffering capacities, may alter the bioavailability of protein-bound drugs, and might have immunologic effects. After a period of recommendations against its use, there now seems to be growing evidence supporting the use albumin (particularly 20% solutions) in specific, critically ill patients and those with proved hypoalbuminemia, where the possible advantages compared with other colloids possibly offset the much higher price [12–15].

BLOOD AND BLOOD PRODUCTS

To provide the brain with a sufficient amount of oxygen, a minimum hemoglobin (Hb) concentration of 4 mmol/L (6 g/dL) is necessary, especially when a patient is breathing room air. Major blood loss may occur during neurosurgery. The accidental opening of a venous sinus during craniotomy, bleeding from an aneurysm or arteriovenous malformation, damage to the internal carotid artery during transsphenoidal surgery, and resection of vascular brain tumors that have not been embolized (e.g., meningiomas) are just a few examples. At a minimum, therefore, a hemoglobin level and a type and screen should be routinely obtained for all patients undergoing craniotomy, and at least 1 cross-matched unit of packed red blood cells (PRBCs) should be available at the beginning of the procedure.

Proper handling of blood loss from the skin and skull can be expected of any dedicated neurosurgeon. However, the venous blood loss from damaged vessels inside the brain is difficult to manage surgically, and therefore the anesthesiologist has to support the neurosurgeons' efforts by optimizing coagulation and preventing fibrinolysis. Performing thrombelastography can be useful in determining the needs of the patient with an evident coagulation problem. The decision to treat bleeding with coagulation factors is driven by the prothrombin time (PT), the international normalized ratio (INR), fibrinogen levels, and the platelet count, if thrombelastography is not available. However, these tests take more time and their results might be outdated, when they arrive on the operating room. Anesthesiologists should strongly consider infusing plasma products, platelets, fibrinogen, and other coagulation factors like recombinant factor VIIa during periods of major blood loss.

On the other hand, one should be aware of the fact that many neurosurgical diseases produce activated coagulation states and a higher risk of perioperative deep venous thrombosis. Therefore, at least mechanical thrombosis prophylaxis by compression stockings is recommended in practically all neurosurgical patients.

CLINICAL PRACTICE

Due to a lack of clinical evidence about the best fluid regimen for most neurosurgical patient subgroups, this paragraph will address the pathophysiologic principles and clinical issues under special circumstances and make some well-founded recommendations. These aim to assist the anesthesiologist who takes care of patients in such situations in choosing a safe, efficient, and practical fluid management strategy.

THE "NORMAL" NEUROSURGICAL PATIENT

Maintaining normovolemia has the highest priority in these patients: the fluid regimen begins with preoperative fasting. In neurosurgical patients without an increased risk of regurgitation and aspiration, drinking clear fluids is allowed up to 2 hours before induction of anesthesia, and eating up to 6 hours before induction. There is no evidence that preoperative use of carbohydrate enriched nutritional drinks have additional values in neurosurgical patients (they may have in neuroanesthetists!), so water, tea, or apple juice will do just fine.

If the patient must be fasted completely for much longer than 2 hours for any reason, intravenous fluids (NaCl 0.9%) should be given to maintain normovolemia.

Patients prepared that way will not arrive in the operating room with volume deficit and will show a less pronounced blood pressure drop after induction of anesthesia.

However, if a patient does arrive fluid depleted due to overnight fasting, it is not effective to attempt to compensate this with a bolus of 1000 mL of crystalloid. It may even be detrimental, as the major part of this bolus will be distributed to tissue, where it may contribute to interstitial and cerebral edema [16].

There is no "best maintenance fluid" for the "normal" neurosurgical patient: too much NaCl 0.9% may cause hyperchloremic acidosis [17], whereas too much RL and other "balanced solutions" are slightly hypotonic and will also produce higher $PaCO_2$ levels. Alternating between both types of fluids (1:1) is a reasonable option.

The amount of maintenance fluid should not be overestimated: In neurosurgery, there is normally a small surgical field with minimal insensible losses [18]. Urine output and gastric losses should be compensated 1:1 with crystalloids, and blood loss should be compensated 1:1 with colloids or blood products, depending on the Hb level and comorbidity of the patient. In general, the preoperative net fluid balance of a "normal" neurosurgical patient should not be more than 1000 mL positive, which in most cases means intravenous drip rates should be slow.

In the postoperative period, patients may start with drinking as soon as they are awake enough to do so safely, and when all coughing and swallowing reflexes have recovered. Low-flow infusion (20–25 mL/h) will be sufficient to keep the intravenous lines open and will avoid hypervolemia. If no thalamic or pituitary damage has occurred during the procedure, patients' thirst drive will help them to stay normovolemic and no additional measures are necessary.

THE PATIENT WITH INCREASED ICP

Fluid management in patients with increased ICP has three major goals, which might be contradictory:

1. To keep the brain perfused

2. To prevent further increase of the ICP

3. To reduce interstitial edema and ICP by osmotically active agents

To achieve these goals as good as possible, several factors must be considered. CPP is defined as the difference between the mean arterial pressure (MAP) and the ICP:

$$CPP = MAP - ICP$$

As mentioned above, the ICP can be decreased by venous drainage. So, if MAP is maintained with a high central venous pressure, venous drainage will become compromised, and the ICP will stay elevated, ultimately resulting in reduced cerebral perfusion. Therefore, normovolemia should be maintained in patients with increased ICP.

To prevent further increase of the ICP by extravasation of water, hypotonic fluids like glucose 5% are obsolete.

Treating interstitial edema by infusion of hyperosmolar fluids like mannitol or hypertonic saline solution is a therapeutic option in patients with increased ICP [19]. However, some aspects must be taken into consideration, when using these fluids:

1. To produce the desired effect, these fluids should be administered as a high-flow bolus within a short time. This may irritate peripheral blood vessels.

2. In case of a disturbed BBB, applying these fluids might be detrimental, because they might pass through the disturbed barrier and increase interstitial edema. However, this concept of "rebound intracranial hypertension" is not based on strong scientific evidence.

3. If these fluids produce the desired effect, they will induce polyuria, which may lead to intravascular hypovolemia and hypotension, resulting in reduced CBF. This effect will be much more pronounced after mannitol than after hypertonic saline administration.

4. Both agents will—at least temporarily—increase the circulating intravascular volume. This may promote or aggravate the occurrence of heart failure in predisposed patients. With mannitol, this effect will last only very short, as rapid diuresis follows administration, and the volume effect of hypertonic saline may last much longer.

5. These fluids may induce significant shifts in plasma sodium concentration. A 320–mOsmol/L ceiling is frequently recommended for the use of mannitol; however, this seems to be based more on popular belief

than scientific evidence. On the other hand, patients with a sodium above 160 mmol/L treated with mannitol have an increased mortality risk. With such a high sodium level, osmolality may be as high as 335 to 340 mOsmol/L.

Considering all this, one can conclude that applying osmotically active agents in case of increased ICP must be a well-indicated therapeutic decision, which in most cases works better in early stages of the underlying disease where the BBB is still intact (trauma, subarachnoid hemorrhage, etc.) than in the later phases, and that such agents can produce serious adverse effects.

THE PATIENT WITH SUBARACHNOID OR INTRACEREBRAL HEMORRHAGE

After intracerebral or subarachnoid hemorrhage, fluid management requires the consideration of two apparently contradictory goals:

1. CPP must be high enough to enable sufficient CBF to the primary area of damage and the penumbra and to counteract vasospasm.

2. CPP must not become so high as to risk rebleeding.

Once the bleeding source has been controlled by coiling or clipping, the risk of rebleeding is minimal, and one can aim for higher blood pressures. In the past, this "triple-H therapy" (hypertension, hypervolemia, hemodilution) has been strongly supported. However, recent study results on the benefit of overfilling these patients to prevent vasospasm have been contradictory [20–22]. Avoiding hypovolemia (maintaining normovolemia) and the administration of a calcium antagonist (nimodipine) seem to be equally effective but with less adverse effects [23]. Keeping the patient slightly hypertensive is recommended by several authors.

During neurovascular surgery, major blood loss may occur, and packed cells and plasma products should be readily available.

THE PATIENT WITH TRAUMATIC BRAIN INJURY

Trauma patients should be resuscitated following an ATLS-like algorithm [24]. Fluid management in these algorithms is part of "C" for circulation. Maintaining blood pressure and oxygenation on the one side, and the prevention of acidosis, hypothermia, and coagulation disturbances on the other side are the major goals in caring for trauma patients, regardless of whether they have traumatic brain injury [25].

In patients with traumatic brain injury, management principles might be different (and less conflicting) in cases where the patient is suffering from isolated brain injury compared with patients suffering from traumatic brain injury as part of a polytrauma.

In both cases, patients need an adequate CPP, but it is much easier to establish this in patients with isolated brain injury: an isolated brain injury almost never (except in children or in cases of severe skin lesions) will be the cause of a hypovolemic shock and administering some intravenous fluids and (if necessary) catecholamines to maintain systolic blood pressure can be done quite easily.

In the case of a patient with, for example, liver rupture and pelvic fracture, as well as severe closed-head injury, increasing the blood pressure by fluid and catecholamine resuscitation can be disastrous, as long as the bleeding source has not been controlled. Permissive hypotension can be applied to limit the ongoing blood loss and to prevent hemodilution from intravenous fluids before blood products can be given, which threatens adequate cerebral perfusion and oxygenation. Evidence does not currently point toward the best approach to these conflicting priorities, and it seems difficult to perform a good, prospective randomized trial to solve these open questions.

It is clearly proved that every episode of hypotension (systolic blood pressure <90 mm Hg) and hypoxemia (SaO_2 <90%), and especially combinations of both, worsens the clinical outcome of patients with traumatic brain injury by increasing secondary brain damage. Above these limits, which should be kept strictly, there is no evidence that aiming for much higher or even supranormal values will further improve the outcome.

Especially in the early period after trauma, when the BBB is still intact, the administration of hypertonic fluids seems to be advantageous [26, 27]. Their small volume prevents excessive hemodilution and blood pressure increases, whereas their hyperosmolar properties will lead to a decrease in intracranial volume, reduced brain edema formation, and ultimately lower ICP. The high sodium content of hypertonic fluids limits their dose.

One should be aware that the detrimental effects of hypotension and hypoxia are pronounced in the presence of anemia. To provide adequate oxygen supply to the brain, Hb should be kept greater than 4 mmol/L (6.5 g/dL), even in young patients without comorbidity, and greater than 6 mmol/L (9.7 g/dL) in older patients with cardiopulmonary comorbidity.

Considering the use of blood products in trauma patients, "damage control transfusion" regimens have been introduced next to "damage control surgery." These protocols support the early use of blood—and coagulation products (including fibrinogen and recombinant factor VII) in case of major blood loss [28], which may finally lead to less use of these products compared with patients in whom resuscitation is first attempted with crystalloids and/or colloids [29, 30]. Monitoring coagulation with laboratory studies and/or thrombelastography is recommended if a "damage control transfusion" regimen is followed.

THE PATIENT WITH DIABETES INSIPIDUS

Cerebral (central) diabetes insipidus is common in neurosurgical patients, especially with pituitary or hypothalamic pathology, but can also occur after any kind of brain injury including any type of intracranial surgery [31, 32].

Due to a lack of antidiuretic hormone (ADH), these patients develop a syndrome of polyuria with low urinary sodium and low urine specific gravity, combined with hypernatremia. These patients can be treated with intravenous desmopressin. The most common intravenous dosage is 1 to 2 µg either daily or in divided doses. The therapy should also include a careful fluid regimen, because it has been shown that, especially in case of intranasal application, severe hyponatremia may result if a patient is overloaded with hypotonic fluids, such as NaCl 0.45%–glucose 2.5%, which is recommended by some authors.

In the general population, renal diabetes insipidus is much more frequent. In renal diabetes insipidus, the ADH level is normal, but the kidney does not properly respond to it. In these patients, sodium and fluid intake must be restricted and hydrochlorothiazide diuretics can be useful.

THE PATIENT WITH HYPONATREMIA

In neurosurgery, but even more in neurocritical care, hyponatremia is frequently seen. It can be caused by the syndrome of inappropriate antidiuretic hormone secretion (SIADH), which can have a wide variety of causes [33]. Examples include the perioperative stress response, pain, and ectopic [(para)neoplastic] ADH secretion. The typical clinical picture of these patients consists of hyponatremia (due to excretion of highly concentrated urine) with hypervolemia (due to water retention). Patients with SIADH are treated with fluid restriction and hypertonic saline solutions in the case of severe hyponatremia (with neurologic symptoms).

Another common cause of hyponatremia is cerebral salt wasting due to the increased release of atrial natriuretic factor, which is part of the cerebral sympathetic stress response frequently seen after subarachnoid hemorrhage or traumatic brain injury.

The condition results in the production of large volumes of sodium-rich urine and must not be confused with diabetes insipidus. Patients with (renal) diabetes insipidus are treated with fluid restriction, whereas patients with cerebral salt wasting should receive intravenous fluids to maintain plasma volume and correct total body sodium. In general, normal saline (0.9% = 154 mmol/L) solutions should be preferred over hypertonic saline.

By now, it will have become obvious that electrolyte and water imbalances in neurosurgical and neurocritical care patients should be thoroughly analyzed before therapy is initiated, as the signs and symptoms of hypernatremia and hyponatremia may seem similar but require a completely different therapeutic approach [34].

Blood and urine sodium and osmolarity measurements should be repeated frequently to prevent overcorrection. Correct osmolarity slowly and carefully to avoid (potentially irreversible) pontine demyelinization [35]

CONCLUSION

Fluid management is one of the cornerstones of neuroanesthesia and neurocritical care. A good regimen will help the neurosurgeon by trying to avoid brain edema formation and venous congestion while optimizing the patient's volume status to maintain adequate brain perfusion and oxygenation. The type and volume of fluids used should be carefully chosen, based on the understanding of the pathophysiologic processes of the individual patient. Just because no sound evidence is available which therapy is the best, at least those measures that are proved to be bad should be strictly avoided [36]. A good goal seems to be "normo-everything": normovolemia, normoglycemia, and normonatremia.

REFERENCES

1. Tommasino C. Fluids and the neurosurgical patient. *Anesthesiol Clin N Am* 2002;20:329–346.
2. Engelhardt B, Sorokin L. The blood-brain and the blood-cerebrospinal fluid barriers: function and dysfunction. *Semin Immunopathol* 2009;31:497–511.
3. Kimelberg HK. Water homeostasis in the brain: basic concepts. *Neuroscience.* 2004;129:851–860.
4. Tommasino C, Picozzi V. Volume and electrolyte management. *Best Pract Res Clin Anaesthesiol.* 2007;21:497–516.
5. Oddo M, Levine JM, Frangos S, et al. Effect of mannitol and hypertonic saline on cerebral oxygenation in patients with severe traumatic brain injury and refractory intracranial hypertension. *J Neurol Neurosurg Psychiatry.* 2009;80:916–920.
6. Rockswold GL, Solid CA, Paredes-Andrade E, et al. Hypertonic saline and its effect on intracranial pressure, cerebral perfusion pressure, and brain tissue oxygen. *Neurosurgery.* 2009;65:1035–1041.
7. Diringer MN, Zazulia AR. Osmotic therapy—fact and fiction. *Neurocrit Care.* 2004;1;219–233.
8. Paczynski RP. Osmotherapy. Basic concepts and controversies. *Crit Care Clin.* 1997;13:105–129.
9. Wakai A, Roberts I, Schierhout G. Mannitol for acute traumatic brain injury. *Cochrane Database Syst Rev.* 2007:CD001049.
10. Schortgen F, Lacherade JC, Bruneel F, et al. Effects of hydroxyethylstarch and gelatin on renal function in severe sepsis: a multicentre randomised study. *Lancet.* 2001;357:911–916.
11. Jungheinrich C, Scharpf R, Wargenau M, et al. The pharmacokinetics and tolerability of an intravenous infusion of the new hydroxyethyl starch 130/0.4 (6%, 500 mL) in mild-to-severe renal impairment. *Anesth Analg* 2002;95:544–551.
12. Vincent JL. Relevance of albumin in modern critical care medicine. *Best Pract Res Clin Anaesthesiol.* 2009;23:183–191.
13. Exo JL, Shellington DK, Bayir H, et al. Resuscitation of traumatic brain injury and hemorrhagic shock with polynitroxylated albumin, hextend, hypertonic saline, and lactated Ringer's: effects on acute hemodynamics, survival, and neuronal death in mice. *J Neurotrauma.* 2009;26:2403–2408.
14. Baker AJ, Park E, Hare GM, et al. Effects of resuscitation fluid on neurologic physiology after cerebral trauma and hemorrhage. *J Trauma* 2008;64:348–357.
15. Caironi P, Gattinoni L. The clinical use of albumin: the point of view of a specialist in intensive care. *Blood Transfus* 2009;7:259–267.
16. Chappell D, Jacob M, Hofmann-Kiefer K, et al. A rational approach to perioperative fluid management. *Anesthesiology.* 2008;109:723–740.
17. Kim JY, Lee D, Lee KC, et al. Stewart's physicochemical approach in neurosurgical patients with hyperchloremic metabolic acidosis during propofol anesthesia. *J Neurosurg Anesthesiol.* 2008;20:1–7.
18. Jacob M, Chappell D, Rehm M. The "third space"—fact or fiction? *Best Pract Res Clin Anaesthesiol.* 2009;23:145–157.
19. Bhardwaj A. Osmotherapy in neurocritical care. *Curr Neurol Neurosci Rep* 2007;7:513–521.
20. Dankbaar JW, Slooter AJ, Rinkel GJ, et al. Effect of different components of triple-H therapy on cerebral perfusion in patients with aneurysmal subarachnoid haemorrhage: a systematic review. *Crit Care* 2010;14:R23.
21. Keyrouz SG, Diringer MN. Clinical review: prevention and therapy of vasospasm in subarachnoid hemorrhage. *Crit Care* 2007;11:220.
22. Muench E, Horn P, Bauhuf C, et al. Effects of hypervolemia and hypertension on regional cerebral blood flow, intracranial pressure, and brain tissue oxygenation after subarachnoid hemorrhage. *Crit Care Med* 2007;35:1844–1851.
23. Treggiari MM, Deem S. Which H is the most important in triple-H therapy for cerebral vasospasm? *Curr Opin Crit Care.* 2009;15:83–86.
24. Rhoney DH, Parker D Jr. Considerations in fluids and electrolytes after traumatic brain injury. *Nutr Clin Pract.* 2006;21:462–478.
25. Fletcher JJ, Bergman K, Blostein PA, et al. Fluid balance, complications, and brain tissue oxygen tension monitoring following severe traumatic brain injury. *Neurocrit Care* 2010;13:47–56.
26. Kerwin AJ, Schinco MA, Tepas JJ 3rd, et al. The use of 23.4% hypertonic saline for the management of elevated intracranial pressure in patients with severe traumatic brain injury: a pilot study. *J Trauma* 2009;67:277–282.
27. Himmelseher S. Hypertonic saline solutions for treatment of intracranial hypertension. *Curr Opin Anaesthesiol.* 2007;20:414–426.
28. McQuay N Jr, Cipolla J, Franges EZ, et al. The use of recombinant activated factor VIIa in coagulopathic traumatic brain injuries requiring emergent craniotomy: is it beneficial? J Neurosurg. 2009;111:666–671.
29. Heindl B, Spannagl M. [Fresh plasma and concentrates of clotting factors for therapy of perioperative coagulopathy: what is known?] *Anaesthesist* 2006;55:926, 928–936.
30. Stein DM, Dutton RP, Kramer ME, et al. Reversal of coagulopathy in critically ill patients with traumatic brain injury: recombinant factor VIIa is more cost-effective than plasma. *J Trauma.* 2009;66:63–72; discussion 73–75.
31. Schrier RW. Body water homeostasis: clinical disorders of urinary dilution and concentration. *J Am Soc Nephrol.* 2006;17:1820–1832.
32. Moore K, Thompson C, Trainer P. Disorders of water balance. *Clin Med.* 2003;3:28–33.
33. Ellison DH, Berl T. Clinical practice. The syndrome of inappropriate antidiuresis. *N Engl J Med.* 2007;356:2064–2072.
34. Palmer BF. Hyponatremia in patients with central nervous system disease: SIADH versus CSW. *Trends Endocrinol Metab.* 2003;14:182–187.
35. Vaidya C, Ho W, Freda BJ. Management of hyponatremia: providing treatment and avoiding harm. *Cleve Clin J Med.* 2010;77:715–726.
36. Randell T, Niskanen M. Management of physiological variables in neuroanaesthesia: maintaining homeostasis during intracranial surgery. *Curr Opin Anaesthesiol* 2006;19:492–497.

12.
INTRACRANIAL TUMORS

Ira J. Rampil and Stephen Probst

INTRODUCTION

Planning the anesthetic for a patient with an intracranial tumor provides an opportunity to practice a bit of translational medicine, combining basic science with clinical observations to optimize patient care and outcome. Neuroanesthesia practice is an area where one must consider the traditional goals of anesthetic management (i.e., unconsciousness, immobility, and amnesia) as well as the effects that drugs and other interventions have on the surgical field. Brain volume most directly impacts the surgical field, and therefore this chapter departs from most other texts in its emphasis on volume control rather than intracranial pressure (ICP). The chapter also reviews the most current in vivo data on compartment volumes in humans and their sensitivity to therapeutic maneuvers. Circumstances and timing play a role in choosing therapy. As treatment protocols for closed head trauma move away from hyperventilation and mannitol as long-duration therapies, they remain bulwarks of treatment in elective surgery for neoplastic disease. There are very few randomized, controlled clinical trials to guide decision-making for the neurosurgical patient, so most thoughtful practitioners use a combination of hypothesis, theory, and expert consensus to inform their care.

EPIDEMIOLOGY AND PATHOPHYSIOLOGY

A basic understanding of the tumor type for which surgery is planned is important to optimize the anesthetic management of the patient. The most common histologic types in adults are meningioma (35%), glioblastoma (16%), pituitary adenoma (14%), and astrocytoma (7%). The median age of patients at diagnosis is 57 years. *Supratentorial* tumors are located above the tentorium of the dura (i.e., the cerebral hemispheres). *Infratentorial* lesions involve the cerebellum and brain stem. Neoplasms in the *infratentorial* region

will generally elicit symptoms at a smaller size. The Central Brain Tumor Registry of the United States (http://www.cbtrus.org/) reports that an estimated 64,530 new cases of primary nonmalignant and malignant brain and central nervous system (CNS) tumors were diagnosed in the United States in 2011. Over 80% of these are supratentorial and about half are malignant. These tumors are responsible for significant morbidity and approximately 12,000 deaths per year in the United States.

Astrocytes are the most common cell in the CNS and are responsible for supratentorial and infratentorial tumors. Tumors derived from astrocytes often present in young adults as new-onset seizures and range in histology from low-grade gliomas (the least aggressive tumor) to glioblastoma multiforme, which is highly aggressive and expands rapidly, outstripping their blood supply, which ultimately results in a central necrosis. These tumors also impair the blood–brain barrier (BBB). These tumors frequently present with symptoms of high ICP. Metastatic tumors in the brain (e.g., from breast or lung) also behave in this fashion. Low-grade astrocytomas are treated with surgical resection or radiation therapy, which results in long-term, symptom-free survival. Treatment of high-grade astrocytomas (e.g., anaplastic astrocytoma) and glioblastoma multiforme centers on palliation and usually involves surgical debulking followed by chemotherapy or radiation.

Meningiomas are derived from meningeal cells and frequently arise from tissues outside of the brain. The majority of meningeal tumors are histologically benign; they are usually well-circumscribed and grow very slowly. They rarely produce a rapid increase in ICP. They can be located near the sagittal sinus, falx cerebri, and cerebral convexity. Treatment is usually with surgical resection, and prognosis is usually very good. Acoustic neuromas are usually a benign schwannoma that involves the vestibular component of cranial nerve VIII within the internal auditory canal. Although these tumors usually occur on only one side, bilateral tumors may occur in patients with neurofibromatosis type 2. Treatment includes surgical resection with auditory evoked potential and facial nerve monitoring or radiation therapy.

Less common tumors include ependymomas, which arise from the cells that line the ventricles and occur in young children; pituitary tumors, which are discussed elsewhere; oligodendrocytomas; and CNS lymphomas.

GOALS OF ANESTHETIC MANAGEMENT

Anesthetic management of patients with an intracranial mass requires knowledge of the pharmacology of anesthetic agents and the pathophysiology of brain tumors. An understanding of the multiple interactions between the circulatory and respiratory systems and the cerebral circulation is also required but, again, is not sufficient. The anesthesiologist must consider several explicit therapeutic goals that sometime compete to successfully optimize care. These goals include optimization of surgical exposure while minimizing brain injury and maximizing patient safety while providing patient comfort.

Hippocrates is said to have created the dictum "first, do no harm" 2500 years ago. The processes of neuroanesthesia and neurosurgery may both lead to brain injury. Surgeons must sometimes exert mechanical pressure on brain tissue to expose a lesion. That pressure may cause injury by tearing axons and synapses, and increasing tissue pressure, preventing blood from traversing capillaries. Anesthetics may also reduce systemic blood pressure below the critical cerebral perfusion pressure (CPP) or may increase ICP, which also reduces CPP to a critical value. Anesthesiologists can also be therapeutic, reducing the bulk of the brain so less surgical retraction is needed to obtain the required exposure. Anesthesiologists can select an anesthetic and monitoring plan that use less in the way of vasodilatory drugs yet maintain good blood pressure control.

Occasionally, the anatomic site of a neoplasm is adjacent to, or intermixed with, the *eloquent cortex*, a portion of the brain that is critical for a behavior such as speech or somatic motor control. To minimize the removal of such vital tissue from the brain, a neurosurgeon may need to map the functional areas in real time during surgery. If the tumor is near the primary motor cortex, the patient cannot be paralyzed during mapping, and if the tumor is near a language center, the patient must be conscious, cooperative, and able to speak during the surgery. These requirements add an extra burden to the anesthesiologist to customize the anesthetic plan to meet both the surgeon's and the patient's needs.

RELEVANT PHYSIOLOGY

The cranium of an adult human is shared by three major anatomic components we model as "compartments": brain tissue, blood, and cerebrospinal fluid. The precise volumes of the cranial vault and its contents vary with age, with gender, and, aside from the bones, with physiologic state. For reasons that will be clear shortly, it is useful to review these individual components.

A large study of American military personnel estimated the cranial vault to have a mean volume of 1442 cm^3 in men and 1332 cm^3 in women. A smaller study using magnetic resonance imaging (MRI) in volunteers found volumes of 1469 ± 102 cm^3 in men and 1289 ± 111 cm^3 in women [1].

In the past two decades, postmortem data on intracranial compartment volumes has begun to be replaced by in vivo data from MRI, single-photon emission computed tomography (SPECT), and positron emission tomography (PET). A recent in vivo MRI study of healthy adults found the brain volume of adults to be 1273 ± 115 cm^3 (±SD for men) and 1131 ± 100 for women [70]. These brain volumes exclude the approximately 14 mL of cerebrospinal fluid (CSF) in the lateral ventricles. Brain volume decreases after age 40, faster in men than in women. These volume estimates include intracellular and extracellular spaces plus the embedded blood volumes. Total CSF is 109 ± 21 mL in men and 95 ± 21 mL in women in the age range of 20 to 40 years and increases thereafter as the brain shrinks. CSF volume is dynamic because it depends not only on its anatomically determined space but also on the relative rate of CSF production versus rate of absorption.

The blood inside the cranial vault is located in one of three physiologic compartments: arteries, capillaries, and veins, and each one has different volume control mechanisms. The brain is extremely heterogeneous in distribution of blood: The cortex has a far higher blood volume and flow than does the white matter. There is instantaneous redistribution of blood in response to changing levels of metabolic activity. It is possible to use simple time averaged values to derive an approximate single value for cerebral blood flow (CBF). In healthy adult volunteers, cortical blood volume was reported as 3.1 ± 0.3 mL blood/100 cm^3 of brain [2], of which the arterial portion was 37% as determined by PET. In another study using tagged red blood cells, a cranial blood volume of 4.17 ± 0.56 mL/100 cm^3 tissue [3] was determined. Using an MRI technique known as dynamic susceptibility contrast, Engvall and colleagues determined a value of 4.5 ± 0.9 mL/100 g of brain [4]. Averaging the results of the three studies yields approximately 3.9 mL/100 g of brain or about 62 mL in a male brain. The three compartments together have a total volume of 1382 cm^3 [1211 (1273 brain – 62 mL of blood) plus 62 mL of blood plus 109 mL]. This estimate is about 60 cm^3 less than the current best estimate of cranial vault volume given here, but then the volume of the meninges and some of the large, conducting, but nonreactive blood vessels are not accounted for. For the purposes of anesthetic management, we will use the new in vivo derived volumes in Table 12.1.

Table 12.1 THERAPEUTIC SENSITIVITY MATRIX

INTRACRANIAL COMPARTMENT	VOLUME (CM³)	FRACTION OF TOTAL	THERAPY	MECHANISM	COMPARTMENT IMPACT	TOTAL IMPACT	NOTES	REFERENCE
Brain	1211	87.6%						
			Mannitol	Osmotic Gradient	2%	1.40%	electrolyte imbalance	Videen 2001
			Steroids	↓ Vasogenic Edema	3%	2.63%	hyperglycemia	Meinig 1980
			Steroid & Furosemide		5%	3.94%		Meinig 1980
			NSAIDs	↓ Vasogenic Edema			↓ hemostasis	Ting 1990
			Barbiturates	↓ Vasogenic Edema			↓ MAP	Harbaugh 1979
CSF	109	7.9%						
			Posture	Translocation	5%	0.39%	↓ MAP & CPP	
			CSFDrain	remove CSF	10%	0.79%	herniation risk	
			Mannitol	↓ production (by 50%)	5%	0.39%	electrolyte imbalance	Donato 1994
Blood	62	4.5%						
			Posture	HeadUp; ↓ JVP	13%	0.58%		
			Hypocapnea	vasocontriction	30%	1.35%		Engvall 2008
			Barbiturates	vasocontriction	17%	0.76%		
			Propofol	vasocontriction	17%	0.76%		Kaisti 2003
			Mannitol	↓ viscosity	6%	0.27%		Muizelaar 1983

Since the skull is not elastic and the contents of those compartments inside the skull are mostly water (which is not compressible), any change in the volume of one component must be matched by a complementary change in the volume of one or both of the other two. This is the *Monro-Kellie doctrine*, and it must be considered when a neoplasm increases brain tissue volume. In this case, both CSF and blood volume must be shifted out of the cranium to compensate for the space occupied by the tumor. The volumes can shift by a small amount, after which the pressure inside the cranium increases sharply with any further increase in brain volume. Patients with a mass effect from a brain tumor are at particular risk for cerebral ischemia because of this volume–pressure effect. The increase in brain volume compresses the vascular tree, which increases resistance to flow and decreases CPP. Pushing the brain parenchyma around the edges of the dura can further compromise perfusion while also causing shear injury and microhemorrhage. Once ischemic, these compromised areas become edematous, which can lead to a cycle of worsening conditions.

To preserve brain function while providing an optimal surgical field, anesthesiologists have evolved a series of therapeutic maneuvers that mitigate the effects of increased intracranial volume and ICP. Table 12.1 reviews the relative effectiveness of each technique and its associated risks.

BLOOD COMPARTMENT

Hypocapnea has long been used to produce a rapid but transient [5] reduction in the intracranial blood volume. Hypocapnea induces vasoconstriction by producing cerebrospinal fluid alkalosis and reducing hydrogen ion concentration on the neuronal side of the BBB. This effect lasts between 4 and 12 hours before bicarbonate buffering restores the original hydrogen ion balance, which terminates the vasoconstriction. Artru [6] suggests that hypocapnea may also mildly reduce CSF compartment volume by increasing rate of CSF absorption. When $Paco_2$ is in the normal range ($Paco_2$ 40 ± 10 mm Hg), the cerebral blood volume (CBV) in awake humans changes by approximately 1.5% for each 1–mm Hg change in $Paco_2$ [7]. Thus, at a $Paco_2$ of 30 mm Hg, CBV would be about 15% less than at baseline. A later trial using similar techniques found a somewhat smaller effect, about 10% less than baseline [4]. Essentially all of the change in volume occurs in the arterial fraction of the vascular space. The use of hypocapnea to reduce CBV has practical limits: In some patients, arterial vasoconstriction caused by hyperventilation may cause neuronal ischemia. The $Paco_2$ at which this might occur in an individual is unpredictable, but a $Paco_2$ of about 25 mm Hg is generally considered to be the safe lower limit. Hypocapnea may also exacerbate injury in the setting of excessive glutamate release by lowering the seizure threshold [8].

Barbiturates and propofol anesthesia decrease CBV. In volunteers, propofol infusion sufficient to depress the electroencephalographic (EEG) bispectral index (BIS) value to 40 (i.e., surgical anesthesia) during normocapnea will reduce CBV in the frontal lobe from 4.2% ± 0.87% to 3.5% ± 0.59% [9], a change of 17%. Like propofol, barbiturates are thought to decrease CBV by decreasing cerebral metabolic rate ($CMRO_2$) while preserving flow–demand coupling, thus shrinking the diameter of arterial supply vessels. Since there are no human studies of the effects of barbiturates on CBV, it is reasonable to assume the magnitude of the arterial resistance changes and thus the CBV are similar. In clinical practice, these intravenous anesthetics provide a useful reduction in CBV and ICP. However, adding hypocapnea to anesthetic-induced vasoconstrictors cannot much decrease the CBV beyond what is safe with anesthetics alone because ischemia can result.

Mannitol decreases blood viscosity and reduces brain water content (discussed later). The decrease in viscosity has been hypothesized to allow vasoconstriction while maintaining required blood flow, and indeed this is seen experimentally [10]. Rosner and Coley [11] hypothesized that this vasoconstrictive effect would only occur in the setting of low CPP, because at CPP values above about 70 mm Hg, autoregulatory cerebral artery vasoconstriction is already present. A recent study in patients with head injury found that while mannitol significantly decreased ICP, neither CBV or CBF appeared to be affected after 1 g/kg intravenous mannitol [12]; therefore, the effects of change in blood viscosity remain controversial.

Manipulation of systemic arterial blood pressure can also be used to change cerebral arterial volume. Cerebral autoregulation causes a reduction in blood volume with increasing blood pressure because resistance arterioles constrict as the mechanism to regulate flow. When CPP rises above 150 mm Hg, CBF increases with pressure as autoregulation fails. Volatile anesthetics impair cerebral autoregulation. Using the Hagen-Poiseuille equation, one may estimate that the arterial component of the blood space decreases by 40% when mean arterial pressure (MAP) is increased from 50 to 150 mm Hg, assuming laminar constant flow and a constant capillary pressure of 30 mm Hg. This amounts to a total of about 7 mL of reduced blood volume.

The capillaries and veins compose roughly 70% of CBV, or 40 cm^3 of blood compartment. They are relatively insensitive to ventilation or pharmacologic agents. Head-up posture can, however, reduce the venous volume by increasing drainage into the central venous circulation. Thus far, this effect has been confirmed by near-infrared analysis [13], which is not a quantitative measurement. A 2.5-cm elevation of the head relative to the heart will reduce cerebral venous pressure by about 1.8 mm Hg, or by approximately 20% of normal. If one assumes the veins start with no wall tension and therefore that volume is linearly proportional to filling pressure, then roughly 8 mL of venous blood (13%

of CBV) will shift out of the intracranial cavity. The venous change is independent of the prior arterial reduction and will not produce ischemia as long as the systemic arterial pressure is sufficient to maintain adequate CPP.

The vascular component of large neoplasms frequently has disturbed regulation of flow [14, 15] due to angioneogenesis, regional hypermetabolism and hypometabolism, and other factors. The blood volume of this tissue is not likely to respond to either hypocapnea or anesthetic-mediated vasoconstriction (e.g., with propofol).

CSF COMPARTMENT

Simple physical maneuvers can be used to reduce CSF volume. Elevating the head will drain some CSF into the spinal arachnoid space, reducing intracranial volume. In the setting of an outflow obstruction, ventriculostomy may be necessary before opening the dura to prevent uncontrolled herniation. For example, ventriculostomy may be necessary if there has been an acute hemorrhage into a necrotic area of the tumor. Artru and colleagues discovered that anesthetic drugs could modulate CSF production and absorption to a small degree in animal models [16–18]. Once the dura has been incised and CSF may freely drain, however, the clinical consequences of these drug-induced changes are unclear.

PARENCHYMAL COMPARTMENT

Brain parenchyma is composed of approximately 80% water in gray matter and 70% in white matter [19]. The volume of parenchyma can be reduced by removing excess water (i.e., edema), which is the major factor in brain swelling. Brain edema has three potential etiologies [20] commonly seen in the operating room; these are summarized in Table 12.2. In the case of brain tumors, a combination of vasogenic and cytotoxic edema frequently coexists.

Mannitol causes an osmotic dehydration of brain tissue by drawing water across an intact BBB and functional cell membranes. It should, therefore, be able to extract from the cranium both extracellular and intracellular water, where it is eliminated by the kidneys. In theory [21], a difference in osmolality across a semipermeable membrane should lead to a free water flux and thus a volume shift proportional to the difference as given by:

$$\frac{V_{new}}{V_{orig}} = \frac{C_{orig}}{C_{new}}$$

For example, if the normal plasma osmolality is 290 mOsm, and a dose of mannitol of 1 g/kg intravenous is given to achieve a peak osmolality of 310 mOsm [22], then the brain should shrink to approximately 94% of its starting volume. This theoretical 6% decrease is, however, not seen in vivo. Where there is no functional BBB, the osmotic gradient is not maintained, so there would be no pressure gradient

Table 12.2 ETIOLOGIES OF CEREBRAL EDEMA

ETIOLOGY	CLINICAL CONDITION	MECHANISM	EXCESS WATER LOCATION	IMAGING
Cytotoxic	Ischemia Metabolic toxins	Cell membrane ATPase pump failure in glia, neurons	intracellular	Grey matter
Vasogenic	Neoplasms Inflammation Trauma High Altitude Malignant Hypertension	↑ meability of Blood-Brain Barrier mediated by VEGF, *etc.*	extracellular	White matter
Interstitial	Hydrocephalus	Obstruction of CSF flow	extracellular	Diffusion MRI

to dehydrate the tissue. Donato [23] found that mannitol decreased brain water in rabbits by 2.06%. In patients with large hemispheric strokes, Videen and colleagues found this dehydration volume loss only in the normal hemisphere and not in the infarcted region, presumably due to BBB disruption [24]. The magnitude of the volume change was 0.8% of the normal hemisphere. Extrapolation to 1.6% for a complete brain should be used with caution in patients with a neoplasm because rapidly growing tumors may have areas of necrosis and BBB disruption. A single dose of mannitol 1 g/kg reduces ICP for 4 to 6 hours. Figure 12.1 illustrates the time-dependent onset of the effect as measured in the study of Videen and colleagues. An earlier study using MRI T1 relaxation as a marker of water content in the brain found a comparable reduction of 1.4% ± 0.3% at 30 minutes after mannitol [25]. This same study found no detectable change in water content due to dexamethasone for up to 6 days after dosing (see later). Intraoperatively, it is obvious that mannitol reduces brain volume, but the literature remains quite sparse regarding optimal dosing, timing, or even outcomes. Intra-arterial injection of mannitol disrupts the BBB and may allow better access to brain tumors for chemotherapeutic agents. Interestingly, without a BBB, the volume behavior of rat glioma cells in vitro is somewhat counterintuitive. When individual cells are exposed to mannitol in vitro, these cells rapidly shrank, but their volume then increased to well above the initial value [26]. A review of the mechanisms [27] of osmotic volume control of cells suggests that mannitol's effect may be limited by compensatory intracellular uptake of sodium, potassium, and chloride ions. Because rapidly growing tumors disrupt the BBB within themselves, osmotic agents may have a reduced effect and may promote a localized volume rebound [39]. Drugs such as furosemide, which inhibit this active transport, potentiate the effect of mannitol [28, 29]. By itself, the ability of furosemide to reduce brain volume is unclear but appears to be limited [30–34]. Finally, mannitol has some other interesting properties that may have benefit: Mannitol is a free radical scavenger [35], which may reduce reperfusion injury [36] in tissue that became ischemic during surgical retraction. Mannitol was also found to reduce apoptosis in rats following transient ischemia [37]. A Cochrane meta-analysis in 2007 concluded that there were insufficient data to prove mannitol's benefit in clinical brain ischemia [38].

Hypertonic saline (3%) has also been proposed as an agent that can reduce brain volume in patients with a brain tumor [40, 41]. A recent study of patients with a supratentorial tumor suggests that hypertonic saline may produce a somewhat larger reduction in brain volume than does mannitol. The dose of osmotic agents that were used may not have been equipotent, however; the mannitol dose was low at less than 0.5 g/kg. This study also did not match extent of cerebral edema in the two treatment groups [41]. Further study may identify the better osmotic agent in the care of patients with brain tumor.

Glucocorticoids are a mainstay treatment of cerebral edema in patients with brain tumors [42–44] and have been widely accepted as a standard of care for decades. A recent meta-analysis confirmed the lack of strong evidence for their use [45], but the introduction of steroids led to a reduction in perioperative mortality from glioma resection from 21% to 3% [46]. The authors did not find any similar effect from the introduction of mannitol. The mechanism by which glucocorticoids reduce edema by is unclear but is thought

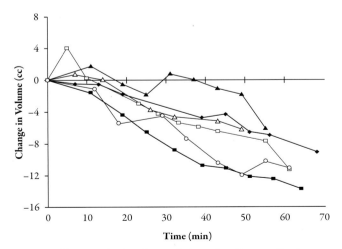

Figure 12.1   Change in brain volume relative to baseline scan for six patients with large hemispheric infarction with mass effect given 1.5 g/kg mannitol following a baseline scan. Dark bar on the X-axis indicates the approximate duration of infusion. Filled triangles represent the patient who received multiple doses of mannitol before the study. The change in volume is seen only in the non-infarcted hemisphere.

to involve reduction of the permeability enhancer VEGF [47] and depression of the inflammatory arachidonic acid cascade. The reduction in permeability due to steroids is relatively rapid [48], but clinical reduction in ICP may take 6 hours, with peak effect occurring between 24 and 72 hours [49]. Corticosteroids provide the largest therapeutic effect on ICP of any maneuver in Table 12.1 ($\approx$ 2.6% of total intracranial volume given a 3% reduction in brain volume [50]) (Table 12.1). If a patient is already being treated with steroids before surgery, there is little incremental benefit to a parenteral dose during induction of anesthesia. Dexamethasone is the most common choice because of its long duration and its minimal mineralocorticoid effect. The side effects of steroids include hyperglycemia, sodium wasting, infection, gastrointestinal irritation and ulceration, and occasionally psychiatric disturbances. It is, therefore, prudent to use the smallest dose that will reduce ICP in an individual patient.

Nonsteroidal anti-inflammatory drugs (NSAIDs) can also reduce brain edema via suppression of the arachidonic acid pathway, and drugs such as indomethacin [51] and ibuprofen [52, 53] have been proposed for this purpose. Although NSAIDs are effective in reducing vasogenic edema, they are contraindicated in the perioperative period and typically for 7 to 10 days after surgery due to the inhibitory effect on platelet function.

APPLIED PRACTICE

This section describes a physiologic approach to anesthetic planning for craniotomy and resection of a neoplasm.

PREOPERATIVE EVALUATION AND THERAPY

Like all preoperative patients, a directed history and physical examination provides important information about whether the patient is adequately prepared for surgery and the relative risk of a craniotomy. In addition to the usual cardiopulmonary and airway assessments, special attention should be placed on the neurologic history and physical examination, including an assessment of the patient's neurologic status. It is particularly important to elicit signs of intracranial hypertension and preexisting neurologic deficits. Patients scheduled for elective tumor resection who present on the day of surgery with signs of high ICP or impending herniation (i.e., headache, nausea, blurred vision, etc.) are now rare because aggressive tumors that increase ICP are usually treated with a course of preoperative dexamethasone. Preexisting deficits should be noted in the record so that the patient is not referred for urgent imaging studies if a longstanding deficit is suddenly "discovered" after surgery. If the patient has a seizure disorder, the antiepileptic therapy should be evaluated. Older antiepileptic drugs such as phenytoin, carbamazepine, phenobarbital, and valproic

acid may induce hepatic enzymes (CYP2C, CYP3A4, and others). These enzymes can dramatically alter the kinetics of drugs that are commonly administered in the perioperative period, such as neuromuscular blocking agents and narcotics. It is also useful to inquire about any preictal aura that a patient may have experienced previously so that a similar complaint before induction can be responded to rapidly.

INTRAOPERATIVE MONITORING

Intraoperative monitoring for patients undergoing a craniotomy includes the American Society of Anesthesiologists' standard monitors. Required monitors include a means of assessing oxygenation, circulation, ventilation, and temperature. Continuous respiratory gas measurement is particularly useful since, as noted earlier, CO_2 is frequently manipulated as a means of controlling brain volume.

Intra-arterial catheters for monitoring of blood pressure was until recently considered to be a "standard of care." Although continuous pressure monitoring is in some cases desirable, it may no longer be essential, and a decision should be made based on each patient's clinical situation. Arterial sampling for blood gas analysis has reliably been replaced by continuous airway gas analysis for all, but patients with severe pulmonary disease markedly altering the alveolar-arterial gradient of CO_2. Most patients undergoing an elective craniotomy for tumor excision are hemodynamically stable during the procedure. Blood loss to an extent causing hemodynamic instability or requiring transfusion is uncommon and can frequently be predicted from a preoperative discussion with the neurosurgeons and a review of the diagnostic imaging. There are always exceptions, of course. For example, the resection of large, nonembolized meningioma or an arteriovenous malformation presenting as a mass lesion may be associated with significant blood loss. For similar reasons, placement of central venous access is rarely indicated. Central venous access via the jugular vein is relatively contraindicated for somewhat impeding venous drainage of the brain and for limiting surgical positioning options.

EEG monitoring is frequently used as an aid to titrating anesthetic effect and may be useful in procedures performed with total intravenous anesthesia, opioids, and neuromuscular blockade. Commercially available systems such as the BIS Monitor Covidien Inc. (Mansfield, MA), M-Entropy GE Healthcare–DatexOhemda (Madison, Wi), and Sedline Masimo (Irvine, Ca) use a forehead-based electrode array. The use of these devices during craniotomy may be questionable in cases where the sensors must be moved to accommodate surgery because they were all developed and calibrated based on data from a frontal electrode montage.

INDUCTION

The primary goals of anesthetic induction include maintaining ICP as low as possible, prevention of coughing on intubation, maintenance of hemodynamic stability, and mild hypocarbia. One possible approach to accomplishing these goals includes administration of fentanyl 3 to 10 µg/kg, which will blunt the hemodynamic response to airway manipulation. The patient is then preoxygenated with voluntary hyperventilation for a few minutes while the opioid reaches the effect compartment. In a hemodynamically stable patient, induction is then accomplished with propofol 75 to 1.5 mg/kg, followed by a neuromuscular blocking agent, which will allow rapid control of the airway. The use of succinylcholine is considered controversial in patients with brain tumors. The controversy is rooted in several dog model studies that demonstrated a small, transient increase in ICP, which appeared to be related to the onset of fasciculations. The ICP increase is blocked with the use of a "defasciculating" dose of a nondepolarizing neuromuscular antagonist. In the absence of contraindication, the use of succinylcholine can be considered a reasonable choice for rapid control of the airway. Bolus doses of esmolol can be given if increased sympathetic activity is anticipated during intubation, especially if a lower dose of opioid is used. Intubate swiftly and smoothly when patient is completely relaxed, confirm placement via exhaled carbon dioxide, and reliably secure the endotracheal tube. Antibiotics, additional steroids and mannitol may be requested by the surgical team.

Rigid head fixation is required for many intracranial surgical procedures. Attachment of the head holder involves the use of pins that penetrate the outer table of the skull. This is extremely noxious, causing a similar amount of pain as surgical incision. It is, therefore, necessary to ensure that the patient has an adequate anesthetic depth and that there is complete neuromuscular blockade. This protects against patient movement and abrupt hypertension, both of which may be hazardous. Incremental boluses of propofol are a reasonable choice when administered 30 seconds before pinning. Small boluses of esmolol may also be used to blunt the hemodynamic response to pinning; this should also be started approximately 30 seconds before the head holder is applied. If rigid head fixation is used, neuromuscular blockade should be used throughout the procedure unless it is specifically contraindicated (e.g., if motor mapping is planned).

MAINTENANCE

The primary goals of anesthetic maintenance include providing the surgeons with good operating conditions by reducing brain volume and maintaining hemodynamic stability. A variety of techniques exist to accomplish these goals, such as nitrous oxide—opioid, volatile anesthetic (≤0.5 MAC and fentanyl infusion 1–3µg/kg/h), total intravenous anesthesia with propofol and fentanyl, neuroleptic anesthetic, as well as many others. Todd and colleagues [54] demonstrated in a prospective, blinded study that propofol or isoflurane or nitrous-narcotic anesthetic techniques all provided acceptable results with similar outcomes.

Neuromuscular blockade is typically maintained using an agent with intermediate duration such as vecuronium or rocuronium. When available, pancuronium may also used for long cases provided that it is discontinued well before emergence in order to ensure complete recovery from neuromuscular blockade. Patients who are being treated with anticonvulsants (e.g., phenytoin, carbamazepine) have altered responses to many drugs and may be resistant to the effects of nondepolarizing muscle relaxants. Mild hypocarbia (end-tidal CO_2 approximately 30 mm Hg) is reasonable for reducing brain volume in most patients. Systemic arterial blood pressure should be well controlled and is typically maintained in the low-normal range for the patient during the scalp incision through lifting the cranial flap (for hemostasis), followed by normal pressure during the intracranial phase (to prevent cerebral vasodilation). Mannitol 0.5 to 1.0 g/kg may be requested by the surgeon to reduce cerebral swelling; in most cases, it is started at the time of surgical incision. The goal of fluid management should be to maintain normovolemia or a slight negative fluid balance. Some tumor types (e.g., meningioma) may be highly vascular and extensive blood loss may occur during the procedure. The relative vascularity of the tumor and the possibility for intraoperative hemorrhage should, therefore, be discussed with the surgeon in advance of the procedure, and the entire team should agree on the fluid management strategy.

TIGHT DURA

The combination of a supratentorial mass lesion and increased intracranial volume complicates surgery for several reasons. Most patients are routinely treated with dexamethasone for at least several days before surgery. Propofol, mannitol, and hyperventilation all act to further decrease brain volume. If, however, the dura is still tense after removal of the bone flap, further decompression must be achieved before opening the dura. Otherwise, the cortex may rapidly herniate through the dural incision, causing bleeding and shearing the brain tissue. While anesthesiologists cannot palpate the dura, visual observation will reveal whether the dura is gently pulsing with ventilation, a reassuring sign that intracranial volume is well controlled. If the dura is not pulsatile, maneuvers to decrease ICP should be started in consultation with the surgical team. At this point, one should check that the jugular veins are not compressed by rotation of the neck and that the head is elevated at least a few centimeters above the left atrium. Adding furosemide 10 to 20 mg will usually enhance the mobilization of water from the brain by mannitol. Remove positive end-expiratory pressure if present to decrease venous back-pressure. Reduce end-tidal CO_2 to a minimal range of 20 to 25 mm Hg by increasing minute ventilation, preferentially by increasing tidal volume rather than rate. If potent volatile anesthetics or other vasodilators are present, they should be discontinued. In severe cases, the surgeon may elect to insert a drain into a lateral ventricle to drain CSF.

BRAIN RETRACTION

Retraction of brain tissue to create or improve surgical exposure is a common cause of injury [57]. This type of injury is not always apparent because the clinical examination may not be sensitive to ischemic injury in noneloquent areas. Serial computed tomography scans may be required over several days to detect the lesion. The basic mechanism of injury is thought to be the creation of tissue pressure greater than capillary perfusion pressure (≈ 25 mm Hg) by the retractor blade [58]. The tissue pressure is proportional to the brain volume displaced by the retractor blade. It is initially at its maximum and then declines as interstitial water is squeezed out of the area (Figure 12.2). Therapeutic interventions that decrease the volumes of the intracranial compartments help also to decrease the pressure required for a surgeon to achieve the view and access needed for surgery. Hyperventilation-induced arterial vasoconstriction may, however, worsen ischemia caused by retraction [57, 59, 60]. Some authors recommend relaxation of retraction pressure at intervals of roughly 10 minutes [57], but the translocation of interstitial water may reduce the need for this. Mannitol and nimodipine have both been shown to be helpful in preserving function in a porcine model of brain retraction [59].

CORTICAL MAPPING

Functional mapping of the brain with electrical stimulation can be used to identify eloquent cortex. This technique may be used when a tumor is in close proximity to known functional areas such as the motor cortex or the language and speech areas; a patient's quality of life would be impacted by resection or inadvertent injury to those areas. Localization of the motor areas allows the surgeon to tailor the area of resection in order to minimize the chance of neurologic deficit. This technique is discussed in depth in Chapter 16 but is briefly discussed here.

The ideal anesthetic technique for patients undergoing cortical mapping during tumor surgery should allow expression of the behaviors associated with the cortex adjacent to the tumor. In the case of tumor resection, the anesthetic requirements are not nearly so stringent are they are of surgical treatment of epilepsy where one must consider the anesthetic effects on the electrophysiology on the seizure foci. For example, if the tumor is involved with area of the motor cortex that supports movement of the face, the face must be visible during the surgical procedure, and the patient should be allowed to recover from neuromuscular blockade during the mapping phase. Electrical stimulation of the associated cortical area will then produce a twitch in the muscles of the face that will be visible to the surgeon or an assistant. Electrical stimulation of the cortex rarely induces a seizure through a phenomenon called *kindling*. These seizures frequently start as localized twitching and may rapidly progress to generalized tonic-clonic seizures. A syringe of propofol should therefore be kept attached to the intravenous line; seizures usually respond to a small dose. Alternatively, the seizure may be terminated by asking the surgeon to irrigate the brain with cold solution.

EMERGENCE

Anesthetic emergence should be smooth and rapid, without coughing, straining, or other phenomena that could raise ICP. The patient should be ready for neurologic assessment as quickly as possible after emergence. The patient's blood pressure should be well controlled at a level that has been agreed on by the surgical and anesthetic teams because there is an association between emergence hypertension and postoperative intracerebral hemorrhage [55]. When the surgeons begin to close, a fentanyl infusion should be discontinued. Remifentanil may be continued throughout closure and discontinued when the dressing is in place. The concentration of potent volatile anesthetics should be reduced, and the $PaCO_2$ should be returned to the normal range. This stage of the procedure requires extra caution because the endotracheal tube and head holder in combination with a decrease in anesthetic depth may rapidly cause hypertension or sudden patient movement. β-Adrenergic blockers such as labetalol or esmolol or calcium channel blockers such as nicardipine or clevidipine are perhaps the best choices for dealing with this hypertension as they can be titrated to effect as the patient awakens and then dissipate rapidly as the blood pressure returns to normal [56].

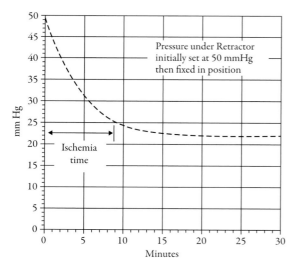

Figure 12.2 This graph, redrawn from the work of Albin58, illustrates the transient response of tissue pressure to retractor pressure on the cerebral cortex. Tissue pressure above 25 mmHg will impede capillary blood flow and cause ischemia in a volume of tissue under the retractor. Under normothermic conditions, ischemia longer than 3–5 minutes is likely to result in neuronal necrosis

PERIOPERATIVE HYPERTENSION

Perioperative hypertension is commonly encountered in patients undergoing intracranial surgery, particularly during emergence. Acute elevation of arterial blood pressure in this population is associated with intracranial bleeding, cerebral edema, increased ICP, and prolonged hospital stays [55, 61, 62], necessitating immediate treatment.

Any one of a number of antihypertensive drugs can be used to treat perioperative hypertension, depending on its etiology. Esmolol is a β_1-selective adrenergic blocker with a short half-life of less than 10 minutes that may be useful in treating elevated blood pressure that is associated with tachycardia but may be only mildly effective in treating hypertension related to increased systemic vascular resistance [63]. Labetalol is an α/β-adrenergic blocker [64] with a peak effect in 10 minutes and a relatively prolonged duration of action (3–5 hours). It is a useful drug for acute hypertension, particularly when used to treat emergence or postprocedure hypertension [65]. Sodium nitroprusside, nitroglycerin, and hydralazine all dilate cerebral capacitance vessels and can increase ICP [66]. They are therefore rarely used to treat hypertension in patients with neurosurgical tumor. Nicardipine is a highly selective dihydropyridine calcium channel blocker that has several advantages for treatment of neurosurgical hypertension [67]. It has a rapid onset of action (1–2 minutes) and an elimination half-life of 30 to 50 minutes [65]. Nicardipine is rapidly distributed, metabolized by the liver, and rapidly eliminated. Nicardipine has a potent dilatory effect and has been proposed as a treatment for cerebral vasospasm [68]. Clevidipine is another relatively new, rapidly acting, vascular-selective, L-type calcium channel antagonist. It has a high clearance (0.05 L/min/kg) and is rapidly hydrolyzed by ubiquitous plasma esterases. Clevidipine elimination is independent of the liver and kidney. It has a very rapid onset and offset (half-life <1 minute), making it easy to titrate to effect. This provides effective, rapidly adjustable blood pressure management [56]. Short-acting drugs are, in general, preferred during the perioperative period due to rapidly changing conditions such as fluid shifts, surgical stress, variable responses to pain, blood loss, and anxiety.

COUGHING

Coughing around the time of awakening is detrimental because freshly incised brain tissue is susceptible to bleeding. Hemostasis produced by themocoagulation and the presence of new clots is tenuous, making the neurosurgical patient especially susceptible to hemorrhage due to hypertension and increases in venous pressure; this may require reoperation. Coughing is induced by many factors, and prevention is most effective when multiple etiologies are dealt with. The noxious stimulation caused by a foreign body in the trachea (i.e., an inflated endotracheal tube cuff) can be reduced by the application of lidocaine ointment 5% (Fougera) to the cuff before intubation. The very viscous ointment is absorbed slowly and desensitizes the trachea for hours, whereas lidocaine spray has a fast onset but provides analgesia for only 14 minutes [69]. Other effective techniques for prolonged neurosurgical procedures include preextubation injection of intravenous lidocaine or filling the endotracheal cuff with a lidocaine solution. Another source of coughing is due to normalization or elevation of CO_2 allowed during closing to encourage spontaneous ventilation. Once spontaneous ventilation begins, asynchrony with the mechanical ventilator may generate coughing and high airway pressures. Maintenance of neuromuscular blockade and ventilation to maintain a $PaCO_2$ less than 40 mm Hg until the end of surgery is helpful. Opioids not only reduce the drive to breathe but also are potent antitussives; an anesthetic technique that incorporates opioids may therefore produce a smoother emergence.

CONCLUSION

Anesthetic management of patients with an intracranial mass requires knowledge of the pharmacology of anesthetic agents and the pathophysiology of brain tumors and offers an opportunity to combine basic science with clinical observations to maximize the possibility of a good neurologic outcome. There are very few evidence-based guidelines to aid decision-making for the neurosurgical patient, so most practitioners base their management strategy on a combination of hypothesis, theory, and expert consensus.

A basic understanding of the tumor type for which surgery is planned is important to optimize the anesthetic management of the patient. An understanding of the multiple interactions between the circulatory and respiratory systems and the cerebral circulation is also required but, again, not sufficient. The anesthesiologist must consider several explicit therapeutic goals that sometime compete to successfully optimize care. These goals include optimization of surgical exposure while minimizing brain injury and maximizing patient safety while providing patient comfort. Management of brain volume is a critical component of the anesthetic management of the patient undergoing intracranial tumor resection. Although hyperventilation and mannitol are no longer used as long-duration treatment, they are still commonly used during surgery for neoplastic disease.

Surgeons must sometimes exert mechanical pressure on brain tissue to expose a lesion. That pressure may cause injury by tearing axons and synapses and increasing tissue pressure, preventing blood from traversing capillaries. Anesthetics may also reduce systemic blood pressure below the critical CPP or may increase ICP, which also reduces CPP to a critical value. Anesthesiologists can also be therapeutic, reducing the bulk of the brain so less surgical retraction is needed to obtain the required exposure. Anesthesiologists can select an anesthetic and monitoring plan that avoids drugs that increase CBV and yet maintain good blood pressure control. These requirements add an extra burden to the anesthesiologist to customize the anesthetic plan to meet both the surgeon's and the patient's needs.

REFERENCES

1. Matsumae M, Kikinis R, Morocz IA, et al. Age-related changes in intracranial compartment volumes in normal adults assessed by magnetic resonance imaging. *J Neurosurg.* 1996;84:982–991.
2. Ito H, Kanno I, Iida H, et al. Arterial fraction of cerebral blood volume in humans measured by positron emission tomography. *Ann Nucl Med.* 2001;15:111–116.
3. Reinstrup P, Ryding E, Ohlsson T, et al. Cerebral blood volume (CBV) in humans during normo- and hypocapnia: influence of nitrous oxide (NO). *Anesthesiology.* 2001;95:1079–1082.
4. Engvall C, Ryding E, Wirestam R, et al. Human cerebral blood volume (CBV) measured by dynamic susceptibility contrast MRI and 99mTc-RBC SPECT. *J Neurosurg Anesthesiol.* 2008;20:41–44.
5. Raichle ME, Posner JB, Plum F. Cerebral blood flow during and after hyperventilation. *Arch Neurol.* 1970;23:394–403.
6. Artru AA. Reduction of cerebrospinal fluid pressure by hypocapnia: changes in cerebral blood volume, cerebrospinal fluid volume, and brain tissue water and electrolytes. *J Cereb Blood Flow Metab.* 1987;7:471–479.
7. Ito H, Kanno I, Ibaraki M, et al. Changes in human cerebral blood flow and cerebral blood volume during hypercapnia and hypocapnia measured by positron emission tomography. *J Cereb Blood Flow Metab.* Jun 2003;23:665–670.
8. Laffey JG, Kavanagh BP. Hypocapnia. *N Engl J Med.* Jul 4 2002;347:43–53.
9. Kaisti KK, Langsjo JW, Aalto S, et al. Effects of sevoflurane, propofol, and adjunct nitrous oxide on regional cerebral blood flow, oxygen consumption, and blood volume in humans. *Anesthesiology.* 2003;99:603–613.
10. Muizelaar JP, Wei EP, Kontos HA, et al. Mannitol causes compensatory cerebral vasoconstriction and vasodilation in response to blood viscosity changes. *J Neurosurg.* 1983;59:822–828.
11. Rosner MJ, Coley I. Cerebral perfusion pressure: a hemodynamic mechanism of mannitol and the postmannitol hemogram. *Neurosurgery.* 1987;21:147–156.
12. Diringer MN, Scalfani MT, Zazulia AR, et al. Effect of mannitol on cerebral blood volume in patients with head injury. *Neurosurgery.* 2012;70:1215–1218.
13. Lovell AT, Marshall AC, Elwell CE, et al. Changes in cerebral blood volume with changes in position in awake and anesthetized subjects. *Anesth Analg.* 2000;90:372–376.
14. Arbit E, DiResta GR, Bedford RF, et al. Intraoperative measurement of cerebral and tumor blood flow with laser-Doppler flowmetry. *Neurosurgery.* 1989;24:166–170.
15. Holodny AI, Schulder M, Liu WC, et al. The effect of brain tumors on BOLD functional MR imaging activation in the adjacent motor cortex: implications for image-guided neurosurgery. *AJNR Am J Neuroradiol.* 2000;21:1415–1422.
16. Artru AA. Dose-related changes in the rate of CSF formation and resistance to reabsorption of CSF during administration of fentanyl, sufentanil, or alfentanil in dogs. *J Neurosurg Anesthesiol.* 1991;3:283–290.
17. Artru AA. Rate of cerebrospinal fluid formation, resistance to reabsorption of cerebrospinal fluid, brain tissue water content, and electroencephalogram during desflurane anesthesia in dogs. *J Neurosurg Anesthesiol.* 1993;5:178–186.
18. Artru AA, Momota T. Rate of CSF formation and resistance to reabsorption of CSF during sevoflurane or remifentanil in rabbits. *J Neurosurg Anesthesiol.* 2000;12:37–43.
19. Fatouros PP, Marmarou A. Use of magnetic resonance imaging for in vivo measurements of water content in human brain: method and normal values. *J Neurosurg.* 1999;90:109–115.
20. Fishman RA. Brain edema. *N Engl J Med.* 1975;293:706–711.
21. Cserr HF, DePasquale M, Patlak CS. Volume regulatory influx of electrolytes from plasma to brain during acute hyperosmolality. *Am J Physiol.* 1987;253(3 Pt 2):F530–F537.
22. Rudehill A, Gordon E, Ohman G, et al. Pharmacokinetics and effects of mannitol on hemodynamics, blood and cerebrospinal fluid electrolytes, and osmolality during intracranial surgery. *J Neurosurg Anesthesiol.* 1993;5:4–12.
23. Donato T, Shapira Y, Artru A, et al. Effect of mannitol on cerebrospinal fluid dynamics and brain tissue edema. *Anesth Analg.* 1994;78:58–66.
24. Videen TO, Zazulia AR, Manno EM, et al. Mannitol bolus preferentially shrinks non-infarcted brain in patients with ischemic stroke. *Neurology.* 2001;57:2120–2122.
25. Bell BA, Smith MA, Kean DM, et al. Brain water measured by magnetic resonance imaging. Correlation with direct estimation and changes after mannitol and dexamethasone. *Lancet.* 1987;1:66–69.
26. McManus ML, Soriano SG. Rebound swelling of astroglial cells exposed to hypertonic mannitol. *Anesthesiology.* 1998;88:1586–1591.
27. McManus ML, Churchwell KB, Strange K. Regulation of cell volume in health and disease. *N Engl J Med.* 1995;333:1260–1266.
28. Thenuwara K, Todd MM, Brian JE Jr. Effect of mannitol and furosemide on plasma osmolality and brain water. *Anesthesiology.* 2002;96:416–421.
29. Pollay M, Fullenwider C, Roberts PA, et al. Effect of mannitol and furosemide on blood-brain osmotic gradient and intracranial pressure. *J Neurosurg.* 1983;59:945–950.
30. Todd MM, Cutkomp J, Brian JE. Influence of mannitol and furosemide, alone and in combination, on brain water content after fluid percussion injury. *Anesthesiology.* 2006;105:1176–1181.
31. Kimelberg HK, Barron KD, Bourke RS, et al. Brain anti-cytoxic edema agents. *Progr Clin Biol Res.* 1990;361:363–385.
32. Plangger C, Volkl H. Effect of furosemide, bumetanide and mannitol on intracranial pressure in experimental brain edema of the rat. *Zentralblatt Neurochir.* 1989;50(3–4):142–144.
33. Cascino T, Baglivo J, Conti J, et al. Quantitative CT assessment of furosemide- and mannitol-induced changes in brain water content. *Neurology.* 1983;33:898–903.
34. Gaab M, Knoblich OE, Schupp J, et al. Effect of furosemide (lasix) on acute severe experimental cerebral edema. *J Neurol.* 1979;220:185–197.
35. Alvarez B, Radi R. Peroxynitrite decay in the presence of hydrogen peroxide, mannitol and ethanol: a reappraisal. *Free Rad Res.* 2001;34:467–475.
36. Ferreira R, Burgos M, Llesuy S, et al. Reduction of reperfusion injury with mannitol cardioplegia. *Ann Thorac Surg.* 1989;48:77–83; discussion 83–74.
37. Korenkov AI, Pahnke J, Frei K, et al. Treatment with nimodipine or mannitol reduces programmed cell death and infarct size following focal cerebral ischemia. *Neurosurg Rev.* 2000;23:145–150.
38. Bereczki D, Fekete I, Prado GF, et al. Mannitol for acute stroke. *Cochrane Database Syst Rev.* 2007:CD001153.
39. Palma L, Bruni G, Fiaschi AI, et al. Passage of mannitol into the brain around gliomas: a potential cause of rebound phenomenon. A study on 21 patients. *J Neurosurg Sci.* 2006;50:63–66.
40. KhitryiGp. [The intensive therapy of brain edema by using clofelin and a hypertonic solution of sodium chloride in neurosurgical patients]. *Likars'ka sprava / Ministerstvo okhorony zdorov'ia Ukrainy.* 1997;May-Jun:127–131.
41. Wu CT, Chen LC, Kuo CP, et al. A comparison of 3% hypertonic saline and mannitol for brain relaxation during elective supratentorial brain tumor surgery. *Anesth Analg.* 2010;110:903–907.
42. Galicich JH, French LA, Melby JC. Use of dexamethasone in treatment of cerebral edema associated with brain tumors. *Lancet.* 1961;81:46–53.

43. Wissinger JP, French LA, Gillingham FJ. The use of dexamethasone in the control of cerebral oedema. *J Neurol Neurosurg Psychiatry*. 1967;30:588.

44. Gutin PH. Corticosteroid therapy in patients with cerebral tumors: benefits, mechanisms, problems, practicalities. *Semin Oncol*. 1975;2:49–56.

45. Ryken TC, McDermott M, Robinson PD, et al. The role of steroids in the management of brain metastases: a systematic review and evidence-based clinical practice guideline. *J Neurooncol*. 2010;96:103–114.

46. Jelsma RK, Bucy PC. The treatment of glioblastoma multiforme. *Trans Am Neurol Assoc*. 1967;92:90–93.

47. Heiss JD, Papavassiliou E, Merrill MJ, et al. Mechanism of dexamethasone suppression of brain tumor-associated vascular permeability in rats. Involvement of the glucocorticoid receptor and vascular permeability factor. *J Clin Investig*. 1996;98:1400–1408.

48. Shapiro WR, Hiesiger EM, Cooney GA, et al. Temporal effects of dexamethasone on blood-to-brain and blood-to-tumor transport of 14C-alpha-aminoisobutyric acid in rat C6 glioma. *J Neurooncol*. 1990;8:197–204.

49. Kaal EC, Vecht CJ. The management of brain edema in brain tumors. *Curr Opin Oncol*. 2004;16:593–600.

50. Meinig G, Reulen HJ, Simon RS, et al. Clinical, chemical, and CT evaluation of short-term and long-term antiedema therapy with dexamethasone and diuretics. *Adv Neurol*. 1980;28:471–489.

51. Ting P. Indomethacin attenuates early postischemic vasogenic edema and cerebral injury. *Adv Neurol*. 1990;52:119–126.

52. Del Maestro RF, Megyesi JF, Farrell CL. Mechanisms of tumor-associated edema: a review. *Can J Neurol Sci*. 1990;17: 177–183.

53. Bundgaard H, Jensen K, Cold GE, et al. Effects of perioperative indomethacin on intracranial pressure, cerebral blood flow, and cerebral metabolism in patients subjected to craniotomy for cerebral tumors. *J Neurosurg Anesthesiol*. 1996;8:273–279.

54. Todd MM, Warner DS, Sokoll MD, et al. A prospective, comparative trial of three anesthetics for elective supratentorial craniotomy. Propofol/fentanyl, isoflurane/nitrous oxide, and fentanyl/nitrous oxide. *Anesthesiology*. 1993;78:1005–1020.

55. Basali A, Mascha EJ, Kalfas I, et al. Relation between perioperative hypertension and intracranial hemorrhage after craniotomy. *Anesthesiology*. 2000;93:48–54.

56. Bekker A, Didehvar S, Kim S, et al. Efficacy of clevidipine in controlling perioperative hypertension in neurosurgical patients: initial single-center experience. *J Neurosurg Anesthesiol*. 2010;22:330–335.

57. Andrews RJ, Bringas JR. A review of brain retraction and recommendations for minimizing intraoperative brain injury. *Neurosurgery*. 1993;33:1052–1063; discussion 1063–1054.

58. Albin MS, Bunegin L, Dujovny M, et al. Brain retraction pressure during intracranial procedures. *Surg Forum*. 1975;26:499–500.

59. Andrews RJ, Muto RP. Retraction brain ischaemia: cerebral blood flow, evoked potentials, hypotension and hyperventilation in a new animal model. *Neurol Res*. 1992;14:12–18.

60. Ravussin P, Mustaki JP, Boulard G, et al. Neuro-anesthetic contribution to the prevention of complications caused by mechanical cerebral retraction: concept of a chemical brain retractor. *Annales Francaises d'Anesthesie et de Reanimation*. 1995;14:49–55.

61. Bruder N, Pellissier D, Grillot P, et al. Cerebral hyperemia during recovery from general anesthesia in neurosurgical patients. *Anesth Analg*. 2002;94:650–654; table of contents.

62. Hatashita S, Koike J, Sonokawa T, et al. Cerebral edema associated with craniectomy and arterial hypertension. *Stroke*. 1985;16: 661–668.

63. Bilotta F, Lam AM, Doronzio A, et al. Esmolol blunts postoperative hemodynamic changes after propofol-remifentanil total intravenous fast-track neuroanesthesia for intracranial surgery. *J Clin Anesth*. 2008;20:426–430.

64. Kanto JH. Current status of labetalol, the first alpha- and beta-blocking agent. *Int J Clin Pharmacol Ther Toxicol*. 1985;23:617–628.

65. Kross RA, Ferri E, Leung D, et al. A comparative study between a calcium channel blocker (nicardipine) and a combined alpha-beta-blocker (labetalol) for the control of emergence hypertension during craniotomy for tumor surgery. *Anesth Analg*. 2000;91:904–909.

66. Van Aken H, Cottrell JE, Anger C, et al. Treatment of intraoperative hypertensive emergencies in patients with intracranial disease. *Am J Cardiol*. 1989;63:43C–47C.

67. Gaab MR, Czech T, Korn A. Intracranial effects of nicardipine. *Br J Clin Pharmacol*. 1985;20(Suppl 1):67S–74S.

68. Flamm ES. The potential use of nicardipine in cerebrovascular disease. *Am Heart J*. 1989;117:236–242.

69. Schonemann NK, van der Burght M, Arendt-Nielsen L, et al. Onset and duration of hypoalgesia of lidocaine spray applied to oral mucosa—a dose response study. *Acta Anaesthesiol Scand*. 1992;36:733–735.

70. Allen JS, Damasio H, Grabowski TJ. Normal Neuroanatomical Variation in the Human Brain: An MRI-Volumetric Study. *Am J Phys Anthro*. 2002;118:341–358.

13.

PITUITARY AND NEUROENDOCRINE SURGERY

Patricia Fogarty-Mack

INTRODUCTION

Anesthetic management of the patient undergoing surgery for a tumor of the pituitary presents unique challenges. Surgical access is frequently through the nose, meaning that the anesthesiologist and surgeon must share a portion of the airway. Surgical access to the operative site is restricted to a narrow endoscope, limiting options if unexpected hemorrhage occurs. The surgical site is very close to multiple fragile, critical structures, including the cavernous sinus and the optic chiasm. A patient with a pituitary mass may have a hormone-secreting tumor (a *functional adenoma*), which in turn causes an endocrine disease. Functional adenomas may affect the patient's airway, cardiovascular system, and various metabolic pathways. Such alterations require specific preoperative attention and consideration throughout the perioperative period. Although there are many subtypes of functional adenoma, the two that have the most impact on anesthetic management are those that secrete growth hormone (GH), leading to acromegaly, and adrenocorticotrophic hormone (ACTH), leading to Cushing's disease.

The endonasal endoscopic approach is a widely used alternative to the traditional microscopic approach to the sella turcica, and offers numerous advantages over an open approach [1, 2]. One investigation comparing perioperative parameters between the two techniques found that patients who underwent the endoscopic endonasal approach had shorter operative times, lower estimated blood loss, less pain, and a shorter hospital stay. A lumbar drain is also required less frequently for this approach [3]. The endonasal endoscopic approach does have several disadvantages: Surgical access to the pituitary is limited, and it may be difficult or impossible to completely resect a large tumor. It is also possible to break through the very thin bone that comprises the sella turcica, which can result in rapid blood loss from the cavernous sinus. This chapter offers a brief review of the anesthetic considerations associated with each pituitary disorder.

PREOPERATIVE CONSIDERATIONS

ACROMEGALY

Airway Considerations

Acromegaly manifests with enlargement of the facial bones, especially the mandible [4, 5], as well as hypertrophy of the laryngeal and pharyngeal soft tissue [6, 7]. Hypertrophy of the periepiglottic folds and calcinosis of the larynx may be seen, as may recurrent laryngeal nerve paresis [8]. These anatomic changes may serve to make intubation technically difficult. In two large reviews, the incidence of difficult intubation in patients with acromegaly was 10% [4] and 9.1% [5], respectively. (In contrast, the incidence of difficult intubation in the general population is between 1% and 4% [5].) Changes in airway anatomy also predispose patients with acromegaly to obstructive sleep apnea (OSA). OSA occurs in 25% of female patients and 70% of male patients and may manifest as snoring or daytime somnolence [9]. This may make mask ventilation extremely difficult during induction of anesthesia. The presence of OSA places these patients at an increased risk of postoperative respiratory failure [10].

Four grades of airway involvement in acromegaly have been described:

- Grade 1: No airway involvement
- Grade 2: Soft tissue hypertrophy of the nasopharynx without glottic involvement
- Grade 3: Glottic stenosis or vocal cord paresis
- Grade 4: Soft tissue hypertrophy and glottic stenosis [11]

Difficult intubation and ventilation were so commonly encountered in Grade 3 and 4 patients that routine tracheostomy had been recommended in the past [11]. The increasing use of fiberoptic bronchoscopy and the introduction of alternative intubating devices such as the videolaryngoscope have, however, rendered the preoperative tracheostomy a rare occurrence [12]. Twenty percent of patients may be difficult to intubate, even when the airway anatomy does not appear to be "difficult" on examination, i.e., patients with a Mallampati Class 1 or 2 airway [13]. In Nemergut and Zuo's review, 50% of Mallampati Class I and II patients were ultimately difficult to intubate [5]. Over time, there may be regression of hypertrophied tissues in the acromegalic patient, and impaired vocal cord function may improve within 10 days of surgery [14, 15].

Cardiovascular Concerns

The leading cause of death in patients with untreated acromegaly is cardiac dysfunction [16]. Cardiac manifestations of acromegaly include endothelial dysfunction, left ventricular (LV) dysfunction and dysrhythmias [17]. Small vessel coronary artery disease has been described [18], and endothelium-dependent vasodilation is impaired [19]. Symptoms of angina should therefore be treated as evidence of myocardial ischemia, even in a patient who has no independent risk factors for cardiovascular disease.

Acromegalic cardiomyopathy is defined as a cardiomyopathy presumed to be caused by chronically elevated growth hormone in the absence of other causes. The incidence of acromegalic cardiomyopathy is 3 to 4 cases per million people per year, and findings include concentric hypertrophy and an increase in LV mass with normal LV dimensions. In many cases, the heart may weigh up to 1300 grams (a normal heart typically weighs less than 250 g) [18]. The severity of the hypertrophy is related to the duration of disease, and the prognosis is worse in the presence of LV dilatation. Left untreated, acromegalic cardiomyopathy progresses through three stages. In the early stage, increased contractility and decreased systemic vascular resistance cause an increase in cardiac output [20, 21]. LV diastolic dysfunction may be significant despite normal LV mass [20]. In the intermediate stage, biventricular hypertrophy develops and diastolic dysfunction becomes evident [22]. Although systolic function is preserved at rest, the patient will have impaired exercise tolerance. The late stage of acromegalic cardiomyopathy is marked by dilatation of the ventricles, decreased systolic function, and congestive heart failure [20, 21, 23, 24].

Acromegalic patients experience a significantly greater frequency and severity of ventricular dysrhythmia is significantly greater in acromegalics than do patients without acromegaly. Dysrhythmias in this population appear to be correlated with LV mass [25]. About 18% to 60% of acromegalic patients also have hypertension [16, 26–29]. Contributing factors appear to be a direct effect of growth hormone as well as an increase in sympathetic tone, cardiac hyperkinesis, an increase in plasma volume, a reduction in

atrial naturetic peptide secretion, and hyperinsulinemia [30, 31, 32, 33, 34, 35]. Even in those patients with normal blood pressure, half have LV hypertrophy [36]. Not surprisingly, many have diastolic dysfunction, with preserved systolic function.

If the underlying disease is treated in the early or intermediate stage, ventricular hypertrophy may resolve but diastolic dysfunction may persist, which is consistent with the histologic finding of interstitial fibrosis. Ten percent of patients diagnosed with acromegaly have signs of high output heart failure and decreased ejection fraction, while 3% have significant systolic dysfunction [24, 36]. In view of these potentially severe cardiac abnormalities, it may be prudent to obtain a resting electrocardiogram and echocardiogram in all patients with regardless of the patient's age.

CUSHING'S DISEASE

Airway

Although the incidence of difficult intubation in the patient with Cushing's disease does not differ from that of the general population (1% to 4%) [5], airway management may still be difficult in this population [23]. Thirty-three percent of patients with Cushing's disease suffer from OSA, and 18% of patients have severe sleep apnea [37]. Many patients with Cushing's disease are morbidly obese and may suffer from gastroesophageal reflux and delayed gastric emptying. Many anesthesiologists consider rapid sequence or awake intubation in this population for these reasons.

Patients with Cushing's disease may lose weight after surgery, with subsequent improvement in airway anatomy and respiratory function.

Cardiovascular

Patients with Cushing's disease are predisposed to significant hypertension. Up to 80% of Cushing's patients have hypertension, and 50% have diastolic pressures greater than 100 mm Hg if untreated [38]. This propensity for hypertension is the direct result of excessive levels of corticosteroids [39, 40]. Hydrocortisone increases hepatic production of angiotensinogen, which activates the renin-angiotensin system, increasing plasma volume [40]. Glucocorticoids increase the number of angiotensin II receptors on vascular smooth muscle cells [41]. This, in turn, augments the response to both endogenous and perhaps exogenous catecholamines. Finally, glucocorticoid inhibition of vascular smooth muscle phospholipase A_2 reduces the production of vasodilatory prostaglandins [42].

LV hypertrophy is far more severe in patients with Cushing's disease than in those with essential hypertension, suggesting a direct effect of elevated cortisol levels upon the myocardium. The incidence of asymmetric LVH, with greater hypertrophy of the intraventricular septum, is also higher [43]. Diastolic dysfunction occurs in at least 40% of patients with Cushing's disease [44]. ECG changes include LV strain pattern, which returns to normal, as do echocardiographic findings, within 1 year after resection of ACTH secreting adenoma [45]. For these reasons, it may be prudent to obtain a resting electrocardiogram and echocardiogram in patients with Cushing's disease regardless of the patient's age.

OTHER PITUITARY MASSES AND MACROADENOMA

Other functional pituitary adenomas include thyrotropic adenoma, prolactinoma, and gonadotropin secreting adenoma. Thyrotropic adenomas comprise only 2.8% of all pituitary tumors and may cause hyperthyroidism [46]. The signs and symptoms of hyperthyroidism are usually present in these patients, and a goiter may even be observed. Because patients are often treated for another presumed cause of hyperthyroidism first, the pituitary tumor can be large at time of presentation, and 60% of tumors are locally invasive. Patients should receive medical treatment for hyperthyroidism prior to surgery.

Patients who have a prolactinoma or gonadotropin secreting ademona often present with nonspecific symptoms. There are no specific airway or cardiovascular concerns in these patients [5, 23]. Women with a prolactinoma usually present with amenorrhea, galatorrhea, and infertility [23]. Men who have a prolactinoma present with erectile dysfunction, premature ejaculation, and loss of libido. Ninety percent of patients with these tumors respond to bromocriptine, a dopamine agonist, and do not require surgery. These nonspecific symptoms may lead to a delayed diagnosis and the patient may develop symptoms of a macroadenoma (a tumor greater than 10 mm) [47].

Patients with a macroadenoma may present with symptoms of a sellar mass including headache, bitemporal hemianopsia (due to compression of the optic chiasm), and hypopituitarism (from compression of the anterior pituitary) [47]. Massive pituitary tumors may cause obstructive hydrocephalus and symptoms of increased intracranial pressure, especially if the tumor obstructs the third ventricle. If symptoms of intracranial hypertension are present, the anesthetic should be tailored to prevent further increases in the ICP.

HEMATOLOGIC AND METABOLIC CONCERNS

Although most patients presenting with pituitary tumors will have had an extensive hematologic, metabolic, and endocrinologic evaluation, several studies are of particular importance to the anesthesiologist and should be obtained as close as practical to the time of surgery. Patients with panhypopituitarism should be given thyroid replacement and hydrocortisone and these medications should be continued on the morning of surgery [23, 48].

Laboratory studies should include baseline hemoglobin level because significant hemorrhage can occur during pituitary surgery. Coagulation studies are not indicated, however, unless the patient has a history consistent with an increased risk of bleeding. Serum electrolytes should be obtained to rule out hyponatremia, which may result from diabetes insipidus (DI) caused by posterior pituitary dysfunction. Sixty percent of patients with Cushing's disease are glucose intolerant and 33% have diabetes mellitus [49], and blood glucose may be increased in acromegaly due to insulin resistance [50]. Measuring serum glucose and hemoglobin A1c may therefore be helpful in patients with Cushing's disease. The "tightness" of perioperative glucose control is controversial, but there is clear evidence that hyperglycemia is undesirable during periods of neuronal ischemia [51–53]. A thyroid panel should also be obtained to ensure that the patient is euthyroid. A pregnancy test should also be obtained, especially in amenorrheic women. Prior to surgery, an active type and screen is should be drawn to ensure that blood products are readily available if needed [23, 48].

INTRAOPERATIVE MANAGEMENT

MONITORING AND VASCULAR ACCESS

The requirements for invasive physiologic monitoring depend on the extent of pituitary disease, the presence of comorbidities, and the planned surgical procedure. Because the patient's head and most of the patient's body will be inaccessible during the surgical procedure, any technical problems with the monitors should be resolved before the surgery begins. Some neuronavigation systems use infrared light, which may interfere with the pulse oximeter waveform. Covering the pulse oximeter probe with foil (e.g., a wrapper from an alcohol swab) to isolate it from the navigation system may cause the waveform to return to normal [54].

Not all anesthesiologists consider invasive monitoring of systemic arterial pressure to be necessary for transsphenoidal pituitary surgery. An intra-arterial catheter has typically been reserved for patients who had significant cardiovascular disease or cardiovascular sequelae of acromegaly. An intra-arterial catheter may, however, be useful because it allows rapid detection and treatment of hemodynamic changes associated with the intranasal injection of vasoactive substances. Continuous monitoring of arterial blood pressure is essential if massive hemorrhage should occur after perforation of the carotid or another artery, a rare but potentially catastrophic occurrence. An arterial line also allows frequent sampling of blood for laboratory analysis, which may be useful in the management of diabetes mellitus and diabetes insipidus. Radial artery catheterization may have a higher risk of complications in patients with acromegaly, especially if symptoms of carpal tunnel syndrome are present. Fifty percent of these patients have may have diminished ulnar blood flow [55], making an Allen's test a recommended procedure in acromegalic patients prior to insertion of an intra-arterial catheter.

Adequate intravenous access is important because abrupt, massive hemorrhage may occur if the carotid artery is perforated or if the surgeons enter the cavernous sinus. All patients scheduled for pituitary surgery should have cross-matched blood available for the same reasons. Central venous pressure monitoring is rarely indicated in these patients and is usually reserved for those with significant compromise in cardiac function. A central venous catheter may, however, be necessary in a patient who does not have adequate peripheral venous access.

AIRWAY MANAGEMENT

Patients with either acromegaly or Cushing's disease may be challenging to mask ventilate and to intubate. In patients with abnormal anatomy, especially those with acromegaly, the anesthesiologist should therefore consider an awake intubation. If an awake intubation is not indicated, it is prudent to have an alternative airway device available in the event that direct laryngoscopy is more difficult than anticipated. Such devices include but are not limited to the gum elastic bougie [5], intubating laryngeal mask airway [56], the Glidescope (Verathon, Bothell, WA), the Airtraq (Prodol Meditec, Bueons Aires, Argentina), McGrathMAC (Aircraft Medical, Edinburgh, Scotland) and the fiberoptic bronchoscope. The choice of a specific device is to be determined based on the airway anatomy and the anesthesiologist's experience.

Patients undergoing pituitary surgery are generally intubated orally because the use of an endonasal approach precludes a nasal intubation. An preformed oral RAE (Ring, Adair and Elwyn, inventors) endotracheal tube may reduce the risk of dislodgement by the surgical team during the procedure. The depth of the oral RAE tube (centimeters) at the lip is determined by the diameter of the tube, which complicates appropriate size selection. Acromegalic patients have a large tongue, which may require that the preformed bend in the tube to be at a greater depth, while the presence of laryngeal or subglottic stenosis may preclude the diameter of tube necessary. An additional disadvantage of the RAE tube is that the preformed bend may make insertion of a fiberoptic bronchoscope through the tube more difficult.

MAINTENANCE OF ANESTHESIA AND PLANNING FOR EMERGENCE

The goals of any anesthetic technique for pituitary surgery include hemodynamic stability and rapid emergence from anesthesia at the end of the procedure. The patient should be pain-free and alert with a patent airway and should be able to comply with a postoperative neurologic exam promptly after awakening. A remifentanil infusion combined with either a potent volatile anesthetic or a propofol infusion is one technique commonly used for pituitary surgery. Remifentanil is an esterase metabolized narcotic that is almost completely eliminated within a few minutes after the infusion is discontinued; its duration of action is unaffected by the duration of the infusion. It is particularly well suited to this procedure because it can be rapidly titrated to accommodate the constantly changing levels of surgical stimuli and it will produce relatively little respiratory depression in immediate postoperative period when there is minimal pain. The use of remifentanil for intraoperative analgesia may reduce the risk of airway obstruction in patients who may already have sleep apnea and whose nasal passages are now packed with gauze and further obstructed because of postsurgical edema. In a clinical comparison of remifentanil to isoflurane anesthesia, patients in the remifentanil group emerged more rapidly and required less labetalol in the perioperative period [57]. Another study comparing infusions of remifentanil and propofol to a remifentanil infusion combined with inhaled sevoflurane revealed that patients in the sevoflurane group emerged more rapidly than did those in the propofol group [58].

The use of neuromuscular blocking agents (NMBs) during pituitary surgery is somewhat controversial. Many anesthesiologists do not use NMBs when the head is fixated in a rigid pin fixation device [57], while others routinely administer these drugs. Many surgeons position the patient with his or her head on a "donut" and do not use a head fixation device. The endoscope may, however, be fixed to a rigid arm, which is secured to the operating table. If the patient moves during surgery, the surgeon might not be able to remove the endoscope rapidly and this could potentially injure the patient. Neuromuscular blockade may be accomplished using either an infusion or administering repeated boluses of a NMB while monitoring the neuromuscular junction. Upon removal of the endoscope from the nasal cavity, the patient can be allowed to recover from neuromuscular blockade, and the residual NMB can be reversed at the conclusion of surgery.

METABOLIC/ENDOCRINE CONCERNS

Because nearly all procedures involve surgical manipulation of the anterior pituitary, dexamethasone 10 mg or hydrocortisone 50 to 100 mg is usually administered at the beginning of the surgery and as indicated throughout the procedure. Some surgeons prefer not to administer steroids to patients with Cushing's disease during the surgery so that serial cortisol levels can be monitored in the postoperative period [48].

Diabetes insipidus (DI) is a common complication of transphenoidal pituitary surgery that is characterized as an inability to concentrate the urine despite systemic hypovolemia. 31% of patients experience transient DI in the perioperative period [59]. In one cohort of patients who had undergone minimally invasive endoscopic pituitary resection, 13.6% rate experienced transient DI after surgery and 2.7% had permanent DI [60]. In most cases the onset occurs within 24 to 48 hours after surgery and resolves within 7 days. Infrequently, however, DI occurs during surgery and is usually diagnosed by a sudden increase in urine output that is out of proportion to intravenous fluid administration. Laboratory findings consistent with DI include low urine specific gravity, a urine osmolality lower than plasma osmolality and serum sodium greater than 145 meq/liter. It is necessary to ensure that the increase in urine output is not caused by overhydration or hyperglycemia. Administration of DDAVP (Desmopressin®) is rarely required in the operating room, but the initial dose of is two to four micrograms intravenously. Patients with acromegaly may have a brisk diuresis in the postoperative period but early treatment with DDAVP is not recommended in this patient population [61].

INTRAOPERATIVE EMERGENCIES

HEMODYNAMIC INSTABILITY AND MYOCARDIAL ISCHEMIA

Hemodynamic variability is common during transphenoidal surgery because of the cardiovascular response to stimulation of the trigeminal nerve [62] and infiltration or topical application of vasoactive agents that are used to decrease bleeding. Multiple studies have been performed in patients undergoing otorhinolaryngology surgery to determine the safety and efficacy of various combinations of drugs for vasoconstriction and analgesia [63–67]. Institutional and surgeon preferences often determine the selection of vasoconstricting agents. The most commonly used agents are alpha agonists and cocaine.

Phenylephrine, oxymetazoline, and a combination of lidocaine or bupivacaine with epinephrine are commonly used to provide hemostasis and analgesia during the endonasal approach to the pituitary. Plasma catecholamine levels may increase by up to 400% within minutes of intranasal epinephrine infiltration, causing profound hypertension and tachycardia [68, 69]. Complications including visual loss [70, 71] and profound hypertension [72, 73] have been attributed to the intranasal injection of local anesthetic in combination with epinephrine. A review of 100 patients at the Mayo Clinic revealed an average increase in systolic and diastolic blood pressures of 60 and 23 mmHg respectively following intranasal injection of local anesthetic with

epinephrine [74]. No relationship was found between dose of epinephrine and severity of hypertension, nor was there any episode of cardiac dysrhythmia, persistent myocardial ischemia or myocardial infarction noted in this cohort [74].

Cocaine (in solutions with concentrations between 4% and 10%) has long been used for both vasoconstriction and analgesia in endoscopic sinus surgery. There are several case of myocardial ischemia and infarction, perhaps secondary to coronary artery spasm, that has even occurred in young adults. The ischemia in these cases was attributed to intraoperative use of topical cocaine [75–78]. The use of cocaine has also been proposed as a cause of postoperative delirium [79] and acute glaucoma [80].

Patients with Cushing's disease and elevated levels of cortisol are predisposed to hypertension that is caused by activation of the angiotensin system. These patients may have an exaggerated response to topical vasoconstrictors [72]. An increase in afterload caused by oxymetazoline (Afrin®), phenylephrine or cocaine may cause acute decompensation in patients with acromegalic cardiomyopathy.

Hypertension caused by injection of alpha agonists should treated by administration of vasodilators. Alpha induced vasoconstriction preferentially shifts blood from the peripheral to the pulmonary circulation, increasing LV end-diastolic volume and pressure. Maintaining adequate contractility is critical in order to prevent severe pulmonary edema in this setting. Theoretically, the negative inotropic effects of calcium channel blockers or an increase in volatile anesthetic agent concentration may have the same untoward effects as beta blockade [66]. Cardiogenic shock and pulmonary edema leading to cardiac arrest and death have been reported in both children and adults who were given beta blockers to treat alpha agonist induced hypertension [81, 82].

A high index of suspicion should be maintained for myocardial ischemia during the time when local anesthetic and vasoconstrictive agents are injected into or applied to the endonasal mucosa. If ST segment monitoring and alarms are available, the baseline levels of the PR segment and ST segment should be obtained and appropriate alarms should be activated, even in patients who are not otherwise at risk for myocardial ischemia. If extreme tachycardia, severe hypertension or myocardial ischemia is detected, cocaine soaked pledgets should be removed from the nasal cavity or injection of other vasoconstricting agents suspended.

Profound hypotension has also been observed following administration of epinephrine. Hemodynamic instability and one to two minutes of profound hypotension has been observed after infiltration with a local anesthetic containing epinephrine [83]. Studies in patients undergoing craniotomy and sinus surgery suggest that hypotension after injection of epinephrine is usually self limited and is often followed by hypertension [84, 85]. It has been further suggested that light general anesthesia is more effective than a fluid bolus in ameliorating this effect [86].

Arterial Injury

Arterial injury, either to the internal carotid artery or to other vessels (e.g., the ophthalmic artery) is a rare but serious complication of transphenoidal resection of pituitary or an intracranial mass. [87–89]. If such an injury should occur, prompt resuscitation with crystalloid solutions and blood products is essential. The anesthesiologist must therefore obtain adequate venous access before the surgery begins in the event that rapid fluid administration is required. The availability of a sufficient amount of cross-matched packed red blood cells should also be ensured. If the surgeon is unable to repair the arterial injury, it may be necessary to pack the bleeding vessel and transport the patient to the interventional radiology suite for an embolization procedure.

POST-OPERATIVE MANAGEMENT

EMERGENCE FROM ANESTHESIA

Patients undergoing transphenoidal resection are generally allowed to emerge from general anesthesia and are extubated at the conclusion of surgery. Patients should be awake and alert and able to maintain their airway. Patients should be hemodynamically stable with an appropriate respiratory rate and tidal volume during spontaneous ventilation before extubation. Neuromuscular blocking agents should be reversed and the adequacy of muscle strength should be established. A leak around the endotracheal tube when the cuff is deflated should be present.

Because nasal packing may render postoperative mask ventilation less effective, additional extubation criteria may be considered. For example, a patient with preexisting sleep apnea may be unable to maintain adequate ventilation and should be monitored overnight in an intensive care or step-down unit.

Postoperative placement of a nasal airway is contraindicated, and continuous positive airway pressure (CPAP) or bilevel positive airway pressure (BiPAP) via facemask may disrupt the surgical closure and cause pneumocephalus. Blind placement of any type of nasal airway, nasogastric tube or nasal endotracheal tube is absolutely contraindicated in the immediate postoperative period [90].

Patients undergoing endoscopic pituitary procedures generally do not require significant doses of narcotics for pain control in the postoperative period. As the local anesthetic wears off, however, patients will have pain that requires judicious management with narcotic analgesics, especially in the patient with sleep apnea. Patients undergoing transphenoidal surgery typically require an average of 5.2 to 6.7 mg of morphine in the post anesthesia care unit (PACU) [88], and bilateral infraorbital nerve blocks have been reported to decrease postoperative narcotic usage [91, 92].

POSTOPERATIVE NAUSEA AND VOMITING PROPHYLAXIS

Single agent antiemetic prophylaxis was not found to reduce the incidence of postoperative emesis (7.5%) in a

Table 13.1   COMMON PERIOPERATIVE CONCERNS IN PITUITARY SURGERY

	ACROMEGALY	CUSHING'S DISEASE	OTHER
Airway Features	Bony enlargement	Buffalo hump	
	Macroglossia	Obesity	
	Laryngeal calcinosis	Reflux	
	Periepiglottic fold hypertrophy		
Difficult ventilation	+	+	No increased incidence
Difficult intubation	+++	No increased incidence	No increased incidence
HTN	+	++ (glucocorticoid excess: rennin-angiotensin effects)	
Cardiac considerations	Concentric LVH	Severe eccentric LVH	
	Diastolic dysfunction followed by systolic dysfunction	Diastolic dysfunction	
	Small vessel coronary artery disease		
	Dysrhythmias related to LV mass	LV strain	
Metabolic	Increased glucose due to insulin resistance	60% with hyperglycemia, 33% frank diabetes mellitus	Thyroid abnormalities

retrospective cohort of transphenoidal surgery patients [993] but the need for rescue medication in the PACU for either nausea or emesis was significantly reduced. It is, however, important to preemptively treat post-operative nausea and vomiting in patients undergoing transphenoidal surgery. Even if a throat pack is used to prevent blood from draining into the stomach, post-operative oozing may continue and even a small amount of swallowed blood may cause nausea and vomiting. This may produce a vicious circle in which the straining from vomiting may lead to further venous oozing, which then exacerbates the problem. Aggressive prophylaxis against nausea and vomiting with drugs with different mechanisms of action may help to prevent this complication. Gentle orogastric suctioning immediately upon conclusion of the surgery also helps to minimize the amount of blood in the stomach, but nasogastric suction is contraindicated.

CONCLUSIONS

The patient with pituitary mass or functional adenoma resected via the endoscopic endonasal approach presents unique challenges for the anesthesiologist. A careful review of the particular medical effects of the tumor as well as the specific perioperative concerns of the surgical approach are essential in guiding perioperative care (Table 13.1).

REFERENCES

1. Comer BT, Young AB, Gal TJ. Impact of endoscopic techniques on efficiency in pituitary surgery. *Otolarygol Head Neck Surg.* 2011;145: 732–736.
2. de Divitiis E. Endoscopic transphenoidal surgery: stone-in-the-pond effect. *Neurosurgery.* 2006;59:512–520.
3. Higgins TS, Courtemanche C, Karakla D, et al. Analysis of transnasal endoscopic versus transseptal microscopic approach for excision of pituitary tumors. *Am J Rhinol.* 2008;22:649–652.
4. Schmitt H, Buchfelder M, Radespiel-Troger M, et al. Difficult intubation in acromegalic patients: Incidence and predictability. *Anesthesiology.* 2000;93:110–114.
5. Nemergut EC, Zuo Z. Airway management in patients with pituitary disease: a review of 746 patients. *J Neurosurg Anesthesiol.* 2006;18:73–77.
6. Kitahata LM. Airway difficulties associated with anesthesia in acromegaly: three case reports. *Br J Anaesth.* 1971;43:1187–1190.
7. Williams RG, Richards SH, Mills RG, et al. Voice changes in acromegaly. *Laryngoscope.* 1994;104:484–487.
8. Edge WG, Whitwam JG. Chondro-calcinosis and difficult intubation in acromegaly. *Anaesthesia.* 1981;36:677–680.
9. Fatti LM, Scacchi M, Pincelli Al, et al. Prevalence and pathogenesis of sleep apnea and lung disease in acromegaly. *Pituitary* 2001;4:259–262.
10. Piper JG, Dirks BA, Traynelis VC, et al. Perioperative management and surgical outcome of the acromegalic patient with sleep apnea. *Neurosurgery.* 1995;36:70–74.
11. Southwick JP, Katz, J. Unusual airway obstruction in the acromegalic patient-indications for tracheostomy. *Anesthesiology.* 1979;51:72–73.
12. Ovassapian A, Doka JC, Romsa DE. Acromegaly—use of fiberoptic laryngoscopy to avoid tracheostomy. *Anesthesiology.* 1981;54:429–430.
13. Hakala P, Randell T, Valli H. Laryngoscopy and fiberoptic intubation in acromegalic patients. *Br J Anaesth..* 1998;80:345–347.
14. Pellitari L, Polo O, Rauhala E, et al. Nocturnal breathing abnormalities in acromegaly after adenomectomy. *Clin Endocrinol* (Oxf). 1995;43:175–182.
15. Wilson CB. Role of surgery in the management of pituitary tumors. *Neurosurg Clin N Am..* 1990;1:139–159.
16. Rajasoorya C, Holdaway IM, Wrightson P, et al. Determinants of clinical outcome and survival in acromegaly. *Clin Endocrinol. (Oxf).* 1994;41:95–102.
17. Clayton RN. Cardiovascular function in acromegaly. *Endocrine Rev.* 2003;24:272–277.
18. Lie JT, Grossman SJ. Pathology of the heart in acromegaly: Anatomic findings in 27 autopsied patients. *Am. Heart J.* 1980;100:41–52.
19. Maison P, Demolis P, Young J, Schaison G, et al. Vascular reactivity in acromegalic patients: preliminary evidence for regional endothelial dysfunction and increased sympathetic vasoconstriction. *Clin Endocrinol (Oxf).* 2000;53:445–451.
20. Herman BL, Bruch C, Saller B et al. Acromegaly: evidence for a direct relation between disease activity and cardiac dysfunction in patients without ventricular hypertrophy. *Clin Endocrinol (Oxf).* 2002;56:595–602.
21. Rossi L, Thiene G, Caregaro L, et al. Dysrhthmias and sudden death in acromegalic heart disease: a clinicopathologic study. *Chest.* 1977;72:495–498.
22. Fazio S, Cittadini A, Sabtini D, et al. Evidence for biventricular involvement in acromegaly: a Doppler echocardiographic study. *Eur Heart J.* 1993;14:26–33.
23. Nemergut EC, Dumont AS, Barry UT, et al. Perioperative management of patients undergoing transsphenoidal pituitary surgery. *Anesth Analg..* 2005;101:1170–1181.
24. Schwarz ER, Jammula P, Gupta R, et al. A case and review of acromegaly-induced cardiomyopathy and the relationship between growth hormone and heart failure: cause or cure or neither or both? *J Cardiovasc PharmacolTher.* 2006;11:232–244.
25. Kahaly G, Olshausen KV, Mohr-Kahaly S, et al. Arrhythmia profile in acromegaly. *Eur Heart J.* 1992;13:51–56.
26. Colao A, Ferone D, Marzullo P, et al. Systemic complications of acromegaly: epidemiology, pathogenesis, and management. *Endocr Rev.* 2004;25:102–152.
27. Colao A, Baldelli R, Marzullo P, et al. Systemic hypertension and impaired glucose tolerance are independently correlated to the severity of the acromegalic cardiomyopathy. *J Clin Endocrinol Metab.* 2000;85:193–199.
28. McGuffin WL, Sherman BM, Roth J, et al. Acromegaly and cardiovascular disorders: a prospective study. *Ann Intern Med.* 1974;81:11–18.
29. Bondanelli M, Ambrosio MR, Degli Uberti EC. Pathogenesis and prevalence of hypertension in acromegaly. *Pituitary.* 2001;4:239–249.
30. Theussen L, Christensen SE, Weeke J, et al. A hyperkinetic heart in uncomplicated acromegaly: explanation of hypertension in acromegalic patients. *Acta Med Scand.* 1988;223:337–343.
31. Ho KY, Kelly JJ. Role of growth hormone in fluid homeostasis. *Horm Res.* 1991;36:44–48.
32. Moller J, Moller N, Frandsen E, et al. Blockade of the rennin-angiotensin-aldosterone system prevents growth hormone-induced fluid retention in humans. *Am J Physiol.* 1997;272: E803–E808.
33. Ikeda T, Terasawa H, Ishimura M, et al. Correlation between blood pressure and plasma insulin in acromegaly. *J Intern Med.* 1993;234:61–63.
34. Bondanelli M, Ambrosio MR, Franceschetti P, et al. Diurnal rhythm of plasma catecholamines in acromegaly. *J Clin Endocrinol Metab.* 1999;84:2458–2467.
35. Wickman A, Friberg P, Adams MA, et al. Induction of growth hormone receptor and insulin-like growth factor-I mRNA in aorta and caval vein during hemodynamic challenge. *Hypertension.* 1997;29:123–130.

36. Lopez-Velasco R, Escobar-Morreale HF, Vega B, et al. Cardiac involvement in acromegaly: specific myocardiopathy or consequence of systemic hypertension. *J Clin Endocrinol Metab.* 1997;82:1047–1053.

37. Shipley JE, Schteingart DE, Tandon R, et al. Sleep architecture and sleep apnea in patients with Cushing's disease. *Sleep.* 1992;15:514–518.

38. Ross EJ, Marshall-Jones P, Friedman M. Cushing's syndrome: diagnostic criteria. *Q J Med.* 1966;35:149–192.

39. Pirpiris M, Yeung S, Dewar E, et al. Hydrocortisone-induced hypertension in men: the role of cardiac output. *Am J Hypertens.* 1993;6:287–294.

40. Mantero F, Boscardo M. Glucocorticoid-dependent hypertension. *J Steroid Biochem Mol Biol.* 1992;43:409–413.

41. Sato A, Suzuki H, Murakam M, et al. Glucocorticoid increases angiotensin II type 1 receptor and its gene expression. *Hypertension.* 1994;23:25–30.

42. Sato A, Suzuki H, Iwaita Y, et al. Potentiation of inositol trisphosphate production by dexamethasone. *Hypertension.* 1992;19:109–115.

43. Sugihara N, Shimizu M, Shimizu K, et al. Disproportionate hypertrophy of the interventricular septum and its regression in Cushing's syndrome: report of three cases. *Intern Med.* 1992;31:407–413.

44. Muiesan ML, Lupia M, Salvetti M, et al. Left ventricular structural and functional characteristics in Cushing's disease. *J Am Coll Cardiol.* 2003;41:2275–2279.

45. Sugihara N, Shimizu M, Kita Y, et al. Cardiac characteristics and postoperative courses in Cushing's syndrome. *Am J Cardiol.* 1992;69:1475–1480.

46. Mindermann T, Wilson CB. Thyrotropin-producing pituitary adenomas. *J Neurosurg.* 1993;79:521–527.

47. Melmed S, Braunstein GD, Chang RJ, et al. Pituitary tumors secreting growth hormone and prolactin. *Ann Intern Med.* 1986;105:238–253.

48. Vance ML. Perioperative management of patients undergoing pituitary surgery. *Endocrinol Metab Clin North Am.* 2003;32:355–365.

49. Smith M, Hirsch NP. Pituitary disease and anaesthesia. *Br J Anaesth.* 2000;85:3–14.

50. Seidman PA, Kofke WA, Policare R, et al. Anaesthetic complications of acromegaly. *Br J Anaesth.* 2000;84:79–82.

51. Baird TA, Parsons MW, Phanh T, et al. Persistent poststroke hyperglycemia is independently associated with infarct expansion and worse clinical outcome. *Stroke.* 2003;34:2208–2214.

52. Lindsberg PJ, Roine RO. Hyperglycemia in acute stroke. *Stroke.* 2004;35:363–364.

53. Sieber FE. The neurologic implications of diabetic hyperglycemia during surgical procedures at increased risk for brain ischemia. *J Clin Anesth.* 1997;9:334–340.

54. Mathes AS, Kreuer S, Schneider SO, et al. The performance of six pulse oximeters in the environment of neuronavigation. *Anesth Analg.* 2008;107:541–544.

55. Campkin TV. Radial artery cannulation: potential hazard in patients with acromegaly. *Anaesthesia.* 1980;35:1008–1009.

56. Law-Koune JD, Liu N, Szekely B, et al. Using the intubating laryngeal mask airway for ventilation and endotracheal intubation in anesthetized and unparalyzed acromegalic patients. *J Neurosurg Anesthesiol.* 2004;16:11–13.

57. Gemma M, Tommasino C, Cozzi S, et al. Remifentanil provides hemodynamic stability and faster awakening time in transsphenoidal surgery. *Anesth Analg.* 2002;94:163–168.

58. Cafiero T, Cavallo LM, Frangiosa A, et al. Clinical comparison of remifentanil-sevoflurane-propofol for endoscopic endonasal transsphenoidal surgery. *Eur J Anaesthesiol.* 2007;24:441–446.

59. Hensen J, Henig A, Fahlbusch R, et al. Prevalence, predictors and patterns of postoperative polyuria and hyponatraemia in the immediate course after transsphenoidal surgery for pituitary adenomas. *Clin Endocrinol.* 1999;50:431–439.

60. Sigounas DG, Sharpless JL, Cheng DM, et al. Predictors and incidence of central diabetes insipidus after endoscopic pituitary surgery. *Neurosurgery.* 2008;62:71.

61. Jane JA, Thapar K, Maartens N, et al. Pituitary surgery: the transsphenoidal approach. *Neurosurgery.* 2002;51:435–444.

62. Abou-Madi MN, Trop D, Barnes J. Aetiology and control of cardiovascular reactions during transsphenoidal resection of pituitary microadenomas. *Can Anaesth Soc J.* 1980;27:491–495.

63. Katz RI, Hovagim AR, Finkelstein HS, et al. A comparison of cocaine, lidocaine with epinephrine, and oxymetazoline for prevention of epistaxis on nasotracheal intubation. *J. Clin. Anesth.* 1990;2:16–20.

64. Dunlevy TM, O'Malley TP, Postma GN. Optimal concentration of epinephrine for vasoconstriction in neck surgery. *Laryngoscope.* 1996;106:1412–1414.

65. Moore MA, Weiskopf RB, Eger EI, et al. Arrhythmogenic doses of epinephrine are similar during desflurane or isoflurane anesthesia in humans. *Anesthesiology.* 1993;79:943–947.

66. Drivas EI, Hajiioannou JK, Lachanas VA, et al. Cocaine versus tetracaine in septoplasty: a prospective, randomized, controlled trial. *J Laryngol Otol.* 2007;121:130–133.

67. Benjamin E, Wong DKK, Choa D. "Moffett's" solution: a review of the evidence and scientific basis for the topical preparation of the nose. *Clin Otolaryngol.* 2004;29:582–587.

68. Taylor S, Achola K, Smith G. Plasma catecholamine concentrations. The effects of infiltration with local analgesics and vasoconstrictors during nasal operations. *Anaesthesia.* 1984;39:520–523.

69. John G, Low JM, Tan PE, et al. Plasma catecholamine levels during functional endoscopic sinus surgery. *Clin Otolaryngol.* 1995;20:213–215.

70. Savino PJ, Burde RM, Mills RP. Visual loss following intranasal anesthetic injection. *J Clin Neuro-ophthalmol.* 1990;10:140–144.

71. Maaranen TH, Mantyjarvi MI. Central retinal artery occlusion after a local anesthetic with adrenaline on nasal mucosa. *J Neuro-ophthalmol.* 2000;20:234–235.

72. Keegan MT, Atkinson JLD, Kasperbauer JL, et al. Exaggerated hemodynamic responses to nasal injection and awakening from anesthesia in a cushingoid patient having transsphenoidal hypophysectomy. *J Neurosurg Anesthesiol.* 2000;12:225–229.

73. Chelliah YR, Manninen PH. Hazards of epinephrine in transsphenoidal pituitary surgery. *J Neurosurg Anesthesiol.* 2002;14:43–46.

74. Pasternak JJ, Atkinson JL, Kasperbauer JL, et al. Hemodynamic responses to epinephrine containing local anesthetic injection and to emergence from general anesthesia in trans-sphenoidal hypophysectomy patients. *J Neurosurg. Anesthesiol.* 2004;16:189–195.

75. Kara CO, Kaftan A, Atalay H, et al. Cardiovascular safety of cocaine anaesthesia in the presence of adrenaline during septal surgery. *J Otolaryngol.* 2001;30:145–148.

76. Makaryus JN, Makaryus AN, Johnson M. Acute myocardial infarction following the use of intranasal anesthetic cocaine. *Southern Med J.* 2006;99:759–761.

77. Ross GS, Bell J. Myocardial infarction associated with inappropriate use of topical cocaine as treatment for epistaxis. *Am J Emerg Med.* 1992;10:219–222.

78. Laffey JG, Neligan P, Ormonde G. Prolonged perioperative myocardial ischemia in a young male: due to topical intranasal cocaine. *J Clin Anesth.* 1999;11:419–424.

79. Audu PB, Curtis N, Armstead V. An unusual case of emergence delirium. *J Clin Anaesth.* 2004;16:545–547.

80. Hari CK, Roblin DG, Clayton MI, et al. Acute angle closure glaucoma precipitated by intranasal application of cocaine. *J Laryngol Otol.* 1999;113:250–251.

81. Schwalm J-D, Hamstra J, Mulji A, et al. Cardiogenic shock following nasal septoplasty: a case report and review of the literature. *Can J Anesth.* 2008;55:6.

82. Groudine SB, Hollinger I, Jones J, et al. New York State guidelines on the topical use of phenylephrine in the operating room. Medical Intelligence Article. *Anesthesiology.* 2000;92:859–864.

83. Yang JJ, Li WY, Jil Q, et al. Local anesthesia for functional endoscopic sinus surgery employing small volumes of epinephrine-containing solutions of lidocaine produces profound hypotension. *Acta Anestheiol Scand*. 2005;49:1471–1476.

84. Yang J, Zheng J, Liu H, et al. Epinephrine infiltration on nasal field causes significant hemodynamic changes: hypotension episode monitored by impedance-cardiography under general anesthesia. *J Pharm Pharmaceut Sci*. 2006;9:190–197.

85. Yang J, Cheng H, Shang R, et al. Hemodynamic changes due to infiltration of the scalp with epinephrine-containing lidocaine solution. *Neurosurg Anesthesiol*. 2007;19:31–37.

86. Li W, Zhou Z, Ji J, et al. Relatively light general anesthesia is more effective than fluid expansion in reducing the severity of epinephrine-induced hypotension during functional endoscopic sinus surgery. *Chin Med J*. 2007;120:1299–1302.

87. Pepper J-P, Wadhwa AK, et al. Cavernous carotid injury during functional endoscopic sinus surgery: case presentations and guidelines for optimal management. *Am J Rhinol*. 2007;109:105–109.

88. Weidenbecher M, Huk WJ, Iro H. Internal carotid artery injury during functional endoscopic sinus surgery and its management. *Eur Arch Otorhinolaryngol*. 2005;262:640–645.

89. Gadhinglajkar SV, Sreedhar R, Bhattacharya RN. Carotid artery injury during transsphenoidal resection of pituitary tumor: anesthesia perspective. *J Neurosurg Anesthesiol*. 2003;15:323–326.

90. Paul M, Dueck M, Kampe S, et al. Intracranial placement of a nasotracheal tube after transnasal trans-sphenoidal surgery. *Br J Anaesth*. 2003;91:601–604.

91. McAdam D, Muro K, Suresh S. The use of infraorbital nerve block for postoperative pain control after transsphenoidal hypophysectomy. *Reg Anesth. Pain Med*. 2005;30:572–573.

92. Higashizawa T, Koga Y. Effect of infraorbital nerve block under general anesthesia on consumption of isoflurane and post operative pain in endoscopic endonasal maxillary sinus surgery. *J Anesth*. 2001;15: 136–138.

93. Flynn BC, Nemergut EC. Postoperative nausea and vomiting and pain after transphenoidal surgery: a review of 877 patients. *Anesth Analg*. 2006;103:162–167.

14.

ANESTHESIA FOR SKULL BASE AND NEUROVASCULAR SURGERY

Jess Brallier

SKULL BASE TUMOR SURGERY

INTRODUCTION

Skull base tumor surgery has changed significantly to become less invasive, moving from predominantly open procedures to endoscopic techniques. Anesthetic techniques for these procedures have evolved to accommodate changes in surgical technique. In the past, the anesthesiologist was most concerned with complications such as intraoperative blood loss and venous air embolism. The focus has now shifted to providing an optimal, bloodless surgical field and using an anesthetic technique that permits the use of neurophysiologic monitoring. Older, medically complicated patients are now candidates for skull base surgery, and management of these patients has become an important consideration. Finally, patients are usually positioned with the head away from the anesthesiologist and his or her arms tucked at the side, complicating airway management and vascular access. While surgery for skull base tumors has become less invasive, it is clear that anesthetic management of these patients requires a profound understanding of the procedure to ensure a smooth perioperative course.

PREOPERATIVE MANAGEMENT

Preoperative anesthetic evaluation should occur before the day of surgery in patients scheduled for an elective procedure. This provides the opportunity for further work-up when necessary, minimizing the possibility of a delay on the day of surgery. An understanding of the surgical procedure and of the tumor type are the primary preoperative considerations in patients presenting for endoscopic skull base surgery. Each surgical procedure varies in terms of the neurovascular structures at risk, operative time, and potential for conversion to open surgery. The most common skull base tumors include chondrosarcoma, chordoma, craniopharyngioma, meningioma, various pituitary tumors, and

schwannoma. These are often histologically benign lesions but require surgical treatment because they can cause nerve and tissue compression.

A thorough but focused history and physical examination is a critical component of the preoperative assessment. Emphasis should be placed on evaluating the neurologic status, airway, cardiovascular system, pulmonary system, endocrine system, and fluid–electrolyte balance. A careful history includes questions regarding the type and location of the lesion, preoperative deficits, and symptoms of elevated intracranial pressure (ICP). The patient should be questioned specifically about headache (often worse in the morning), vomiting, drowsiness, seizures, focal deficits, balance, vision changes, hearing loss, speech difficulties, bulbar symptoms, facial pain and paralysis, and personality changes. If the preoperative assessment has been completed in advance, a careful review of the neurologic system should be performed on the day of surgery to screen for new symptoms and exacerbation of previous ones.

Airway

Careful attention to airway management is imperative when anesthetizing patients for skull base tumor resection. Patients with acromegaly caused by a pituitary tumor may be difficult to ventilate and to intubate because production of excess growth hormone causes soft tissue hypertrophy of the mouth, nose, tongue, turbinates, soft palate, and epiglottis and aryepiglottic folds. Bony proliferation also results in prognathism and malocclusion. Twenty-five percent of patients with a pituitary adenoma have a coexisting goiter, which may cause tracheal compression. These patients may also have sleep apnea, which further complicates airway management [1]. Patients should be asked about intubation history and, when available, prior anesthetic records reviewed. Compared with other individuals, patients with elevated ICP have a low tolerance for apnea (apnea leads to increases in $PaCO_2$ to increases in cerebral blood flow [CBF] to increases in ICP), highlighting the need for adequate ventilation and efficiency when securing the airway. A complete airway examination should include the thyromental distance, mouth opening, and the Mallampati score. The examination should also include head and neck movement and an evaluation of the patient's ability to prognath. If the history and physical examination suggest that airway management will be difficult, the anesthetic plan should include consideration of an awake intubation. Emergency and adjunctive airway equipment should also be readily available.

Cardiac

The cardiac evaluation is an essential part of any preoperative assessment and is particularly important in patients with certain types of skull base pathology. Patients with acromegaly, for example, often present with myocardial hypertrophy, decreased cardiac performance, and increased cardiovascular mortality. Cardiovascular complications cause a 5-fold increase in mortality in patients with Cushing's disease compared with the normal population [2, 3]. A preoperative cardiac evaluation is guided by the 2007 American College of Cardiology (ACC)/American Heart Association (AHA) algorithm for perioperative evaluation of the patient for noncardiac surgery and the patient's symptoms, exercise tolerance, medical history, and tumor type. Most patients presenting for endoscopic skull-based procedures present an intermediate risk. Acromegaly and Cushing's disease may increase the risk of structural and electrical cardiac pathophysiology leading to QT interval prolongation [4, 5]. Ordering preoperative electrocardiograms in these patients may therefore be appropriate and further evaluation may be warranted in patients with functional adenomas.

Respiratory

Preoperative respiratory considerations for the patient presenting for skull base tumor resection are essentially the same as those for individuals presenting for general surgery. However, special attention must be given to patients with Cushing's disease and acromegaly. Patients with Cushing's disease can present with moon facies and truncal obesity, potentially making airway management more difficult. These patients are also at a higher risk for aspiration. Acromegalic patients may also present with a number of respiratory challenges. These patients have a high incidence of obstructive sleep apnea, which can complicate airway management and respiratory status throughout the perioperative period [6].

Laboratory/Endocrine Evaluation

Patients presenting for skull base tumor resection may have metabolic abnormalities as a result of their intracranial pathology. Hyponatremia is frequently associated with tumors of the posterior pituitary. Hypercalcemia may indicate a diagnosis of multiple endocrine neoplasia, type I. Pituitary adenomas generally present with symptoms of anterior pituitary hormone excess. On the other hand, a subgroup of patients presenting for transsphenoidal surgery may have hypopituitarism and will receive hormone replacement therapy guided by laboratory studies. Some patients may have adrenal insufficiency and stress dose steroid administration should also be considered in the perioperative period [7]. Men with pituitary tumors and low testosterone levels are at risk for anemia [7].

Basic laboratory studies should include a complete blood count, electrolytes, and a metabolic profile. Coagulation studies are not usually necessary unless the patient has a known bleeding disorder. Additional studies are guided by the tumor type and location. In patients with a tumor of the anterior pituitary, laboratory tests should include a thyroid panel, serum levels of cortisol, adrenocorticotropic hormone, insulin-like growth factor 1, testosterone, luteinizing hormone, follicle-stimulating hormone, and prolactin [7].

INTRAOPERATIVE MANAGEMENT

Induction

Premedication should be avoided in patients presenting for skull base tumor surgery because administration of benzodiazepines or opioids may cause patients with elevated ICP to deteriorate rapidly. Administering an antisialogogue such as glycopyrrolate is also prudent when anticipating a difficult airway. Oversedation may cause hypoventilation and the resulting increase in $PaCO_2$ may increase CBF and exacerbate intracranial hypertension (HTN). If premedication is required (e.g., for a child or an extremely nervous patient) sedatives should be given by the anesthesiologist in a monitored setting.

American Society of Anesthesiologists (ASA) standard monitors (electrocardiogram, noninvasive blood pressure cuff, pulse oximetry, respiratory gas monitoring, and temperature) should be used in all patients. Invasive monitoring of systemic arterial pressure should be considered in patients with skull base tumors, especially if intracranial HTN, significant heart disease, or other underlying comorbidities are present. Although central venous pressure monitoring is not usually necessary for skull base surgery, it should be considered if large fluid shifts are suspected or large-bore peripheral intravenous catheters cannot be inserted. The patient is usually positioned with his or her head away from the anesthesiologist with the arms tucked at the side. This makes the airway, intravenous catheters, and intra-arterial catheter relatively inaccessible. During induction, however, the patient should be positioned toward the anesthesia machine and personnel and turned away after the airway is secured. Longer circuits, intravenous extensions, and sufficiently longer monitoring cables will also be required.

If a difficult airway is anticipated, then consideration should be given to an awake intubation, especially if problems with mask ventilation are anticipated. Thorough topicalization should be performed with local anesthesia via atomization and combination of transtracheal and superior laryngeal nerve blocks. Careful, sedation can also be administered using small amount of benzodiazepines such as midazolam or dexmedetomidine. Dexmedetomidine, an α_2-agonist, provides effective sedation without the hypoventilation that often accompanies other agents. However, hypotension and bradycardia are common side effects of this drug, making careful titration essential. If a difficult airway is anticipated (e.g., in an acromegalic patient), appropriately large oral airways, laryngeal mask airways (LMAs), and backup intubation devices (e.g., fiberoptic bronchoscope and/or video laryngoscopes) should be readily available [8]. Should subglottic stenosis be anticipated, a range of endotracheal tube sizes should be ready and available. If available, a second anesthesia provider can help with ventilation or intubation if the airway is lost during induction. If the patient is at risk for aspiration (e.g., a morbidly obese patient with Cushing's disease), a rapid sequence induction and extubation only when the patient is fully conscious may help to prevent aspiration.

The presence of cardiac disease, the projected length of surgery, the underlying pathology, and the presence or absence of intracranial HTN all guide the selection of an induction agent. Propofol, etomidate, and thiopental decrease ICP by decreasing CBF, which makes them appropriate choices for induction of general anesthesia. Propofol must be used discriminately in patients with cardiac disease due to the potential for precipitous decreases in blood pressure and myocardial depression. Similarly, it must be carefully titrated in patients with intracranial HTN as sustained drops in blood pressure can lead to dangerous decreases in CPP. Etomidate may be an appropriate alternative in many of these patients due to its ability to maintain hemodynamic stability. However, it can cause adrenal suppression which might prove to be problematic in patients undergoing pituitary surgery. Thiopental is no longer available in the United States and may be less appealing because of its longer half-life and its tendency to cause nausea and vomiting. Etomidate may maintain hemodynamic stability in patients with decreased left ventricular function. Ketamine should be avoided in patients with intracranial tumors because it increases ICP and $CMRo_2$.

The choice of a muscle relaxant at induction is guided by anticipated ability to manage the airway and whether the patient is considered to have a full stomach. Should a rapid sequence induction be necessary, succinylcholine may be the most appropriate drug. However, this drug should be administered with caution in patients who have known motor weakness or critical intracranial HTN due to its potential to precipitate a hyperkalemic arrest or further increase ICP, respectively. The perceived risk of aspiration

must be balanced against these risks. If neurophysiologic monitoring is planned (somatosensory evoked potentials [SSEPs] or motor evoked potentials [MEPs]), a compatible anesthetic will have to be administered. Inhalational agents cause a dose-dependent decrease and increase in evoked potential amplitude and latency, respectively. This necessitates either decreasing the concentration of inhalational agent used or avoiding it entirely. Alternatively, using a total intravenous anesthetic (TIVA) provides excellent anesthesia with negligible effect on neurophysiologic monitoring. Similarly, when MEPs or electromyography (EMG) (in this case facial nerve monitoring) is to be used, muscle relaxants must be avoided once surgery has started [9, 10]. However, using an intermediate-acting, nondepolarizing muscle relaxant such as rocuronium is usually appropriate for intubation and during line placement. In any case, the anesthesiologist should discuss the intended use of neuromuscular blocking agents with the surgeon and the monitoring staff.

Maintenance

The anesthetic plan should provide analgesia, amnesia, patient immobility, and hemodynamic stability while managing ICP and providing a "bloodless" surgical field. Potent volatile anesthetics, intravenous anesthetics such as propofol, and narcotic techniques have all been used successfully. Narcotics do not cause cerebral vasodilation and may therefore provide an optimal surgical field. Use of a narcotic with an ultra-short half-life, such as remifentanil, provides analgesia during the procedure and a rapid emergence after the surgery has ended. Regardless of the chosen technique, the agents used should promote rapid awakening on surgical conclusion to allow for prompt, neurologic assessment.

Blood loss during surgery for skull base tumors results from injury to various vascular structures near the operative site. Slow, intermittent venous bleeding is the most common cause of blood loss during these procedures. However, more serious bleeding has resulted from injury to the internal carotid artery (ICA) and smaller vessels at the anterior skull base. These complications have resulted in range from blindness, pituitary apoplexy, and stroke with permanent neurologic sequelae [11]. Intraoperative bleeding tends to be more significant in patients with large tumors extending into the suprasellar region. Endoscopic surgery is generally not associated with large amounts of blood loss or intraoperative fluid shifts. However, should it occur it can become substantial as the surgeon operates and attempts to get hemostatic control in a very small field. Adequate intravenous access in the form of two large-bore intravenous catheters should be obtained when risk of significant bleeding is present. Fluid maintenance with an iso-osmotic crystalloid is generally adequate for intraoperative fluid replacement and usually osmotic diuresis is not necessary. Iso-osmotic crystalloid solutions such as Plasma-Lyte or 0.9% normal saline are usually adequate for fluid replacement. Care must be taken not too administer large volumes of lactated Ringer's (LR) solution as it is not truly iso-osmolar with respect to the plasma. Consequently, the administration of large volumes of LR can result in decreased plasma osmolality and increased brain water content and ICP [12]. Hypo-osmolar fluids and dextrose containing solutions should also be avoided for similar reasons [12].

Diabetes insipidus (DI) is not uncommon in patients undergoing skull base surgery. Factors found to increase the risk of postoperative DI include young age, male sex, large intrasellar mass, cerebrospinal fluid (CSF) leak, and resection of certain types of lesions (craniopharyngioma, Rathke-cleft cysts, and adrenocorticotropic hormone–secreting pituitary adenomas. The onset of DI is usually heralded by large volumes of dilute urine in the absence of mannitol administration or other inciting factors. A urine electrolyte panel will demonstrate hyponatremia and low specific gravity, while plasma sodium and specific gravity are elevated. Should DI be detected intraoperatively, an intravenous infusion of aqueous ADH should be administered along with an isotonic crystalloid solution [13, 14]. Serum sodium and plasma osmolality are measured at frequent, regular intervals and therapy altered as needed. Postoperatively, DI is treated with subcutaneous injections of aqueous vasopressin. One dose is often all that is required, but additional injections can be administered as needed. Additionally, patients with an intact thirst mechanism should be allowed access to free water and intravenous fluids restricted [15].

Postoperative pain is generally limited in these patients so large doses of long-acting opioids are usually not necessary. A few studies have illustrated the benefits of specific nerve blocks during sinus surgery by reducing the amount of anesthetic and antihypertensives needed during surgery [16]. Bilateral sphenopalatine ganglion blocks were shown in one study to decrease immediate postoperative opioid requirements and PACU stay [17]. Such blocks are safe, effective, and easily administered at the start of the anesthetic. Additionally, the utilization of nonopioid analgesics such as intravenous acetaminophen are also valuable postoperative adjuncts.

Emergence

The anesthetic plan in most patients should permit the patient to awaken rapidly and be able to cooperate with a neurologic examination as soon as possible after surgery. Barring any untoward intraoperative events, immediate extubation is usually appropriate in patients who do not have extensive preoperative deficits. The choice of sedatives and narcotics with relatively short half-lives is an important part in accomplishing this goal. Straining and coughing during emergence may lead to venous bleeding or a cerebrospinal fluid leak. The use of narcotics (either careful boluses of fentanyl or a longer-acting narcotic or a low-dose remifentanil infusion) will help the patient to be comfortable and alert. Nausea and vomiting are very common in this patient population and its detrimental effects on ICP are well documented [7]. Aggressive pharmacologic prophylaxis and treatment with 5-HT$_3$ antagonists (e.g., ondansetron) should therefore be used. Additional antiemetics may be administered as necessary, but droperidol should be avoided because of its sedative effects and the possibility of QT prolongation. Due to patient positioning, the patient's airway may not be immediately available to the anesthesia care provider until all surgical drapes and barriers have been removed. Coordinating emergence and extubation with the surgical team are important determinants of successful emergence. Ensuring that the patient is fully conscious and following commands prior to extubation is generally preferred. However, deep extubation may be appropriate in carefully selected candidates. If a previously neurologically intact patient fails to awaken and residual anesthetic agents have been excluded as a cause, immediate diagnostic imaging should be obtained to exclude the possibility of an intracranial hematoma.

POSTOPERATIVE MANAGEMENT

The level of care required in the postoperative period depends on the type of surgery performed, the potential for postoperative complications, and the patient's medical comorbidities. Most patients are transferred to the neurosurgical intensive care unit for postoperative management, but those having less extensive surgery may be admitted to the PACU and subsequently transferred to a medical-surgical floor. Patients with a history of obstructive sleep apnea or other cardiopulmonary comorbidities, for example, should be transferred to a monitored bed in the immediate postoperative period.

Postoperative complications may occur soon after surgery or may be delayed. Early complications include CSF leak, bleeding, DI, and visual loss. Late complications include hormone deficits (particularly with transphenoidal pituitary surgery), prolonged problems with electrolyte and water balance, and meningitis [7, 18, 19]. Headache is common after skull base surgery, and acute postoperative pain is usually treated with opioids and Nonsteroidal anti-inflammatory drugs (NSAIDs). However, if postoperative bleeding is a concern, avoiding NSAIDs and relying on short-acting opioids or intravenous acetaminophen may be prudent.

CONCLUSIONS: SKULL BASE
TUMOR SURGERY

Skull base tumor surgery has undergone significant evolution over the past 30 years. The advent of minimally invasive surgical technique has decreased the incidence of complications such as massive hemorrhage and venous air embolism. The challenges presented by this surgery include providing a relatively "bloodless" surgical field and managing complicated patients with multiple medical comorbidities. Each stage of the perioperative period requires the anesthesiologist to make careful decisions to provide optimal management of these patients.

ANESTHESIA FOR NEUROVASCULAR PROCEDURES

INTRACRANIAL ANEURYSMS

Introduction

Despite improvements in the treatment of intracranial aneurysms, the morbidity and mortality associated with aneurysmal rupture remain high. The incidence of intracranial aneurysms (IAs) varies between countries but has been reported to be present on autopsy in 0.2% to 9.9% of the general population. Subarachnoid hemorrhage (SAH) due to rupture of an aneurysm affects 30,000 Americans per year and is responsible for approximately 5% of all strokes [13, 14]. Furthermore, an estimated 6700 in-hospital deaths occur each year as a result of aneurysmal SAH in the United States, and this is associated with a 30-day mortality rate of 45% [14]. A large proportion of patients with a ruptured aneurysm suffer from additional morbidity in the form of rebleeding or vasospasm. Although the clinical prognosis remains disappointing after a ruptured aneurysm, careful anesthetic management during surgical clipping or endovascular coiling is paramount to good outcomes.

Preoperative Management

Treatment of intracranial aneurysms in the twenty-first century consists of either surgical clipping or endovascular coiling. The anesthetic considerations for patients undergoing clipping or coiling are often the same and are partially based on the preoperative condition of the patient.

Assessing the severity of the patient's SAH (if any) is an important part of the preoperative evaluation of these patients. Although many methods of objectively grading the clinical findings associated with aneurysmal bleeding have been proposed, the most commonly used scoring systems are the modified Hunt and Hess grading scale and the Glasgow Coma Scale (Tables 14.1 and 14.2). The Hunt and Hess score correlates not only with surgical risk and prognosis but also with the degree of associated cerebral pathophysiology and likelihood of vasospasm [15]. Patients with lower Hunt and Hess scores are likely to have relatively normal ICP and intact CBF autoregulation, while those with a higher score will probably have more aberrant pathophysiology, including intracranial HTN, impaired autoregulation, and cerebral edema. Other classifications, such as the Fisher grading scale, are used to predict the risk and severity of cerebral vasospasm after SAH [16] (Table 14.3).

Table 14.1 **THE HUNT AND HESS CLINICAL GRADES FOR SAH**

GRADE	CRITERIA
0	Unruptured aneurysm
1	Asymptomatic or minimal headache and nuchal rigidity
2	Moderate to severe headache, nuchal rigidity; no neurologic deficit other than cranial nerve palsy
3	Drowsiness, confusion, or mild focal deficit
4	Stupor, hemiparesis, possible early decerebrate rigidity, vegetative disturbance
5	Coma, decerebrate rigidity, moribund

Table 14.2 **THE GLASGOW COMA SCALE**

FEATURE	SCORE
Eye opening	
Spontaneous	4
To speech	3
To pain	2
None	1
Verbal response	
Oriented	5
Confused conversation	4
Inappropriate words	3
Incomprehensible sounds	2
None	1
Best motor response	
Obeys commands	6
Localizes to pain	5
Flexion or withdrawal	4
Abnormal flexion (decorticate)	3
Abnormal extension (decerebrate)	2
No response (flaccid)	1

It is also important to assess the patient's neurologic status with particular attention to the presence of preoperative focal deficits. Patients with lower Hunt and Hess clinical grades are less likely to present with cerebral pathophysiology (e.g., intracranial HTN, impairment of cerebral autoregulation) than are patients with higher-grade pathology

Table 14.3 **FISHER GRADES IN SAH**

GRADE	CT FINDING(S)
1	No blood detected
2	Diffuse thin layer of subarachnoid blood (vertical layers <1 mm thick)
3	Localized clot or thick layer of subarachnoid blood (vertical layers ≥1 mm thick)
4	Intracerebral or intraventricular blood with diffuse or no subarachnoid blood

[17–19]. The presence of vasospasm has important prognostic implications and will influence intraoperative hemodynamic management as well.

Evaluation of the airway should include a history of prior intubations and a review of previous anesthetic records when available. If the patient is unable to provide the history, it may be possible to obtain this information from family or friends. A thorough airway examination will guide the choice of a specific airway management technique. This information is particularly important in this patient population because an unexpected difficult airway and its associated hemodynamic effects may potentially lead to rupture in patients with untreated aneurysms. Moreover, the patient with compromised CBF may be especially sensitive to hypoxia. If a difficult airway is anticipated, adjunct airway equipment and additional anesthesia personnel should be available during induction of anesthesia. If an awake intubation is indicated, topical anesthesia should be used and superior laryngeal nerve blocks considered. A transtracheal block is probably best avoided in this clinical situation due to its potential to cause coughing resulting in elevated blood pressure and ICP.

If time permits, the patient's cardiovascular status should be optimized before surgery. Electrocardiographic abnormalities, elevation of cardiac biomarkers (i.e., troponins), and wall motion abnormalities are common in patients who have had an SAH [20, 21]. The majority of patients with these findings have normal coronary artery anatomy; the cardiac dysfunction seen after SAH is neurogenic in origin. Although the exact mechanism of these changes is unknown, it is generally accepted that sympathetic stimulation induces catecholamine release in the myocardium, which leads to impaired systolic and diastolic function, repolarization abnormalities, and myocardial damage [22]. In most cases, surgical intervention need not be delayed for further cardiac workup in patients without a known cardiac history, but patients who have an established cardiac history and in whom concomitant ischemic heart disease is suspected, briefly postponing the surgery or intervention may be necessary to obtain additional information or suggestions from a cardiologist about optimizing the patient's cardiac status. Use of invasive monitoring such as transesophageal echocardiography may help to optimize intraoperative management in patients with tenuous cardiovascular status.

Patients may also present with compromised pulmonary function. Neurogenic pulmonary edema (NPE) is common in patients after SAH, and pneumonia has also been described. NPE is associated with poor-grade SAH and is thought to be due to massive catecholamine release (mainly norepinephrine) after aneurysmal rupture. These catecholamines consequently cause endothelial damage, vasoconstriction, and vascular permeability [23]. In cases of severe pulmonary edema in which oxygen exchange is compromised, treatment with diuretics may be considered.

Patients with aneurysmal SAH often have electrolyte and volume disturbances, which may contribute to a poor outcome [24]. The most common electrolyte disturbance is hyponatremia and is usually due to the syndrome of inappropriate antidiuretic hormone secretion (SIADH) and cerebral salt wasting (CSW). In SIADH, an excessive amount of ADH is released in the absence of increased serum osmolality or arterial blood volume depletion. The increase in ADH levels results in diminished water excretion with normal sodium excretion. These patients are therefore normovolemic or hypervolemic. In contrast, patients with CSW are hyponatremic due to active urinary sodium excretion, not water retention. They are therefore hypovolemic. Normally, the treatment for SIADH is fluid restriction, and for CSW, salt and fluid replacement. However, fluid restriction in the context of SAH is potentially dangerous as it increases the risk of delayed cerebral ischemia and thus poor outcome [24]. Maintaining volume status and correcting electrolyte abnormalities are important parts of preoperative optimization.

Timing of Intervention

The timing of cerebral aneurysm surgery has been the subject of extensive debate. Definitive surgical treatment was historically delayed to allow cerebral edema to resolve, subarachnoid blood to be resorbed, and aneurysmal clot to stabilize. There is a growing trend toward early intervention (generally within 72 hours of SAH) with prevention of rebleeding and facilitation of vasospasm treatment as the primary reasons. In 1990, the International Cooperative Study on the Timing of Aneurysm Surgery study evaluated the surgical and medical management of 3251 patients suffering from SAH. Overall, mortality and neurologic outcome were similar in patients who underwent early surgery (0 to 3 days after bleed) or late surgery (11 to 14 days after bleed). The highest morbidity and mortality rates were found among patients who underwent operations 7 to 10 days after SAH [25], likely due to the fact that the incidence of cerebral vasospasm also peaks during this time interval. Furthermore, a subgroup analysis of patients admitted to the North American centers involved in the trial showed that results were best in this population when surgery was performed between 0 and 3 days. These findings argue strongly for early diagnosis and referral for surgical intervention in this patient population [26]. Others have argued that early surgery decreases the risk of rebleeding and facilitates optimal treatment of vasospasm by permitting a higher degree of blood pressure augmentation [27–29].

Intraoperative Management

Premedication

Premedication may be used with caution in select patients to mitigate preoperative anxiety in patients presenting for cerebral aneurysm surgery. If anxiolysis or sedation is necessary before bringing the patient to the operating room, small doses of short-acting benzodiazepines or opioids may be carefully titrated in a monitored setting. Administering a sedative to a patient may exacerbate intracranial HTN if the patient is allowed to hypoventilate, which increases $PaCO_2$. Sedation should also be administered only after consulting with the neurosurgical team, as the patient may no longer be able to comply with a neurologic examination.

Anesthesia Induction and Endotracheal Intubation

The induction of anesthesia and management of the airway are critical events in the patient with an untreated cerebral aneurysm. The objectives are to attain loss of consciousness and prevent further aneurysmal bleeding while preserving adequate cerebral perfusion. Very tight control of systemic blood pressure is therefore critical during this stage of the procedure and should be guided with continuous invasive monitoring. While the incidence of rupture during induction is rare, it is a devastating complication and is usually avoidable with careful hemodynamic management. In patients with allow grade aneurysm (Hunt-Hess scores of 0 to 2), ICP is usually normal and cerebral autoregulation is generally preserved. Lowering the MAP during induction and intubation decreases the transmural pressure (TMP) across the wall of the aneurysm, lowering the risk of subsequent bleeding. A moderate decrease in CPP does not usually produce acute cerebral ischemia in this group of patients. TMP is defined as:

$$TMP = MAP - ICP$$

Assuming ICP remains relatively constant, pressure across the aneurysmal wall decreases with the MAP. Thus, lowering the MAP slightly below the patient's baseline and avoiding acute increases in MAP help to prevent aneurysmal rupture. This is the same equation used to represent cerebral perfusion pressure (CPP):

$$CPP = MAP - ICP$$

Patients who have a higher-grade lesion (i.e., Hunt-Hess 4 or 5) are more likely to have aberrant cerebral pathophysiology and require a different strategy for managing the hemodynamic response to induction of anesthesia and airway management. These patients may have intracranial HTN and decreased CPP. A large decrease in MAP may therefore compromise cerebral perfusion. Although decreasing MAP decreases TMP, it also decreases CPP, placing these patients at risk for further ischemic insult. MAP should therefore be maintained at or close to the patient's preoperative baseline. Monitoring ConsiderationsIn addition to monitors recommended by the ASA basic monitoring standards, additional modalities should include an intra-arterial catheter to monitor blood pressure on a beat-to-beat basis. This should be inserted before induction so that untoward fluctuations in blood pressure can be rapidly treated. Although central

venous access is usually not indicated as an independent invasive monitor, it may be considered in patients with poor intravenous access or if prolonged vasopressor use is anticipated. Otherwise, two large-bore intravenous catheters should be inserted for fluid resuscitation in the event of excessive surgical bleeding or an intraoperative aneurysm rupture. A urinary catheter should be inserted after induction to measure urine output. Core temperature can be monitored with either the urinary catheter or an esophageal temperature probe.

Evoked potential monitoring is being used more and more frequently during cerebral aneurysm clipping as a means of measuring perfusion, particularly when temporary clipping is to be used. Although such monitoring is potentially valuable, the anesthetic plan must be modified to allow the neurophysiologists to record the signals. Potent volatile anesthetic agents decrease the amplitude and increase the latency of evoked potential signals (MEPs are more affected than are SSEPs) when their concentration exceeds 0.5 MAC. Total intravenous anesthesia (TIVA) or partial TIVA (augmented with less than 0.5 MAC of a potent volatile anesthetic agent) can be used to provide an appropriate level of anesthesia while preserving the evoked potential signals. If monitoring with MEPs is planned, neuromuscular blocking agents should be avoided.

Anesthesia Maintenance

As with induction, the anesthesiologist should focus on maintaining hemodynamic stability, an optimal surgical field, and normal cerebral physiology while ensuring a timely emergence at the conclusion of the procedure.

A variety of anesthetic techniques can be used to meet these stated objectives and the choice of a specific drug matters less than how that drug is used. A variety of drugs, including thiopental, propofol, and etomidate, can be used to induce a state of unconsciousness while simultaneously decreasing CBF and cerebral metabolic rate ($CMRO_2$). Ketamine should be avoided because it tends to increase ICP and $CMRO_2$. Induction with a potent volatile anesthetic will produce a dose-dependent increase in CBF and should be avoided. A variety of agents can also be used to blunt the sympathetic response of laryngoscopy and prevent unacceptable elevations in blood pressure. At the top of the list are potent, short-acting opioid agents such as fentanyl and remifentanil, which can be easily titrated to effect. One should also ensure the ready availability of vasopressors (phenylephrine-ephedrine) and short-acting antihypertensives (esmolol-nitroglycerin) in the case of undesirable decreases or increases in MAP.

Many patients presenting for cerebral aneurysm surgery are hypovolemic, particularly after an SAH. Restoration of adequate intravascular volume is critical to maintaining hemodynamic stability in these patients. Fluid administration prior to application of the vascular clip is guided by intraoperative blood loss and urine output while taking into consideration the need for a relaxed brain. Overzealous fluid administration may cause brain swelling and make operating conditions more difficult. Patients with a high-grade aneurysm may require administration of vasopressors to maintain an adequate CPP.

The end result of interventions that reduce intracranial volume and improve surgical conditions is to decrease the volume of one of the components of the cranium: cerebral tissue, blood, or CSF. A variety of strategies can be used during the procedure to improve cerebral perfusion while providing an optimal surgical field. Patient positioning is a quick, safe, and effective means of lowering ICP. Even 10 degrees of head elevation has been shown to dramatically decrease ICP while maintaining CPP [30].

Mannitol, an osmotic diuretic, is commonly used to decrease brain tissue volume.. When 0.5 to 1 g/kg is given over 30 minutes, mannitol creates an osmotic gradient that shifts intracellular water to the intravascular space. After a brief initial rise in CBF, cerebral blood volume (CBV), and ICP, mannitol decreases CBV and ICP. Complications of mannitol administration include electrolyte abnormalities, including hyponatremia, hypochloremia, and hyperkalemia and transient volume overload and pulmonary edema in patients with compromised cardiac function. Recently, 3% hypertonic saline (HTS) has gained favor as a means of relaxing the brain. One randomized controlled study showed that HTS provided better brain relaxation than did mannitol in patients undergoing elective supratentorial craniotomy [31]. A meta-analysis of the randomized trials comparing HTS to mannitol for treating elevated ICP also found HTS to be more effective in this regard [32]. It is customary at our institution to use mannitol as first-line therapy for brain relaxation.

Hyperventilation to induce moderate hypocapnea (Paco$_2$ between 25 and 35 mm Hg) has long been used to decrease ICP during neurosurgical procedures. Hypocapnea decreases CBV by causing cerebral vasoconstriction in areas of the brain with preserved autoregulation. Although the safety and effectiveness of this technique are controversial, a recent randomized controlled trial of hypocapnea during supratentorial brain tumor resection showed that surgical conditions are improved when moderate hypocapnea is used. ICP was measured in both groups, and the surgeon was asked to evaluate brain bulk using a 4-point scale. Intraoperative hyperventilation in this setting improved surgeon-assessed brain bulk and was associated with a decrease in ICP [33].

Drainage of cerebrospinal fluid (CSF) through a ventriculostomy catheter or during the surgical procedure is a safe and effective in lowering ICP and promoting a relaxed brain, even when other maneuvers have failed [34]. CSF drainage should not exceed 5 mL/min because rapid withdrawal may cause bradycardia or precipitate herniation.

A variety of factors play a role in the choice of anesthetic agents for neurovascular procedures. The ideal anesthetic technique provides a hemodynamically stable patient who awakens rapidly at the end of the procedure to facilitate early postoperative neurologic assessment. Excluding unexpected intraoperative events, most patients with grade 0 to 3 aneurysms are allowed to emerge from anesthesia and will be ready for extubation at the conclusion of surgery. Even if extubation of the trachea is not planned, the anesthetic technique should permit a brief neurologic examination prior to leaving the operating room. The primary anesthetic agent should preserve coupling between CBF and CMRO$_2$, maintain cerebrovascular autoregulation, and minimize increases in CBF and CMRO$_2$. The choice of TIVA over potent volatile anesthetics [35–37] is controversial, and careful titration of the anesthetic is probably more important than the choice of a specific agent. Controversy has long surrounded the use of nitrous oxide in the neurosurgical population. Opponents of its use suggest that it has unfavorable effects on cerebral hemodynamics and that it can exacerbate ischemic neurologic injury. However, recent data obtained from patients undergoing cerebral aneurysm surgery demonstrate that no long-term, adverse effects on gross neurologic or cognitive function existed after the use of nitrous oxide. Thus, its global avoidance in the neurosurgical population seems unwarranted in most circumstances [38].

Opioids, which have been used for decades, decrease CMRO$_2$ and ICP while producing only negligible changes in CBF [35]. A short-acting narcotic such as remifentanil will facilitate rapid emergence at the end of surgery. High doses of morphine should be avoided during the procedure because it is more sedating and has a longer half-life, but morphine may be administered in small incremental doses at the end of the procedure to manage postoperative pain.

Controlled hypotension and temporary artery occlusion are commonly used to decrease the risk of rupture while the aneurysm is being manipulated. The stress on the aneurysmal wall (TMP) is directly proportional to blood pressure, and controlled hypotension may decrease the chance of rupture during microdissection and clip application. Controlled hypotension also helps to control hemorrhage and decrease blood loss if the aneurysm ruptures during surgery. It also improves visualization during surgical dissection should routine bleeding or even aneurysmal rupture occur. Prolonged systemic hypotension may, however, cause end-organ (e.g., kidney) damage or global cerebral ischemia and the lowest safe pressure is unclear in patients with medical comorbidities. The lower limit of cerebral autoregulation has been defined as an MAP of 50 mm Hg in healthy individuals but is probably higher in patients with conditions such as chronic HTN. In patients with HTN, therefore, the lower limit of cerebral autoregulation may be closer to 65 or 70 mm Hg; an MAP in the low 50s may produce cerebral ischemia. Moreover, autoregulation is impaired in patients who have had SAH, placing them at risk for cerebral vasospasm and a poor neurologic outcome.

The artery feeding the aneurysm can be temporarily occluded to reduce the risk of aneurysm rupture. This technique has been used extensively as an alternative to controlled hypotension. Although the risks of global cerebral ischemia and end-organ damage are potentially avoided, temporary artery occlusion carries the risk of focal ischemia/infarction in the area supplied by the occluded vessel. To optimize cerebral perfusion and minimize the risk of regional ischemia, the blood pressure is often increased to a level above baseline during temporary clipping to ensure adequate collateral flow. The risk of focal ischemia increases with longer temporary occlusion times. EEG and evoked potential monitoring has been used as a means to monitor and detect changes consistent with cerebral ischemia during surgical clipping and is useful particularly when operating on giant aneurysms. Although deliberate hypothermia and reduction of cerebral metabolic rate with anesthetic agents such as propofol and thiopental have been used frequently during long periods of ischemia, little evidence exists to support their use [39].

Despite all precautions, the risk of aneurysmal rupture still exists. Should aneurysmal rupture occur, the primary objective is to quickly get control of the bleeding. If rupture occurs after craniotomy and during clip placement, the blood pressure should be temporarily decreased to provide a visually optimal surgical field. Ipsilateral carotid compression may also be helpful for controlling bleeding proximal to the aneurysm. Resuscitation with fluids and blood products during this time will require large-bore intravenous access. Isotonic crystalloid solutions such as Plasmalyte or normal saline are reasonable choices, as are some colloids. Avoidance of hetastarch, however, is advisable due to its tendency to promote coagulopathy.

EMERGENCE   As with skull base tumor surgery, emergence from cerebral aneurysm surgery requires careful planning. Facilitating rapid emergence, preventing HTN, and minimizing coughing on the endotracheal tube are important. The use of short-acting anesthetics facilitates rapid emergence and allows timely neurologic assessment. The decision to extubate the patient should be based on the patient's preoperative neurologic status, extent of surgery, and intraoperative course. Failure to emerge following discontinuation of anesthesia in a previously neurologically intact patient should prompt immediate diagnostic imaging.

Postoperative Period

Proper care for the patient undergoing cerebral aneurysm surgery extends beyond the operating room and into the postoperative period. All patients undergoing a neurovascular procedure should be admitted to the neurosurgical intensive care unit (or similar monitored setting) for management by a critical care team. Regardless of the postoperative are clinical status, such patients will have neurologic, respiratory, and fluid and electrolyte needs best managed by a specialist in a controlled, monitored setting.

PAIN MANAGEMENT   Pain after craniotomy remains a clinical dilemma for both patients and physicians and remains poorly managed and undertreated. Often, clinicians erroneously believe that craniotomies cause little pain and that liberal use of opioid medications will preclude neurologic evaluation and cause neurologic deterioration [40, 41]. Postcraniotomy pain has been shown to worsen perioperative morbidity and mortality because it activates the sympathetic nervous system. Such sympathetic stimulation increases the risk of cardiac complications and secondary intracranial hemorrhage (ICH) [42]. Current recommendations for analgesia after craniotomy include a comprehensive strategy that includes a combination of opioids, acetaminophen, anticonvulsants, and possibly NSAIDs [40]. Although scalp infiltration with local anesthesia has not been shown to consistently reduce acute postoperative pain, one group recently showed its value in decreasing the incidence of chronic pain [43].

CEREBRAL ARTERIOVENOUS MALFORMATIONS

Introduction

Arteriovenous malformations (AVMs) are the most common intracranial vascular malformation with an approximate incidence of one per 5000 people [44]. Clinical symptoms generally appear in the second decade of life with half of all patients suffering a spontaneous ICH, which may be associated with significant morbidity. Surgical resection of these lesions can be quite challenging, making a thorough understanding of their anatomy and pathophysiology and potential problems associated with the surgical procedure paramount to a successful outcome.

Pathophysiology

An AVM is a mass of blood vessels that shunts blood directly from the high-pressure arterial circulation to the low-pressure venous circulation without passing through a defined capillary bed. An AVM typically consists of a vascular core (the *nidus*) that consists of a complex network of abnormal, dilated vessels. The resultant hemodynamic pathophysiology includes venous HTN and high-velocity blood flow through the feeding arteries, the nidus, and the draining veins. The resultant changes in cerebral circulation have two primary characteristics: A rapid shunt flow increases the total amount of blood passing through the AVM and causes cerebral arterial hypotension along the shunt pathway. There is a progressive decrease in arterial pressure proceeding from the cerebral arterial circle (of Willis) to the nidus of the AVM [45]. The circulatory beds in parallel with the shunt system are therefore perfused at lower-than-normal pressures despite relatively normal flow [46]. Even though there is significant cerebral arterial hypotension, most patients do not experience ischemic symptoms, which implies the presence of some adaptive change in total cerebrovascular resistance [46]. One explanation may be a phenomenon known as *adaptive autoregulatory displacement*, which occurs in vascular areas adjacent to the AVM [47]. In these areas, the lower limit of the autoregulatory curve appears to be shifted to the left, which is the opposite the response to chronic, systemic HTN (characterized by a rightward shift). The chronic hypotension caused by the AVM does not usually result in ischemia because of this adaptive leftward shift, which places the lower limit of autoregulation below that of the normal brain [48, 49]. The vascular response to $Paco_2$ is preserved before and after resection of an AVM, providing further evidence of a physiologically intact autoregulatory capacity.

Cerebral steal has long been proposed as an explanation for preoperative focal neurologic deficits in patients who have a cerebral AVM. It has been suggested that the arterioles in tissue adjacent to the AVM are maximally dilated. This may result in cerebral steal in the setting of decreased perfusion pressure. Arterial hypotension in the distribution of normal brain tissue is relatively common in patients with AVMs, however, and focal neurologic deficits are rare. An alternative explanation is that the local mass effect produced by the abnormal vessels of the AVMs is probably responsible for preoperative focal findings unrelated to ICH.

Just as cerebral steal has been blamed for preoperative focal deficits, normal perfusion pressure breakthrough (NPPB) has been postulated to cause intraoperative appearance bleeding and edema and postoperative hemorrhage and swelling [46]. Hyperemic complications occur in only 5% of patients and the criteria used to study them vary considerably among investigators [45]. NPPB is attributed to cerebral hyperemia caused by the sudden exposure of previously hypotensive regions to normal blood pressure. This theory assumes that chronic dilation of vessels in hypotensive/ischemic territory leads to a loss of autoregulation [49]. Several observations contradict this theory, however. First, cerebral hyperemia that develops after resection of an AVM is global and is not limited to the side of the AVM. Second, there is no relationship between changes in cerebral blood flow after resection and the degree of arterial hypotension induced by AVM shunts. Third, autoreulatory response is not impaired in hypotensive regions but is intact and shifted to the left. Finally, cerebrovascular reactivity to $Paco_2$ is preserved after AVM resection, suggesting that the vessels in previously hypotensive territories are not plegic [45, 50-52]. Therefore, much of the concern related to bleeding and edema caused by NPPB seems theoretical and less clinically relevant.

Clinical Presentation

Patients with a cerebral AVM may present with or without bleeding. More than half of all patients develop spontaneous ICH, which is associated with the greatest morbidity. Hemorrhagic presentation is thought to be more likely for several reasons. Increasing age, deep AVM location and exclusive deep venous drainage have been found to be independent predictors that are associated with hemorrhagic manifestations [53]. Other studies have found that additional risk factors include deep and infratentorial location, small AVM diameter, the presence of a single arterial feeder, exclusive venous drainage, combined deep and superficial venous drainage, and coexisting arterial aneurysms [54]. Although the majority of patients are diagnosed with AVM after an ICH, 20% present with seizures and another 15% are asymptomatic at the time of presentation [46]. The varied clinical presentations of cerebral AVMs reflect the heterogeneity of these lesions and their outcomes.

Treatment

Cerebral AVMs are treated with either microsurgical resection or radiosurgery. The objective of each treatment is complete obliteration of the lesion to prevent bleeding or other neurologic complications such as seizures or focal neurologic deficits. Although surgery is probably the most definitive option, it is invasive and requires general anesthesia and admission to the intensive care unit. Stereotactic radiosurgery is usually reserved for patients with deep, small AVMs who are unable to tolerate general anesthesia [55]. Many patients with an AVM undergo endovascular embolization prior to surgical resection, although this is less important in patients who are scheduled for radiosurgery. Embolization decreases blood flow through the AVM, which decreases the possibility of intraoperative hemorrhage and postoperative hyperperfusion bleeding. Preoperative embolization is particularly beneficial in the 10% of patients who have arterial aneurysms in addition to the AVM. The AVM is generally embolized with polyvinyl alcohol particles, microcoils, cyanoacrylate monomers, or ethylene vinyl alcohol [55].

Preoperative Management

Treatment of a cerebral AVM is rarely an emergency. Unless a massive hemorrhage requires urgent management, there is usually an opportunity to ensure that the patient's medical management is optimal. A thorough preoperative evaluation should include a history and physical examination, a review of the imaging, and a discussion with the operative team. The goal of the preoperative assessment is to rule out the presence of other comorbidities, such as cardiac or vascular disease, that may require further workup. Laboratory studies should a chemistry panel, complete blood count, and a coagulation panel. Because there is a risk of hemorrhage during AVM resection, the patients should be typed and cross-matched for blood products.

Intraoperative Management

Monitoring and Vascular Access

In addition to ASA standard monitors (electrocardiography, pulse oximetry, capnography, and temperature), invasive monitoring, including an intra-arterial catheter, should be considered. An intra-arterial catheter is routinely used in AVM resection and permits continuous monitoring and tight control of blood pressure. It also facilitates intraoperative blood sampling to measure oxygenation, ventilation, an electrolyte panel, and hemoglobin level. In contrast to cerebral aneurysms, brief periods of systemic HTN rarely cause an AVM to rupture, so an intra-arterial catheter may be inserted after anesthesia has been induced. Because rapid bleeding may occur during the procedure, large-bore intravenous access is imperative during AVM resection. A central venous catheter should be considered in patients who have poor peripheral venous access or if prolonged treatment with vasoactive drugs is predicted. Evoked potential monitoring has been used to monitor the central nervous system during AVM resection. Although no clinical trials exist, case reports and smaller observational studies suggest that neurophysiologic monitoring may be effective during cerebral AVM resection [56]. Monitoring of the jugular venous saturation has also been proposed as a means to managing normal perfusion pressure breakthrough and hyperemia, which can occur during AVM resection [57].

Anesthetic Technique

The primary goals of anesthetic management are to provide immobility and unconsciousness, to maintain adequate oxygenation and ventilation, and to ensure hemodynamic stability and cerebral perfusion. A variety of anesthetic techniques may be used to accomplish these goals; there is no single specific agent that must be used for AVM treatment. In general, intracranial HTN is less common in patients scheduled for elective AVM resection than with other neurosurgical lesions, but some patients may present with moderate intracranial HTN. It may therefore be prudent to avoid maneuvers that cause cerebral vasodilation.

INDUCTION   Premedication with incremental small doses of benzodiazepines and/or an opioid is reasonable in the anxious, neurologically intact patient. In many cases, insertion of an intra-arterial catheter may be deferred until after induction is complete. If, however, the patient has an untreated cerebral aneurysm in addition to the AVM or is hemodynamically unstable, it may be safer to insert the arterial catheter before induction. General anesthesia can be induced with propofol, etomidate, or thiopental (if available), followed by a nondepolarizing neuromuscular blocking agent after adequate ventilation has been demonstrated. After induction, intubation, and line insertion, the patient may be positioned. Patient positioning varies depending on the location of the lesion but is often supine with both arms tucked at the patient's sides. Access to the patient is limited during the procedure, so intravenous and arterial catheters should be inspected for kinks and tension on the tubing before the surgical drapes are applied.

MAINTENANCE   AVM resection may present the anesthesiologist with a variety of intraoperative challenges, including hemodynamic instability, rapid blood loss, management of intracranial HTN, and multiple comorbidities. Important objectives include providing an adequate surgical field in which to operate safely and efficiently while maintaining hemodynamic stability, controlling ICP, preserving cerebral perfusion, and providing an anesthetic that is conducive to neurophysiologic monitoring. The patient should be awake and alert at the end of the procedure to facilitate a neurologic examination.

Longer-acting drugs should therefore be avoided whenever possible to expedite emergence. High concentrations of potent volatile anesthetic (greater than 0.5 MAC) generally decrease the amplitude of SSEPs and may ablate or significantly impair recording of motor evoked potentials, so their use should be limited; a TIVA may therefore be most appropriate. If MEPs will be monitored, it may be necessary to forego the use of neuromuscular blocking agents after the patient is intubated. The combination of a potent volatile agent or propofol and short-acting opioid agonists such as remifentanil will provide analgesia, unconsciousness, and immobility. If an opioid other than remifentanil is administered as an infusion, it should be discontinued during the last hour of surgery to facilitate a timely emergence.

A relaxed brain is important because it allows the surgeons to use retraction and gentle manipulation to expose the AVM. In addition to improving the visual field and facilitating resection, brain relaxation helps to minimize ischemia associated with retraction. A number of maneuvers can be used to relax the brain. Mannitol (0.5 to 1 g/kg) is commonly administered for this purpose but should be used with caution in patients who are hypovolemic or who have compromised left ventricular function. Positioning the patient in a 30-degree "head-up" position is also effective, but raising the head more than 30 degrees may cause a venous air embolism. Drainage of CSF via a lumbar or ventricular drain is also effective but should be done slowly to avoid overdrainage and possible herniation. Finally, careful selection of anesthetic agent also facilitates this goal. Relying less on potent volatile anesthetics, which tend to increase CBF and more on intravenous agents may help to promote a more relaxed, retractable brain.

A hemodynamically stabile patient is critical to a successful procedure. Systemic arterial blood pressure should be kept as close as possible to preoperative pressure, unless a higher or lower value has been agreed on with the surgical team. Although induced hypotension may be desired during certain parts of the operation, particularly when rapid bleeding is encountered, some patients may not tolerate long periods of sustained hypotension, particularly those with chronic HTN. A safe rule of thumb is to maintain systemic blood pressure similar to the patient's baseline when feasible and to decrease blood pressure during periods of rapid blood loss.

Fluid management is centered around maintaining euvolemia while avoiding dehydration to maintain stable systemic and cerebral hemodynamics. Successful fluid resuscitation and maintenance of adequate intravascular volume are accomplished with an isotonic crystalloid solution (e.g., normal saline or PlasmaLyte) or a colloid solution. Although no conclusive evidence exists as to whether crystalloid is preferred over colloid, it is probably best to avoid administration of large volumes of hetastarch because of the theoretical concerns about coagulopathy [58, 59]. Hypo-osmolar crystalloid solutions such as lactated Ringer's solution and hypotonic saline should also be avoided because they can exacerbate cerebral edema, making brain retraction more difficult. Control of blood glucose has long been a controversial topic in neurosurgery and there are few concrete guidelines. A recent publication reviewed the topic of perioperative glucose control in neurosurgical patients and had this to report: "Recently a systematic review was published from a meta-analysis of 21 trials in heterogenic populations of critically ill patients, including stroke and head trauma…. On the basis of this systematic review, the American College of Physicians recommended not using IIT [intensive insulin therapy] under any circumstances in hospitalized patients…. Actually, tight blood glucose control does not have any solid evidence for its implementation in the perioperative neurosurgical period or in victims of any cerebral injury from any cause…" [60]. Nevertheless, excessively high (and extremely low) blood glucose levels should be avoided because hyperglycemia is known to be responsible for perioperative complications such as poor wound healing, longer hospital stays and increased morbidity and mortality. Although little evidence exists to support the benefits of tight glucose control, glucose-containing crystalloid solutions should be avoided and blood levels maintained between 140 and 180 mg/dL [60].

Temperature regulation and the theoretical benefits of hypothermia have been debated for years in both the neurosurgery and neurosurgical anesthesia literature. It has been postulated that mild hypothermia (34° to 35°C) provides cerebral protection against ischemia in patients undergoing craniotomy. Although this concept has been supported in numerous animal studies and has been shown to be helpful in patients with traumatic brain injury, little has been published to support this finding in patients undergoing craniotomy. Results of the IHAST investigation were published in 2005 illustrating that mild hypothermia conferred no cerebral protective benefit on good-grade patients (World Federation of Neurological Surgeons score of I, II, and III) undergoing craniotomy for SAH. Furthermore, perioperative hypothermia is associated with many adverse perioperative outcomes. Hypothermia prolongs the effects of potent volatile and intravenous anesthetics and those of neuromuscular blocking agents. Hypothermia prolongs anesthetic recovery, increases the risk of perioperative bleeding, increases the incidence of wound infection, and prolongs hospital stay. Mild hypothermia triples the incidence of adverse perioperative myocardial events due to the increase in myocardial demand caused by shivering [61]. There is, therefore, no evidence to suggest that patients undergoing surgical or endovascular treatment of an AVM will benefit from hypothermia, and temperature management should be optimized to maintain normothermia.

Most patients who undergo cerebral AVM resection are allowed to emerge from anesthesia extubated at the end of the procedure. If the patient is to remain intubated after the procedure, the patient may be briefly awakened so that the neurosurgeons can perform an abbreviated examination to rule out a major vascular injury or postoperative bleed. In this case, the patient can be resedated after the surgeons are satisfied with the examination and the patient is then transported asleep, intubated, and mechanically ventilated to the ICU. In either case, the goal of emergence is rapid, smooth awakening and hemodynamic stability.

At a minimum, the purpose of the postoperative neurologic examination is to ensure that the patient is moving all extremities and following simple commands before leaving the operating room. Factors that can alter the examination include true emergencies such as bleeding; patient morbidity such as edema, excessive retraction, and intraoperative seizures; and residual anesthetic agents. Using anesthetic agents with a short half-life minimizes the likelihood of a delayed emergence, which could confound the examination. If a longer-acting opioid infusion is used, it should be discontinued 1 hour before emergence. Straining and coughing are always undesirable after craniotomy. Strategies that mitigate the risk of coughing include continuing a remifentanil infusion until the dressing is in place and administering antiemetics to prevent nausea and vomiting. Multimodal antiemetic therapy (e.g., ondansetron and metoclopramide) should be considered. Management of emergence HTN helps to prevent bleeding after hemostasis has been established. Antihypertensive agents can include β-blockers (e.g., labetalol) and peripheral vasodilators such as nicardipine or hydralazine. If hydralazine is used, it should be administered in small, incremental doses because of its prolonged onset time and duration of action. Nitroglycerine is a cerebral vasodilator and its use should be avoided in neurosurgical patients.

Postoperative Management

Patients who have undergone a cerebral AVM resection should be transferred to a neurosurgical intensive care unit (NSICU) after surgery for management of NPPB, hyperemia, seizures, edema, and hemorrhage. Systemic blood pressure should be maintained in a relatively narrow range to minimize the risk of postoperative bleeding. Because blood pressure may be labile in this patient population, shorter-acting drugs (e.g., nicardipine) may be easier to titrate. Pain management is also a concern in patients who have undergone a craniotomy for AVM resection. A narcotic such as morphine or hydromorphone may be used in small, incremental doses to achieve postoperative analgesia, and PCA may be considered when the patient is lucid and able to participate in his or her own pain management. Non-narcotic analgesics such as intravenous acetaminophen are useful adjuncts in managing acute, postcraniotomy pain.

Endovascular Embolization

Endovascular procedures are covered extensively in another chapter. Patients may undergo preoperative embolization of an AVM either as part of preoperative management or as the sole treatment. The objective is to eliminate as many fistulas and feeding arteries as possible to decrease the risk of spontaneous hemorrhage. Embolization may be the only intervention in patients who are poor surgical candidates but is most often used as a preoperative adjunct in patients presenting for microsurgical resection as a means to decrease intraoperative hemorrhage. Because the patient must not move during the procedure, general anesthesia is the technique of choice. Although the risk of bleeding during these cases is much less than for surgical resection, at least one large-bore intravenous line should be inserted and blood should be available in the event that bleeding does occur. Insertion of an intra-arterial catheter is generally preferred to carefully monitor and control blood pressure and can be used to draw blood samples should substantial bleeding occur. Finally, these procedures are further complicated by the fact that they often are performed in remote locations sometimes devoid of backup supplies and personnel.

Conclusions: Neurovascular Procedures

Despite advances in the treatment of cerebral aneurysms, the morbidity and mortality for patients experiencing SAH remain high. Many neurosurgical centers are moving towards endovascular coiling as a means of treatment. However, many aneurysms are still clipped surgically. Characteristics that often preclude neurointerventional treatment include location and the size of the aneurysmal base.

Regardless of whether the lesion is to be treated surgically or in the endovascular suite, preoperative knowledge of the aneurysmal grade is critical to proper anesthetic management. Patients with low-grade aneurysms (Hunt-Hess grades 1 and 2) compared with those with higher-grade lesions tend to have less pathophysiologic derangement, are less prone to vasospasm. and have better outcomes. Perioperative considerations for aneurysm surgery are many. The anesthesiologist is challenged to provide a hemodynamic milieu that avoids aneurysmal rupture but also cerebral ischemia. He or she must also tailor the anesthetic to accommodate for evoked potential monitoring (if performed) and quickly alter patient hemodynamics in the face of temporary artery occlusion or aneurysmal rupture. Diligent postoperative management in an ICU setting is also imperative in preventing and treating aneurysmal rebleeding and cerebral vasospasm. Meticulous, thoughtful care throughout the perioperative period is essential to ensuring quality care for patients with cerebral aneurysms. Treatment teams who are familiar with the challenges and potential complications should manage these patients. Finally, deliberate and ongoing communication between all members of the care team is necessary to achieving successful outcomes in this challenging area of neurosurgery.

REFERENCES

1. Lim M, et al. Anaesthesia for pituitary surgery. *J Clin Neurosci.* 2006;13:413–418.
2. Palmeiro C, et al. Growth hormone and the cardiovascular system. *Cardiol Rev.* 2012;20:197–207.
3. Miljic P, et al. Pathogenesis of vascular complications in Cushing's syndrome. *Clin Hematol.* 2012;11:21–30.
4. Fatti L, et al. Effects of treatment with somatostatin analogues on QT interval duration in acromegalic patients. *Clin Endocrinol.* 2006;65:626–630.
5. Alexandraki K, et al. Specific electrocardiographic features associated with Cushing's disease. *Clin Endocrinol.* 2011;74:558–564.
6. Vannucci L, Luciani P, Gagliardi E, Paiano S, Duranti R, Forti G, Peri A. Assessment of sleep apnea syndrome in treated acromegalic patients and correlation of its severity with clinical and laboratory parameters. *J Endocrinol Invest.* 2013;36:237–242.
7. Nemergut EC, et al. Perioperative management of patients undergoing transsphenoidal pituitary surgery. *Anesth Analg.* 2005;101:1170–1181.
8. Nemergut EC, et al. Airway management in patients with pituitary disease: a review of 746 patients. *J Neurosurg Anesthesiol.* 2006;18:73–77.
9. Sloan T, Heyer E. Anesthesia for intraoperative neurophysiologic monitoring of the spinal cord. *J Clin Neurophysiol.* 2002;19:430–443.
10. Deiner S, et al. Patient characteristics and anesthetic technique are additive but not synergistic predictors of successful motor evoked potential monitoring. *Anesth Analg.* 2010;111:421–425.
11. Ransom ER, Chiu AG. Prevention and management of complications in intracranial endoscopic skull base surgery.. *Otolaryngol Clin North Am* 2010;43:875–895.
12. Tommasino, C. Fluids and the neurosurgical patient. *Anesthesiol Clin North Am* 2002;20:329–346.
13. Loh JA, Verbalis JG. Disorders of water and salt metabolism associated with pituitary disease. *Endocrinol Metab Clin North Am* 2008;37: 213–234.
14. Kincaid BMS, Lam AM. Anesthesia for neurosurgery. In Barash PG, Cullen BF, Stoelting RK, Cahalan M, Shock MC, eds. Clinical Anesthesia. 6th edition. Philadelphia: Lippincott Williams and Wilkins; 2009;1020.
15. Devin JK. Hypopituitarism and central diabetes insipidus: perioperative diagnosis and management. *Neurosurg Clin N Am* 2012;23:679–689.
16. Higashizawa T, et al. Effect of infraorbital nerve block under general anesthesia on consumption of isoflurane and postoperative pain in endoscopic endonasal maxillary sinus surgery. *J Anesth.* 2001;15:136–138.
17. DeMaria S Jr, Govindaraj S, Chinosorvatana N, Kang, S, Levine AI. Bilateral sphenopalatine ganglion blockade improves posoperative analgesia after endoscopic sinus surgery. *Am J Rhinol Allergy* 2012;26:e23–27.

18. Kristof RA, et al. Incidence, clinical manifestations, and course of water and electrolyte metabolism disturbances following transsphenoidal pituitary adenoma surgery: a prospective observational study. *J Neurosurg*. 2009;111:555–562.

19.. Armengot M, et al. Transphenoidal endoscopic approaches for pituitary adenomas: a critical review of our experience. *Acta Otorrinolaringol Esp*. 2011; 62:25–30.

20. Rinkel GJ, et al. Prevalence and risk of rupture of intraranial aneurysms: a systematic review. *Stroke*. 1998;29:251–256.

21. Bederson JB, et al. Guidelines for the mangement of aneurysmal subarachnoid hemorrhage: a statement for healthcare professionals from a special writing group of the Stroke Council, American Heart Association. *Stroke*. 2009;40:994–1025.

22. Rosen DS, et al. Subarachnoid hemorrhage grading scales: a systematic review. *Neurocrit Care*. 2005;2:110–118.

23. Frontera JA, et al. Prediction of symptomatic vasospasm after subarachnoid hemorrhage: the modified fisher scale. *Neurosurgery*. 2006;59:21–27.

24. Heuer GG, et al. Relationship between intracranial pressure and other clinical variables in patients with aneurysmal subarachnoid hemorrhage. *J Neurosurg*. 2004;101:408–416.

25.. Zweifel C, et al. Continuous assessment of cerebral autoregulation with near-infrared spectroscopy in adults after subarachnoid hemorrhage. *Stroke*. 2010;41:1963–1968.

26. Urrutia VC, et al. Blood pressure management in acute stroke. *Neurol Clin* 2008;26:565–568.

27. Rose JT, et al. Subarachnoid hemorrhage with neurocardiogenic stunning. *Rev Cardiovasc Med*. 2010;11:254–263.

28. Hakeem A, et al. When the worst headache becomes the worst heartache! *Stroke*. 2007;38:3292–3295.

29. van der Bilt IA, et al. Impact of cardiac complications on outcome after aneurysmal subarachnoid hemorrhage: a meta-analysis. *Neurology*. 2009;72:635–642.

30. Inamasu J, et al. Subarachnoid hemorrhage complicated with neurogenic pulmonary edema and takotsubo-like cardiomyopathy. *Neurol Med Chir (Tokyo)*. 2012;52():49–55.

31. Dorhout Mees SM, et al. Brain natriuretic peptide concentrations after aneurysmal subarachnoid hemorrhage: relationship with hypovolemia and hyponatremia. *Neurocrit Care*. 2011;14:176–178.

32. Kassell NF, et al. The International Cooperative Study on the Timing of Aneurysm Surgery. Part 1: overall management results. *J Neurosurg*. 1990;73:18–36.

33. Haley EC Jr, et al. The International Cooperative Study on the Timing of Aneurysm Surgery. The North American experience. *Stroke*. 1992;23(2:205–214.

34. Ross N, et al. Timing of surgery for supratentorial aneurysmal subarachnoid haemorrhage: report of a prospective study. *J Neurol Neurosurg Psychiatry*. 2002;72:480–484.

35.. McLaughlin N, et al. Aneurysmal surgery in the presence of angiographic vasospasm: an outcome assessment. *Can J Neurol Sci*. 2006;33:181–188.

36. Baltsavias GS, et al. Effects of timing of coil embolization after aneurysmal subarachnoid hemorrhage on procedural morbidity and outcomes. *Neurosurgery*. 2000;47:1320–1329.

37. Haure P, et al. The ICP-lowering effect of 10 degrees reverse Trendelenburg position during craniotomy is stable during a 10-minute period. *J Neurosurg Anesthesiol*. 2003;15:297–301.

38. Wu CT, et al. A comparison of 3% hypertonic saline and mannitol for brain relaxation during elective supratentorial brain tumor surgery. *Anesth Analg* 2010;10:903–907.

39. Kamel H, et al. Hypertonic saline versus mannitol for the treatment of elevated intracranial pressure: a meta-analysis of randomized clinical trials. *Crit Care Med*. 2011;39:554–559.

40. Gelb AW, et al. Does hyperventilation improve operating condition during supratentorial craniotomy? A multicenter randomized crossover trial. *Anesth Analg*. 2008;106:585–594.

41. Murad A, et al. Role of controlled lumbar CSF drainage for ICP control in aneurysmal SAH. *Acta Neurochir Suppl*. 2011;110:183–187.

42. Cole CD, et al. Total Intravenous Anesthesia: Advantages for Intracranial Surgery. *Neurosurgery*. 2007;61:369–378.

43. Engelhard K, et al. Inhalational or intravenous anesthetic for craniotomies? Pro inhalational. *Curr Opin Anaesthesiol*. 2006;19:504–508.

44. Schifilliti D, et al. Anaesthetic-related neuroprotection: intravenous or inhalational agents? *CNS Drugs*. 2010;24:893–907.

45. Pasternak J, Lanier W. Is nitrous oxide use appropriate in neurosurgical and neurologically at-risk patients? *Curr Opin Anesthesiol*. 2010;23:544–550.

46. Todd M, et al. Mild intraoperative hypothermia during surgery for intracranial aneurysm. *N Engl J Med*. 2005;352:135–145.

47. Flexman, , et al. Acute and chronic pain following craniotomy. *Curr Opin Anaesthesiol*. 2010;23:551–557.

48. Mordhors C, et al. Prospective assessment of postoperative pain after craniotomy. *J Neurosurg Anesthesiol*. 2010;2010:202–206.

49. Basali A, Mascha E, Kalfas I. Relationship between perioperative hypertension and intracranial hemorrhage after craniotomy. *Anesthesiology*. 2000;93:48–54.

50. Batoz H, et al. The analgesic properties of scalp infiltrations with ropivacaine after intracranial tumoral resection. *Anesth Analg*. 2009;109:240–244.

51. Saleh O, et al. Arteriovenous Malformation, Complications, and Perioperative Anesthetic Management. *Middle East J Anesthesiol* 2008;19:737–756.

52. Fogarty-Mack P, et al. The effect of arteriovenous malformations on the distribution of intracerebral arterial pressures. *AJNR Am J Neuroradiol* 1996;17:1143–1149.

53. Hashimoto T, Young WL. Anesthesia-related considerations for cerebral arteriovenous malformations. *Neurosurg Focus*. 2001;11:e5.

54. Kader A, Young WL. The effects of intracranial arteriovenous malformations on cerebral hemodynamics. *Neurosurg Clin N Am*. 1996;7:767–781.

55. Nornes H, Grip A. Hemodynamic aspects of cerebral arteriovenous malformations. *J Neurosurg*. 1980;53:456–464.

56. Spetzler RF, et al. Normal perfusion pressure breakthrough theory. *Clin Neurosurg*. 1978;25:651–672.

57. Young WI, et al. Pressure autoregulation is intact after arteriovenous malformation resection. *Neurosurgery*. 1993;32:491–496; discussion 496–497.

58. Young WL, et al. Evidence for adaptive autoregulatory displacement in hypotensive cortical territories adjacent to arteriovenous malformations. Columbia University AVM Study Project. *Neurosurgery*. 1994;34:610–611.

59. Young WL, et al. The effect of arteriovenous malformation resection on cerebrovascular reactivity to carbon dioxide. *Neurosurgery*. 1990;27:266–267.

60. Stapf C, et al. The New York Islands AVM Study: design, study progress, and initial results. *Stroke*. 2003;34:e29–e33.

61. Lv X, et al. Angioarchitectural characteristics of brain arteriovenous malformations with and without hemorrhage. *World Neurosurg*. 2011;76(1-2):95–99.

62. Zacharia BE, et al. Management of ruptured brain arteriovenous malformations. *Curr Atheroscler Rep*. 2012;24. [Epub ahead of print].

63. Anastasian ZH, et al. Radiation exposure of the anesthesiologist in the neurointerventional suite. *Anesthesiology*. 2011;114:512–520.

64. Wilder-Smith OH, et al. Jugular venous bulb oxygen saturation monitoring in arteriovenous malformation surgery. *J Neurosurg Anesthesiol*. 1997;9:162–165.

65. Barron ME, Wilkes MM, Navickis RJ. A systematic review of the comparative safety of colloids. *Arch Surg*. 2004;139:552–563.

66. Hartog CS, Kohl M, Reinhart K. A systematic review of third-generation hydroxyethyl starch (HES 130/0.4) in resuscitation: safety not adequately addressed. *Anesth Analg*. 2011;112:635–645.

67. Godoy DA, et al. Perioperative glucose control in neurosurgical patients. *Anesthesiol Res Pract*. 2012;. Article ID 690362, 13 pages, doi:10.1155/2012690362.

68. Reynolds L, Beckmann J, Kurz A. Perioperative complications of hypothermia. *Best Pract Res Clin Anaesthesiol* 2008;22:645–657.

15.

ANESTHESIA FOR STEREOTACTIC RADIOSURGERY AND INTRAOPERATIVE MAGNETIC RESONANCE IMAGING

Armagan Dagal and Arthur M. Lam

A number of different systems are now available for stereotactic radiosurgery, and the anesthetic requirements for these procedures vary according to each patient as well as the systems used. This chapter briefly reviews the development and functional applications of stereotactic surgery and then discusses the anesthetic implications of this procedure.

BACKGROUND

Two British scientists, Sir Victor Horsley (a pioneer neurosurgeon) and Robert Henry Clarke, described the stereotaxic apparatus and its applications for the first time in 1908 [1]. The name "stereotaxic" was adopted from the Greek words *stereos,* meaning "solid," and *taxis,* meaning "arrangement." (In the United States, the word "stereotactic" is preferred, combining the Greek word *stereos* with the Latin word *tactis,* the pluperfect passive form of the verb *tangere* meaning "to touch.") Based on the Cartesian coordinate system, this device enabled them to map the brain in great detail, and they described procedures in which they were able to ablate intracranial targets using electrocoagulation. Three decades later, two American neurosurgeons, Ernest A. Spiegel and Henry T. Wycis, modified the design for use in stereotactic neurosurgical procedures in humans [2]. They created a molded frame for an individual patient's head using a plaster cranial cap. They aligned their frame not just to the cranium but also to brain landmarks such as the calcified pineal gland and the foramen of Monroe by means of intraoperative pneumoencephalography, hence naming their device "stereoencephalotome." By 1952, they had developed a stereotactic atlas of the human brain.

In the 1950s, surgical incision of the extrapyramidal system to treat movement disorders (MDs) such as Parkinson's disease (PD) started to emerge as a treatment option, and Russell Meyers, a neurosurgeon at the University of Iowa, reported that his open neurosurgical techniques carried a 15.7% mortality rate. By 1958, Spiegel and colleagues had reported a 2% mortality rate for stereotactic surgery for MDs (3), and an estimated 25,000 functional stereotactic procedures were ultimately performed before the introduction of L-dopa in the 1960s [4].

Lars Leksell (1907–1986), a Swedish neurosurgeon, attempted to reduce the high morbidity and mortality associated with invasive neurosurgery. He translated the Horsley-Clarke stereotaxy principle into arc centered stereotactic apparatus in 1947, using polar coordinates instead of Cartesian coordinates. The device enabled the precise placement of a needle or electrode into a desired location within the human brain [5].These efforts used an orthovoltage x-ray tube attached to a stereotactic frame to produce converging beams, which intersected at the treatment target. Physicists Liden and Larsson of Uppsala University in Sweden used a stereotactic target localization to direct proton beams at a target. The device used 201 sources of cobalt-60 distributed with collimators to create a sharply circumscribed disc-shaped lesion, and the device was initially used during functional neurosurgery [6–8]. Further development of this concept culminated in 1968 with the introduction of the first Gamma Knife unit at the Sophiahemmet Hospital.

In 1972, Steiner and Leksell used radiosurgery to treat arteriovenous malformation (AVM) [9] for the first time.

Target localization improved dramatically when computed tomography (CT) was used in conjunction with the stereotactic apparatus [10]. Leksell described the application of CT during radiosurgery and noted the technique enabled rapid and accurate target localization. With the advent of better imaging methods, solid tumors like vestibular schwannomas became radiosurgical targets [11]. By 1985, Leksell and colleagues reported the potential application of magnetic resonance imaging (MRI) to radiosurgery. Today CT, MRI, and angiography are used commonly during radiosurgical planning [12].

After 4.5 years of intensive review, the first Gamma Knife unit was installed in the United States at the University of Pittsburgh in 1987 under the leadership of L. Dade Lunsford, a neurosurgeon [13].

Alternative technologies continue to be developed. Linear accelerator (LINAC) radiosurgery was introduced in the early 1980s. The first report on LINAC based radiosurgery was published in 1983 by Betti and Derechinsky. It was Lutz and Winston, however, who created the technology to quantify and calculate dosimetry and improve the accuracy of the LINAC- based system. Their system delivers focused collimated x-ray beam on a stereotactically identified target. Since linear accelerators are more available and less expensive than the Gamma Knife, the LINAC became a popular radiosurgery system [14–16].

John R. Adler at Stanford University developed the Cyberknife technology, combining a linear particle accelerator with a robotic arm, thus creating a frameless system that adjusts for patient movement using real-time x-ray images (Accuray Inc., Sunnyvale, CA). Cyberknife system received Food and Drug Administration clearance in 2001 for the treatment of tumors in any location of the body [17, 18].

TYPES OF STEREOTACTIC RADIOSURGERY

GAMMA KNIFE

The Leksell Gamma Unit is both the simplest and the oldest currently used device (Figure 15.1). The radiation source consists of 201 cobalt-60 sources that are enclosed within a hemispheric vault. During the decay process, gamma rays with energies of 1.17 and 1.33 MeV are emitted; this energy is then directed through precisely machined portals so as to converge at a single target with high precision. This technique allows the energy to be delivered with high accuracy but comes at the cost of generating "hot spots" sometimes as high as twice the marginal prescription dose within the

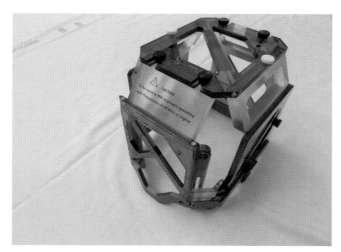

Figure 15.2   Leksell stereotactic head frame.

treatment volume. The hemispheric configuration of the Gamma Knife limits its use to intracranial targets, and treatment is largely limited to single-fraction radiosurgery applications. A rigid head frame is used to help direct the beams (Figure 15.2).

LINEAR ACCELERATORS

Linear accelerator (LINAC) radiosurgery uses customized, general-purpose linear accelerators to obtain high-conformity treatment where radiation energy is focused so that the treatment volume receives a high therapeutic dose while surrounding normal tissue is given a relatively low dose [14, 19–21]. These devices use a magnetron to accelerate electrons that then collide with a target to generate photons. These photons are then focused through a portal to achieve a collimated beam of gamma radiation.

Cyberknife is a frameless stereotactic radiosurgery (SRS) system that uses a lightweight LINAC that is mounted on a highly mobile robotic arm directed by a real-time guidance system (Figure 15.3). This obviates the need for rigid fixation as used in frame-based systems such as the Gamma Knife. The Cyberknife system determines the

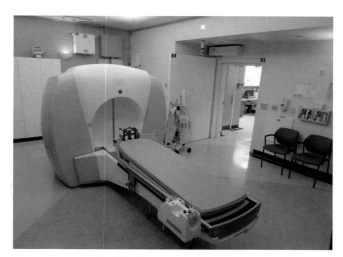

Figure 15.1   Gamma Knife Perfexion

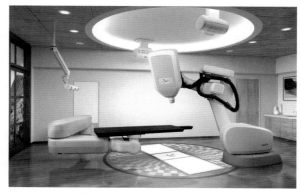

Figure 15.3   Cyberknife.   (Image used with permission from Accuray Incorporated.)

location of the skull or spine in the coordinate frame of the radiation delivery system by comparing digitally reconstructed CT phantoms obtained from the patient's treatment planning images with real-time oblique radiographs obtained during the procedure. When the patient (target) moves, the system detects the change, and the robot makes appropriate adjustments to maintain accurate targeting. The system also uses sophisticated infrared tracking to accommodate for motion caused by respiration. This innovative system has enabled SRS to be expanded to include the head, spine, chest, abdomen, and pelvis.

PROTON BEAM RADIOSURGERY

Proton radiotherapy is as effective as conventional linear accelerator or Gamma Knife. As ionized particles travel through matter, most of their energy is lost immediately before the particles come to rest. As a result, when protons move through human tissue, most of their energy dissipate within a discrete band of spatial depth measuring roughly 12 to 16 mm. To treat a large tumor, varying amounts of energy must be delivered; this is usually accomplished by placing a variable thickness attenuator into the beam path.

There is no current evidence exists to show the superiority of this technique in the clinical setting over photon-based techniques, either from the standpoint of disease control or toxicity [22, 23].

INDICATIONS
SRS for Oncological Pathology

- Malignant glioma
- Meningioma
- Acoustic schwannoma
- Pituitary and pineal tumors
- Skull base tumors
- Acoustic neuroma
- Metastatic brain tumors
- Head and neck tumors
- Primary and metastatic spinal tumors

SRS for Functional Disorders

- AVMs
- Trigeminal neuralgia
- Movement disorder
- Psychiatric disorders
- Pain disorders
- Epilepsy

SRS for Neurosurgical Guidance

- Biopsy
- Catheter placement
- Cysts/abscess drainage
- Electrode placement
- Evacuation of intracerebral hemorrhage
- Map a lesion for open craniotomy (AVM, deep tumor)

Experimental

- Stereotactic clipping of aneurysms
- Stereotactic laser surgery
- CNS transplantation
- Foreign body removal

The main use of radiosurgery is to change the biology of the tumor cells so as to inhibit proliferation. A successful outcome of radiosurgical treatment is therefore the arrest of tumor growth, not disappearance of the tumor. Radiosurgery is generally inappropriate for patients who have a large tumor or are symptomatic from tumor mass effects. Because external beam techniques can achieve only a limited degree of conformity, radiosurgical treatment of larger tumors may expose normal tissue to an unacceptably high level of radiation. Large tumors may therefore require surgical debulking (i.e., to reduce tumor volume) or fractionated treatments.

Overall postradiosurgical complication rates are reported to be between 3% and 40%.

Less severe neurological symptoms are thought to be due to transient swelling that begins 12 to 48 hours after therapy. Patients may develop nausea, dizziness or vertigo, seizures, or new headache as a result. Long-term complications include cranial nerve dysfunction and neurological deficits. Among published series involving 100 patients or more, rates of these significant long-term complications range from 0% to 16% in centers utilizing median doses of 12 to 15 Gy. Radiosurgery-induced cancers (mainly glioblastomas) have a reported incidence of between 0 and 3 cases per 200,000 patients, and this does not appear to be above the natural incidence of cancer in the general population [24, 25].

SRS for Oncological Pathology

Vestibular schwannoma (VS) is the most extensively studied disease in which SRS is applied as a standalone treatment with adjusted efficacy of stabilization around 91.1% ("efficacy of stabilization" refers to the tumors that either decrease in size or remain stable as a result of the treatment).

VS is a benign tumor that usually presents with impaired hearing and balance because of direct compression of the acoustic nerve. Facial motor dysfunction, brainstem compression, and hydrocephalus are late symptoms. If left untreated, continued growth causes symptoms that are progressively more severe. Although no randomized controlled studies have firmly established a maximum permissible size, a tumor that is larger than 3 cm in diameter is generally considered suitable for SRS.

Nonvestibular intracranial schwannomas have also been successfully treated with SRS with good tumor control and minimal risk of complications.

Complication and deterioration rates related to SRS treatment remain low: postradiation facial dysfunction rate of 7.1% and non–cranial nerve complications of 5.6%. Hearing preservation can be achieved in 60% of the patients if diagnosis is made prior to the unilateral loss of hearing. This is a higher rate than that which can be achieved in patients undergoing surgical resection, but the beneficial effects of treatment do not occur immediately [26, 27].

Glioblastoma multiforme (GBM) is the most highly malignant primary intracranial tumor. Survival after diagnosis ranges from 12 to 24 months, and there are no treatments that extend long-term survival to a significant extent. Volume of the initial surgical resection has been shown to provide a significant survival benefit, and radiotherapy, brachytherapy, and chemotherapy have been evaluated as adjuvant therapy for GBM [28].

Meningiomas arise from arachnoidal cap cells commonly associated with arachnoid granulations at the dural venous sinuses, cranial nerve foramina, cribriform plate, and medial middle fossa. This tumor is most commonly benign but may exhibit atypical or malignant features and behavior. The lesion may arise anywhere along the dura, including the convexity and base of the skull. SRS is primarily used for adjuvant therapy of meningiomas that have undergone previous resection, particularly for histologically atypical or anaplastic tumors [29]. SRS has an overall stabilization rate of 89.0%, with a low complication rate of 7% [30, 31].

The most common intracranial tumor is a metastatic lesion with an extracranial primary origin. About 20% to 40% of patients with cancer develop intracranial metastases [32]. The Joint AANS/CNS (American Association of Neurological Surgeons and Congress of Neurological Surgeons) group made the following evidence-based recommendations.

Level 1: Single-dose SRS with whole brain radiation therapy (WBRT) leads to longer survival for patients with single metastatic brain tumors who have a Karnofsky Performance Scale (KPS) ≥70.

Level 2: Single-dose SRS along with WBRT is superior in terms of local tumor control and maintaining functional status when compared to WBRT alone for patients with 1–4 metastatic brain tumors who have a KPS ≥70.

Level 3: Single-dose SRS and WBRT may lead to significantly longer patient survival for patients with 2–3 metastatic brain tumors.

Level 4: Single-dose SRS and WBRT is superior to WBRT alone for improving patient survival for patients with single or multiple brain metastases and a KPS < 70.

Level 2: Surgical resection plus WBRT and SRS plus WBRT represent effective treatment strategies, resulting in relatively equal survival rates [33–36].

SRS has been evaluated in the treatment of intracranial oncological pathologies other than metastases and primary brain tumors. Kobayashi et al. and Chung et al. studied SRS in craniopharyngioma with long-term follow-up. They reported 77% and 87% tumor control rate, respectively [37, 38]. Sheehan et al. found that SRS resulted in tumor stabilization or regression in 88% of 26 patients with trigeminal schwannoma [39]. Further studies are needed to fully elucidate the role of radiosurgery as a tool for treating these intracranial pathologies [40].

Arteriovenous Malformation

The goals of brain AVM treatment are typically to prevent hemorrhage, control seizures, or stabilize progressive neurological deficits. AVMs may be suitable for one or more of four management strategies: observation, surgical excision, SRS, endovascular embolization, or a combination. Management decision depends on the risk of subsequent hemorrhage. Young age, prior hemorrhage, small AVM size, deep venous drainage, and high flow make subsequent hemorrhage more likely [41]. Procedural risk of complications leading to permanent neurological deficits or death has been reported to be 7.4% (range, 0%–40%) after microsurgery, 5.1% (range, 0%–21%) after SRS, and 6.6% (range, 0%–28%) after embolization. Success rates are 96% (range, 0%–100%), 38% (range, 0%–75%), and 13% (range, 0%–94%) respectively. SRS can be effective for malformations that are smaller than 3.5 cm, but complete obliteration requires approximately 1 to 3 years after treatment and cure is not always obtained. Delayed complications include hemorrhage in the latency period and radiation edema or necrosis can occur as late complications [42–46].

SRS FOR FUNCTIONAL DISORDERS

SRS is used in the treatment of functional disorders including pain syndromes, epilepsy and behavioral disorders. Targets include the trigeminal nerve (for trigeminal neuralgia), cingulate gyrus and internal capsule (for pain disorders and obsessive compulsive disorder), globus pallidus (for relief of PD), and the corpus callosum and medial temporal lobe (for epilepsy).

TRIGEMINAL NEURALGIA

Ablative techniques and microvascular decompression may be used to treat trigeminal neuralgia (TN) that has become refractory to medical management. Microvascular decompression is highly invasive and carries with it the risks associated with a craniotomy. Trigeminal radiosurgery is a noninvasive technique that ablates the segment of the trigeminal nerve within the prepontine cistern. It can also be described as a retrogasserian radiosurgical rhizolysis. Outcomes are considered to be good to excellent in approximately 80% of patients who receive the procedure [47–50]. Paresthesia or numbness of varying degrees has been observed in 6% to 70% of patients following radiosurgical treatment. Those who developed sensory loss reported to have a better long-term pain control. Risk of recurrent pain is reported to be around 40% to 45% and retreatment may become necessary [51–55].

EPILEPSY

SRS can be used to treat epilepsy in patients where the seizures arise in the medial temporal lobe. When mesial temporal lobe epilepsy (hippocampus, parahippocampal gyrus, and amygdala) is treated with SRS, complete seizure freedom can be achieved in 60% to 65% of these patients [56, 57]. These results are comparable to outcomes from microsurgery [58].

MOVEMENT DISORDERS

Most patients with MDs are treated effectively with medical management. Some patients who have limited relief from pharmaceuticals or experience bothersome side effects of the drugs may benefit from deep brain stimulation (DBS). DBS and surgical lesioning of the thalamus and basal ganglia have a high success rates and a very low incidence of complications. Despite these positive outcomes, however, DBS and procedures that create a surgical lesion are contraindicated in some patients. SRS has been used for a noninvasive treatment alternative and for medication-intolerable patients, who are unable to undergo DBS or lesioning due to medical comorbidities [59].

PARKINSON'S DISEASE

Deep brain stimulation of the subthalamic nucleus and the globus pallidus internus has become the preferred stereotactic technique for PD. Surgery is usually performed under local anesthesia, which permits patient cooperation and intraoperative evaluation of tremor and dyskinesia during trial stimulation.

Monitored anesthesia care for DBS implantation is challenging because of the long duration of the procedure, the extremely claustrophobic conditions, the nature of the patient's illness, and the requirement for the patient's cooperation during the procedure [60]. Some surgical teams prefer the use of sedation during the periods of nonintervention "silent" time either with propofol [61] or remifentanil infusion [62]. Nevertheless, temporary suppression of PD tremor has been described with both drugs [63, 64]. General anesthesia is rarely used but can be used when patients are unable to tolerate the procedure under local anesthesia. Maltete et al. [65] compared the outcomes on patients who received general anesthesia versus local anesthesia for DBS implantation and found that bilateral targeting of the subthalamic nucleus was less precise in patients who received general anesthesia.

PSYCHIATRIC DISORDERS

Electrical stimulation via stereotactically implanted quadripolar electrodes in both anterior limbs of the internal capsules in patients with obsessive–compulsive disorder provides reversible and adjustable treatment. This method has been used in patients who are refractory to other treatments [66–68]. Either general or local anesthesia may be used for its application.

INTRAOPERATIVE MRI

The first nuclear resonance studies in condensed matter were carried out in the laboratories of Bloch and Purcell in 1946 [69–71]. These experiments did not produce any images, but they laid the foundations of the MRI and magnetic resonance spectroscopy (MRS) applied to biomedical sciences. Approximately 21 years later, two pioneering articles by Lauterbur and Mansfield and Granell independently proposed to use nuclear magnetic resonance to form an image [72]. MRI offers the advantages of being noninvasive and sensitive to a broad range of tissue properties while producing extremely high-resolution images. Intraoperative MRI (iMRI) has been recently introduced as a tool to improve the accuracy of stereotactic targeting and to help surgeons visualize the extent of their resection [73–75].

PHYSICAL PRINCIPLES OF MRI

The process that underlies the acquisition of an MR image can very simply be explained as follows: All atomic nuclei possess a charge (protons) and mass (neutrons and protons]. Some nuclei also possess a property known as "spin." The rotation of neutrons and protons in a nucleus creates a local magnetic field and the nucleus behaves like a miniature magnet.

MRI of the human body is possible because a large proportion of human tissue contains water, and water molecules contain hydrogen. Hydrogen molecules are dipoles and behave like small magnets. When placed in a magnetic field, the nuclei align with the field, and their resonant frequency increases by approximately 42.58 MHz/1.0 T of magnetic field. If a pulse of radiofrequency (RF) energy is delivered at the resonant frequency of the hydrogen nuclei, the dipoles will start to spin around the magnetic field as a result. When the RF pulse is discontinued, the dipoles realign with the magnetic field, losing energy to their surroundings. Some of this energy is picked up by receiver coil oriented in various axes and used to generate an MR image. The rate at which the energy is lost to the surroundings is dependent on the chemical composition of the tissues. Combined with the density of water, this gives rise to the contrast in the image.

The scan technique can be modified to highlight or suppress the echo in various tissues by varying the "relaxation rate." "T" refers to the relaxation time constant, and images may be T1 weighted (generated a few milliseconds after the electromagnetic field is removed) or T2 weighted (generated later than T1]. Nuclei in hydrogen take a long time to decay to their original position, so fluid will appear dark (minimal signal) in a T1-weighted (early) image, but white in the later T2 image as the signal appears.

Magnetic fields are measured in units of Gauss and Tesla. The Earth's magnetic field varies between 0.5 and 1.0 Gauss; 1 Tesla is equivalent to 10,000 Gauss. MRI requires extremely strong magnetic fields (between 0.2 and 3.0 T) to increase the resonant frequency of the nuclei to a level that can be measured by the scanner. In most high-field MRIs, this field is generated by a superconducting electromagnet in which an alloy (usually titanium-niobium) is immersed in liquid helium and cooled to below 4.2 degrees Kelvin. Because the signal that makes up the final MR image is very weak, any external radiofrequency sources can greatly interfere with its detection by the gradient coils. To prevent this, the MRI machine is contained within a radiofrequency shield called a Faraday cage. This is built into the walls of the MR room or provided as mobile cage [76].

Intraoperative MRI can be used in a fixed location MRI-OR (operating room) (more suitable for high-field MRI technology) or as a mobile MRI unit (generally using low-field MRI scanners]. Portable MRI units also require portable shields or Faraday cage to be used. This design enables the OR to be used as a standard OR if required. Open MRI scanners use a Helmholtz pair of superconductive magnets instead of one single solenoid. The two magnets are separated by a 60-cm gap where the magnetic field is homogeneous, thus providing access to the patient during scanning. To save space and weight, portable MRI units do not use liquid helium; cyclic cryo-coolers are used to cool the coils to 9 degrees K.

Intraoperative MRI has a number of applications in neurosurgery. Cerebral structures may move when the cranium is opened and cerebrospinal fluid is lost; this is referred to as *brain shift*. MRI allows the surgeon to dynamically alter the surgical approach to compensate for the movement. It can be used intermittently to update the data for navigational systems or continuously to provide real-time guidance of surgical tools [77–80]. In addition, MRI can be used to detect intraoperative complications (e.g., hemorrhage or a large pneumocranium) at the end of surgery.

ANESTHESIA AND MRI

Dedicated OR suites are required to provide adequate space for the required equipment, provisions for the portable shields (if a low-field, portable MRI unit is used), surgical equipment, and personnel. The size of the room is dictated by the size of the magnetic field, which is determined by the field strength and shielding. All ferromagnetic objects must be located outside the 5 Gauss line. A portable Faraday cage is used around the low-field scanner to prevent the low energy electrical noise emitted from infusion pumps, electronic display units, monitoring units, and CPUs from degrading the quality of images obtained [81].

Preoperative assessment of patients undergoing MRI includes a determination of whether the patient can safely be positioned within a strong magnetic field. Implanted medical devices and other contraindications to scanning require further evaluation and consultation with the MRI safety personnel.

Implantable medical devices fall into two main categories:

- *Active implantable medical devices.* These include pacemakers, defibrillators, neurostimulators, cochlear implants and drug pumps, where functionality is dependent on an energy source. Active implants contain metal components, which may suffer damage during exposure to MR. In addition, the implant may be attracted and moved by the magnetic field. Sensing/stimulation lead electrodes may inappropriately sense electrical energy induced by either the magnetic or RF fields, resulting in modified therapy or dysfunction. A potential may exist for tissue damage from induced current especially RF, where high current density flows through very small surface electrodes. Larger metallic components may also suffer temperature increase.

- *Nonactive implantable medical devices.* They require no power source for their function. For example: hip/knee joint replacements, heart valves, aneurysm clips, coronary stents and dental work. Some clips and implants are ferromagnetic; they can be displaced by the magnetic field, may result in heat generation, may create noise as well as degrade image quality.

- *Tissue expanders, implants, transdermal patches, tattoos, and make-up.* Burns due to the presence of metallic components have been reported to the MHRA (Medicines and Healthcare product Regulatory Agency) in the United Kingdom. Transdermal medicinal patches containing metal should be removed and replaced after scanning if this can be done without affecting patient treatment. Tattoos may contain iron oxide or other ferromagnetic substances that are conductive. During scanning, patients should be asked to report any discomfort immediately. The ACR (American College of Radiology) recommends that cold compresses or ice packs be placed on the tattooed areas and kept in place throughout the MRI process if these tattoos are within the volume in which the body coil is being used for RF transmission. All make-up, particularly eye make-up should be removed as it may also contain metallic fibers.

Anesthetic considerations for patients undergoing iMRI are much the same as for other neurosurgical procedures. Both inhalational and intravenous agents can be used successfully for delivery of anesthesia. iMRI-specific management issues should be considered, which includes access to the OR (especially during the scan, when the doors may be locked), the use of MRI-compatible equipment, patient monitoring, and patient and personnel safety.

Aspects of the room setup that affect the anesthesiologist include patient positioning, portable shield positioning, and monitoring equipment placement. Commercially available gas delivery equipment, monitors, and infusion pumps have been designed for use outside of a specified distance from the MRI scanner [82]. MRI conditional monitoring equipment incorporates fiberoptic and wireless technologies to reduce electrical noise. Monitors should be set up to allow viewing both inside and outside the MRI suite.

Because the patient will be relatively inaccessible and heavy equipment will be moving around the patient, precautions should be taken against the accidental disconnection of the breathing circuits, infusion lines, or monitoring cables. There is also lack of direct patient observation and high-level acoustic noise impeding monitoring alarms, which may delay decision-making and management of emergencies.

The patient is usually positioned with his or her head well away from the anesthesiologist, requiring extension tubing for the breathing circuit, intravenous (IV) lines, and intra-arterial catheter. The extension tubing on the IV lines require that additional fluid be used to flush medications into the patient.

INSPIRED OXYGEN CONCENTRATION

The MRI technologists and radiologists should be advised if 100% O_2 is administered to the patient during the scan. High concentrations of inspired oxygen may produce an artifact in the form of an abnormally high signal in cerebrospinal fluid (CSF) spaces in the T2-weighted fluid-attenuated inversion recovery (FLAIR) sequence.

SPECIFIC ISSUES RELATED TO MRI SAFETY

Specific terminology is used to describe whether equipment is safe to use around an MRI scanner and how close to the scanner a specific piece of equipment may be brought. The term *MRI Safe* refers to an item that does not contain any ferromagnetic material and poses no known hazards in all MRI environments. For example, an aluminum IV pole or plastic tubing holders may be safely brought into the magnetic field. An item that has been demonstrated to pose no known hazards in a specified MRI environment and under specified conditions is referred to as *MRI Conditional*. Many items now are marked as MRI conditional, and the conditions under which they can be safely used are listed and attached to the device [83]. For example, an infusion pump might safely be exposed to a magnetic field of 1.0 T, but its power supply must remain outside of the 1000 Gauss line. *MRI Unsafe* items (e.g., a steel oxygen tank) cannot be brought into the MRI environment [84–89].

Implanted devices may pose one of several hazards to patients in the MRI environments.

The time-varying magnetic field and radiofrequency energy may produce heating and burns. Injury may occur due to effects of the static magnetic field that causes movement or twisting of a ferromagnetic object, projectile effect, artifacts, and device malfunction [85, 90, 91]. For example, the pressure setting of programmable hydrocephalus shunts may be inadvertently changed by the magnetic field leading to overdrainage or underdrainage of CSF.

An estimated 50% to 75% patients with implanted cardiac devices are expected to need a MR scan during the lifetime of their device [92]. Until recently, however, the use of MRI scanners in patients with an implanted pacemaker was contraindicated because of the possibility that a relatively weak magnetic field of 5 Gauss could cause a fatal device malfunction. Concerns include:

- pacemaker or lead wires movement
- unexpected programming changes (e.g., resetting to default parameters)
- inhibition of pacemaker output
- inappropriate sensing of fast transients and elevated cardiac rates
- transient asynchronous pacing
- pacemaker reed switch malfunction
- rapid cardiac pacing
- the induction of ventricular fibrillation
- local thermogenic cardiac tissue destruction

Sudden deaths have in fact been reported in patients with pacemakers during or shortly after MRI investigations [93].

Presence of a permanent pacemaker no longer represents a strict contraindication to MR in carefully selected clinical circumstances provided that specific strategies are followed [94, 95], and several new devices have been approved for use in magnetic fields of up to 1.5 T.

Patients with aneurysm clips or cardiac/intracranial stents may or may not be able to undergo MRI depending on the type of device and the manufacturer, and the strength of the MRI magnetic field. When in doubt, the specifications should be obtained from the manufacturer of the device for compatibility before MRI is performed.

Patients with implanted neurostimulators should not undergo MR according to current recommendations. The primary concern is that the RF and gradient fields may interfere with the operation of these devices or cause thermal injury. Some manufacturers are, however, suggesting that MR examinations of specific devices may be safe if strict guidelines relating to scanning parameters, in particular to RF exposure, are followed [96].

HIGH-LEVEL ACOUSTIC NOISE

Extremely high noise levels above 85 decibels (the sound pressure level generally considered to be safe) can be produced during MRI due to rapid switching of the gradient coils. Staff working in MRI units should protect themselves by remaining in the MR control room during sequence acquisition or by wearing earplugs in the examination room. All patients must be given ear protection, regardless of whether they are awake or anesthetized. High ambient noise levels may mask monitor alarms or the sound of partial airway obstruction in an unintubated patient. It is also very difficult to communicate with other staff members during the scanning procedure. Vigilance and attention to visual cues are therefore essential [97].

CRYOGEN SAFETY (ZONE IV: THE ZONE WHERE THE MRI SCANNER IS LOCATED)

Liquid helium and liquid nitrogen are the most commonly used cryogens in high field MR environments.

- *Asphyxiation in oxygen-deficient atmospheres*—if exposed to room air or if the magnet is quenched, these cryogenic liquids will rapidly boil off and expand into a gaseous state, potentially replacing the air in the room. This may cause asphyxiation, which is why the oxygen content of room air is monitored in the MRI environment. One potential safety precaution is to connect a Jackson-Rees circuit and mask to supply of oxygen with long tubing. This could then be used if the room air becomes hypoxic.

- *Cold burns, frostbite, and hypothermia*—transient exposure to very cold gas produces discomfort in breathing and can provoke an attack of asthma in susceptible individuals.

- *Combustion and explosion hazard from oxygen enrichment of atmosphere*—liquid nitrogen can condense air from the atmosphere, which can lead to production of liquid containing a higher oxygen content than that of normal air. This higher oxygen content increases the combustibility of many materials, creating potentially explosive conditions.

CONTRAST REACTIONS

Gadolinium-based contrast agents (Gd-CAs) are used in MRI to improve visualization of vascular structures or to increase the contrast resolution of tissues. In comparison with other radiological contrast agents, Gd-CAs are relatively safe with a high therapeutic ratio and low incidence of anaphylaxis (approximately 1:100,000). Other side effects are mild and include headache, nausea and vomiting, local burning, skin wheals (2%) itching, sweating, facial swelling, and thrombophlebitis [98].

Patients with renal failure are at risk of developing a rare, potentially life-threatening condition with Gd-CAs called nephrogenic systemic fibrosis or nephrogenic fibrosing dermopathy (NSF or NFD). Patients at greatest risk for developing NSF after receiving GBCAs (gadolinium-based contrast agents) are those with impaired elimination of the drug, including patients with acute kidney injury (AKI) or chronic, severe kidney disease (with a glomerular filtration rate [GFR] <30 mL/min/1.73 m^2). Higher than recommended doses or repeat doses of GBCAs also appear to increase the risk for NSF. Use of the three of the GBCA drugs—Magnevist, Omniscan, and Optimark—are contraindicated in patients with AKI or with chronic, severe kidney disease [99].

Otherwise, the risk of Gd-CAs should be carefully considered, and the smallest possible dose of Gd-CAs should be administered only if an unenhanced scan proves insufficient. If repeated administration is planned, there should be a period of at least seven days between doses. The Gd-CAs are not recommended in pregnancy unless absolutely necessary [100, 101].

ANESTHETIC CONSIDERATIONS

SRS and stereotactic surgical procedures are complex, and the anesthesiologist plays a critical role throughout the perioperative period. The first step of a stereotactic procedure is usually application of the stereotactic frame with skull pins. The patient then undergoes CT or MRI to determine the exact three-dimensional position of the region of interest. After imaging, the patient is transported from the radiology suite back to the OR. This is a critical period because it involves transporting a sedated patient through the hospital with marginal access to the airway. The next step is the surgical procedure, which may include resection of a lesion, a partial or complete lobectomy, corpuscallosotomy, or a hemispherectomy (for seizure disorders), thalamotomy, pallidotomy, deep brain stimulator insertion (for MDs), or tumor resection for the localized tumor etc. In a patient with an MD (e.g., PD), a DBS electrode is inserted through a burr hole for microelectrode recordings (MER) and testing of the subthalamic nucleus stimulation in an awake patient. The electrode is secured to the skull and then connected to a lead that is tunneled to a pulse generator in the chest or abdomen.

The management of a specific patient will depend on the nature of the surgical procedure, coexisting medical problems, and other factors and varies from keeping the patient awake with monitored anesthesia care, conscious sedation, to general anesthesia. Details of the suggested anesthetic management options are described next. The anesthetic goals for SRS and stereotactic surgery include patient comfort and immobility (by providing adequate analgesia and sedation), all the while attempting to have an alert, cooperative patient to obtain appropriate intraoperative neurological assessments.

Anesthetics and sedatives should be chosen so as not to interfere with electrophysiological brain mapping and clinical testing. Many common GABAergic sedative drugs, including propofol and midazolam, ameliorate tremor or rigidity in patients undergoing functional neurosurgery. They also interfere with brain mapping and electroencephalography or testing of the implanted DBS electrode lead in these patients. Moreover, these medications easily impair the level of consciousness and may cause disinhibition or inability to cooperate with intraoperative testing, as well as respiratory depression, which can be very challenging to manage, especially with the patient's head fixed inside a metal head frame [91].

PREOPERATIVE EVALUATION

A detailed anesthestic assessment should be done prior to surgery. Preanesthesia workup should include the assessment of the surgical condition and any comorbidities, a review of imaging, as well as requisition of laboratory studies as needed. Patients with dystonia or torticollis may present difficulties in airway management and require careful assessment and planning. Although patients who are scheduled to undergo MRI during their procedure will be screened by the technologist performing the procedure, it is not unreasonable for the anesthesiologist to screen for the presence of implants or other contraindications to a strong magnetic field.

Psychological preparation of the patient is important for the long and potentially difficult awake procedures. It is therefore critically important to establish a rapport with the patient if the procedure will be done with the patient awake. At a minimum, positioning during the surgical procedure and details of planned invasive monitors should be discussed and informed consent should be obtained. The preanesthesia visit should also include an assessment of the

patient's anxiety level and reassurance that he or she will be made as comfortable as possible.

Patients with neurodegenerative disorders are often elderly and may have respiratory, cardiovascular, and autonomic system compromise. In general, medications used for treatment of motor symptoms should not be taken on the night before or on the morning of surgery, and this should be discussed with the patient's neurosurgeon. Other medications, such as antihypertensive agents, should be continued. Specific anesthetic considerations will apply to patients with different disorders, but in general preoperative benzodiazepines, opioids, and other sedatives can make the patient uncooperative or mask a tremor and therefore should be avoided.

Potential drug interactions and adverse effects from anti-Parkinson's medications may also occur during anesthesia. Ergot-derived dopamine agonists are associated with a higher incidence of cardiac valvular disorders [102]. Selective monoamine oxidase inhibitors may have serious interactions with meperidine and sympathomimetic agents, and the possibility of discontinuing these drugs should be discussed with the patient's treating physician [103]. Patients with psychiatric, epileptic and chronic pain disorders will present with their own set of challenges and will need special consideration in the management of their medications perioperatively [60, 63, 64, 104].

INTAROPERATIVE MANAGEMENT

At a minimum, intraoperative monitoring must comply with American Society of Anesthesiologists guidelines and should include an electrocardiogram, noninvasive arterial blood pressure, pulse oximetry, and respiratory gas monitoring. In most cases, tight control of systemic arterial blood pressure will require invasive blood pressure monitoring. Supplemental oxygen is delivered through a nasal cannula or via a mask with an outlet for end-tidal CO_2 and respiratory rate monitoring.

Proper positioning of the patient on the operating table is critical to ensuring patient comfort and cooperativeness. The head and neck should be positioned with a small degree of neck flexion and extension at the atlanto-occipital junction. This helps to improve airway patency and facilitates airway management if the airway must be secured during the procedure. The patient's legs should be flexed and supported under the knees to maintain stability when the head and back are elevated to a sitting position. Direct visual and verbal contact with the patient should be maintained throughout the procedure. The environment should be kept quiet, calm, and comfortable and the room temperature and humidity adjusted to make the patient comfortable. The decision to insert a urinary catheter is based on the characteristics of each patient and duration of the surgical procedure. It may be possible to omit a urinary catheter for shorter procedures if careful fluid balance is maintained.

LOCAL ANESTHESIA AND MONITORED ANESTHESIA CARE

Monitored anesthesia care with or without conscious sedation is generally preferred in patients who are undergoing insertion of a DBS using a stereotactic frame. This technique relies on local anesthesia augmented with judicious use of narcotics or other analgesics for pain relief in the beginning of the procedure. Infiltration of the subcutaneous tissue or placement of a scalp nerve block (supraorbital and occipital nerves) provides adequate surgical anesthesia. Bupivacaine, ropivacaine, and lidocaine can be used with or without epinephrine. Careful attention to the volume of local anesthetic that has been injected will minimize the risk of toxicity in patients who may already be prone to seizures. The maximum permissible dose is based on the patient's weight. The maximum dose of lidocaine is 5 mg/kg and up to 7 mg/kg with epinephrine, for bupivacaine 2 mg/kg (without epinephrine) and 3 mg/kg with epinephrine, and for ropivacaine 3.6 mg/kg with epinephrine. Repeated administration of local anesthesia may be required for prolonged procedures.

CONSCIOUS SEDATION TECHNIQUE

The use of conscious sedation (CS) aims to have a patient with a minimally depressed level of consciousness but one who is able to maintain his or her own airway and respond to verbal stimulation. Generally, there is no manipulation of the airway other than the administration of supplemental oxygen via a nasal cannula or a facemask. Sedation may be given throughout the whole procedure or can be administered intermittently during painful parts of the procedure. Frequently used drugs for CS include propofol, opioids such as fentanyl or remifentanil, and dexmedetomidine [105–107]. Benzodiazepines are usually avoided because they alter the threshold for stimulation and may inhibit accurate clinical assessment of the patient [108].

Propofol is one of the most frequently used drugs for both CS and general anesthesia in stereotactic procedures either alone or in combination with remifentanil. Propofol provides titratable sedation and a rapid, smooth recovery and minimizes interference with electrocorticographic recordings, lead placement, and stimulation testing. However, it will decrease the incidence of seizures, and has to be discontinued at least 15 to 30 minutes prior to electrocorticographic recordings [109, 110]. Propofol may also cause tonic–clonic movements mimicking seizures but will also effectively stop seizures. Retrospective analysis of an asleep-awake-asleep (AAA) technique using propofol and remifentanil showed that adequate conditions were obtained in 98% of patients, with a median wake-up time of 9 minutes [111]. The mean infusion rates of propofol reported in the literature are approximately 50 µg/kg/min. Propofol has been reported to reduce tremors, as well as to produce myoclonus movements [104, 112–114]. The possibility of propofol-induced dyskinesia and the suppression of tremors with remifentanil should be taken into consideration in the management of patients with PD.

Remifentanil, a potent ultra short-acting synthetic opioid, is commonly used to provide analgesia and sedation during neurosurgical procedures in awake patients. It offers the advantages of rapid titration and an ability to awaken the patient quickly for a neurological evaluation. It has, however, been reported to decrease tremors in patients with PD [63]. Opioids have been reported to produce epileptiform activity in patients with epilepsy, and at high doses may also produce myoclonic movements that may clinically resemble seizure-like activity. However, this does not appear to be a problem during awake craniotomies as the doses of opioids used are generally very low [111, 115, 116].

Dexmedetomidine, a centrally acting α_2-agonist that offers sedation and anxiolysis, may be the ideal sedative for stereotactic or awake procedures [112, 117–120]. Light sedation is generally achieved with a low-dose infusion (0.3–0.6 µg/kg/h). Because it is not mediated by GABA receptors, dexmedetomidine usually provides ideal conditions for MER, while maintaining hemodynamic stability and analgesia [119, 121, 122], although some neurosurgeons continue to prefer complete "sedation-free" environment during MER. In addition to its sedative effects, dexmedetomidine helps to prevent hypertension through its central α-agonist activity. Dexmedetomidine does not cause respiratory depression, even with infusions at the higher end of the dose range, and has an anesthetic-sparing effect. The cerebral effects are consistent with a desirable neurophysiological profile, including neuroprotective characteristics [123–125]. It is particularly useful when it is necessary to map areas of the brain responsible for language and an awake, cooperative patient must be capable of undergoing neurocognitive testing. Dexmedetomidine can be used as a sole agent, an adjunct, or a rescue drug for the awake craniotomy [119, 126, 127].

THE ASLEEP-AWAKE-ASLEEP AAA TECHNIQUE

The AAA anesthesia technique is frequently used for epilepsy surgery or tumor resection. It is especially useful when a tumor or epileptic focus is located near a critical area of the brain. Prior to resection, the epileptic focus is identified or the function of the brain cortex is mapped usually by MRI. Despite their rapid development and precision in imaging technologies, these methods may be complemented or superseded by the intraoperative mapping of cortical functions in the awake patient. After the brain is exposed, the neurosurgeon applies electrical stimulation to the exposed cortex of the awake patient and the patient is evaluated for sensory, motor, and speech effects as well as any effects on more complex cognitive functions. Additional testing can also be performed during resection of the lesion, and the resection is stopped if symptoms emerge. This allows maximal tumor resection while minimizing neurological deficits, hopefully offering improved postoperative quality of life, and a better chance of survival [128].

After the patient arrives in the OR, routine physiological monitors are applied and general anesthesia is induced. Airway patency can be maintained with an oral or nasopharyngeal airway, a cuffed oropharyngeal airway, a laryngeal mask airway (LMA), or an endotracheal tube. In general, a LMA is the preferred technique. Either an inhalation or an IV anesthetic technique may be used, with or without controlled ventilation. A continuous infusion of propofol is one widely accepted technique. After induction of general anesthesia, the patient is positioned, the head is fixed into the head holder and the surgical procedure begins. Skin infiltration with local anesthetic at pin insertion sites and the skin incision, or performance of a scalp nerve block, provides pain relief during the awake portion of the procedure and reduces opiate requirements.

When the neurosurgeon is ready to begin brain mapping, the patient is allowed to emerge from general anesthesia and the airway is removed. The transition from the "asleep" to the "awake" phase is one of the most challenging portions of the anesthetic because of the possibility of complications while awakening the patient and manipulating the airway while the brain is exposed. Coughing, a Valsalva maneuver, vomiting, and movement during LMA removal or tracheal extubation may cause life-threatening complications such as bleeding, brain swelling, and venous air embolism. Many anesthesiologists therefore try to minimize airway instrumentation whenever feasible. In this regard, a supraglottic airway such as LMA is preferred to an endotracheal tube.

After the testing is completed, general anesthesia or heavy sedation may be resumed and the airway may or may not be reinserted. When mapping is completed, patient can be returned to the "asleep" phase. Airway instrumentation when the patient's head is in pins and covered by the surgical drapes may be difficult, especially if emergency intubation of the trachea is required [118, 126, 129, 130].

The advantages of the AAA technique include increased patient comfort, a secured airway (which also offers the ability to use hyperventilation if necessary), and improved ability to tolerate the surgery, especially for longer procedures.

GENERAL ANESTHESIA

Patients groups more likely to require general anesthesia [65, 131, 132] are

- Infants and children
- Patients with learning difficulties
- Patients with certain seizure or continuous MDs
- Patients with severe pain
- Patients with claustrophobia
- Critically ill patients
- Patients undergoing neurological examinations, particularly where raised intracranial pressure is a concern (sedation is contraindicated as it can be potentially dangerous)

Intraoperative mapping and stimulation testing are difficult or impossible under general anesthesia. Awake craniotomy has been a well-established neurosurgical technique to minimize complications for lesions involving eloquent cortex. Recent clinical trials reported that the patients with supratentorial lesions in proximity to the eloquent cortex had better neurological outcome, maximal tumor removal and overall patient satisfaction with awake craniotomy (AC) than surgery under general anesthesia [133, 134]. However, these results have not always been consistent and have been challenged. Difference in series by Gupta et al. favoring general anesthesia over AC could be explained in part by the nonutilization of electrophysiological study/ brain mapping. Interestingly, in this series, surgical and KPS outcomes become statistically insignificant at 3-month follow-up [135].

General anesthesia has nonetheless been used in patients unable to tolerate awake DBS insertion [65, 131, 136, 137]. Yamada et al. found that the use of general anesthesia in 15 patients with PD did not adversely affect postoperative improvements in motor and daily activity scores, except for "off-medication" bradykinesia, compared with 10 patients treated under local anesthesia [131]. Lefaucheur et al. published a retrospective analysis of 54 patients undergoing DBS implantation. General anesthesia was induced by a propofol and remifentanil infusion with mechanical ventilation. During the electrophysiological recording time, propofol was reduced to a level that maintained the bispectral index at 60. In the retrospective analyses, the mode of anesthesia (general anesthesia versus local anesthesia) had no influence on the clinical outcome after DBS in patients with PD [136].

Schulz et al. analyzed the effects of bispectral index monitoring during general anesthesia for DBS in patients with MDs. Interestingly, they did not find a reduction in propofol use, nor did the patients wake up more rapidly during the test period [138]. General anesthesia also can be maintained with a potent volatile anesthetic (e.g., desflurane). As long as the minimal alveolar concentration (MAC) level was kept below 1, it did not drastically interfere with microelectrode mapping [139].

General anesthesia has several disadvantages in functional neurosurgery. For example, surgery for PD is associated with intraoperative respiratory and cardiovascular complications, as well as neurological exacerbations including rigidity, confusion, and prolonged recovery time

[60, 64, 140]. The ability to perform neurological evaluations during the procedure is lost, as is the ability to identify collateral effects of stimulation such as dysarthria and motor responses. For epilepsy surgery, if intraoperative localization of an epileptic focus is planned, the influence of anesthetic agents should be kept to a minimum. (It is, however, also important to be cognizant of the risk of awareness.) The preoperative discussion should include a discussion of the possibility of awareness and recall during electrocorticographic recording, and should also include reassurance that if awareness occurs, it will be brief and painless. All anesthetics affect electrocorticography, but the use of the shorter-acting anesthetic agents, either inhalation agents and/or intravenous agents, will allow for more rapid changes in the depth of anesthesia. During the time of recording, all or most of the anesthetic agents should be stopped or kept to a minimum. Long-term anticonvulsant therapy may lead to increased dosage requirements of opioids and neuromuscular blocking agents [115], and these effects should be taken into account. If the patient has had a recent craniotomy or burr holes for electrode placement, intracranial air might still be present and nitrous oxide should be avoided to prevent complications from an expanding pneumocephalus. Complications that may occur during epilepsy surgery are similar to those for any craniotomy, but severe bradycardia is a common occurrence during resection of the amygdalohippocampus [141].

COMPLICATIONS

A high level of suspicion and vigilance are required for detection of complications during stereotactic surgery. Intraoperative respiratory complications are common and may result from patient positioning, excessive sedation, and restrictive pulmonary dysfunction associated with PD. The presence of the fixed stereotactic frame makes airway management difficult and potentially dangerous. Slipping downward on the table while head is fixed has resulted in complete upper airway obstruction even in non-sedated patients. Should it become necessary to secure the airway but the patient is not in distress, intubating the patient without removing the head frame will allow the surgery to proceed. If, however, urgent intubation is required, the frame should be removed from the patient so that the airway can be rapidly secured. Appropriate airway equipment such as oral and nasal airways, LMAs, endotracheal tubes, laryngoscope, and fiberoptic bronchoscope should be immediately available [142].

The incidence of intracerebral hemorrhage after DBS is about 2% to 4%. Possible risk factors include a history of chronic hypertension or acute intraoperative hypertension. Hypertension occurs frequently, especially when the patient is awake. Tight blood pressure control is therefore required because intracranial hemorrhage, particularly along the electrode trajectory, has been associated with

arterial hypertension. Evidence suggests that maintaining a systolic blood pressure of less than 140 mm Hg may be protective. Judicious use of sedation will help to prevent hypertension. Other useful vasoactive agents may include labetalol, hydralazine, nitroglycerine, sodium nitroprusside, and esmolol [143–145].

Venous air embolism may occur during creation of a burr hole in awake patients; the first sign is frequently sudden vigorous coughing. Other signs are unexplained chest pain, nausea, hypoxemia, and hypotension. Earlier detection may be possible with precordial Doppler monitoring. The incidence of venous air embolism in the recumbent position is estimated at around 3% to 4.5% [146]. Management is largely supportive and includes flooding the surgical field with fluid, cauterization of open veins, and liberal application of bone wax to the exposed bone. If the airway is not secured but the patient requires immediate ventilation, an LMA may be inserted as a rescue maneuver until the head frame can be removed. N_2O should be immediately discontinued and replaced with 100% O_2. The blood pressure should be supported with fluid and vasopressors. If possible, the patient should be put into the Trendelenberg position to bring the operative site below the level of the heart. If available, a central venous catheter may be advanced into the right atrium in order to aspirate air. Preventive measures include avoidance of hypovolemia (as hydration increases central venous pressure [CVP]), which in turn decreases the pressure gradient between the surgical site and CVP. Furthermore, adequate volume status is associated with increased left atrial pressure, which minimizes the risk of paradoxical air embolism to the left side of the circulation [147].

Neurological complications may occur during or after the procedure [34, 35, 41]. Seizures may occur especially during stimulation testing. Most seizures are focal and do not require treatment. In cases of tonic–clonic seizures prior to electrocorticographic recordings, seizures can be treated with a small dose of thiopental or propofol; afterward, benzodiazepines or longer-acting anticonvulsants may be used. A sudden loss of consciousness due to an intracranial bleed or from a major neurological injury will require rapid treatment. This would usually include aborting the surgical procedure and the implementation of the full resuscitation regimen of supporting airway, breathing, and circulation.

CONCLUSION

The neurosurgical scope of SRS and stereotactical surgical procedures is ever-expanding, and other than Gamma Knife and cyberknife, many of these procedures require sedation or general anesthesia or both. Recognition of the neurosurgical demands and the procedures involved would allow the anesthesiologist to design the optimal sedation/anesthetic regimen for the patient involved, with the ultimate goal of improving patient safety.

REFERENCES

1. Horsley V, Clarke RH. The structure and functions of the cerebellum examined by a new method. *Brain.* 1908;31:45–124.
2. Spiegel EA, Wycis HT, Marks M, et al. Stereotaxic apparatus for operations on the human brain. *Science.* 1947;106:349–350.
3. Spiegel EA, Wycis HT, Baird HW 3rd. Long-range effects of electropallidoansotomy in extrapyramidal and convulsive disorders. *Neurology.* 1958;8:734–740.
4. Spiegel EA. Methodological problems in stereoencephalotomy. *Confin Neurol.* 1965;26:125–132.
5. Leksell L. The stereotaxic method and radiosurgery of the brain. *Acta Chir Scand.* 1951;102:316–319.
6. Larsson B, Leksell L, Rexed B, et al. The high-energy proton beam as a neurosurgical tool. *Nature.* 1958;182:1222–1223.
7. Leksell L, Larsson B, Andersson B, et al. Lesions in the depth of the brain produced by a beam of high energy protons. *Acta Radiol.* 1960;54:251–264.
8. Larsson B, Leksell L, Rexed B. The use of high energy protons for cerebral surgery in man. *Acta Chir Scand (Sweden).* 1963;125: 1–5.
9. Steiner L, Leksell L, Greitz T, et al. Stereotaxic radiosurgery for cerebral arteriovenous malformations. Report of a case. *Acta Chir Scand.* 1972;138:459–464.
10. Bergstrom M, Greitz T. Stereotaxic computed tomography. *AJR Am J Roentgenol.* 1976;127:167–170.
11. Leksell L, Jernberg B. Stereotaxis and tomography. A technical note. *Acta Neurochir (Wien).* 1980;52(1-2):1–7.
12. Leksell L, Leksell D, Schwebel J. Stereotaxis and nuclear magnetic resonance. *J Neurol Neurosurg Psychiatry.* 1985;48:14–18.
13. Lunsford LD, Maitz A, Lindner G. First United States 201 source cobalt-60 gamma unit for radiosurgery. *Appl Neurophysiol.* 1987;50:253–256.
14. Lutz W, Winston KR, Maleki N. A system for stereotactic radiosurgery with a linear accelerator. *Int J Radiat Oncol Biol Phys.* 1988;14:373–381.
15. Winston KR, Lutz W. Linear accelerator as a neurosurgical tool for stereotactic radiosurgery. *Neurosurgery.* 1988;22:454–464.
16. Rahman M, Murad GJ, Bova F, et al. Stereotactic radiosurgery and the linear accelerator: accelerating electrons in neurosurgery. *Neurosurg Focus.* 2009;27:E13.
17. Adler JR Jr, Chang SD, Murphy MJ, et al. The Cyberknife: a frameless robotic system for radiosurgery. *Stereotact Funct Neurosurg.* 1997;69:124–128.
18. Lasak JM, Gorecki JP. The history of stereotactic radiosurgery and radiotherapy. *Otolaryngol Clin North Am.* 2009;42:593–599.
19. Gehring MA, Mackie TR, Kubsad SS, et al. A three-dimensional volume visualization package applied to stereotactic radiosurgery treatment planning. *Int J Radiat Oncol Biol Phys.* 1991;21:491–500.
20. Colombo F, Benedetti A, Pozza F, et al. External stereotactic irradiation by linear accelerator. *Neurosurgery.* 1985;16:154–160.
21. Betti O, Derechinsky V. [Multiple-beam stereotaxic irradiation]. *Neurochirurgie.* 1983;29:295–298.
22. Seifert V, Stolke D, Mehdorn HM, et al. Clinical and radiological evaluation of long-term results of stereotactic proton beam radiosurgery in patients with cerebral arteriovenous malformations. *J Neurosurg.* 1994;81:683–689.
23. Weber DC, Chan AW, Bussiere MR, et al. Proton beam radiosurgery for vestibular schwannoma: tumor control and cranial nerve toxicity. *Neurosurgery.* 2003;53:577–586; discussion 86–88.
24. Rowe J, Grainger A, Walton L, et al. Risk of malignancy after gamma knife stereotactic radiosurgery. *Neurosurgery.* 2007;60:60–65; discussion 5–6.
25. Starke RM, Williams BJ, Hiles C, et al. Gamma Knife surgery for skull base meningiomas. *J Neurosurg.* 2012;116:588–597.
26. Karpinos M, Teh BS, Zeck O, et al. Treatment of acoustic neuroma: stereotactic radiosurgery vs. microsurgery. *Int J Radiat Oncol Biol Phys.* 2002;54:1410–1421.
27. Pollock BE. Vestibular schwannoma management: an evidence-based comparison of stereotactic radiosurgery and microsurgical resection. *Prog Neurol Surg.* 2008;21:222–227.
28. Keles GE, Anderson B, Berger MS. The effect of extent of resection on time to tumor progression and survival in patients with glioblastoma multiforme of the cerebral hemisphere. *Surg Neurol.* 1999;52:371–379.
29. Johnson WD, Loredo LN, Slater JD. Surgery and radiotherapy: complementary tools in the management of benign intracranial tumors. *Neurosurg Focus.* 2008;24:E2.
30. Sekhar LN, Sen CN, Jho HD, et al. Surgical treatment of intracavernous neoplasms: a four-year experience. *Neurosurgery.* 1989;24:18–30.
31. De Jesus O, Sekhar LN, Parikh HK, et al. Long-term follow-up of patients with meningiomas involving the cavernous sinus: recurrence, progression, and quality of life. *Neurosurgery.* 1996;39:915–919; discussion 9–20.
32. Patchell RA. The management of brain metastases. *Cancer Treat Rev.* 2003;29:533–540.
33. Muacevic A, Wowra B, Siefert A, et al. Microsurgery plus whole brain irradiation versus Gamma Knife surgery alone for treatment of single metastases to the brain: a randomized controlled multicentre phase III trial. *J Neurooncol.* 2008;87:299–307.
34. Patchell RA, Tibbs PA, Walsh JW, et al. A randomized trial of surgery in the treatment of single metastases to the brain. *N Engl J Med.* 1990;322:494–500.
35. Vecht CJ, Haaxma-Reiche H, Noordijk EM, et al. Treatment of single brain metastasis: radiotherapy alone or combined with neurosurgery? *Ann Neurol.* 1993;33:583–590.
36. Linskey ME, Andrews DW, Asher AL, et al. The role of stereotactic radiosurgery in the management of patients with newly diagnosed brain metastases: a systematic review and evidence-based clinical practice guideline. *J Neurooncol.* 2010;96:45–68.
37. Kobayashi T, Kida Y, Hasegawa T. Long-term results of gamma knife surgery for craniopharyngioma. *Neurosurg Focus.* 2003;14:e13.
38. Chung WY, Pan DH, Shiau CY, et al. Gamma knife radiosurgery for craniopharyngiomas. *J Neurosurg.* 2000;93(Suppl 3):47–56.
39. Sheehan J, Yen CP, Arkha Y, et al. Gamma knife surgery for trigeminal schwannoma. *J Neurosurg.* 2007;106:839–845.
40. Pannullo SC, Fraser JF, Moliterno J, et al. Stereotactic radiosurgery: a meta-analysis of current therapeutic applications in neuro-oncologic disease. *J Neurooncol.* 2011;103:1–17.
41. van Beijnum J, van der Worp HB, Buis DR, et al. Treatment of brain arteriovenous malformations: a systematic review and meta-analysis. *JAMA.* 2011;306:2011–2019.
42. Colombo F, Pozza F, Chierego G, et al. Linear accelerator radiosurgery of cerebral arteriovenous malformations: an update. *Neurosurgery.* 1994;34:14–20; discussion -1.
43. Friedman WA. Radiosurgery for arteriovenous malformations. *Clin Neurosurg.* 1995;42:328–347.
44. Pollock BE. Stereotactic radiosurgery for arteriovenous malformations. *Neurosurg Clin N Am.* 1999;10:281–290.
45. Lunsford LD, Kondziolka D, Flickinger JC, et al. Stereotactic radiosurgery for arteriovenous malformations of the brain. *J Neurosurg.* 1991;75:512–524.
46. Farhat HI. Cerebral arteriovenous malformations. *Dis Mon.* 2011;57:625–637.
47. Pollock BE, Phuong LK, Gorman DA, et al. Stereotactic radiosurgery for idiopathic trigeminal neuralgia. *J Neurosurg.* 2002;97: 347–353.
48. Huang CF, Kondziolka D, Flickinger JC, et al. Stereotactic radiosurgery for trigeminal schwannomas. *Neurosurgery.* 1999;45:11–16; discussion 6.
49. Regis J, Manera L, Dufour H, et al. Effect of the Gamma Knife on trigeminal neuralgia. *Stereotact Funct Neurosurg.* 1995;64(Suppl 1):182–192.
50. Fountas KN, Smith JR, Lee GP, et al. Gamma Knife stereotactic radiosurgical treatment of idiopathic trigeminal neuralgia: long-term outcome and complications. *Neurosurgical Focus.* 2007;23:E8.

51. Pollock BE, Foote RL, Stafford SL, et al. Results of repeated gamma knife radiosurgery for medically unresponsive trigeminal neuralgia. *J Neurosurg.* 2000;93(Suppl 3):162–164.

52. Kondziolka D, Zorro O, Lobato-Polo J, et al. Gamma Knife stereotactic radiosurgery for idiopathic trigeminal neuralgia. *J Neurosurg.* ;2010;112:758–765.

53. Kano H, Kondziolka D, Niranjan A, et al. Gamma Knife stereotactic radiosurgery in the management of cluster headache. *Curr Pain Headache Rep.* 2011;15:118–123.

54. Lazzara BM, Ortiz O, Bordia R, et al. Cyberknife radiosurgery in treating trigeminal neuralgia. *J Neurointerv Surg.* 2013;5:81–85.

55. Elaimy AL, Hanson PW, Lamoreaux WT, et al. Clinical outcomes of gamma knife radiosurgery in the treatment of patients with trigeminal neuralgia. *Int J Otolaryngol.* 2012;2012:919186.

56. Bartolomei F, Hayashi M, Tamura M, et al. Long-term efficacy of gamma knife radiosurgery in mesial temporal lobe epilepsy. *Neurology.* 2008;70:1658–1663.

57. Regis J, Rey M, Bartolomei F, et al. Gamma knife surgery in mesial temporal lobe epilepsy: a prospective multicenter study. *Epilepsia.* 2004;45:504–515.

58. Malikova H, Vojtech Z, Liscak R, et al. Microsurgical and stereotactic radiofrequency amygdalohippocampectomy for the treatment of mesial temporal lobe epilepsy: different volume reduction, similar clinical seizure control. *Stereotact Funct Neurosurg.* 2010;88:42–50.

59. Elaimy AL, Arthurs BJ, Lamoreaux WT, et al. Gamma knife radiosurgery for movement disorders: a concise review of the literature. *World J Surg Oncol.* 2010;8:61.

60. Nicholson G, Pereira AC, Hall GM. Parkinson's disease and anaesthesia. *Br J Anaesth.* 2002;89:904–916.

61. Fabregas N, Rapado J, Gambus PL, et al. Modeling of the sedative and airway obstruction effects of propofol in patients with Parkinson disease undergoing stereotactic surgery. *Anesthesiology.* 2002;97:1378–1386.

62. Gray H, Wilson S, Sidebottom P. Parkinson's disease and anaesthesia. *Br J Anaesth.* 2003;90:524; author reply 525.

63. Bohmdorfer W, Schwarzinger P, Binder S, et al. [Temporary suppression of tremor by remifentanil in a patient with Parkinson's disease during cataract extraction under local anesthesia]. *Anaesthesist.* 2003;52:795–797.

64. Burton DA, Nicholson G, Hall GM. Anaesthesia in elderly patients with neurodegenerative disorders: special considerations. *Drugs Aging.* 2004;21:229–242.

65. Maltete D, Navarro S, Welter ML, et al. Subthalamic stimulation in Parkinson disease: with or without anesthesia? *Arch Neurol.* 2004;61:390–392.

66. Nuttin BJ, Gabriels LA, Cosyns PR, et al. Long-term electrical capsular stimulation in patients with obsessive-compulsive disorder. *Neurosurgery.* 2003;52:1263–1272; discussion 72–74.

67. Friehs GM, Park MC, Goldman MA, et al. Stereotactic radiosurgery for functional disorders. *Neurosurg Focus.* 2007;23:E3.

68. Greenberg BD, Price LH, Rauch SL, et al. Neurosurgery for intractable obsessive-compulsive disorder and depression: critical issues. *Neurosurg Clin N Am.* 2003;14:199–212.

69. Purcell EM, Torrey HC, Pound RV. Resonance absorption by nuclear magnetic moments in a solid. *Am Phys Soc.* 1946;69:37–38.

70. Bloembergen N, et al. Relaxation effects in nuclear magnetic resonance absorption. *Am Phys Soc.* 1948;73:679–712.

71. Bloch F, et al. The nuclear induction experiment. *Am Phys Soc.* 1946;70:474–485.

72. Lauterburg P. Image formation by induced local interactions: examples employing nuclear magnetic resonance. *Nature.* 1973;242:190–191.

73. Jolesz FA. 1996 RSNA Eugene P. Pendergrass New Horizons Lecture. Image-guided procedures and the operating room of the future. *Radiology.* 1997;204:601–612.

74. Kahn T, Schmidt F, Modder U. [MR imaging-guided interventions]. *Radiologe.* 1999;39:741–749.

75. Jolesz FA. Future perspectives in intraoperative imaging. *Acta Neurochir Suppl.* 2003;85:7–13.

76. Davis PD, Kenny GNC. *Basic physics & measurement in anaesthesia.* 5th ed. Elsevier Butterworth-Heinemann; 2003.

77. Dorward NL, Alberti O, Velani B, et al. Postimaging brain distortion: magnitude, correlates, and impact on neuronavigation. *J Neurosurg.* 1998;88:656–662.

78. Berger MS, Deliganis AV, Dobbins J, et al. The effect of extent of resection on recurrence in patients with low grade cerebral hemisphere gliomas. *Cancer.* 1994;74:1784–1791.

79. Laws ER, Parney IF, Huang W, et al. Survival following surgery and prognostic factors for recently diagnosed malignant glioma: data from the Glioma Outcomes Project. *J Neurosurg.* 2003;99:467–473.

80. Hill DL, Maurer CR Jr, Maciunas RJ, et al. Measurement of intraoperative brain surface deformation under a craniotomy. *Neurosurgery.* 1998;43:514–526; discussion 27–28.

81. Bergese SD, Puente EG. Anesthesia in the intraoperative MRI environment. *Neurosurg Clin N Am.* 2009;20:155–162.

82. Guidance for industry and FDA staff: establishing safety and compatibility of passive implants in the magnetic resonance (MR) environment. 2008. http://www.fda.gov/downloads/MedicalDevices/DeviceRegulationandGuidance/GuidanceDocuments/UCM107708.pdf

83. Farling P, McBrien ME, Winder RJ. Magnetic resonance compatible equipment: read the small print! *Anaesthesia.* 2003;58:86–87.

84. Shellock FG, Crues JV 3rd. MR safety and the American College of Radiology White Paper. *AJR Am J Roentgenol.* 2002;178:1349–1352.

85. Shellock FG, Crues JV. MR procedures: biologic effects, safety, and patient care. *Radiology.* 2004;232:635–652.

86. Shellock FG, Spinazzi A. MRI safety update 2008: part 2, screening patients for MRI. *AJR Am J Roentgenol.* 2008;191:1140–1149.

87. Woods TO. Standards for medical devices in MRI: present and future. *J Magn Reson Imaging.* 2007;26:1186–1189.

88. Guidance for industry and FDA staff: establishing safety and compatibility of passive implants in the magnetic resonance (MR) environment 2008 [updated August 21, 2008. http://www.fda.gov/downloads/MedicalDevices/DeviceRegulationandGuidance/GuidanceDocuments/ucm107708.pdf

89. Farling PA, Flynn PA, Darwent G, et al. Safety in magnetic resonance units: an update. *Anaesthesia.*2010;65:766–770.

90. Chung SM. Safety issues in magnetic resonance imaging. *J Neuroophthalmol.* 2002;22:35–39.

91. Stecco A, Saponaro A, Carriero A. Patient safety issues in magnetic resonance imaging: state of the art. *Radiol Med.* 2007;112:491–508.

92. Kalin R, Stanton MS. Current clinical issues for MRI scanning of pacemaker and defibrillator patients. *Pacing Clin Electrophysiol.* 2005;28:326–328.

93. Ferris NJ, Kavnoudias H, Thiel C, et al. The 2005 Australian MRI safety survey. *AJR Am J Roentgenol.* 2007;188:1388–1394.

94. Martin ET, Coman JA, Shellock FG, et al. Magnetic resonance imaging and cardiac pacemaker safety at 1.5-Tesla. *J Am Coll Cardiol.* 2004;43:1315–1324.

95. Martin ET. Can cardiac pacemakers and magnetic resonance imaging systems co-exist? *Eur Heart J.* 2005;26:325–327.

96. Device Bulletin Safety Guidelines for Magnetic Resonance Imaging Equipment in Clinical Use DB2007(03) December 2007 http://www.mhra.gov.uk/Publications/Safety guidance/DeviceBulletins/CON2033018 (accessed May 21, 2013).

97. Sesay M, Tauzin-Fin P, Jeannin A, et al. Audibility of anaesthesia alarms during magnetic resonance imaging: should we be alarmed? *Eur J Anaesthesiol.* 2009;26:117–122.

98. Li A, Wong CS, Wong MK, et al. Acute adverse reactions to magnetic resonance contrast media—gadolinium chelates. *Br J Radiol.* 2006;79:368–371.

99. FDA Drug Safety Communication. New warnings for using gadolinium-based contrast agents in patients with kidney dysfunction. 2010. http://www.fda.gov/Drugs/DrugSafety/ucm223966.htm

100. Shellock FG, Spinazzi A. MRI safety update 2008: part 1, MRI contrast agents and nephrogenic systemic fibrosis. *AJR Am J Roentgenol.* 2008;191:1129–1139.

101. Agarwal R, Brunelli SM, Williams K, et al. Gadolinium-based contrast agents and nephrogenic systemic fibrosis: a systematic review and meta-analysis. *Nephrol Dial Transplant.* 2009;24:856–863.

102. Zanettini R, Antonini A, Gatto G, et al. Valvular heart disease and the use of dopamine agonists for Parkinson's disease. *N Engl J Med.* 2007;356:39–46.

103. Gillman PK. Monoamine oxidase inhibitors, opioid analgesics and serotonin toxicity. *Br J Anaesth.* 2005;95:434–441.

104. Krauss JK, Akeyson EW, Giam P, et al. Propofol-induced dyskinesias in Parkinson's disease. *Anesth Analg.* 1996;83:420–422.

105. Erickson KM, Cole DJ. Anesthetic considerations for awake craniotomy for epilepsy. *Anesthesiol Clin.* 2007;25:535–555, ix.

106. Skucas AP, Artru AA. Anesthetic complications of awake craniotomies for epilepsy surgery. *Anesth Analg.* 2006;102:882–887.

107. Manninen PH, Balki M, Lukitto K, et al. Patient satisfaction with awake craniotomy for tumor surgery: a comparison of remifentanil and fentanyl in conjunction with propofol. *Anesth Analg.* 2006;102:237–242.

108. Davies A. Midazolam-induced dyskinesia. *Palliat Med.* 2000;14: 435–436.

109. Samra SK, Sneyd JR, Ross DA, et al. Effects of propofol sedation on seizures and intracranially recorded epileptiform activity in patients with partial epilepsy. *Anesthesiology.* 1995;82:843–851.

110. Herrick IA, Craen RA, Gelb AW, et al. Propofol sedation during awake craniotomy for seizures: patient-controlled administration versus neurolept analgesia. *Anesth Analg.* 1997;84:1285–1291.

111. Keifer JC, Dentchev D, Little K, et al. A retrospective analysis of a remifentanil/propofol general anesthetic for craniotomy before awake functional brain mapping. *Anesth Analg.* 2005;101:502–508, table of contents.

112. Khatib R, Ebrahim Z, Rezai A, et al. Perioperative events during deep brain stimulation: the experience at cleveland clinic. *J Neurosurg Anesthesiol.* 2008;20:36–40.

113. Lotto M, Boulis NM. Intrathecal opioids for control of chronic low back pain during deep brain stimulation procedures. *Anesth Analg.* 2007;105:1410–1412, table of contents.

114. Deiner S, Hagen J. Parkinson's disease and deep brain stimulator placement. *Anesthesiol Clin.* 2009;27:391–415, table of contents.

115. Kofke WA, Tempelhoff R, Dasheiff RM. Anesthetic implications of epilepsy, status epilepticus, and epilepsy surgery. *J Neurosurg Anesthesiol.* 1997;9:349–372.

116. Herrick IA, Craen RA, Blume WT, et al. Sedative doses of remifentanil have minimal effect on ECoG spike activity during awake epilepsy surgery. *J Neurosurg Anesthesiol.* 2002;14:55–58.

117. Souter MJ, Rozet I, Ojemann JG, et al. Dexmedetomidine sedation during awake craniotomy for seizure resection: effects on electrocorticography. *J Neurosurg Anesthesiol.* 2007;19:38–44.

118. Ard JL Jr, Bekker AY, Doyle WK. Dexmedetomidine in awake craniotomy: a technical note. *Surg Neurol.* 2005;63:114–116; discussion 6–7.

119. Rozet I, Muangman S, Vavilala MS, et al. Clinical experience with dexmedetomidine for implantation of deep brain stimulators in Parkinson's disease. *Anesth Analg.* 2006;103:1224–1228.

120. Talke P, Stapelfeldt C, Garcia P. Dexmedetomidine does not reduce epileptiform discharges in adults with epilepsy. *J Neurosurg Anesthesiol.* 2007;19:195–199.

121. Rozet I. Anesthesia for functional neurosurgery: the role of dexmedetomidine. *Curr Opin Anaesthesiol.* 2008;21:537–543.

122. Elias WJ, Durieux ME, Huss D, et al. Dexmedetomidine and arousal affect subthalamic neurons. *Mov Disord.* 2008;23:1317–1320.

123. Kuhmonen J, Pokorny J, Miettinen R, et al. Neuroprotective effects of dexmedetomidine in the gerbil hippocampus after transient global ischemia. *Anesthesiology.* 1997;87:371–377.

124. Kuhmonen J, Haapalinna A, Sivenius J. Effects of dexmedetomidine after transient and permanent occlusion of the middle cerebral artery in the rat. *J Neural Transm.* 2001;108:261–271.

125. Dahmani S, Paris A, Jannier V, et al. Dexmedetomidine increases hippocampal phosphorylated extracellular signal-regulated protein kinase 1 and 2 content by an alpha 2-adrenoceptor-independent mechanism: evidence for the involvement of imidazoline I1 receptors. *Anesthesiology.* 2008;108:457–466.

126. Mack PF, Perrine K, Kobylarz E, et al. Dexmedetomidine and neurocognitive testing in awake craniotomy. *J Neurosurg Anesthesiol.* 2004;16:20–25.

127. Moore TA 2nd, Markert JM, Knowlton RC. Dexmedetomidine as rescue drug during awake craniotomy for cortical motor mapping and tumor resection. *Anesth Analg.* 2006;102:1556–1558.

128. Sanai N, Berger MS. Operative techniques for gliomas and the value of extent of resection. *Neurotherapeutics.* 2009;6:478–486.

129. Bekker AY, Kaufman B, Samir H, et al. The use of dexmedetomidine infusion for awake craniotomy. *Anesth Analg.* 2001;92:1251–1253.

130. Huncke K, Van de Wiele B, Fried I, et al. The asleep-awake-asleep anesthetic technique for intraoperative language mapping. *Neurosurgery.* 1998;42:1312–1316; discussion 6–7.

131. Yamada K, Goto S, Kuratsu J, et al. Stereotactic surgery for subthalamic nucleus stimulation under general anesthesia: a retrospective evaluation of Japanese patients with Parkinson's disease. *Parkinsonism Relat Disord.* 2007;13:101–107.

132. Hertel F, Zuchner M, Weimar I, et al. Implantation of electrodes for deep brain stimulation of the subthalamic nucleus in advanced Parkinson's disease with the aid of intraoperative microrecording under general anesthesia. *Neurosurgery.* 2006;59:E1138; discussion E.

133. Manchella S, Khurana VG, Duke D, et al. The experience of patients undergoing awake craniotomy for intracranial masses: expectations, recall, satisfaction and functional outcome. *Br J Neurosurg.* 2011;25:391–400.

134. Sacko O, Lauwers-Cances V, Brauge D, et al. Awake craniotomy vs surgery under general anesthesia for resection of supratentorial lesions. *Neurosurgery.* 2011;68:1192–1198; discussion 8–9.

135. Gupta DK, Chandra PS, Ojha BK, et al. Awake craniotomy versus surgery under general anesthesia for resection of intrinsic lesions of eloquent cortex—a prospective randomised study. *Clin Neurol Neurosurg.* 2007;109:335–343.

136. Lefaucheur JP, Gurruchaga JM, Pollin B, et al. Outcome of bilateral subthalamic nucleus stimulation in the treatment of Parkinson's disease: correlation with intra-operative multi-unit recordings but not with the type of anaesthesia. *Eur Neurol.* 2008;60:186–199.

137. Machado A, Rezai AR, Kopell BH, et al. Deep brain stimulation for Parkinson's disease: surgical technique and perioperative management. *Mov Disord.* 2006;21(Suppl 14):S247–S258.

138. Schulz U, Keh D, Barner C, et al. Bispectral index monitoring does not improve anesthesia performance in patients with movement disorders undergoing deep brain stimulating electrode implantation. *Anesth Analg.* 2007;104:1481–1487, table of contents.

139. Lin SH, Chen TY, Lin SZ, et al. Subthalamic deep brain stimulation after anesthetic inhalation in Parkinson disease: a preliminary study. *J Neurosurg.* 2008;109:238–244.

140. Mason LJ, Cojocaru TT, Cole DJ. Surgical intervention and anesthetic management of the patient with Parkinson's disease. *Int Anesthesiol Clin.* 1996 Fall;34:133–150.

141. Sato K, Shamoto H, Yoshimoto T. Severe bradycardia during epilepsy surgery. *J Neurosurg Anesthesiol.* 2001;13:329–332.

142. Venkatraghavan L, Manninen P, Mak P, Lukitto K, et al. Anesthesia for functional neurosurgery: review of complications. *J Neurosurg Anesthesiol.* 2006;18:64–67.

143. Santos P, Valero R, Arguis MJ, et al. [Preoperative adverse events during stereotactic microelectrode-guided deep brain

surgery in Parkinson's disease]. *Rev Esp Anestesiol Reanim.* 2004;51:523–530.

144. Binder DK, Rau GM, Starr PA. Risk factors for hemorrhage during microelectrode-guided deep brain stimulator implantation for movement disorders. *Neurosurgery.* 2005;56:722–732; discussion -32.

145. Gorgulho A, De Salles AA, Frighetto L, et al. Incidence of hemorrhage associated with electrophysiological studies performed using macroelectrodes and microelectrodes in functional neurosurgery. *J Neurosurg.* 2005;102:888–896.

146. Hooper AK, Okun MS, Foote KD, et al. Venous air embolism in deep brain stimulation. *Stereotact Funct Neurosurg.* 2009;87:25–30.

147. Balki M, Manninen PH, McGuire GP, et al. Venous air embolism during awake craniotomy in a supine patient. *Can J Anaesth.* 2003;50:835–838.

16.

AWAKE CRANIOTOMY

John Ard

INTRODUCTION

Awake craniotomy may be new to most anesthesiologists, but it has its beginning in antiquity. Trephined skulls dating back thousands of years have been found in South America and other parts of the world (Figure 16.1). Not much is known about these ancient neurosurgical patients, but it seems likely that the anesthesia provided was rudimentary at best.

Thierry de Martel (1876–1940), a leading neurosurgeon in France, was the first modern neurosurgeon to advocate for awake craniotomy [1]. And in an attempt to avoid deaths due to improper ether anesthesia, Harvey Cushing, the father of modern neurosurgery, began to experiment with nerve blocks using cocaine [2]. Cushing first used local anesthesia while caring for patients with traumatic injuries during World War I, and subsequently applied it to all other cranial work. From 1917 to 1932, local anesthesia was used almost universally in neurosurgical suites [1].

Eventually, better general anesthetics, better trained anesthesia providers, and better monitoring and equipment led to the replacement of local anesthesia with general endotracheal anesthesia as the predominant anesthetic technique. Awake craniotomy is still performed and may be the technique of choice when an awake patient is the best monitor of neurological function.

INDICATIONS FOR AWAKE CRANIOTOMY

The usual indication for an awake craniotomy is the surgical resection of a lesion near eloquent areas of the brain, including language, motor, and sensory areas as well as the visual cortex. The lesion may be a seizure focus, tumor, or vascular malformation. If the lesion is distant from the identified area, the surgeon can be aggressive with the resection. If the lesion is near or part of eloquent area, the surgeon can perform a partial resection and avoid causing a neurological deficit in the patient.

An awake, cooperative patient allows the surgeon to perform intraoperative cortical mapping to identify critical areas before starting a resection. The mapping is done using direct cortical electrical stimulation. While the surgeon stimulates the cortex, another doctor (neurologist or neuropsychologist) asks the patient to perform language, perceptual, motor, or sensory tasks that are disrupted when the cortex associated with that area is stimulated. This procedure is repeated until the eloquent areas are delineated.

Additionally, functional neurosurgical procedures like deep brain stimulator insertion for Parkinson's disease often require an awake patient [3]. The awake state is preferred by many neurosurgeons because intraoperative testing and patient feedback can help the surgeon place the deep brain stimulator. Stereotactic brain biopsies and other small, superficial procedures may be done awake as well. Some neurosurgeons have advocated awake craniotomy in a wider range of cases [4]. The purported benefits of awake craniotomy beyond delineating eloquent brain areas are shorter intensive care unit (ICU) stays, shorter hospital stays, and the avoidance of general anesthesia [4].

CONTRAINDICATIONS TO AWAKE CRANIOTOMY

It is difficult to overstate the importance of patient selection in awake craniotomy. Proper patient selection and preparation will greatly improve the chances of success.

Since the purpose of an awake craniotomy is to perform intraoperative cortical mapping, it is imperative that the patient be highly motivated and able to communicate. Patients in whom communication is impaired (e.g., altered mental status, difficulty hearing, or inability to speak) would be poor candidates for awake craniotomy. Patients must also have the emotional maturity and coping mechanisms to handle the anxiety and discomfort of being awake during this procedure; although older children have successfully undergone awake craniotomy. There are case reports and

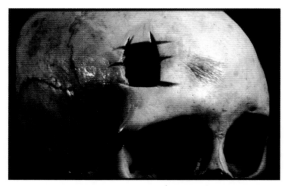

Figure 16.1 Prehistoric Peruvian skull. (Photograph provided by the San Diego Museum of Man.)

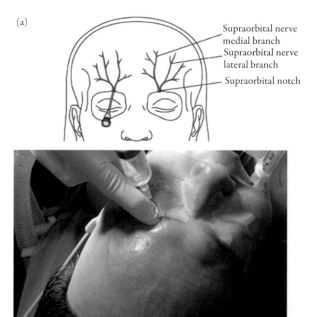

(a)

Supraorbital nerve medial branch
Supraorbital nerve lateral branch
Supraorbital notch

(b)

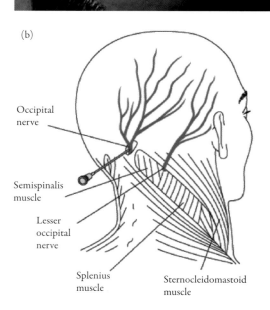

Occipital nerve

Semispinalis muscle

Lesser occipital nerve

Splenius muscle

Sternocleidomastoid muscle

Figure 16.2 Sensory innervation of the scalp.

case series of patients as young as 9 years tolerating awake craniotomy [5, 6]. A decision to proceed with such a case would require a careful examination of risks and benefits as well as careful preparation of the patient and his or her family. In general, however, patients who are very young or who have emotional issues or anxiety disorders may be poorly suited to this technique.

Factors other than the neurologic status of the patient may prohibit the use of local anesthesia with sedation. Surgery in the prone position is poorly suited to an awake technique because of the inherent problems associated with emergency airway management. The prone position would also be difficult for a patient who is awake to tolerate for any extended period of time. Sleep apnea, obesity, or a difficult airway could make emergency airway management problematic. Airway management in the middle of surgery is liable to be difficult even under the best conditions. These risks must be weighed against the benefit of doing the craniotomy awake.

LOCAL ANESTHESIA

Adequate local anesthesia is critical to the success of an awake craniotomy, and a variety of drugs and techniques are effective. Some authors prefer a full scalp block [7], while others prefer a field block at the incision site [8]. If rigid head fixation (pins) is used, then local anesthetic must be placed under the pins. Once the craniotomy is performed, additional local anesthesia may be needed to anesthetize the dura mater. Bupivacaine 0.25% to 0.5% is a common choice for scalp block because of its long duration of action. It appears to be safe in doses up to 2.0 mg/kg [9]. At this dose, blood levels of bupivacaine used for a scalp block were well below those associated with convulsions.

Harvey Cushing described his technique for infiltrating the incision site with local anesthetic [10]. The scalp block, a more recent innovation, was first described by Girvin in 1986 [11]. This technique usually [12] involves blocking the six nerves that supply sensory innervations to the scalp (Figure 16.2) Recent articles on awake craniotomy

have used the scalp block to improve intraoperative patient comfort [13]. The scalp block has also been shown to decrease the hemodynamic response to craniotomy [14] and improve postoperative pain control [15].It is important to use long-acting agents because these procedures normally take several hours. The addition of epinephrine (1:200.00) will increase the intensity and duration of the block. This is particularly important in the highly vascular scalp.

The safety of the scalp block using levobupivacaine 0.5% (1.6 to 3.2 mg/kg) and ropivacaine 0.75% (2.18 to 4.38 mg/kg) has recently been confirmed in two published articles [16, 17]. In these studies, bilateral scalp blocks were performed without signs or symptoms of systemic toxicity. Plasma levels peaked about 15 minutes after the local was injected and peak blood levels were below those associated with toxicity. The volume of local anesthesia administered at each site can vary from 2 to 5 mL of bupivacaine, ropivacaine, or levobupivacaine [10–13]. The only episodes of local anesthetic toxicity after scalp infiltration were reported by Archer et al. [18], who reported seven episodes of toxicity of a total of 354 patients. The local anesthetic used was dibucaine and the doses were not recorded.

Here is a description of the scalp block technique by Osborn and Sebeo [12], reprinted with permission:

See Figure 16.3.

1) Supraorbital Nerve

The supraorbital nerve can be blocked as it emerges from the orbit. The supraorbital notch is palpated by the finger, and the needle is inserted along the upper orbital margin, perpendicular to the skin, approximately 1 cm medial to the supraorbital foramen.

2) Supratrochlear Nerve

Emerging from the superiomedial angle of the orbit, and running up on the forehead parallel to the supraorbital nerve a finger's breadth medial to it, the supratrochlear nerve can either be blocked as it emerges above the eyebrow or can be involved by a medial extension of the supraorbital block.

3) Auriculotemporal Nerve

The auriculotemporal nerve can be blocked by infiltration over zygomatic process, with an injection 1 to 1.5 cm anterior to the ear at the level of the tragus. The superficial temporal artery is anterior to the auriculotemporal nerve at the level of the tragus, and should always be palpated and its course identified before blockade.

4) Zygomaticotemporal Nerve

The zygomaticotemporal nerve is blocked by infiltration from the supraorbital margin to the posterior part of the zygomatic arch. Arising midway between auriculotemporal and supraorbital nerves where it emerges above the zygoma, the zygomaticotemporal nerve ramifies as it pierces temporalis fascia. Both deep and superficial injection plains are thus recommended.

5) Greater Occipital Nerve

The greater occipital nerve can be blocked by infiltration approximately halfway between the occipital protuberance and the mastoid process, 2.5 cm lateral to the nuchal median line. The best landmark is to palpate the occipital artery, and inject medially after careful aspiration. This should avoid potential intra-arterial injection.

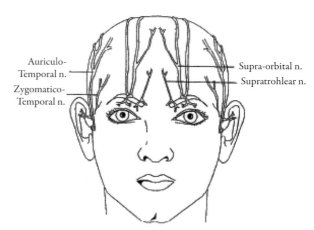

Auriculo-Temporal n.
Zygomatico-Temporal n.
Supra-orbital n.
Supratrohlear n.

Figure 16.3   Scalp block.

6) Lesser Occipital Nerve

The lesser occipital nerve can be blocked by infiltration along the superior nuchal line, 2.5 cm lateral to the greater occipital nerve block.

ANESTHETIC TECHNIQUE

Patients may experience a different level of pain during each stage of the surgical procedure. Incision of the scalp, bone flap removal, and opening of the dura are the most painful parts of the procedure. The patient may experience little or no pain during brain mapping and resection, which is the portion of the surgery during which the patient must be awake and cooperative. The amount of pain will again increase while the dura, skull, and skin are closed.

Patients undergoing awake brain mapping may be managed with local anesthesia and sedation[18, 19, 20], or using an "asleep-awake-asleep" technique[21, 22]. Local anesthesia with sedation, also known as monitored anesthesia care, requires varying the level of sedation quickly at different stages of the surgery. The patient breathes spontaneously throughout the procedure. Supplemental oxygen can be added as needed. The strength of this technique is the lack of airway manipulation. This makes the chance of coughing less likely but makes airway obstruction more likely.. Some means of securing the airway emergently must be immediately available. End-tidal CO_2 monitoring will help identify obstruction before hypoxemia occurs.

The advantage of the "asleep-awake-asleep" technique is that the patient is under general anesthesia and the airway is controlled during the painful parts of the surgery. The patient is awakened when it is time to map the brain, which is the least painful part of the surgery. Airway management can be accomplished with an endotracheal tube [20], an LMA [21] or another airway device [23]. The key to success is a smooth transition from asleep to awake and back again. If the patient coughs or becomes disoriented, bleeding or brain swelling could result.

SEDATIVE AGENTS AND REGIMENS

Providing sedation during an awake craniotomy has two competing goals and therefore requires a considerable amount of planning. The patient should be as comfortable as possible during the procedure, but oversedation may render the patient unable to cooperate or may produce airway obstruction. Over the years, many drugs and combinations of drugs have been used for sedation during awake craniotomy.

In 1954, Penfield and Pasquet [24] used nitrous oxide during the asleep portion of the procedure, but this drug interfered with electroencephalography even after its discontinuation. They settled on sodium thiopental and codeine to provide sedation and analgesia during the most painful parts of the procedure [24]. The sedating effect of the sodium thiopental lasted longer than nitrous oxide, but it allowed for better electroencephalographic studies.

Neuroleptanalgesia became popular in the 1960s. This technique uses a combination of a narcotic and a neuroleptic such as droperidol or haloperidol [25]. Surgeons and anesthesiologists rated the analgesia provided by this technique as good or excellent in the majority of cases [26]. Patients were usually sleepy but able to respond to commands. Respiratory depression did occur, however, as might be expected with any technique reliant on narcotics [26].

Propofol is now the most popular agent for awake craniotomy [27, 28]. This is due in large part to the pharmacokinetics of the drug. Awakening is more rapid and complete than with thiopental and methohexital [29]. The rapid onset and offset of propofol allow the anesthesiologist to change the depth of anesthesia quickly, which is essential during this procedure. Its shorter duration of action after discontinuing an infusion is explained by its very high clearance, coupled with the slow diffusion of drug from the peripheral to the central compartment [30]. Propofol also has antiemetic effects, which is an important consideration during awake brain surgery [31]. Propofol can cause respiratory depression and airway obstruction, however, so adequate monitoring of oxygenation and ventilation are essential [32].

An ideal anesthetic agent for the patient undergoing awake craniotomy would provide anxiolysis and analgesia without respiratory depression or clouding of consciousness. Dexmedetomidine became widely available several years ago, and this drug is now being used as a sedative during awake craniotomy [33, 34]. Dexmedetomidine is a highly selective α_2-agonist with sedative, analgesic, and anesthetic-sparing effects [35]. The primary action of α_2-adrenoreceptor agonists is the inhibition of norepinephrine release that causes attenuation of excitation in the central nervous system. Small-dose infusion of this drug in healthy volunteers provided sedation that could be easily reversed with verbal stimulation [35]. Because dexmedetomidine does not suppress ventilation, using the drug makes apnea much less likely. The anesthetic-sparing effect of dexmedetomidine allows a decreased use of other anesthetics. This facilitates a rapid emergence and greater control of anesthetic depth.

After Zornow et al. [36] published data showing a decrease in cerebral blood flow with dexmedetomidine in humans, there was concern that its use may lead to an increase in cerebral ischemia. Drummond et al. [37], however, recently published data that showed dexmedetomidine produces a concomitant decrease in cerebral metabolic rate and cerebral blood flow.

Even with an adequate local anesthetic block and propofol or dexmedetomidine as a primary sedative, most patients will require at least some narcotics to alleviate pain during this procedure. Because of their potential to cause respiratory depression, narcotics should be used sparingly. Small bolus doses of a rapid-acting narcotic like fentanyl or a narcotic infusion at a low rate are likely to be the safest alternatives. Remifentanil is an ultra short-acting synthetic opioid that is administered as an infusion. It has an ester linkage that undergoes rapid hydrolysis by nonspecific tissue and plasma esterases [38], so that the drug does not accumulate. The context-sensitive half-life is very short (2 to 5 minutes) and is independent of the duration of infusion [39]. This short half-life allows the anesthesiologist to provide improved comfort and safety [40, 41].

MONITORING

All patients undergoing awake craniotomy should at a minimum be monitored according to the American Society of Anesthesiologists (ASA) standards. Capnography is the best way to detect airway obstruction before hypoxemia occurs. A survey of recent articles on awake craniotomy, reveals a spectrum of opinions regarding invasive monitors. Sarang et al. [42] and Berkenstadt et al. [22] placed arterial catheters in all patients, while Blanshard et al. [43] inserted arterial catheters in only 11% of patients. Central venous catheters were inserted infrequently. Blanshard et al. placed central venous catheters in 1.6% of patients. Indications in this group included potentially large blood loss and procedures done with the patient in the sitting position.

An arterial catheter is beneficial because it allows for intraoperative measurement of $PaCO_2$, glucose, and hemoglobin levels. Additionally, precise blood pressure monitoring helps insure adequate cerebral perfusion at all times. A bladder catheter should be placed in patients undergoing an awake craniotomy, especially if diuretics are given, although some groups choose not to insert one if the anticipated surgery time is short [4]. Last, a depth of consciousness monitor may be of help if it is difficult to maintain proper levels of sedation throughout the procedure and facilitate a prompt wake up regardless of anesthetic technique used [44].

The location of the surgical incision may, however, prohibit the use of this monitor.

POSITIONING FOR COMFORT AND SAFETY

Patients should be positioned so as to facilitate surgical access while maximizing patient comfort and accessibility to the airway. Supine and lateral positions with the head turned toward the anesthesiologist allow for emergency airway management as well as functional testing. The prone position is uncomfortable, and access to the airway is nearly impossible; this position should therefore be avoided in awake patients. All pressure points should be well padded, and the patient should be loosely restrained to prevent him or her from reaching into the surgical field. Whenever possible, the patient should be allowed to position him- or herself, and should be included in the process. It should be noted that a position that is slightly uncomfortable at the beginning of the procedure may become intolerable several hours later.

EVIDENCE OF EFFECTIVENESS

Advances in functional MRI and neuronavigation techniques may make cortical mapping and awake craniotomy unnecessary in some cases. There is a lack of studies that directly compare awake craniotomy with intraoperative cortical mapping to general anesthesia with neurophysiologic monitoring. Only one small, randomized prospective study has compared awake craniotomy to general anesthesia for resection of tumors in eloquent cortex [45]. The patients who received general anesthesia had better outcomes, but the study patient numbers were small and cortical mapping was not performed in the awake patients.

There are several retrospective studies that show good results with awake craniotomy and cortical mapping [46–48]. Sanai et al.'s [46] recent retrospective review of 250 patients with tumor near the language center found only 1.6% of patients with persistent language deficit 6 months after tumor resection with awake craniotomy and cortical mapping. The study by Daffau et al. [48] compared two series of patients operated on at the same institution over different time periods. The first group of low-grade glioma patients had their tumors removed under general anesthesia without cortical mapping. The second group underwent awake craniotomy, cortical mapping, and tumor resection when the tumor was located near the language center. The patients in the awake craniotomy group had a greater number of total and subtotal resections with a reduction in severe permanent deficits from 17% to 6.5%. This is increasingly important because extent of tumor resection is an independent prognostic factor for patient survival.

PATIENT PERCEPTION

Most case series of awake craniotomy in the literature report satisfactory results. Very few papers comment on patient perception of the procedure. A few published papers did look specifically at patient perception [49–51]. Danks et al. [50] used a mixture of lidocaine 1% and bupivacaine 0.25% for their scalp block. They performed monitored anesthesia care with midazolam, fentanyl, and sufentanil. Some patients also received propofol. The results of their satisfaction survey appear in Table 16.1.

The majority of patients was satisfied with the procedure and would do it again if they had to. Whittle et al. [49] studied patient satisfaction with awake craniotomy as well. They used an asleep-awake-asleep technique with propofol and remifentanil infusions. Their findings were similar to those of Danks et al., with only 20% of patients experiencing pain, 29% anxiety, and 14% fear. It remains to be seen whether newer drugs and better technique can improve patient satisfaction with this procedure.

COMPLICATIONS

Although some authors have stated that awake craniotomy involves increased operative risk compared to craniotomy under general anesthesia [52], there are limited data directly comparing the two options. It is difficult to improve on the safety offered by general anesthesia. A secure airway as well as an immobile and anesthetized patient goes a long way toward eliminating intraoperative problems. The awake craniotomy offers a chance for better surgical outcomes, including a more complete resection of a lesion or avoidance of severe neurological impairment. There is certainly an increased risk of intraoperative problems that would be unlikely to occur under general anesthesia.

Table 16.1 SATISFACTION WITH ANESTHESIA DURING AWAKE CRANIOTOMY

SATISFACTION RATING	NO. OF PATIENTS	WOULD THEY UNDERGO IT AGAIN?
5	2	1 yes, 1 no
6	1	1 yes
7	3	3 yes
10	15	13 yes, 2 no
Total	21	

a The patients were asked to rate their overall levels of satisfaction with the intraoperative experience on a scale of 0 to 10, where 0 represents complete dissatisfaction and 10 represents complete satisfaction. These patients' responses to the question, "If you needed to undergo another craniotomy, would you agree to have it performed under local anesthesia and monitored conscious sedation if it were indicated?" are correlated with these satisfaction ratings.

From Danks RA, Rogers M, Aglio LS, et al. Patient tolerance of craniotomy performed with the patient under local anesthesia and monitored conscious sedation. *Neurosurgery.* 1998;42: 28–34. Reproduced with permission from Wolters Kluwer Health.

INTRAOPERATIVE NAUSEA AND VOMITING:

Archer et al. [18] retrospectively reviewed 354 cases of awake craniotomy and reported an 8% incidence of nausea and vomiting during awake craniotomy. This study was published in 1988 and a neuroleptic anesthesia technique with droperidol and fentanyl was used. In more recent studies, Blanshard et al. [43] and Skousas and Artru [53] reported rates of 1% in their retrospective reviews. Blanshard et al. cited the use of propofol without narcotics to explain the low rate of nausea and vomiting. Berkenstadt et al. [22] recorded no incidences of intraoperative nausea and vomiting using a technique that included clonidine, propofol, and remifentanil, but this study included only 25 patients. Intraoperative nausea and vomiting can be mitigated with prophylactic administration of serotonin antagonists (e.g., ondansetron), steroids (e.g., dexamethasone), the use of propofol for sedation, and limiting narcotics.

INTRAOPERATIVE SEIZURES

Intraoperative seizures are one of the more common intraoperative complications. Seizures may occur because the patient has a preexisting seizure disorder but may also be due to cortical stimulation. The highest reported incidence was 16% In Archer et al.'s [18] retrospective review, while Skucas and Artu [53] and Sarang and Dinsmore [42] found a lower incidence of 3% and 2%, respectively. None of these patients aspirated gastric contents, and only 2 of the 785 patients from the three studies combined [18, 42, 53] required conversion to general anesthesia after a seizure. One of the patients who seized in the Sarang and Dinsmore study had a prolonged postictal state and the procedure was abandoned.

More recently, Serletis and Bernstein [4] studied 610 patients undergoing awake craniotomy and recorded an intraoperative seizure rate of 4.9% The authors added that the seizures were frequently focal and self-limiting and rarely required conversion to general anesthesia. In a technical note, Sartorius and Berger [54] remarked that seizures are easily terminated with the direct application of iced Ringer's lactate solution onto the cortex. The incidence of intraoperative seizures may be further decreased by prophylactic antiepileptic medication.

HYPOXIA OR RESPIRATORY DEPRESSION

Respiratory depression with or without hypoxia occurred infrequently in the large case series of awake craniotomies. Sarang and Dinsmore [42] reported three incidences of airway obstruction in the early cases of his series. None of the patients developed hypoxemia or required conversion to general anesthesia. Skucas and Artru [53] reported five desaturations among their 332 patients. All of these patients were obese and three required conversion to general anesthesia with an endotracheal tube or an LMA.

CONVERSION TO GENERAL ANESTHESIA

Conversion to general anesthesia was relatively uncommon in all the large retrospective reviews [18, 42, 43, 53]. Only 14 of 1026 patients in all four studies combined required conversion to general anesthesia. The reasons for conversion included over sedation, uncooperative patients, a prolonged postictal state, and poor ventilation resulting in hypoxia. Despite the low rate of conversion to general anesthesia, rapid conversion to general anesthesia may be necessary in any patient undergoing awake craniotomy. This may be necessary not only for the above mentioned reasons, but also in case of hemorrhage, status epileptics, or poor operating conditions.

Other reported intraoperative problems included movement, hypotension, hypertension, tachycardia, and bradycardia. These problems generally did not appear to interfere with the surgery or affect clinical outcome.

CONCLUSION

There is only one small randomized, prospective study comparing awake craniotomy to craniotomy done under general anesthesia, so it is difficult to know if this technique leads to an improvement in patient outcome. It is also difficult to recommend one awake craniotomy technique over another since they have not been compared in a scientific manner. Because of the relative ease of doing craniotomy under general anesthesia, it seems likely that the vast majority of brain surgery will continue to be done under general anesthesia, with awake procedures reserved for those cases where functional cortical mapping is essential to ensuring a good outcome.

Whatever anesthetic technique is used, there are a few details that must be observed to ensure success. Careful patient selection is likely the most important single element necessary for success. This is followed by patient preparation. The patient should understand what will happen during the time he or she is awake in the operating room. An adequate local anesthesia block will allow the patient to be fully awake and cooperative with minimal discomfort. The avoidance of long acting anesthetic agents and polypharmacy will keep patient confusion and agitation to a minimum. Finally, a plan for emergency airway management should be in place at all times.

REFERENCES

1. Sachs E, Hoeber P. *The history and development of neurological surgery*. London: Cassell & Co; 1952:85.

2. Greenblatt S, ed. *A history of neurosurgery*. Park Ridge, IL: American Association of Neurological Surgeons; 1997:217.

3. Kalenka, A, Scharz A. Anesthesia and Parkinson's disease: how to manage the new therapies. *Curr Opin Anaesthesiol*. 2009;22:419–424.

4. Serletis D, Bernstein M. Prospective study of awake craniotomy used routinely and nonselectively for supratentorial tumors. *J Neurosurg* 2007;107:1–6.

5. Klimek M, Verbrugge SJC, Roubos S, et al. Awake craniotomy for glioblastoma in a 9-year-old child. Anaesthesia. 2004;59:607–609.

6. Soriano SG, Eldredge EA, Wang FK, et al. The effect of propofol on intraoperative electrocorticography and cortical stimulation during awake craniotomies in children. Paediatr Anaesth. 2000;10:29–34.

7. Sahjpaul R. Awake craniotomy: controversies, indications and techniques in the surgical treatment of temporal lobe epilepsy. *Can J Neurol Sci*. 2000;27(Suppl 1):S55–S63.

8. Taylor MD, Bernstein M. Awake craniotomy with brain mapping as the routine surgical approach to treating patients with supratentorial intraaxial tumors: a prospective trial of 200 cases. *J Neurosurg* 1999;90:35–41.

9. Colley PS, Heavner JE. Blood levels of bupivacaine after injection into the scalp with and without epinephrine. *Anesthesiology* 1981;54:81–84.

10. Cushing HW. Notes on penetrating wounds of the brain. *Br Med J*. 1918;1:221.

11. Girvin JP. Neurosurgical considerations and general methods for craniotomy under local anesthesia. *Int Anesthesiol Clin*. 1986;24:89–113.

12. Osborn I, Sebeo J. "Scalp block" during craniotomy: a classic technique revisited. *J Neurosurg Anesthesiol* 2010;22:187–194.

13. Costello TG, Cormack JR. Anaesthesia for awake craniotomy: a modern approach. *J Clin Neurosci*. 2004;11:16–19.

14. Pinosky ML, Fishman RL, Reeves ST, et al. The effect of bupivacaine skull block on the hemodynamic response to craniotomy. *Anesth Analg*. 1996;83;1256–1261.

15. Nguyen A, Girard F, Boudreault D, et al. Scalp nerve blocks decrease the severity of pain after craniotomy. *Anesth Analg*. 2001;93:1272–1276.

16. Costello TG, Cormack JR, Mather LE, et al. Plasma levobupivacaine concentrations following scalp block in patients undergoing awake craniotomy. *Br J Anaesth*. 2005;94:848–851.

17. Costello TG, Cormack JR, Hoy C. et al. Plasma ropivacaine levels following scalp block for awake craniotomy. *J Neurosurg Anesthesiol*. 2004;16:147–150.

18. Archer D, McKenna J, Morin L. Conscious-sedation analgesia during craniotomy for intractable epilepsy: a review of 354 consecutive cases. *Can J Anesth* 1988;35:338–344.

19. Hans P, Bonhomme V, Born JD, et al. Target-controlled infusion of propofol and remifentanil combined with bispectral index monitoring for awake craniotomy. *Anaesthesia* 2000;55:255–259.

20. Berkenstadt H, Perel A, Hadani M, et al. Monitored anesthesia care using remifentanil and propofol for awake craniotomy *J Neurosurg Anesthesiol* 2001;13:246–249.

21. Huncke K, Van de Wiele B, Fried I, et al. The asleep-awake-asleep anesthetic technique for intraoperative language mapping. *Neurosurgery*. 1998;42:1312–1316.

22. Ard J, Bekker A, Doyle W. Dexmedetomidine in awake craniotomy: a technical note. *Surg Neurol* 2005;63:114–117.

23. Audu PB, Loomba N. Use of cuffed oropharyngeal airway (COPA) for awake intracranial surgery. *J Neurosurg Anesthesiol*. 2004;16:144–146.

24. Penfield W, Pasquet A. Combined regional and general anesthesia for craniotomy and cortical exploration. *Anesth Analg* 1954;33:145–164.

25. Welling E, Donegon J. Neuroleptanalgesia using alfentanil for awake craniotomy. *Anesth Analg*. 1989;68:57–60.

26. Tasker R, Marshall B. Analgesia for surgical procedures performed on conscious patients. *Can Anaesth Soc J*. 1965;12:29–33.

27. Meyer F, Bates LM. Awake craniotomy for aggressive resection of primary gliomas located in eloquent brain. *Mayo Clin Proc* 2001;76:677–687.

28. Silbergeld DL, Mueller WM, Colley PS, et al. Use of propofol (diprivan) for awake craniotomies: technical note. *Surg Neurol* 1992;38:271–272.

29. Doze VA, Westphal LM, White PF. Comparison of propofol with methohexital for outpatient anesthesia. *Anesth Analg* 1986;65:1189–1195.

30. Evers AS, Crowder CM, Balser JR. General anesthetics. In Brunton LL, Laso JS, Parker KL, eds. *Goodman & Gilman's The pharmacological basis of therapeutics*. 11th ed. http://www.accessanesthesiology.com/content/937527

31. McCollum JS, Milligan KR, Dundee JW. The antiemetic action of propofol. *Anaesthesia*. 1988;43:239–240.

32. Blouin RT, Conard PF, Gross JB. Time course of ventilatory depression following induction doses of propofol and thiopental. *Anesthesiology*. 1991;75:940–944.

33. Rozet I. Anesthesia for functional neurosurgery: the role of dexmedetomidine. *Curr Opin Anaesthesiol*. 2008;21:537–543.

34. Bekker A, Sturaitis MK. Dexmedetomidine in neurological surgery. *Neurosurgery*. 2005;57(Suppl):1–10.

35. Hall J, Uhrich T. Sedative, amnestic, and analgesic properties of small dose dexmedetomidine infusions. *Anesth Analg* 2000;90:699–705.

36. Zornow MH, Maze M, Dyck JB, et al. Dexmedetomidine decreases cerebral blood flow velocity in humans. *J Cereb Blood Flow Metab* 1993;13:350–353.

37. Drummond JC, Dao AV, Roth DM, et al. Effect of dexmedetomidine on cerebral blood flow velocity, cerebral metabolic rate, and carbon dioxide response in normal humans. *Anesthesiology*. 2008;108:225–232.

38. Burkle H, Dunbar S, Van Aken H. Remifentanil: a novel, short-acting μ-opioid. *Anesth. Analg* 1996;83:646–651.

39. Michelsen LG, Hug CC Jr. The pharmacokinetics of remifentanil. *J Clin Anesth*. 1996;8:679–682.

40. Bonhomme V, Franssen C, Hans P. Awake craniotomy. *Eur J Anaesthesiol* 2009;26:906–912.

41. Hol J, Klimek M, van der Heide-Mulder M, et al. Awake craniotomy induces fewer changes in the plasma amino acid profile than craniotomy under general anesthesia. *J Neurosurg Anesthesiol*. 2009;21:98–107.

42. Sarang A, Dinsmore J. Anaesthesia for awake craniotomy: evolution of a technique that facilitates awake neurological testing. *Br J Anaesth* 2003;90:161–165.

43. Blanshard HJ, Chung F, Manninen PH, et al. Awake craniotomy for removal of intracranial tumor: considerations for early discharge. *Anesth Analg* 2001;92:89–94.

44. Gan TJ, Glass P, Windsor A, et al. Bispectral Index monitoring allows faster emergence and improved recovery from propofol, alfentanil, and nitrous oxide anesthesia. Anesthesiology. 1997;87:808–815.

45. Gupta DK, Chandra PS, Ojha BK, et al. Awake craniotomy versus surgery under general anesthesia for resection of intrinsic lesions of eloquent cortex: a prospective randomized study. *Clin Neurol Neurosurg*. 2007;109:335–343.

46. Sanai N, Mirzadeh Z, Berger M. Functional outcome after language mapping for glioma resection. *N Engl J Med* 2008;358:18–27.

47. Kim S, McCutcheon I, Suki D, Weinberg J, et al. Awake craniotomy for brain tumors near eloquent cortex: correlation of intraoperative cortical mapping with neurological outcomes in 309 consecutive patients. *Neurosurgery*. 2009;64:836–846.

48. Daffau H, Lopes M, Arthuis F, et al. Contribution of intraoperative electrical stimulations in surgery of low grade gliomas: a comparative study between two series without (1985-96) and with (1996-2003)

functional mapping in the same institution. *J Neurol Neurosurg Psychiatry*. 2005;76:845–851.

49. Whittle IR, Midgley S, Georges H, et al. Patient perceptions of "awake" brain tumour surgery. *Acta Neurochir (Wien)*. 2005;13:275–277.

50. Danks RA, Rogers M, Aglio LS, et al. Patient tolerance of craniotomy performed with the patient under local anesthesia and monitored conscious sedation. *Neurosurgery*. 1998;42:28–34.

51. Manninen PH, Balki M, Lukitto K, et al. Patient satisfaction with awake craniotomy for tumor surgery: a comparison of remifentanil and fentanyl in conjunction with propofol. *Anesth Analg* 1996;102:237–242.

52. Picht T, Kombos T, Gramm HJ, et al. Multimodal protocol for awake craniotomy in language cortex tumor surgery. *Acta Neurochir (Wien)*. 2006;148:127–137.

53. Skucas A, Artru A. Anesthetic complications of awake craniotomies for epilepsy surgery. *Anesth Analg* 2006;102:882–887.

54. Sartorius CJ, Berger MS. Rapid termination of intraoperative stimulation-evoked seizures with application of cold Ringer's lactate to the cortex. Technical note. *J Neurosurg* 1998;88:349–351.

17.

ANESTHESIA FOR POSTERIOR FOSSA SURGERY

Rashmi N. Mueller

INTRODUCTION

The unique anatomic features of the posterior fossa require special consideration by surgeons and anesthesiologists. Anteriorly, the bony posterior fossa is bordered by the clivus; the floor and sides are made up by the occipital and temporal bones with the foramen magnum in the center while superiorly, the tentorium cerebelli covers the fossa. Vital neuronal and vascular structures, namely, the brainstem, cerebellum, cranial nerves, the vertebral and basilar arteries, and numerous venous sinuses (including the torcula, superior petrosal, transverse and sigmoid sinuses), are tightly confined within this space. Cerebrospinal fluid (CSF) flows out through the aqueduct of Sylvius into the fourth ventricle, through the foramen of Magendie and Luschka into the basal cisterns [1].

Compared with the supratentorial fossa, relatively small masses in the restrictive infratentorial compartment can cause increased local pressure and brain herniation. Secondary hydrocephalus often develops when a mass or edema obstructs CSF outflow. Intraoperative stimulation of the brainstem may cause profound hemodynamic and rhythm disturbances including asystole. Significant injury to the brainstem may result in severe morbidity and mortality including a delay or a failure to emerge from anesthesia after surgery.

As surgeons operate, air can be entrained through open venous sinuses, leading to venous air embolism which can be fatal. Lower cranial nerve injury sustained during the procedure may impair the patient's ability to either maintain an airway or prevent aspiration following extubation of the trachea.

COMMON POSTERIOR FOSSA LESIONS AND THEIR PRESENTING SYMPTOMS

Some of the most common surgical procedures performed in the posterior fossa are resections of cerebellopontine angle tumors (mainly acoustic schwannomas), resection of other cerebellar tumors and vascular lesions, Chiari I decompression, and surgery for petroclival tumors [2].

Patients may present with signs of intracranial hypertension such as headaches, nausea and vomiting and cranial nerve palsies, cerebellar signs, facial pain and spasm, or more devastating neurologic deficits depending on the type, location, size and rate of growth of the lesion. Specific clinical syndromes are described based on the location of cerebellar tumors [1]. Midline lesions of the cerebellum and the fourth ventricle cause disturbances in balance and an unsteady wide-based gait. Nystagmus, hydrocephalus, papilledema, and cranial nerve palsies can occur. Patients with lateral cerebellar lesions (Figure 17.1) may develop typical cerebellar signs. These include ataxia, dysmetria, dysarthria, gaze paresis, dysdiadochokinesia, intention tremor, hypotonia, and scanning speech. Very large lateral tumors can lead to hydrocephalus and brainstem compression. Lesions at the cerebellopontine angle (Figure 17.2) may compress the facial and vestibulocochlear nerves causing facial paresis, hearing loss and vertigo. Hydrocephalus and cerebellar symptoms may occur as the growths enlarge.

Patients with tumors in the brain stem (Figure 17.2) may present with spasticity, contralateral motor and sensory deficits, and ipsilateral cranial nerve palsies. Large, compressive brain stem lesions can cause bradycardia, hypertension, altered respiration, and hyperthermia.

Type I Chiari malformation (Figure 17.3) is associated with an underdeveloped bony posterior fossa and is characterized by descent of the cerebellar tonsils below the foramen magnum ("hindbrain hernia") [3]. Syringomyelia may be present. Patients often have severe headaches, nystagmus, and lower cranial nerve palsies. They may also have other signs of high intracranial pressure (ICP), ataxia, and bulbar dysfunction (e.g., absent gag, which is very common even in the absence of other symptoms). Syringomyelia results in sensory loss and muscle atrophy in the hands. Symptoms of type I Chiari malformation classically appear in adolescence or adulthood. In contrast, type II Chiari malformation is more likely to be discovered in the neonatal period. Frequently, medullary kinking, an elongated fourth ventricle, and "beaking" of the quadrigeminal plate accompany

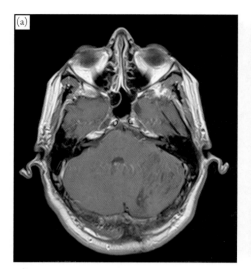
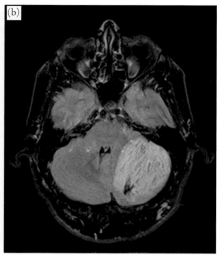

Figure 17.1 *Cerebellar gangliocytoma.* Axial views of MRI with and without contrast showing a large dysplastic cerebellar gangliocytoma occupying the left cerebellum with deformity of the fourth ventricle. (Images courtesy of Srilatha Joglekar, MD.)

the cerebellar descent into the spinal canal. Type II Chiari malformation is associated with spina bifida, hydrocephalus, and syringomyelia. Patients often develop lower cranial nerve deficits, progressive spasticity, and quadriparesis. The surgical treatment is suboccipital craniectomy and upper cervical laminectomy, sometimes with duraplasty. The syrinx usually resolves spontaneously, but sometimes a shunt is necessary [3].

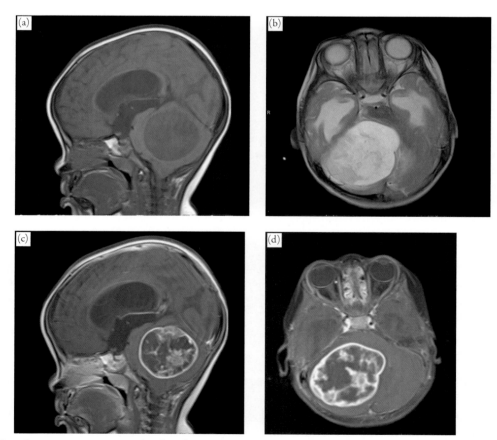

Figure 17.2 *Cerebellar pilocytic astrocytoma.* Sagittal and axial MRI views with and without contrast in a 1-year-old showing a huge pilocytic cerebellar astrocytoma. There is displacement and compression of the brainstem and fourth ventricle with resultant marked dilatation of both lateral and third ventricles and significant transependymal flow. Inferior displacement of cerebellar tonsils through foreman magnum is seen. A right lateral ventriculostomy has been performed. (Images courtesy of Arnold H. Menezes, MD.)

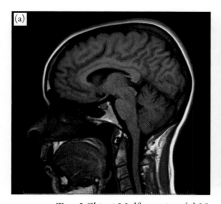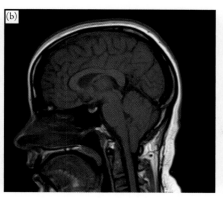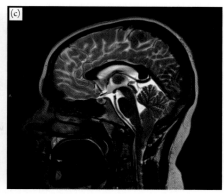

Figure 17.3   *Type I Chiari Malformation.* (a) Normal MRI of the posterior fossa for comparison; (b and c) MRI in two different patients with Type I Chiari malformation with tonsillar herniation ("hindbrain hernia") below the foramen magnum into the cervical spinal space. Syrinx is absent.

SURGICAL APPROACHES AND INTRAOPERATIVE POSITIONING

There are various surgical approaches to the posterior fossa including suboccipital, supracerebellar infratentorial, transtemporal, and transoral approaches. Indirect routes through the supratentorial fossa include combined supratentorial infratentorial, occipital transtentorial, and temporal transtentorial approaches [1]. Patients undergoing posterior fossa surgery are usually positioned intraoperatively in one of the following ways.

THE SITTING POSITION

The sitting position (Figure 17.5) provides optimal surgical access to midline posterior fossa and upper cervical lesions.

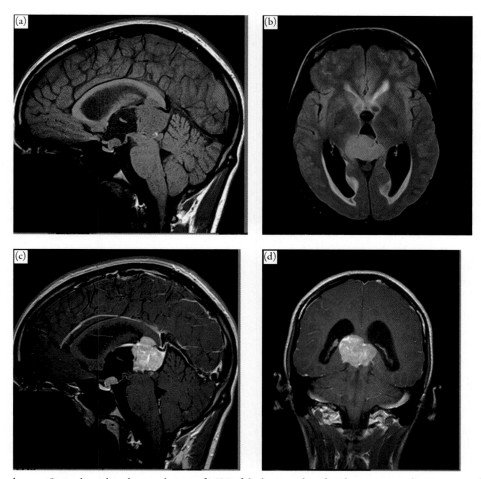

Figure 17.4   *Pineal gland tumor.* Sagittal, axial, and coronal views of MRI of the brain with and without contrast showing a pineal gland germinoma. There is obstructive hydrocephalus with dilatation of the lateral and third ventricles. A smaller suprasellar mass is also present. Pineal gland tumors are often accessed via the supracerebellar infratentorial approach in the sitting position.   (Images courtesy of Kenneth D. Williams, MD, and Srilatha Joglekar, MD.)

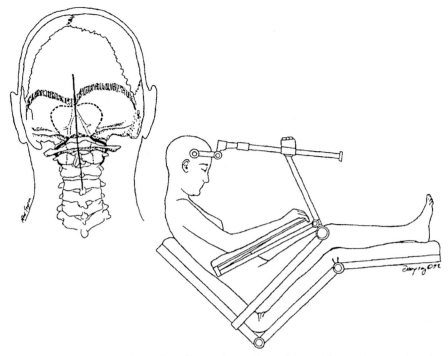

Figure 17.5 *The sitting position.* The sitting position is shown here along with a midline suboccipital surgical approach to the posterior fossa. Note that the head-holder is attached to the upper part of the table so that the back can be quickly lowered in an emergency. (Reproduced from Patel SJ, Wen DY, Haines SJ. Posterior fossa: surgical considerations. In: Cottrell JE and Smith SD, ed. *Anesthesia and Neurosurgery.* St. Louis, MO: Mosby; 2001:277, with permission from Elsevier.)

It also facilitates access to fourth ventricular tumors, tumors at the cerebellopontine angle [3], and to the pineal gland (located in the supratentorial fossa) via the supracerebellar infratentorial approach (Figure 17.4).

There are a number of other advantages to operating in the sitting position. Surgical blood loss is lower. In one report about patients undergoing posterior fossa craniotomy, the number of supine patients [4] who were transfused more than 2 units of blood (13%) was greater than patients in the sitting position who needed transfusion (3%). Gravity ensures better CSF and venous drainage (provided extreme flexion of the neck is avoided). Ventilation is easier, especially in obese patients [5, 6]. The airway and extremities are more accessible during the procedure compared with the prone position, and the patient's face is visible which is useful for facial nerve monitoring. Cranial nerve function may be better preserved after surgery, possibly due to improved surgical exposure in the sitting position [7].

The sitting position has numerous complications associated with it including venous air embolism (VAE), hemodynamic changes, and pneumocephalus. Chiefly due to the danger of VAE, the sitting position is seldom used in most modern neurosurgical centers. In the few centers where surgeons and anesthesiologists are accustomed to managing large numbers of sitting craniotomies, the risk of surgery and anesthesia in this position appears to be low [8]. It is strongly recommended that anesthesia providers who are inexperienced with the use of the sitting position for craniotomy seek guidance from an anesthesiologist who has managed a fair number of such cases.

Venous Air Embolism

Intracranial surgery in the sitting position is associated with a high incidence of venous air embolism. One study using transesophageal echocardiography (TEE) in patients in the sitting position reported that VAE occurred in 76% of patients undergoing posterior fossa surgery compared with 25% of patients having cervical spine surgery [9]. Using precordial Doppler monitoring in sitting patients, 39% of patients undergoing posterior fossa surgery and 12% of patients having cervical spine surgery were found to develop VAE [4]. Pin holder placement and the drilling of burr holes have also been infrequently associated with VAE [10].

Pathophysiology of VAE

Factors that modify the severity of venous air embolism include the position of the patient, the type of ventilation, the volume and rate of air entering the veins, and the central venous pressure [11]. The volume of air and rate of entry into the venous circulation depends on the magnitude of the pressure gradient between the exposed vein and the right side of the heart. Gravitational gradients as small as 5 cm facilitate VAE [12]. In sitting craniotomies, the operative site is usually more than 20 cm above the heart and the resultant subatmospheric pressure in the dural sinuses is ideal for drawing air into the venous circulation. Large and noncollapsible venous sinuses are tethered open by the dura and bone in the posterior fossa and are excellent portals for air entry, particularly in a hypovolemic patient. This explains why VAE is more likely in the sitting position during craniotomies rather than in spine surgery. Careful and meticulous surgical dissection with the liberal use of bone wax and saline irrigation will reduce the chances of air entry.

The cardiovascular response to VAE depends on whether air is entrained in a single large bolus or as a continuous infusion of gas [11]. When a significant amount of air is slowly entrained into a vein, it passes into the lungs and impairs blood flow distal to the pulmonary artery, causing a progressive increase in central venous and pulmonary arterial pressure. Increased dead space, ventilation/perfusion (V/Q) mismatch, pulmonary edema, hypoxia, hypercarbia, and bronchoconstriction can result. Rapid entrainment of a large amount of air may lead to an air lock in the right heart with acute right ventricular failure, arrhythmias, myocardial ischemia, and frank cardiovascular collapse. Children tend to have more severe hemodynamic complications from VAE [13].

Paradoxical air embolism (PAE) occurs when air enters the systemic circulation through a patent foramen ovale (PFO). The incidence of probe patent PFO detected at autopsy in adults is 28% [14]. In one study of 21 patients undergoing neurosurgery in the sitting position, paradoxical air embolism developed only with the entrainment of a large amount of air [15]. Positive end-expiratory pressure (PEEP) was originally thought to reduce air entrainment by increasing venous pressure. However, in the presence of a PFO, the addition of PEEP could facilitate the development of a paradoxical air embolism. Cardiac or cerebral ischemia may result from a paradoxical air embolism. Based on the incidence of a PFO and the apparent need for entrainment of a large magnitude of air to produce a paradoxical air embolism, the actual incidence of neurologic deficits produced by arterial air embolism may be very low. Paradoxical air embolism has been detected by echocardiography even in patients who do not have a PFO. One proposed explanation for this is that air can travel from the right heart through the pulmonary circulation and into the left heart [16]. Percutaneous PFO closure has been recommended by some as a safe and efficacious procedure for the preoperative management of patients scheduled to undergo neurosurgery in the sitting position [17].

Monitoring for VAE

The lethal dose of air is believed to be 3 to 5 mL/kg or a 200- to 300-mL bolus of air in humans [18]. Transesophageal echocardiography (TEE) is the most sensitive monitor for detecting the presence and estimating the amount of embolized air (Figure 17.6). TEE can detect as little as 0.02 mL/kg of air. In the operating room, TEE may be used to identify the presence of a PFO in anesthetized patients before

surgery in the sitting position as it is more sensitive than precordial echocardiography. TEE can also be helpful in monitoring volume status and left ventricular wall motion. However, it is not practical for continuous monitoring during a case. TEE requires near-constant attention from a specially trained practitioner. During sitting craniotomy, a large echocardiography probe in the esophagus may conceivably cause pharyngeal injury by creating pressure at the acute angle created by neck flexion, and may also obstruct venous drainage. A pediatric or a probe with a small diameter is advisable if continuous intraoperative TEE is planned.

Precordial cardiac auscultation by Doppler ultrasound is nearly as sensitive as TEE for the detection of VAE [11]. Doppler can identify as little as 0.05 mL/kg of air [19]. The probe is placed at the third or fourth intercostal space just right of the sternum over the junction of the superior vena cava and the right atrium [20]. Doppler ultrasound can detect VAE before pathophysiologic changes occur [21]. End-tidal carbon dioxide will decrease significantly with a VAE. This decrease may be slow when air is entrained gradually. Venous air embolism accompanied by a decrease in end-tidal carbon dioxide is usually significant (as opposed to detection only by TEE, which is oversensitive) [20]. A combination of precordial Doppler signals for air and a decrease in end-tidal carbon dioxide is the best practical warning that a clinically significant volume of air has entered the venous system.

A central venous catheter enables entrained air to be aspirated from the right atrium. Insertion of a central venous catheter should therefore be considered in patients who are scheduled for a craniotomy in the sitting position. A multiorifice catheter allows retrieval of a larger volume of air compared with a single-lumen catheter [12]. For maximal removal of air, the tip of a multiorifice catheter should be positioned 2.0 cm below the junction of the superior vena cava and the right atrium. For a single-orifice catheter, the best position for aspiration of air is 3 cm above the

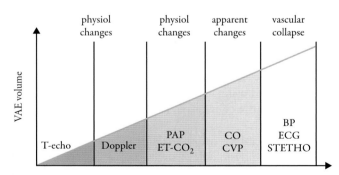

Figure 17.6 *The relative sensitivity of various monitors for VAE.* (VAE); BP, blood pressure; CO, cardiac output; CVP, central venous pressure; ECG, electrocardiogram; ET-CO$_2$, end-tidal carbon dioxide; PAP, pulmonary artery pressure; physiol, physiological; stetho, auscultation; T-echo, transesophageal echocardiogram. (Reproduced from Drummond JC, Patel PM. Neurosurgical anesthesia. In *Miller's Anesthesia.* 7th ed. Philadelphia, PA: Elsevier, 2009:2056, with permission from Elsevier.)

superior vena cava–atrium junction. However, aspiration from the right atrium is poor with either type of catheter. Peripheral central vein catheterization kits are available that allow insertion of a central catheter through the antecubital vein using electrocardiography (ECG) to guide optimal placement. Detecting a change in Doppler signals by injecting agitated saline has also been advocated as a way to guide proper position of the right atrial catheter. This test can be misleading when confirming placement of the central venous catheter. However, injecting agitated saline is a useful method to facilitate proper placement of the precordial Doppler probe [22]. Other routes of central venous cannulation may be used including the internal jugular or subclavian veins. A large hematoma in the neck can interfere with venous drainage, so care should be taken to avoid inadvertent arterial puncture. Patients with elevated ICP should not remain in the Trendelenburg position for a prolonged time as the brain can get engorged with venous blood, further elevating the ICP.

Pulmonary arterial and central venous pressures will increase if VAE occurs, but these are nonspecific signs. The ECG may show ST-segment changes or a right ventricular strain pattern. Bradyarrhythmias or tachyarrhythmias can occur. A millwheel murmur has been traditionally described with air embolism, but it is a late and insensitive sign. End-tidal nitrogen is theoretically increased with a large VAE. However, this is also not a very sensitive sign, is seldom monitored with modern anesthesia machines, and even when monitored, is not a reliable indicator of recovery from VAE [23]. Its role in detecting air embolism is limited at present [20].

Management of VAE

Doppler or TEE can help detect small amounts of embolized air (less than 10 mL). There is usually no change in end-tidal carbon dioxide or the blood pressure when the VAE is small. Surgeons should be warned nevertheless as small emboli may herald subsequent, larger emboli [20]. Moderate-sized air emboli (10-50 mL) are often accompanied by an increase in systemic blood pressure and heart rate, as well as Doppler signals and a drop in end-tidal carbon dioxide. Again, surgeons should be immediately notified so that they can take measures such as flooding the field with saline and using wax to seal open bony edges. If a central venous catheter is in place, an attempt to aspirate air should be made.

Large air emboli (more than 50 mL) will be accompanied by major physiologic changes [20]. A precipitous drop in end-tidal carbon dioxide and Doppler signals may occur together with oxygen desaturation, bronchoconstriction, cardiac dysrhythmias including tachycardia or bradycardia, hypotension, right heart failure, and cardiovascular collapse. In life-threatening cases of VAE, in addition to aspirating air from the central venous catheter, the anesthesiologist

may consider occluding the ipsilateral jugular vein to stop further air entrainment. Care should be taken not to compress the carotid artery as this can cause cerebral ischemia. If cardiopulmonary resuscitation (CPR) is necessary, the head of the bed must be lowered; 100% oxygen should be administered and nitrous oxide discontinued. Fluids, inotropic agents, and vasopressors should be given as necessary. A left lateral position may assist in dispelling an air lock in the right heart but is not a good position for CPR and is effectively impossible to attain in a patient whose head is secured in pins. In cases of PAE, postoperative hyperbaric oxygen (HBO) therapy may be considered. HBO will dissolve air bubbles and improve oxygenation [24, 25].

During less severe episodes of air embolism, the anesthesiologist should confer with the surgical team about the decision to proceed with or discontinue the surgery. Factors such as the urgency of the procedure and the patient's medical condition and age should be taken into account. If there are repeated small air emboli with no apparent entry points or unexplained hemodynamic changes, then halting the surgery should be strongly considered as catastrophic air embolism may occur further into the procedure. At the least, surgery should not continue until the VAE has resolved. Afterward, careful dissection with the liberal use of bone wax and irrigating solutions in the field will reduce the chances of further air embolism.

Other Complications of the Sitting Position

Hemodynamic changes including hypotension, decreased cardiac output, and increased systemic and pulmonary vascular resistance may occur in the unmodified sitting position. Severe hypotension can compromise cerebral perfusion. Hypotension is caused by peripheral venous pooling of blood in the extremities and exacerbated by positive pressure ventilation and the effect of anesthetic agents. There appears to be a relationship between the American Society of Anesthesiologists (ASA) status of the patient and the incidence and degree of hypotension. Patients with a higher ASA status tend to have more severe hypotension [26]. The risk of hypotension can be lowered by a number of measures. These include the administration of volume, avoidance of high airway pressures, application of compression stockings to the legs, and careful positioning. Gradual elevation of the head and torso, flexion at the hips, and knees raised to the level of the heart can all help maintain venous return and alleviate hypotension [27]. In a study of 579 infratentorial craniotomies including 333 in the sitting, and 246 in the horizontal position, the incidence of hypotension (defined as a reduction of systolic blood pressure of 20% or more from the baseline) was found to be similar between the two groups of patients [4–8, 27, 28].

People with degenerative spine disease undergoing craniotomy in the sitting position can develop ischemia of the cervical spinal cord leading to quadriplegia [29]. Neurologic deficits including stroke have also been described after shoulder surgery in the sitting position [30]. It is important to make sure that the transducer for the arterial line is placed at the level of the external auditory canal and that adequate perfusion pressure at the surgical site is maintained. Extreme neck flexion, hypotension, and anemia should be avoided in patients at risk for spinal cord ischemia.

Additional complications in the sitting position include injuries caused by impaired venous drainage, nerve injury, and air entry into the CNS. Exaggerated flexion of the head, especially with a rigid oral airway in place, can compress the base of the tongue leading to obstructed venous drainage. Consequently, macroglossia, necrosis of the tongue, and massive swelling of the head and neck may occur [31–33]. Peripheral neuropathies of the brachial plexus, ulnar, sciatic and common peroneal nerves have been reported after surgery in the sitting position [7, 34, 35]. Careful positioning, adequate padding of pressure points, and prevention of extreme flexion of the hip may reduce the risk of neuropathy. Pneumocephalus is common after surgery in the sitting position and is usually benign. Tension pneumocephalus can be life-threatening (discussed in a later section). Finally, a rare complication of craniotomy in the sitting patient is supratentorial intracerebral hemorrhage in the subcortical white matter [23]. One additional disadvantage of the sitting position for surgeons is that it may lead to neck and arm fatigue due to the angle required for operating [1].

Contraindications to the Sitting Position

The sitting position is traditionally considered contraindicated in patients with an open ventriculoatrial shunt, severe cerebrovascular disease, severe cervical stenosis, and right-to-left cardiac shunts including a probe patent foramen ovale [28]. Markedly hypovolemic or hypotensive patients may not tolerate the sitting position without decompensating further. Venous air embolism is also more likely to occur in extremely hypovolemic patients. Craniotomy in patients with severe hydrocephalus in the sitting position carries an increased risk of pneumocephalus and subdural hemorrhage [1].

THE PRONE POSITION

The prone position (Figure 17.7) is useful for accessing tumors in the posterior fossa, especially tumors that are closer to the midline. The incidence of venous air embolism while prone is lower than in the sitting position but higher than in the supine position. Complications associated with prone positioning include malposition of the endotracheal tube and difficult ventilation, neuropathies or other injuries due to pressure, facial or airway edema, and rarely, blindness due to either retinal artery thrombosis or ischemic optic neuropathy. The adult head is typically secured using three-point fixation while a Mayfield horseshoe headrest is used in children because their thin skull bone often makes

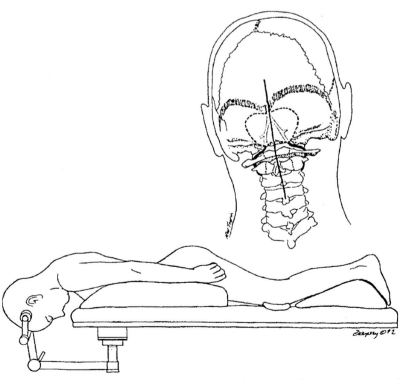

Figure 17.7 *The prone position.* The prone position and the suboccipital approach to the posterior fossa are demonstrated. The head is secured in a moderately flexed position with a skull-fixation device.

(Reproduced from Patel SJ, Wen DY, Haines SJ. Posterior fossa: surgical considerations. In: Cottrell JE and Smith SD, ed. *Anesthesia and Neurosurgery*. St. Louis, MO: Mosby; 2001:278, with permission from Elsevier.)

pin-fixation problematic. The neck is flexed to allow optimal surgical access. The position of the endotracheal tube should be carefully verified in the supine position before turning the patient prone. After intubation, it is helpful to use a fiberoptic bronchoscope to confirm that the tip of the endotracheal tube is at an acceptable distance (approximately 3 cm in average-sized adults) from the carina. If the tip of the tube is too close to the tracheal carina, it could migrate into the right main bronchus after flexion of the neck. Some practitioners prefer to use a wire-reinforced or a nasal endotracheal tube to prevent kinking of the endotracheal tube. If a wire-reinforced tube is used and postoperative intubation desired, it is usually necessary to exchange it with a regular endotracheal tube at the conclusion of the procedure. One should also take care to prevent the patient from biting down on the wire-reinforced tube since this is likely to deform the tube, leading to airway obstruction.

During positioning, one should ensure protection of vulnerable areas such as the elbows, knees, abdomen, genitals, breasts, and superficial peripheral nerves (e.g., the ulnar and tibial nerves). The breasts should be tucked inward to prevent direct pressure on the nipples, which can cause necrosis. The arms are padded and secured at the sides of the patient for posterior fossa or cervical spine surgery. Intravascular catheters and their associated tubing should be checked for patency after positioning is completed. Intraoperatively, surgeons often lean in at the sides of the patient and this can interfere with proper inflation of a blood pressure cuff placed on the upper arm.

THE LATERAL POSITION

The lateral position (Figure. 17.8) provides access to the cerebellopontine angle, cerebellum, and infracerebellar region [3]. In this position, significant bleeding from the superior petrosal venous sinus can occur while dissecting down to the cerebellopontine angle [3]. Access to the airway is superior to that in the prone position. The patient's superior shoulder may, however, get in the surgeon's way, so it is often pulled in a caudal direction using adhesive tape. Too much traction may cause a stretch injury of the brachial plexus, so this should be done with caution. Proper positioning should also emphasize protection of pressure points such as the dependent shoulder. The common peroneal nerve may be injured in the lower leg if the fibula is not padded near it's head. An infra-axillary roll will prevent pressure on the neurovascular bundle in the axilla.

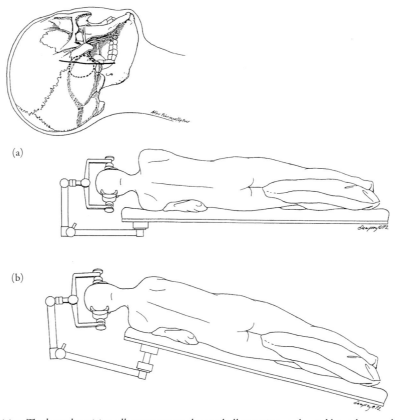

(a)

(b)

Figure 17.8   *A, B, The lateral position.* The lateral position allows access to the cerebellopontine angle, and lateral or cerebellar hemispheric lesions. The legs are padded and an infra-axillary roll has been placed. A. The upper shoulder is in the surgeon's way and may be pulled caudally with tape (carefully to prevent injury to the brachial plexus). B, Minor alteration allows good access to the retromastoid area with the shoulder out of the way.   (Reproduced from Patel SJ, Wen DY, Haines SJ. Posterior fossa: surgical considerations. In: Cottrell JE and Smith SD, ed. *Anesthesia and Neurosurgery.* St. Louis, MO: Mosby; 2001:327, with permission from Elsevier.)

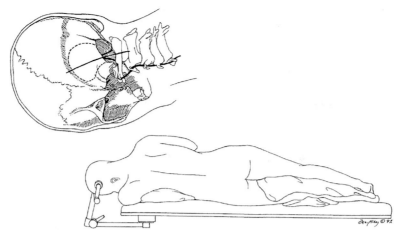

Figure 17.9   *The Park-Bench Position.* The park-bench or semi-prone position allows both lateral and midline approaches to the cerebellum including the cerebellopontine angle. It is quicker to achieve than the prone position and may be used in emergent cases. (Reproduced from Patel SJ, Wen DY, Haines SJ. Posterior fossa: surgical considerations. In: Cottrell JE and Smith SD, ed. *Anesthesia and Neurosurgery.* St. Louis, MO: Mosby; 2001:329, with permission from Elsevier.)

The lower arm is usually placed next to the body while the upper arm can be flexed and supported with pillows or foam. A pillow or blankets should be placed between slightly flexed legs.

PARK-BENCH OR SEMIPRONE POSITION

The park-bench position (Figure 17.9) can be useful for emergent surgery for cerebellar hemorrhage or infarction [3] (although the prone position is often used instead for these procedures). In this position, the patient is midway between the prone and lateral position, with the face turned downward and the ipsilateral shoulder moved out of the surgeon's way. Excessive rotation of the neck may cause venous obstruction, increased brain bulk and venous bleeding [1].

THE SUPINE POSITION

The supine position (Figure 17.10) with the neck laterally rotated is used for surgery at the cerebellopontine angle, particularly for small tumors. This position circumvents the problem of the nondependent shoulder being in the surgeon's way (as occurs in the lateral position) [1]. A roll is placed under the ipsilateral shoulder to prevent stretch of the brachial plexus and the elbows and knees are padded (not shown). Once again care should be taken to prevent extreme neck rotation; it is even more important to do so in patients with spondylosis of the cervical spine and those with severe carotid artery disease [1].

COMPLICATIONS OF POSTERIOR FOSSA SURGERY

Some of the complications related to the various intraoperative positions have been discussed in the preceding sections.

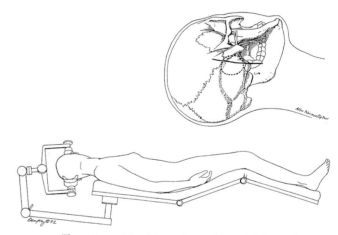

Figure 17.10   *The supine position.* The supine position with the neck laterally rotated and flexed for surgery at the cerebello-pontine angle. This position circumvents the shoulder being in the surgeon's way (as occurs in the lateral position.) (Reproduced from Patel SJ, Wen DY, Haines SJ. Posterior fossa: surgical considerations. In: Cottrell JE and Smith SD, ed. *Anesthesia and Neurosurgery.* St. Louis, MO: Mosby; 2001:331, with permission from Elsevier.)

Other complications associated with infratentorial surgery are presented in the following section.

HEMODYNAMIC CHANGES

In addition to the hemodynamic pertubations associated with the sitting position, there are other inherent hemodynamic changes which can occur with posterior fossa surgery. Lower cranial nerve nuclei and the cardiovascular and respiratory centers are located in close proximity in the brainstem. Dissection in the floor of the fourth ventricle can injure these structures. Cranial nerves V, IX, X, and XII can also be damaged during surgery at the cerebellopontine angle. Decades ago, when intraoperative mechanical ventilation was not in widespread use, posterior fossa tumors were resected in spontaneously breathing patients.

Respiratory disturbances were an early sign of injury to the respiratory centers and the lower cranial nerve nuclei. This sign will not occur, however, in patients who are being mechanically ventilated. At present, cardiovascular abnormalities (such as hypertension and tachycardia, hypotension or hypertension with bradycardia, sinus arrhythmia and ventricular arrhythmias) alone serve to forewarn of imminent, catastrophic injury to the brain stem [36]. If hemodynamic disturbances occur, the surgeon should be immediately notified. Pharmacological agents that can mask these signs should be avoided during these procedures unless the changes are truly life-threatening or do not resolve with the cessation of surgical stimulation. In addition, such patients should be extubated only after the adequate return of respiration and upper airway protective reflexes [36].

PNEUMOCEPHALUS

Pneumocephalus is common after posterior fossa surgery in the sitting position and usually resolves spontaneously [37, 38]. Air can collect at the operative site or layer in the supratentorial fossa during a posterior fossa procedure by an "inverted pop bottle" phenomenon [39, 40]. Less commonly, air entry into epidural or dural spaces in large volumes can cause a mass effect (tension pneumocephalus) and lead to brain herniation [41, 42]. Reduced brain volume, caused by aggressive use of osmotic agents, hypocarbia, and surgical decompression of tumor or blood, facilitates the formation of a tension pneumocephalus [43]. CSF drainage either by a catheter or by gravity in the sitting position further predisposes to the accumulation of intracranial air. Many recommend that nitrous oxide be discontinued (and hyperventilation stopped) before dural closure [27]. Others have suggested that nitrous oxide use does not increase ICP and need not be discontinued following dural closure [44]. In any case, if nitrous oxide has not been used during the case, it should not be introduced after the dura is closed because pockets of trapped air will increase in volume. Overall, it does not appear that nitrous oxide use (before dural closure) per se causes tension pneumocephalus [45]. Although various time intervals for avoiding nitrous oxide for repeat surgery after a craniotomy have been put forth, it may be more prudent to examine computed tomography scans for residual pneumocephalus in patients who return for surgery [40]. Postoperatively, a tension pneumocephalus should be suspected if a patient has seizures, unexplained neurological deficits, confusion or delayed emergence, especially after infratentorial surgery in the sitting position [7]. Hemodynamic changes such as tachycardia or bradycardia, and hypertension may be present. Urgent action such as a diagnostic computed tomography scan followed by drainage of air through a burr hole could be life-saving in such situations.

SURGICAL COMPLICATIONS OF POSTERIOR FOSSA SURGERY

In addition to the complications already mentioned, other surgical complications of posterior fossa surgery include cerebrospinal fluid leaks (most common), meningitis, wound infection, and cranial nerve (III to XII) palsies. Patients undergoing resection of cerebellar tumors may develop cerebellar edema. Hydrocephalus, hematomas and mutism are other complications after surgery on the cerebellum [2]. Damage to the cerebellum during midline posterior fossa tumor (medulloblastomas and other cerebellar tumors) resections may cause transient aphasia, especially in children [46]. Infratentorial craniotomies have a higher incidence of postoperative infection rates compared to supratentorial surgery [2]. Intraoperative contamination, CSF leaks, foreign bodies, long surgery, long-term use of steroids, and diabetes all contribute to postoperative infection. CSF seepage after posterior fossa craniectomy (7% incidence) may be due to poor dural closure or infection causing wound dehiscence [7]. CSF leaks in turn can lead to meningitis. According to some reports [14], a suboccipital craniectomy causes more CSF seepage in children than does a craniotomy for posterior fossa surgery. Infection is also less likely to occur if the bone flap is replaced.

The mortality rate after posterior fossa surgery in one study of 500 patients at a single institution was found to be 2.6% [2]. The patient's age, preexisting medical condition, type of tumor, and neurological impairment were determinants of mortality. Hematoma formation, brain edema with herniation, damage to blood vessels leading to ischemia and infarction, and tumor progression all contribute to poor outcome including death after posterior fossa surgery. Seizures are not common after infratentorial surgery. Deep venous thrombosis prophylaxis is important, especially in patients with cancer.

ANESTHETIC MANAGEMENT OF THE PATIENT UNDERGOING POSTERIOR FOSSA SURGERY

Preoperatively, the patient presenting for elective surgery should have the usual preanesthetic evaluation. Any preexisting neurological deficits should be noted. Brain imaging studies should be reviewed for the location of lesion and any associated hydrocephalus. If the procedure is tumor resection, it should be noted whether the tumor is intra-axial (e.g., gliomas) or extra-axial (e.g., meningioma), if there is a mass effect on the brain, midline shift, enhancement with contrast, surrounding edema, and the tumor's relation to nearby blood vessels and sinuses [47]. Planned operative positioning should be ascertained from surgeons.

If surgery in the sitting position is planned, the patient should be screened for conditions that would make such a position risky (e.g., the presence of a patent foramen ovale, or severe hypovolemia). Preoperative transthoracic echocardiography to screen for a PFO may be performed in patients who will be in the sitting position. Preoperative transthoracic echocardiography (TTE) combined with transesophageal echocardiography (when the images obtained by TTE were poor) detected PFO in 28% of 165 neurosurgical patients. If a PFO was detected, an alternative position to the sitting position was used for the procedure[48]. As discussed previously, the actual incidence of a clinically significant paradoxical air embolism is likely to be relatively low, even in a sitting craniotomy. If a large number of sitting craniotomies are performed at a given center, it may not be cost effective to obtain preoperative echocardiograms in all such patients and practitioners may feel comfortable proceeding without this study.

Patients may be severely hypovolemic before surgery due to hyperosmotic therapy, diuretics, vomiting, decreased intake due to altered mental status, or a condition such as diabetes insipidus. If this or other contraindications to the sitting position are identified, an alternative plan should be discussed with the surgeon and the patient.

A baseline electrocardiogram is useful to compare against any new intraoperative or postoperative rhythm changes. Depending on the type and location of the lesion, the anticipated length of the surgery and expected fluid shifts, as well as the patient's preoperative neurologic status and other medical problems, the possibility of postoperative intubation as well as intensive care unit admission should be discussed with the patient. Coagulation status should always be assessed for craniotomies. Cross-matched blood must be available if intraoperative transfusion is deemed likely. Premedication should be either be withheld or administered extremely cautiously in patients who have abnormal intracranial elastance. Patients with brain tumors are usually on steroids to reduce peritumoral edema; these should be continued in the perioperative period. Antibiotics should be administered before incision and re-dosed at the appropriate interval because of the increased risk of infection.

A patient with a large posterior fossa mass or a pineal gland tumor may have hydrocephalus and an external ventricular drain may have been placed prior to resection of the tumor (Figure 17.2). The anesthesiologist should determine whether the drainage system is open or sealed, its level relative to the patient's head, and the amount of drainage. Overdrainage or under drainage of CSF can have serious consequences such as intracranial bleeding, worsened hydrocephalus and intracranial hypertension. Vigilance is particularly important during patient transport and positioning and when changing the height of the operating room table. It is prudent to close the ventriculostomy drains of most patients during transport to prevent mishaps (for example, if a drainage bag falls to the ground unnoticed, excessive amounts of CSF may be inadvertently drained). Like other catheters and tubes, these catheters can also be accidentally removed.

When the patient is placed in the sitting position, the back is raised approximately sixty degrees and the hips and knees flexed [1]. The arms may be crossed across the chest and the extremities padded to prevent neuropathies. Extreme flexion and rotation of the neck should be avoided. Large and rigid oral airways should be avoided to prevent interference with venous drainage. There should be at least 4 to 5 cm of distance between the chin and the chest. The head-holder should be attached to the table such that the head and upper body can be moved as one unit (Figure 17.5). This will enable rapid, supine repositioning in the case of an emergency.

As discussed previously, a patient undergoing a craniotomy in the sitting position should have a central venous catheter, ideally placed at the junction of the SVC and the right atrium. A precordial Doppler should be positioned over the right atrium and may be tested with agitated saline or a small amount of air (0.1–0.2 mL) injected via the previously placed right atrial catheter. An intra-arterial catheter should be placed.

Nitrous oxide (50%) did not increase either the incidence or the severity of VAE in sitting craniotomies as long as it was discontinued immediately at the first sign of Doppler signals for VAE [19]. (It is reasonable to avoid using nitrous oxide for sitting craniotomies if one is concerned about its potential effect in enlarging air emboli that may not be immediately detected.) Volatile agents and propofol, short- or intermediate-acting narcotics (fentanyl, remifentanil), may be used according to individual preference. Desflurane has a greater tendency to stimulate coughing during extubation and hence may be avoided despite the quicker emergence associated with its use [49, 50]. High doses of volatile agents and nitrous oxide increase cerebral blood flow. This increase in cerebral blood flow is generally not clinically significant, especially when the patient is being mildly hyperventilated (Paco$_2$ 30–35 mm Hg). However, volatile agents and nitrous oxide are best avoided in cases of intractable brain swelling. Neuromuscular blocking agents are usually administered especially if the patient's head will be immobilized in a pin head-holder during the procedure. The use of neuromuscular blocking agents ensures an immobile field, reduces airway pressures and consequently venous bleeding, decreases the chances of injury due to patient movement, and facilitates hyperventilation. Prevention of spontaneous breathing in the sitting position will also reduce the chances of air entrainment caused by negative inspiratory pressure during a sudden respiratory effort.

Surgeons often request that mannitol or hypertonic saline be administered before the dura is opened in order to decrease brain bulk. Mannitol and hypertonic saline increase the osmolality of serum and draw fluid from the brain across an intact blood–brain barrier. In a prospective, randomized blinded study comparing the effects of equimolar doses of mannitol and 3% hypertonic saline during craniotomy, no difference in brain relaxation was found between the two agents [51]. Hyperventilation (an arterial carbon dioxide level of 30 to 35 mm Hg is usually considered safe) also decreases cerebral blood volume and brain bulk and counteracts any vasodilation due to volatile anesthetic agents. Extreme hyperventilation may cause cerebral ischemia. If the neck is excessively rotated or the head of the bed is not elevated, increased cerebral venous volume could contribute toward a potentially difficult and bloody dissection. Hypotonic and glucose-containing fluids are generally avoided during intracranial procedures unless specifically indicated. Normal saline, albumin, and packed red cells (when indicated) are the mainstay of fluids given to neurosurgical patients. Hypotonic solutions will increase cerebral edema while hyperglycemia can aggravate neurologic injury.

EMERGENCE AFTER POSTERIOR FOSSA CRANIOTOMY

After completion of surgery in the posterior fossa, it is important to ascertain that the patient is alert, and has adequate respiration and return of airway reflexes. Injury to cranial nerves IX, X, and XII can jeopardize airway patency and the ability to protect against aspiration. Long-acting sedatives and muscle relaxants should be avoided toward the end of the case, particularly without agreement with the surgical team. Frequently, an expeditious postoperative neurological assessment is desirable even in patients who will be left intubated.

Postoperative intubation and mechanical ventilation should be considered in patients who have had a long procedure, especially near the brainstem, or who have significant brain edema [7]. In one retrospective study of 145 adult patients undergoing infratentorial craniotomy, a higher ASA score, longer surgery, more blood loss, surgery near the brain stem, and an overall longer hospital stay were more common in patients who stayed intubated at the end of surgery [52]. Patients who had intracranial vascular surgery had more intraoperative blood loss and underwent surgery for a longer duration (and hence were more likely to stay intubated postoperatively) compared to those who had surgery for tumor resection. Patients with a poor preoperative neurologic status, those with lower cranial nerve palsy and absence of gag and cough reflexes, and hypothermic patients should also be left intubated [7]. Those with Chiari II may develop respiratory complications and should be carefully monitored postoperatively [3].

The patient should not be allowed to move or to regain consciousness while the head is secured in the head holder. This will increase venous pressure, may lead to cerebral edema and bleeding, as well as cause scalp lacerations from the pins, cervical spine injury, and other injuries. The depth of anesthesia can be reduced once the pins have been removed. Similarly, coughing is undesirable at emergence.

The patient should not be suctioned while lightly anesthetized as this could provoke coughing. Smokers and patients who have received desflurane are more likely to cough vigorously at extubation [49, 50]. Several drugs have been used to decrease the probability of coughing at extubation including narcotics, dexemedetomidine and lidocaine. One technique that may be adapted to neurosurgical patients is a low-dose remifentanil infusion (0.015 µg/kg/min) during emergence and extubation [53, 54]. This dose does not cause respiratory or cognitive depression in most patients but reduces the likelihood of coughing. However, this technique should be used judiciously and with attention to the overall clinical situation. Hypertension at emergence should be avoided as this can cause cerebral edema and intracranial bleeding after craniotomy.

ELECTROPHYSIOLOGICAL MONITORING

During surgery at the cerebellopontine angle, facial nerve conduction is often monitored using electromyography (EMG). Intraoperative monitoring of facial motor evoked potentials has also been described as a reliable technique to help preserve facial nerve function during this procedure [46–55]. Although direct facial nerve stimulation elicits motor activity even in the paralyzed state, surgeons usually request that patients not be intensely pharmacologically paralyzed during facial nerve conduction monitoring [56]. Motor evoked potentials (MEPs) can aid in monitoring corticospinal tract function during brainstem surgery [57]. Intense paralysis should also be avoided when motor evoked potentials are used. Intravenous anesthetics without nitrous oxide can be used if there is trouble obtaining adequate MEPs with volatile agents and nitrous oxide. Fortunately, modern MEP methods using multiple stimuli usually elicit satisfactory responses even in the presence of volatile agents or nitrous oxide.

Somatosensory evoked potentials (SSEPs) are sometimes used to monitor for spinal cord ischemia during cervical spine and posterior fossa procedures in the sitting position [58]. SSEPs may also correlate with neurological outcome after venous air embolism [59]. One obvious problem with relying on SSEPS is that only the sensory tract is monitored. The patient could develop new motor deficits despite intraoperative preservation of SSEPs. An increased risk of failure of SSEP monitoring has been described during infratentorial surgery on tumors with brainstem compression; undetected surgical damage causing postoperative neurological deficits occurred despite intact SSEPs [60]. High concentrations of volatile agents and nitrous oxide, as well as hypothermia, hypoxia, and hypercarbia, can increase the latency and depress the amplitude of SSEPs. Abrupt changes in anesthetic depth or physiologic parameters should be avoided during critical stages of the surgical procedure in order to prevent confusion about the etiology of any alterations in SSEPs.

If evoked potentials deteriorate during surgery, brain retractors and anything else pressing on the brain or vessels (e.g., sponges) should be removed and surgical manipulation ceased. Adequate arterial pressure should be ensured and a high venous pressure, if present, corrected (by elevating the patient's head or reducing PEEP) [57].

Brainstem auditory evoked potentials (BAEPs) may be used during acoustic neuroma or microvascular decompression to help preserve the integrity of CN VIII [61]. BAEPs are robust and resistant to interference by anesthetic agents.

CONCLUSIONS

Surgery in the posterior fossa presents unique challenges to the anesthesiologist. The majority of problems are due to the complex anatomy of the posterior fossa and the position that the patient is in during surgery. As with other challenging cases that anesthesiologists encounter, good communication with the surgical team and the patient, anticipation of likely problems, and careful planning will go a long way toward ensuring a smooth perioperative course for these patients. The author would like to thank Dr. Michael M. Todd for his helpful suggestions on an earlier draft of this chapter.

The author would like to thank Dr. Michael M. Todd for his helpful suggestions on an earlier draft of this chapter.

REFERENCES

1. Porter SS SA, Rengachary SS. Surgery and anesthesia of the posterior fossa. In: MS A, ed. *Textbook of Neuroanesthesia*. New York, NY: McGraw-Hill; 1997:971–1008.
2. Dubey A, Sung WS, Shaya M, et al. Complications of posterior cranial fossa surgery—an institutional experience of 500 patients. *Surg Neurol*. 2009;72:369–375.
3. Patel SJ WD, Haines SJ. Posterior fossa: surgical considerations. In: Cottrell JE, Smith SD, ed. *Anesthesia and Neurosurgery*. St. Louis, MO: Mosby; 2001:319–333.
4. Black S, Ockert DB, Oliver WC Jr, et al. Outcome following posterior fossa craniectomy in patients in the sitting or horizontal positions. *Anesthesiology*. Jul 1988;69(1):49–56.
5. Miller RA. Mechanical or spontaneous ventilation in the sitting position for neurosurgery? *Anaesthesia*. 1971;26:93.
6. Bitte EM, Goebert HW. Anesthesia for neurosurgery in the sitting position. *Pacific Med Surg*. 1966;74:22–24.
7. Rath GP, Bithal PK, Chaturvedi A, et al. Complications related to positioning in posterior fossa craniectomy. *J Clin Neurosci*. 2007;14:520–525.
8. Leonard IE, Cunningham AJ. The sitting position in neurosurgery—not yet obsolete! *Br J Anaesth*. 2002;88:1–3.
9. Papadopoulos G, Kuhly P, Brock M, et al. Venous and paradoxical air embolism in the sitting position. A prospective study with transoesophageal echocardiography. *Acta Neurochir*. 1994;126:140–143.
10. Cabezudo JM, Gilsanz F, Vaquero J, et al. Air embolism from wounds from a pin-type head-holder as a complication of posterior fossa surgery in the sitting position. Case report. *J Neurosurg*. 1981;55:147–148.
11. Albin MS, Carroll RG, Maroon JC. Clinical considerations concerning detection of venous air embolism. *Neurosurgery*. 1978;3:380–384.
12. Albin MS. Venous air embolism: a warning not to be complacent—we should listen to the drumbeat of history. *Anesthesiology*. 2011;115:626–629.
13. Matjasko J, Petrozza P, Cohen M, et al. Anesthesia and surgery in the seated position: analysis of 554 cases. *Neurosurgery*. 1985;17:695–702.
14. Hagen PT, Scholz DG, Edwards WD. Incidence and size of patent foramen ovale during the first 10 decades of life: an autopsy study of 965 normal hearts. *Mayo Clin Proc*. 1984;59:17–20.
15. Mammoto T, Hayashi Y, Ohnishi Y, et al. Incidence of venous and paradoxical air embolism in neurosurgical patients in the sitting position: detection by transesophageal echocardiography. *Acta Anaesthesiol Scand*. 1998;42:643–647.
16. Schlundt J, Tzanova I, Werner C. A case of intrapulmonary transmission of air while transitioning a patient from a sitting to a supine position after venous air embolism during a craniotomy. *Can J Anaesth*. 2012;59:478–482.
17. Fathi AR, Eshtehardi P, Meier B. Patent foramen ovale and neurosurgery in sitting position: a systematic review. *Br J Anaesth*. 2009;102:588–596.
18. Toung TJ, Rossberg MI, Hutchins GM. Volume of air in a lethal venous air embolism. *Anesthesiology*. 2001;94:360–361.
19. Losasso TJ, Muzzi DA, Dietz NM, et al. Fifty percent nitrous oxide does not increase the risk of venous air embolism in neurosurgical patients operated upon in the sitting position. *Anesthesiology*. 1992;77:21–30.
20. Domaingue CM. Anaesthesia for neurosurgery in the sitting position: a practical approach. *Anaesth Intens Care*. 2005;33:323–331.
21. Maroon JC, Albin MS. Air embolism diagnosed by Doppler ultrasound. *Anesth Analg*. 1974;53:399–402.
22. Colley PS, Pavlin EG, Groepper J. Assessment of a saline injection test for location of a right atrial catheter. *Anesthesiology*. 1979;50:258–260.
23. Haines SJ, Maroon JC, Jannetta PJ. Supratentorial intracerebral hemorrhage following posterior fossa surgery. *J Neurosurg*. 1978;49:881–886.
24. Dunbar EM, Fox R, Watson B, et al. Successful late treatment of venous air embolism with hyperbaric oxygen. *Postgrad Med J*. 1990;66:469–470.
25. Torres Martinez FJ, Kuffler DP. Hyperbaric oxygen treatment to eliminate a large venous air embolism: a case study. *Undersea Hyperbaric Med*. 2011;38:297–304.
26. Albin MS, Babinski M, Wolf S. Cardiovascular responses to the sitting position. *Br J Anaesth*. 1980;52:961–962.
27. Porter JM, Pidgeon C, Cunningham AJ. The sitting position in neurosurgery: a critical appraisal. *Br J Anaesth*. 1999;82:117–128.
28. Black S CR. Tumor surgery. In: Cucchiara RF BS, Michenfelder JD, ed. *Clinical Neuroanesthesia*. New York: Churchill Livingstone; 1998:343–366.
29. Wilder BL. Hypothesis: the etiology of midcervical quadriplegia after operation with the patient in the sitting position. *Neurosurgery*. 1982;11:530–531.
30. Papadonikolakis A, Wiesler ER, Olympio MA, et al. Avoiding catastrophic complications of stroke and death related to shoulder surgery in the sitting position. *Arthroscopy*. 2008;24:481–482.
31. Teeple E, Maroon J, Rueger R. Hemimacroglossia and unilateral ischemic necrosis of the tongue in a long-duration neurosurgical procedure. *Anesthesiology*. 1986;64:845–846.
32. McAllister RG. Macroglossia—a positional complication. *Anesthesiology*. 1974;40:199–200.
33. Ellis SC, Bryan-Brown CW, Hyderally H. Massive swelling of the head and neck. *Anesthesiology*. 1975;42:102–103.
34. Wang JC, Wong TT, Chen HH, et al. Bilateral sciatic neuropathy as a complication of craniotomy performed in the sitting position: localization of nerve injury by using magnetic resonance imaging. *Child Nerv Syst*. 2012;28:159–163.

35. Gozal Y, Pomeranz S. Sciatic nerve palsy as a complication after acoustic neurinoma resection in the sitting position. *J Neurosurg Anesthesiol.* 1994;6:40–42.

36. Drummond JC, Todd MM. Acute sinus arrhythmia during surgery in the fourth ventricle: an indicator of brain-stem irritation. *Anesthesiology.* 1984;60:232–235.

37. Di Lorenzo N, Caruso R, Floris R, et al. Pneumocephalus and tension pneumocephalus after posterior fossa surgery in the sitting position: a prospective study. *Acta Neurochir.* 1986;83:112–115.

38. Standefer M, Bay JW, Trusso R. The sitting position in neurosurgery: a retrospective analysis of 488 cases. *Neurosurgery.* 1984;14:649–658.

39. Lunsford LD, Maroon JC, Sheptak PE, et al. Subdural tension pneumocephalus. Report of two cases. *J Neurosurg.* 1979;50:525–527.

40. Sloan T. The incidence, volume, absorption, and timing of supratentorial pneumocephalus during posterior fossa neurosurgery conducted in the sitting position. *J Neurosurg Anesthesiol.* 2010;22:59–66.

41. Azar-Kia B, Sarwar M, Batnitzky S, et al. Radiology of intracranial gas. *Am J Roentgenol Radium Ther Nucl Med.* 1975;124:315–323.

42. Findler G, Hoffman HJ, Munro IR. Tension pneumocephalus complicating craniofacial surgery in a shunted hydrocephalic patient: case report. *Neurosurgery.* 1980;7:525–528.

43. Friedman GA, Norfleet EA, Bedford RF. Discontinuance of nitrous oxide does not prevent tension pneumocephalus. *Anesth Analg.* 1981;60:57–58.

44. Domino KB, Hemstad JR, Lam AM, et al. Effect of nitrous oxide on intracranial pressure after cranial-dural closure in patients undergoing craniotomy. *Anesthesiology.* 1992;77:421–425.

45. Pasternak JJ, Lanier WL. Is nitrous oxide use appropriate in neurosurgical and neurologically at-risk patients? *Curr Opin Anaesthesiol.* 2010;23:544–550.

46. Aguiar PH, Plese JP, Ciquini O, et al. Transient mutism following a posterior fossa approach to cerebellar tumors in children: a critical review of the literature. *Child Nerv Syst.* 1995;11:306–310.

47. Weinghart JD and BRem H. In: RIchard WH, ed. *Youman's Neurological Surgery.* Vol 2, 6th ed. Philadelphia, PA: Elsevier Saunders:1261–1266.

48. Weihs W, Schuchlenz H, Harb S, et al. [Preoperative diagnosis of a patent foramen ovale: rational use of transthoracic and transesophageal contrast echocardiography]. *Der Anaesthesist.* 1998;47:833–837.

49. White PF, Tang J, Wender RH, et al. Desflurane versus sevoflurane for maintenance of outpatient anesthesia: the effect on early versus late recovery and perioperative coughing. *Anesth Analg.* 2009;109:387–393.

50. Arain SR, Shankar H, Ebert TJ. Desflurane enhances reactivity during the use of the laryngeal mask airway. *Anesthesiology.* 2005;103:495–499.

51. Rozet I, Tontisirin N, Muangman S, et al. Effect of equiosmolar solutions of mannitol versus hypertonic saline on intraoperative brain relaxation and electrolyte balance. *Anesthesiology.* 2007;107:697–704.

52. Cata JP, Saager L, Kurz A, et al. Successful extubation in the operating room after infratentorial craniotomy: the Cleveland Clinic experience. *J Neurosurg Anesthesiol.* 2011;23:25–29.

53. Aouad MT, Al-Alami AA, Nasr VG, et al. The effect of low-dose remifentanil on responses to the endotracheal tube during emergence from general anesthesia. *Anesth Analg.* 2009;108:1157–1160.

54. Lee JH, Koo BN, Jeong JJ, et al. Differential effects of lidocaine and remifentanil on response to the tracheal tube during emergence from general anaesthesia. *Br J Anaesth.* 2011;106:410–415.

55. Matthies C, Raslan F, Schweitzer T, et al. Facial motor evoked potentials in cerebellopontine angle surgery: technique, pitfalls and predictive value. *Clin Neurol Neurosurg.* 2011;113:872–879.

56. Macdonald DB. Intraoperative motor evoked potential monitoring: overview and update. *J Clin Monit Comput.* 2006;20:347–377.

57. Sarnthein J, Bozinov O, Melone AG, et al. Motor-evoked potentials (MEP) during brainstem surgery to preserve corticospinal function. *Acta Neurochir.* 2011;153:1753–1759.

58. Urasaki E, Wada S, Matsukado Y, et al. Monitoring of short-latency somatosensory evoked potentials during surgery for cervical cord and posterior fossa lesions—changes in subcortical components. *Neurol Medicochir.* 1988;28:546–552.

59. Reasoner DK, Dexter F, Hindman BJ, et al. Somatosensory evoked potentials correlate with neurological outcome in rabbits undergoing cerebral air embolism. *Stroke.* 1996;27:1859–1864.

60. Wiedemayer H, Sandalcioglu IE, Armbruster W, et al. False negative findings in intraoperative SEP monitoring: analysis of 658 consecutive neurosurgical cases and review of published reports. *J Neurol Neurosurg Psychiatry.* 2004;75:280–286.

61. Moller AR. Monitoring auditory function during operations to remove acoustic tumors. *Am J Otol.* 1996;17:452–460.

18.

SURGERY FOR EPILEPSY

Lorenz G. Theiler, Robyn S. Weisman, and Thomas M. Fuhrman

INTRODUCTION

Surgery for epilepsy includes a variety of procedures such as tissue resection, implantation of a device to prevent or reduce seizures (e.g., a vagal nerve stimulator or deep brain stimulator), or mapping to localize the seizure focus.

These procedures may require a general or local anesthetic for patient safety and comfort. For example, intraoperative mapping requires minimal use of anesthetic agents that may suppress epileptic signals. Surgical resection may require that the patient be awake in order to protect the eloquent areas of the brain or to allow the epileptic focus to be evaluated during the operation. The anesthetic implications may also include the addition of prophylaxis for or treatment of a postoperative seizure.

EPILEPSY

Epilepsy is a chronic neurologic disorder that is defined as two or more unprovoked seizures. Up to 10% of all people have one seizure during their lifetime, and having a single seizure does not constitute a diagnosis of epilepsy. It is more likely to occur in the very young or in people over the age of 65 but may occur at any age. It is estimated that around 50 million people worldwide have epilepsy. Some forms of epilepsy, such as those associated with congenital conditions or those with a genetic component, are more prevalent in childhood. In older patients, traumatic head injuries, tumors, and cerebrovascular disease are the most common etiologies. Other etiologies, such as infection or tumor, may occur at any age. Epilepsy is not a single disorder but rather a constellation of disorders with different signs and symptoms that range from fairly benign to debilitating. A person's epilepsy is said to be medically refractory when it cannot be brought under control after satisfactory test periods of two or more antiepilepsy medications.

Patients with epilepsy have often suffered from social stigmatization. A diagnosis of epilepsy is still a basis to prevent a person from getting married or as a reason to annul a marriage in China and India. It was only in 1970 that the United Kingdom repealed a law making it illegal for those with epilepsy to marry. Even the United States had laws preventing those with epilepsy from entering public buildings such as restaurants or theaters until the 1970s. Social acceptance has taken great strides with the advancements in therapy, treatment, and the understanding of epilepsy. Patients with medically verified seizure control can now drive an automobile and may qualify for a pilot's license if they have been seizure free for at least 10 years.

Epilepsy has been recognized for more than 3000 years. A translation of a cuneiform, from Mesopotamia dated before 1000 years BC, described the falling sickness (epilepsy). The Babylonian term was *miqtu*. "If at the time of his possession, while he is sitting down, his (left) eye moves to that side, a lip puckers, saliva flows from his mouth, and trunk on the left side jerk (or twitch) like a (newly) slaughtered sheep, it is *miqtu*" [1]. Epilepsy received its present name from the Greek *epilepsia* ("to seize"), as was noted in the work of Hippocrates, *Sacred Disease* circa 400 BC. That work discussed the symptoms of eye movements, convulsions, and loss of bowel/bladder function. Over the next 500 to 700 years, tonic and clonic seizures were described, and changes in heart rate and respirations were appreciated [2]. John Hughlings Jackson in 1870 gave an address titled *A Study of Convulsions* in which he described a convulsion as "but a symptom, and implies only that there is an occasional, an excessive, and a disorderly discharge of nerve tissue on muscles. This discharge occurs in all degrees; it occurs with all sorts of conditions of ill health, at all ages, and under innumerable circumstances" [1].

Epilepsy has a wide range of symptoms that include seizures, symptoms of the primary diseases associated with some types of epilepsies, and an increased risk for death. In 2002 a report from the United Kingdom, the National Sentinel Audit of Epilepsy-Related Deaths, noted "1000 deaths occur every year in the UK as a result of epilepsy." Most of them are associated with seizures and 42% of deaths were potentially avoidable [3]. This increased risk may be due to an episode of *status epilepticus* (a prolonged seizure or two or more seizures very close together) and may be related to a lack of compliance with antiepileptic drug (AED) therapy. Traumatic injury may occur during a seizure, resulting in a hospital stay or death. Patients with epilepsy have an increased risk of suicide due to depression that may be secondary to the psychological aspects of the disease or as a side effect of many AEDs. The increased risk of suicide may be up to 5 times higher in patients with epilepsy than the population as a whole and up to 25 times higher in patients with temporal lobe epilepsy [4].

Epilepsy increases a person's risk of premature death by 2 to 3 times that of the general population [5]. Sudden unexpected death in epilepsy (SUDEP) [5] is a rare occurrence for which the etiology remains controversial. There seems to be an association of cardiac disturbances with epileptic seizures, and ictal cardiac arrest has been proposed as one possible mechanism of SUDEP. One report notes that over 55% of patients with refractory epilepsy have autonomic dysfunction [6]. Forty percent of patients with refractory epilepsy have been found to have abnormalities in rhythm or repolarization [7]. Standridge and colleagues reported abnormal QT intervals were seen in 12% of all the patients on a pediatric epilepsy monitoring unit [8]. Cardiac rhythms observed during seizures include atrial fibrillation, supraventricular tachycardia, premature ventricular contractions, bundle-branch block, and atrioventricular block [7]. Another study found a decrease in the incidence of SUDEP in patients who had undergone successful surgery for epilepsy [9]. In general, the patients at highest risk for epilepsy-related deaths are those who often have underlying neurologic impairment or poorly controlled seizures. Patients who have controlled seizures and therefore often have less neurologic impairment are at much lower risk of epilepsy-related death.

Epilepsy has also been associated with obstructive sleep apnea (OSA). One case series describes a small number of patients with epilepsy who were initially screened for OSA and then underwent diagnostic polysomography. Of 13 adults who were screened for possible OSA, 6 were diagnosed with OSA by polysomography. While maintaining their current AED therapy, three of those with OSA were then treated with continuous positive airway pressure (CPAP). The CPAP treatment resulted in at least a 45% decrease in seizure activity [10]. The report did not state whether episodes of sleep apnea coincided with cardiac arrhythmias.

MEDICAL MANAGEMENT

Seizures in many patients can be controlled with medication. One study of patients with newly diagnosed epilepsy found that 47% achieved effective seizure control with the use of a single drug. Another 14% became seizure free after a second or third drug had been added to their treatment regimen. In that study, the use of two drugs simultaneously successfully treated an additional 3% of patients [11]. AED therapy is effective in about 70% of patients with epilepsy [12].

AED's are classified by their effect on sodium channels, calcium channels, γ-aminobutyric acid (GABA), or glutamate receptors. They can also be separated somewhat by the types of seizure symptoms they best treat [13]. Many of the most commonly used AEDs are listed in Table 18.1 along with possible drug interactions and side effects. Some of those patients who suffer significant side effects from AEDs and other patients, from the 30% nonresponsive to medical therapy group, may have conditions that are amenable to surgical therapy. Moreover, AEDs control epileptic seizures but do not treat the underlying condition or halt progression of the disease.

Although AEDs can be used to manage seizures, these drugs have significant side effects that can limit their use in certain patients (Table 18.1). In a study by Baker and colleagues, 88% of patients reported at least one side effect with medication to control their epilepsy. Only 12% of patients in the study had no side effects from the AEDs. During the study period, almost a third of patients required a medication change at least once in that year and 6% required medication change 3 or more times in that year [12]. Side effects may include rash, hypersensitivity, liver failure, gastrointestinal problems, aggravation of seizures, dizziness, and somnolence. Side effects typically appear soon after treatment has started. Neurologic complications of treatment, including sedation, encephalopathy, depression, behavioral problems, psychotic episodes, and cognitive disorders, may be delayed. Possible hematologic side effects include leukopenia, aplastic anemia, thrombocytopenia, and megaloblastic anemia. Some patients have also experienced pancreatitis, nephrolithiasis, and weight loss or weight gain. Teratogencity has also been noted with some of the agents used to control epilepsy [13].

PREANESTHETIC ASSESSMENT OF PATIENTS WITH EPILEPSY

Preanesthetic evaluation of a patient undergoing epilepsy surgery consists of a routine medical evaluation as well as implications of the seizure disorder and its treatment (Table 18.2) [13–16].

The patient should be questioned about side effects of the patient's current AEDs. AEDs have numerous systemic effects and laboratory studies are guided by the specific drugs being used. For example, some medications affect liver function, thyroid function, or blood cell counts. In a study by Verma and colleagues, only 1 of 317 had thyroid function test changes and only 14 of 642 patient had elevated liver function tests [17]. This study conclude that routine liver function tests are not necessary in patients receiving only one AED unless hepatic disease is also present. Patients receiving two or more agents, specifically if they include phenobarbital or valproate, and those requiring very high doses of AEDs should have their liver function tests monitored. Clinicians should be aware that an aspartate aminotransferase (AST) level does not reflect therapy with phenytoin, while alanine aminotransferase (ALT)

Table 18.1 SOME OF THE REPORTED POSSIBLE SIDE EFFECTS OF AEDS

GENERIC NAME	BRAND NAME	ENZYME INDUCER	POSSIBLY DECREASE EFFECT OF	POSSIBLY INCREASE EFFECT OF	OTHER POSSIBLE EFFECTS
Carbamazepine	Tegretol	Yes	Muscle relaxants, methadone, anticoagulants	Diltiazem*	Elevated LFTs Lowered T$_4$ Hyponatremia
Clorazepate	Tranxene	Yes			
Clonazepam	Klonopin	Yes			
Ethosuximide	Zarontin	No			
Felbamate	Felbatol	No			Liver toxicity Aplastic anemia
Fosphenytoin	Cerebyx	Yes			
Gabapentin	Neurontin	No			
Lamotrigine	Lamictal	Yes			Hyponatremia
Levetiracetam	Keppra	No			
Oxcarbazepine	Trileptal	Yes	Nifedipine, nimodipine		Hyponatremia
Phenobarbital	Luminal	Yes	Muscle relaxants, diltiazem, nifedipine, nimodipine, metoprolol Anticoagulants		ALT increase No change in TF Ts or decreased TFTs
Phenytoin	Dilantin	Yes	Muscle relaxants, nifedipine, nimodipine Anticoagulants	Diltiazem	Elevated AL Tlowers T$_4$ and T uptake Gingival hyperplasia**
Pregabalin	Lyrica	No			Hyponatremia
Primidone	Mysoline	Yes			
Topiramate	Topamax	Yes			Nephrolithiasis
Valproate semisodium	Depakote	No		Anticoagulants	AST Increase
Valproic acid	Depakene	No			Thrombocytopenia, lowered T uptake Pancreatitis ALT increase
Zonisamide	Zonegran	No			Nephrolithiasis

Data from References 13–16.

*Diltiazem can inhibit cytochrome P450, which can lead to neurotoxicity through increased levels of carbamazepine. (Nifedipine, as a dihydropyridine calcium channel blocker, does not inhibit cytochrome P450.)

In general, the enzyme-inducing AEDs increase the metabolism of antiarrhythmics, β-blockers, and dihydropyridine calcium antagonists.

†See below for discussion of gingival hyperplasia.

elevations could be related to phenytoin therapy but not to other AEDs. Elevations in both ALT and AST should not be proscribed just to AED therapy alone [17].

The general preanesthetic assessment of a patient with epilepsy should proceed on the same lines as any other preoperative evaluation. Other conditions with higher incidence in people with epilepsy are noted in Table 18.3 [18–20]. Compared with the general population, people with epilepsy have significantly higher prevalence (more than two) of stomach ulcers, urinary incontinence, intestinal disorders, migraine headaches, Alzheimer's disease, and chronic fatigue syndrome [18]. Other conditions with higher incidence in people with epilepsy are noted in Table 18.3 [19]. Some conditions, such as urinary incontinence in a patient with cerebral palsy and epilepsy, or stomach ulcers in a patient severely depressed with his or her condition, have a clear association with epilepsy. Others, like hypertension, asthma, and chronic obstructive pulmonary disease, are more prevalent in patients with epilepsy, but the relationship is not obviously apparent.

Patients with epilepsy may be at increased risk for having a difficult airway. Phenytoin causes gingival hyperplasia in up to 57% of patients within 6 months of initiating phenytoin therapy, although this may also be attributed in part to poorer dental hygiene while taking phenytoin [21]. Phenobarbital rarely causes gingival hyperplasia, as can calcium channel blockers and cyclosporine [22]. A patient with severe gingival hyperplasia may present with a problematic

Table 18.2 SIMPLIFIED PREANESTHETIC CLASSIFICATION OF EPILEPSY

Etiology (Known cause: structural abnormality, disease state or idiopathic)

Signs and symptoms of the seizures (Generalized "full body" seizure or focal seizure)

Structural location in the brain where the seizures originate. (May not be fully appreciated prior to surgery, as some procedures involve detailed mapping [electrocorticography] of the suspected brain area)

Is it part of a syndrome? (What other manifestations may be included in the syndrome)

Triggering event (If applicable, in general it would be prudent to avoid triggering agents/activities although the trigger may be included as provocative test during intraoperative electrocorticography).

difficult airway as the hyperplasia can reduce the oral opening available and the tissue may be prone to bleeding. Even mild cases can result in gingival bleeding that can obscure the view or result in aspiration of blood during routine direct laryngoscopy. Patients who have undergone previous frontotemporal craniotomy may also have a difficult airway as soon as a few days to a week after surgery. There are many reports about patients with a previous normal airway examination only to have a very limited oral opening shortly after a previous surgery [23–27]. In most cases, the anesthesia team relied on the previous preoperative evaluation or the intraoperative anesthesia record, which described an easy intubation. Some patients were able to open their mouths less than two-thirds of what they were previously reported, in some cases, between 0.20 and 2.0 cm [26, 27]. The condition is known as pseudoankylosis of the mandible and it can occur after surgery involving the temporalis muscle following frontotemporal, supratentorial, or pterional craniotomy. These patients' limited oral opening could preclude the use of an laryngeal mask airway (LMA) and may require a fiberoptic intubation.

NEUROSURGICAL EVALUATION

The International League against Epilepsy (ILAE) classification system, which last updated their classification scheme

Table 18.3 CONDITIONS MORE PREVALENT IN PEOPLE WITH EPILEPSY THAN IN THE GENERAL POPULATION [21]

Diabetes	Bronchitis/emphysema
Stroke	Heart disease
Asthma	High blood pressure
Cancer	Thyroid conditions
Arthritis	Back problems
Allergies	Glaucoma
Cataracts	Fibromyalgia

in 1999 [28], has proved to be beneficial for physicians and researchers. This system permits the characteristics of a disease (e.g., incidence, epidemiology, etiologies, and treatments) to be objectively compared. Criteria include general history of the neurologic condition of the patient and seizure history (onset and duration). *Resistant seizures* are defined as a history of more than 1 to 2 years of failed medical therapy with at least two drugs at the maximally tolerated dosages; seizures are incapacitating or significantly interfere with normal activities.

The neurologic evaluation is usually divided into two parts. The first stage is noninvasive and includes neuropsychological evaluation, electroencephalographic (EEG), magnetic resonance imaging (MRI) and functional MRI (fMRI), positron emission tomography (PET), and single-photon emission computerized tomography (SPECT) [29]. Although it is not noninvasive test, a Wada test is usually performed during the initial evaluation.

The intracarotid amobarbital procedure (Wada test) (IAP) was conceived by Juhn A. Wada in 1948 [30]. Amobarbital, a short-acting barbiturate, is injected directly into the carotid artery and anesthetizes that cerebral hemisphere for approximately 5 minutes. The Wada test is currently used to evaluate four areas of concern: prediction of memory function, speech lateralization, seizure foci localization, and predict surgical outcome [31]. In addition to amobarbital, pentobarbital, methohexital, etomidate, and propofol have all been used. There is no standardized dosing protocol. Amobarbital doses in adults range from 60 to 200 mg, and the speed of injection varies between institutions. The best that was determined were two methods that use specific memory testing (named for the cities where the institutions of development are located: Seattle and Montreal) agreed in 70% of the patients, while comparing the Seattle to the Interview method achieved only 45% agreement [32, 33].

Complications of IAP include encephalopathy (7.2%), strokes (1.2%), and transient ischemic attacks (TIAs) (0.6%). Other complications were related to allergic reaction (0.3%) or procedural problems such as carotid artery dissection (0.4%) or bleeding or infection (0.8%). Two other patients were noted to have short periods of apnea described as self-limited [20]. Loddenkemper reviewed the Wada test in 677 consecutive patients and found more than 10% (74 of 677) had complications without any reported deaths [34]. Respiratory complications have been reported in patients with abnormal carotid and basilar circulation. Intracarotid injection of amobarbital in these patients resulted in brainstem perfusion and subsequent respiratory arrest [31]. In other reports, deaths have occurred after strokes during the IAP [35]. However, not all problems during an IAP result in serious complications. English reported a patient who suffered a stroke undergoing an IAP during a presurgical evaluation. The cerebral infarct ablated the seizure focus and resolved the patient's seizure disorder [36]!

Because of the risks involved and the possible inaccuracy of the results, IAP is being supplanted by less invasive studies such as fMRI, PET, SPECT, and transcranial Doppler [37, 38]. Invasive testing should be reserved for situations when the noninvasive tests give equivocal or conflicting results or when the noninvasive testing cannot provide the accuracy required [39].

SURGICAL MANAGEMENT

VAGAL NERVE STIMULATOR

Vagal nerve stimulation (VNS) was first used clinically for treatment of partial-onset seizures in 1988 and was approved for clinical use in the United States in 1997 [40, 41]. VNS may be considered in patients whose seizures are poorly controlled with medication and may be the only option for approximately 40% of patients who are not candidates for more invasive surgical procedures. VNS has also been shown to be efficacious in patients who had already undergone surgical resections in attempts to control their epilepsy. In a comparative study of over 4700 patients, 921 patients after cranial surgery and 3822 patients with only VNS surgical treatment, Amar and colleagues noted a reduction of seizure incidence of 42.5% at 3 months after VNS implantation in the post cranial surgery group [42].

VNS devices typically use a periodic stimulation cycle, although some patients who experience an aura before seizures are able to place a magnet over the VNS to turn it on when they sense an imminent seizure. One study compared "high-stimulation" and "low-stimulation" protocols. The high-stimulus group received a 500-μsec pulse at 30 Hz every 30 seconds on a 5-minute on–off cycle, while the low-stimulus group received a 130-μsec pulse at 1 Hz on for 30 seconds every 3 hours [43]. High stimulation resulted in a 28% reduction in seizures with only a 15% reduction in the low-stimulus group.

By 2004, Guberman estimated over 25,000 VNSs had been implanted with clinical success indicated by reduction of the frequency of seizures by 50% or more in 30% to 40% of patients [44–47]. Follow-up studies of patients have shown continued successful responses over 4 years after VNS implantation [48, 49].

The VNS intermittently stimulates the vagus nerve, indirectly stimulating the brain [49–52. The stimulator itself appears similar to a cardiac pacemaker and is implanted under the skin. An electrode is tunneled under the skin to the neck, where it is wrapped around the vagus nerve. The left vagus nerve is used, because the right side has a greater effect on the sinoatrial node. (The left side seems to have a greater effect on the atrioventricular node [53].) The incidence of reported bradyarrhythmias *is less than* 0.1% if the left vagus nerve is stimulated, but Ali and colleagues reported an incidence of almost 9% (3 of 35 patients) of

complete heart block and transient asystole during the surgical implantations of VNSs [54]. Those patients responded to the initial left VNSs with cardiac arrhythmias; however, the arrhythmias ceased after stopping the stimulations. Of those three patients, only one had an abnormal electrocardiogram (ECG) prior to surgery, a first-degree heart block. Arrhythmias have almost always occurred during implantation of the device, but there was one case in which a patient had syncope attributed to a bradyarrhythmia (coinciding with VNS) over 2 years after his VNS implantation [55]. It would therefore seem prudent to review the preoperative ECG and obtaining a cardiac electrophysiology consult for patients with an abnormal ECG prior to any VNS implantation [56].

After almost 20 years of clinical use, the exact mechanism of inhibition of seizures by the VNS is still unknown. It is the efferent actions of the vagal nerve carrying impulses form the brain to the viscera that is most familiar to clinicians (parasympathetic actions), but those tracts of the vagal nerve comprise only around 20% of the nerve's fibers. The other 80% are afferent sensory fibers that carry signals to the brain in the nucleus tractus solitarius and then on to areas of the brain often associated with seizure activity [40, 49]. EEG synchronization may be either increased or decreased by VNS in animals, but this effect does not occur in humans [50, 51]. Work has been done regarding the levels of neurotransmitters in patients with VNS [50, 51]. Marrosu and colleagues showed that GABA receptor density normalized after 1 year of VNS, while receptors in patients in a control group followed for a similar period did not have the same changes in their receptor density [52].

VNS devices are almost always implanted under general anesthesia. The propensity for significant arrhythmias, even with the reported low rate of occurrence, has been advocated as a reason to make general anesthesia the prudent choice [56]. They have, however, also been implanted under deep and superficial cervical plexus nerves. In one study, 12 patients had the procedure under regional and local anesthesia without any complication, while 10 previous patients underwent placement under general anesthesia. Three of the patients who received general anesthesia suffered postoperative seizures and eight had significant nausea and vomiting [57].

Despite their potential to cause dysrhythmias, even patients who are at risk for SUDEP may benefit from implantation of a VNS. Annegers studied almost 2000 patients for 2 years before and after a VNS was implanted and found no correlation between the VNS and SUDEP. The incidence of SUDEP after VNS was no different than the group for the 2 years before the VNS (4.1 versus 4.5 per 1000 person-years). However, in the next 2-year follow-up period, there was actually a reduction in the incidence of SUDEP at only 1.7 per 1000 person-years [58].

Noncardiac complications of VNS implantation include infection and hematoma. Horner's syndrome, partial left-sided facial paralysis, voice alteration (sometimes only during a stimulus period), and reversible left vocal cord paralysis have also been reported [40, 59]. The true incidence of complications, especially the less severe ones, is probably not known. The VNS device manufacturer had maintained a voluntary patient registry, but only about 40% of patients with a VNS have been added as of 2001 [59].

DEEP BRAIN STIMULATION

Deep brain stimulation (DBS) is used as therapy for seizures. This technology is also used for movement disorders and is being investigated as a treatment for obesity and depression. The DBS has been shown to be of benefit in patients with epileptogenic lesions in the hippocampus, the anterior thalamic nucleus, the centromedian thalamic nucleus, the subthalamic nucleus, the caudate nucleus, or the cerebellum (the cerebellum is the only current noncortical area to be stimulated in the treatment of epilepsy) [60, 61]. Monthly seizures have been reduced from a range of 14% to 76% in clinical studies [62]. Although DBS is not considered to be as invasive as a craniotomy, its complications include hemorrhage and new neurologic deficits during the perioperative period. Late postoperative complications include hardware problems or erosion through skin, etc. [63]. In one case, venous air embolism was reported in a patient who was positioned with the head 30 degrees or more upright, for patient comfort and surgeon preference, and allowed to breathe spontaneously [64]. Although that case report involved DBS implantation in a patient with a movement disorder, this complication may occur in any patient undergoing a DBS under local and monitored anesthesia care (MAC).

DBS implantation is most often accomplished under local anesthesia or MAC in patients with movement disorders because it is necessary to continuously evaluate the patient during the procedure to ensure proper placement. DBS implantation for epilepsy may be performed under local or general anesthesia because the seizure focus may already have been identified, making further intraoperative testing unnecessary. The anesthetic technique should be discussed with the surgeons before bringing the patient to the operating room, and the anesthetic plan should be designed to minimize neurologic effects if the procedure is to be done awake.

GAMMA KNIFE

Gamma knife (GK) radiosurgery uses a series of highly focused beams of radiation that deliver a high dose of radiation to specific area of brain [65]. GK was first used in 1995 and has been used successfully in decreasing or stopping some patient's seizures, especially those of the mesial temporal structures [66, 67]. General anesthesia is rarely used for GK treatment unless a patient's condition requires that level of care. For example, a patient with frequent, poorly controlled seizures or a patient with a significant degree of cognitive impairment might be unable to tolerate the procedure without general anesthesia. Late cognitive problems have been reported in patients undergoing GK; however, these seemed to be tied to postradiation edema and not to the GK procedure itself [68].

ANESTHETIC IMPLICATIONS

Anesthetic agents may have anticonvulsant or proconvulsant properties and may have effects ranging from epileptiform activity on EEG through producing myoclonus or frank seizures. Some anesthetic agents may have both effects, depending on the dose given. Anesthetic agents are classified by their anticonvulsant/proconvulsant activity in Tables 18.4 and 18.5. Use of a specific agent is determined by its anticipated effects during the planned surgery. For example, some agents with proconvulsant activity have been shown to increase activity in eleptogenic foci and are used as an aid to electrocorticographic analysis prior to surgical resection [71, 74, 76, 80–83].

Awake craniotomy and implantation of intracranial electrodes with subsequent monitoring have reduced somewhat the number of craniotomies with intraoperative location of seizure foci. Intraoperative mapping is still commonly used, however, and is directly affected by the anesthetic agents given (see Tables 18.4 and 18.5). Dexmedetomidine, for example, has been used successfully in awake craniotomies and does not interfere with electrocorticographic mapping prior to resection [84, 85].

Many studies describe EEG, electrocorticography, or depth electrode monitoring in patients with epilepsy but do not include control groups of patients. In most cases, the use of general anesthesia and neuromuscular blockade masks the true incidence of intraoperative seizures. In general, the proconvulsant effects of anesthetic agents are seen almost exclusively in patients with a preoperative history of seizures [69, 75]. Proconvulsant doses of alfentanil (30 mg/kg), remifentanil (infusion of 0.1 μg/kg to a total of 1 mg/kg), methohexital (50-mg doses), etomidate (0.1 to 0.15 mg/kg), or propofol (25-mg doses until burst suppression, mean dose to spiking, 88.2 mg) have caused an increase in the incidence of spikes from an eliptogenic foci [76–78, 80–83].

Table 18.4 **INHALATIONAL AGENTS**

PROCONVULSANT	ANTICONVULSANT	NO EFFECT
Enflurane	Halothane	Nitrous oxide*
Sevoflurane	Enflurane	
	Isoflurane	
	Sevoflurane	
	Desflurane	

Data from References 69–73.

*Isolated cases have implicated N$_2$O as proconvulsant [74].

Table 18.5 ELIPTOGENIC ACTIVITY OF INTRAVENOUS ANESTHETIC AGENTS

PROCONVULSANT	ANTICONVULSANT
Etomidate	Diazepam
Propofol	Lorazepam
Methohexital	Midazolam
Morphine	Thiopental
Alfentanil	Propofol
Fentanyl	Etomidate
Sufentanil1	Local Anesthetics
Remifentanil	Ketamine
Meperidine	
Diazepam	
Local Anesthetics	
Clonidine	
Ketamine	

Enflurane, sevoflurane, etomidate, and local anesthetics are the only agents that have been reported to cause seizures in patients without a history of epilepsy [69, 75]. In one retrospective analysis of 81 cases of intraoperative seizures in France, 70 patients did not have a preoperative history of seizures. Thirty patients (43%) experienced generalized, tonic-clonic seizures while 20 patients were described as having "increased tone with twitching and rhythmic movements" and 11 (16%) had only involuntary movements. Of the patients with a history of seizures, seven had generalized seizure activity. Almost 75% of the seizure-like phenomena occurred during either induction or emergence [78]. The study concluded that approximately 2 million patients received intraoperative propofol per year in France, making only 81 episodes of seizures almost insignificant.

In general, halothane and isoflurane slow the EEG frequency with deeper levels of anesthesia. Enflurane (as a historical reference) is more likely to produce spike activity than sevoflurane, which is in turn more active than either isoflurane or desflurane [86–90]. Another study of sevoflurane with other anesthetic agents (fentanyl, droperidol, and N_2O) could suppress spike activity [73]. Kurita and colleagues studied the effect of N_2O on spike activity and found that N_2O significantly reduced the spiking activity, although it did not affect which areas were responsible for the activity [91]. In another study, sevoflurane 2.5% and mild hyperventilation were combined with dexmedetomidine [92]. The median frequency of the electrocorticographic readings was reduced, but there was no effect seen on the spiking activity.

The conflicting results of those and other studies make planning an anesthetic for intraoperative electrocorticographic studies very difficult. For example, sevoflurane, with its propensity to increase spike activity, would seem an ideal agent, but varying the concentration of sevoflurane may

cause different effects on specific areas of the brain [93]. Hyperventilation is frequently requested by neurosurgeons for the purpose of reducing intracranial pressure or improving the surgical field. Hyperventilation has been shown to increase EEG activity, while hypoventilation can reduce epileptogenic activity [86, 87].

The proposed reason for this is that hypoventilation and the resultant increased cerebral blood flow could result in less ischemia to the epileptogenic areas. In a study by Kurita and collagues, the addition of hyperventilation did increase spike activity; however, as with other studies using various levels of sevoflurane, the areas with increased activity did not always correspond to the areas of preoperative EEG seizure recordings.

Even when other methods are used to localize epileptic tissue, the choice of anesthetic agents may cause confusion. 41 patients in one study underwent magnetoencephalography (MEG), a noninvasive functional imaging technique that requires the patients to be immobile for a prolonged period of time [94]. The use of general anesthesia did not significantly alter the ability to record the interictal epileptiform spike activity. A study was performed to look at the results of MEG functional imaging in two groups of patients, with or without general anesthesia. The two groups had comparable results in the percentage of patients having spike activity. However, there was no crossover testing, and

Table 18.6 ANESTHETIC PLANS FOR PATIENTS WITH EPILEPSY SURGICAL PROCEDURES UNDER GENERAL ANESTHESIA

Avoid
(Increased potential for seizure activity)
Etomidate
Methohexital
Sevoflurane
Enflurane
Alfentanil
Hyperventilation
Possibly Useful
(Reduces potential for seizures)
Premedication with benzodiazepines
Pentothal for induction
Normoventilation
To illicit spike activity under general anesthesia, consider use in patients with epilepsy
Etomidate
Enflurane
Sevoflurane
Methohexital
Alfentanil
Hyperventilation

the general anesthetics used (ketamine for induction and then either low-dose propofol, sevoflurane, or etomidate for maintenance) can all increase or decrease spike activity, which may cause errors in interpretation.

These studies suggest that intraperative electrocorticography under general anesthesia may define areas of epileptic activity but should probably be used only to confirm the preoperative EEG results. Electrocorticography without functional mapping or mapping near the motor cortex can be accomplished under general anesthesia (without neuromuscular blockade when stimulating the motor cortex). On the other hand, functional mapping and direct cortical electrical stimulation require patient cooperation and therefore either MAC anesthesia or an "awake" craniotomy [95].

Patients being considered for surgical resection of epileptic foci should have had those areas fully defined prior to surgery. This invasive part of the presurgical resection evaluation requires implantation of intracranial electrodes [39]. The choice of electrode type depends on the goals of the evaluation. Grid electrodes are used to differentiate epileptic foci from eloquent areas. Smaller grid electrodes or strip electrodes and depth electrodes (placed intracerebrally) allow better evaluation of the deep structures of the brain. Foramen ovale electrodes are placed through the skin on the side of the face and radiologically guided through the foramen ovale. Foramen ovale electrodes can record only from the mesial temporal areas and thus are used only when recordings from that area are required. Both the foramen ovale electrodes and the depth electrodes (somewhat similar to a DBS placement) may be positioned under local anesthesia. The grid electrodes require a craniotomy, most often under general anesthesia, to allow direct placement over the area of the brain to be studied. The anesthetic plan should include the possibility of preliminary mapping. This will entail close communication with the neurosurgeon and neurologist involved both preoperatively and intraoperatively. Once the electrodes are implanted, the patient spends several days evaluating the data obtained from subsequent EEG recordings. A second craniotomy under general anesthesia is then required for resection of the epileptic foci.

AWAKE CRANIOTOMY

Craniotomies have been performed in awake patients for eons. Archeologists in Peru have discovered a total of 214 skulls with evidence of early neurosurgical procedures, including trephinations and burr holes, from historical periods long before the era of general anesthesia [96]. Of these, 55% showed evidence of complete healing after the procedures. More recently, Roberts Bartholow electrically stimulated the brain of a patient in 1874 whose skull had been eroded by an ulceration [97]. Horsley performed a surgical craniotomy with local anesthesia in 1886; Davidoff added sedation to local anesthesia in 1934. Penfield used

local anesthesia and sedation in 1937, and he also electrically stimulated the patient's brain. In 1953, Pasquet performed an "awake-asleep" craniotomy for patient comfort. Neuroleptic anesthesia (combination of droperidol and fentanyl) was first used in 1959, signaling the modern era of awake craniotomies [96].

When a surgeon must operate in an eloquent area of the brain, including speech or motor areas, the surgeon might request that the patient be awake for the procedure. Giving the patient the ability to report odd sensations or speak without compromise, or allowing the neurologist to find a small, localized epileptic focus by electrocorticography, can potentially change the surgical outcome. Creating an optimal surgical field while keeping the patient safe and comfortable during a major surgical procedure under local anesthesia is a challenge for the anesthesiologist.

The anesthetic management of the patient undergoing an awake craniotomy begins with preoperative evaluation [98–104]. It is critical for the patient, the surgeon, and the anesthesiologist to form a relationship before the patient enters the operating room. The anesthesiologist should explain everything that the patient might experience and describe how the anesthesia care team will provide for the patient's safety and comfort. The patient will need constant reassurance as his or her level of consciousness is changing throughout the procedure. Management of a "lost" airway, seizures, or other complication must be thoroughly planned before the procedure begins.

The anesthetic plan for an awake craniotomy should provide for adequate analgesia during opening and closing of the surgical site. The patient must be fully consciousness and able to cooperate during functional testing and mapping. The patient should ideally be comfortable throughout the procedure with adequate ventilation and the airway safely maintained [98]. The anesthesia care team must be aware of medications that might interfere with functional testing, whether by direct effect or by altering a patient's consciousness. Such medications should either be avoided or their use must be discontinued at an appropriate time to allow optimal operating conditions (Table 18.7).

Table 18.7 **CURRENT AGENTS FOR AWAKE CRANIOTOMIES**

AGENTS	POSSIBLE SIDE EFFECTS
Dexmedetomidine [105–111]	Rapid onset; sedation without respiratory depression. Has analgesic effect. May lead to bradycardia or hypotension. Must be stopped prior to mapping or stimulation.
Propofol [112–119]	Rapid onset; may promote respiratory depression or hypotension. Must be stopped prior to mapping or stimulation.
Remifentanil (Often paired with propofol)	Rapid on/off effect and good analgesia and some sedative effect, may lead to respiratory depression.

Archer et al., 1988: 354 consecutive patients [120]

Craniotomy under conscious sedation with droperidol and fentanyl. (This technique had been used at the Montreal Neurological Institute and Hospital for over 50 years at the time of the publication.)

Seven patients had conversion to GETA (general endotracheal anesthesia). Eleven patients required reversal of their sedation. End-tidal CO_2 was not monitored (only transcutaneous oxygenation was monitored).

Fifty-five patients (15.5%) had intraoperative seizures and 27 (7.6%) suffered nausea and vomiting. Seven patients had signs of local anesthetic toxicity and 11 patients were sedated to the point of interfering with their assessment.

Sarang et al., 2003: Ninety-nine patients in three groups [121]

Group 1. Patients sedated throughout the procedure. No end-tidal CO_2 monitoring; 7% of patients developed airway obstruction.

Groups 2 and 3; asleep-awake-asleep technique.

Group 2. Patients breathed spontaneously, airway protected with LMA (laryngeal mask airway). Anesthesia provided with propofol infusion and fentanyl. **All** patients with end-tidal CO_2 >45; 70% required additional analgesia.

Group 3. Total intravenous anesthesia with propofol and remifentanil. No patient with an **end-tidal** CO_2 >45, no additional analgesia required.

Skucas et al., 2006: 332 patients; 203 asleep-awake-asleep vs. 129 patients with GETA (general endotracheal anesthesia) [122]

Awake: Propofol infusion and local anesthetic; propofol infusion stopped during language or motor assessment and/or sensory mapping and for electrocorticography. No airways employed originally however 6 patients did require airway intervention.

Statistically higher incidences of hypertension, hypotension, tachycardia, bradycardia, and respiratory depression (**Paco$_2$** mean >47) occurred in the awake craniotomy group. The authors noted the awake craniotomy technique may have contributed to one case with poor clinical outcome.

Sereletis et al., 2007: (Neurosurgical Point of View), prospective series of 610 patients [123]

Report of one surgeon's prospective series of 610 patients who underwent awake craniotomies with "light sedation and application of local anesthetic." Only two patients required conversion to a general anesthesia technique. Intraoperative seizures occurred in only 4.9%. Brain mapping was undertaken in 511 patients, 78 suffered postoperative neurologic deficits. {Of note mapping was considered positive if it identified eloquent cortex, this was accomplished in 115 (22.5%). Negative mapping, seen in 77.5%, did not identify eloquent cortex. This was noted not to have been a dysfunction of the "stimulation apparatus." {However as agents used for sedation were not identified, it is possible that those medications could have influenced the mapping procedures.}

Nausea and vomiting were mentioned only to say the literature suggests a lower incidence with awake craniotomy versus craniotomies under general anesthesia but the incidence in this series was not noted

Hol et al., 2009: Forty patients undergoing craniotomy under either general anesthesia or awake [124]

Patients undergoing craniotomy under general anesthesia had amino acid profiles more consistent with increased stress than those undergoing awake craniotomy. Also pain levels and mean hospitalization time was lower in the awake craniotomy group.

Conte et al., 2010: 238 consecutive procedures [125]

135 described as asleep-awake (LMA and general anesthesia then removal of the LMA for language testing, 57% with complications) and 103 asleep-asleep (patients intubated and "sedated" for motor testing, 41% complications).

Five of the asleep-awake group required LMA removal and subsequent endotracheal intubation.

Hypertension and hypotension were both much more common in the asleep-awake group. Seizures were about equal between the two groups. Vomiting (7%), apnea (4%), and agitation (6%) were only noted in the asleep-awake group.

In this study, the Bispectral Index monitor was used. A BIS index less than 65 was considered general anesthesia; a BIS index of 45 to 65 was used for motor testing, and a BIS index of 80 to 100 for language testing.

In general terms, the anesthetic for an awake craniotomy should start with minimal premedication. It is best to avoid the use of benzodiazepines during the procedure because these agents may later interfere with functional testing. An "asleep-awake ± asleep" craniotomy has been used successfully for many awake procedures (Table 18.8). For this technique, general anesthesia is induced with a short-acting agent such as propofol; the airway is maintained with a mask, LMA, or endotracheal tube. Nerve blocks may help to provide analgesia during the awake portion of the procedure. Surgery then proceeds under general anesthesia, possibly with an potent volatile anesthetic or an intravenous technique consisting of either propofol and remifentanil or dexmedetomidine [100–103, 125–128]. When a neurologic examination is required, the patient is allowed to emerge from anesthesia and any artificial airway is removed. CPAP [129] or bilevel positive airway pressure (BiPAP) may help to support the patient's airway and provide ventilation during these procedures [130, 131]. Use of these devices will support the airway without the need for an artificial airway, which might precipitate coughing or a Valsalva maneuver by the patient, which could have serious consequences on a patients intracranial pressure [99, 109, 111, 117, 132, 133]. After functional testing is completed, the patient may have the sedation restarted or general anesthesia induced depending on anesthesia/surgery preference and patient safety.

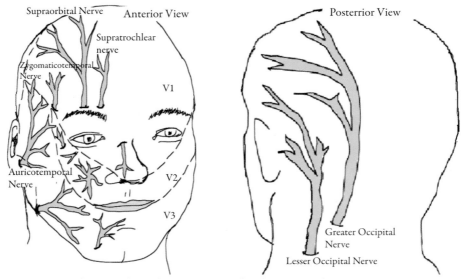

Figure 18.1   The six nerves to be blocked for regional anesthesia/patient comfort during an awake craniotomy.

The first use of the scalp block in the literature for awake craniotomy was by Girvin in which he injected a total of 12 mL of bupivacaine at five nerve locations: the greater and lesser occipital nerves, the auriculotemporal nerve, the zygomaticotemporal nerve, and the supraorbital nerves [134]. Additionally, more local anesthetic may be needed for scalp flaps, Girvin used 60 mL of dilute bupivacaine for this without complications. However, bupivacaine has fallen out of favor for most regional anesthesiologists and has been mainly replaced by ropivacaine, which has less risk of life-threatening cardiotoxicity or neurotoxicity in the event of an accidental intravascular injection or overdose [135]. Central nervous system local anesthetic toxicity may manifest as altered mental status, seizure, or coma, all of which can masquerade the underlying diagnosis or surgical manipulation. The scalp block can be successfully performed by injecting 2 to 3 mL of local anesthetic at six different nerve locations in the scalp [104, 117, 136–138] (see Figure 18.1). The first nerve blocked, in no particular order, is the auriculotemporal nerve, which supplies anterior and superior to the ear. The anatomic landmark for the auriculotemporal nerve is slightly anterior to the ear at the level of the tragus but posterior to the superficial temporal artery [104, 117, 136–138].

The second nerve for this technique is the zygomaticotemporal nerve, which supplies the lateral scalp between the ear, anterior to the auriculotemporal nerve, and the forehead. This nerve is blocked by a deep and superficial field block from the area of scalp innervated by the supraorbital nerve to the area innervated by the auriculotemporal nerve [104, 117, 136–138].

The third and fourth nerves that Costello describes for his block are the supraorbital and supratrochlear nerves, both of which supply the area superior and anterior to the eye along the forehead. The supraorbital nerve can be

blocked by a field block from the supraorbital notch and extending the infiltration medially approximately 1 cm, which will cover the supratrochlear nerve [104, 117, 136–138].

The final nerves that need to be blocked include the greater and lesser occipital nerves, which supply the posterior scalp behind the ear and extend to the top of the skull. The anatomic landmarks for the greater occipital nerve are the halfway point between the mastoid process and the occipital protuberance, medial to the occipital artery. After the landmark for the greater occipital nerve has been found, the lesser occipital nerve can be blocked 2.5 cm lateral to the greater occipital nerve [138]. The lesser occipital nerve courses between the semispinalis muscle medially, the splenius muscle laterally, and the sternocleidomastoid muscle superiorly [138].

CONCLUSIONS

Providing anesthesia for the surgical treatment of epilepsy can be complex and challenging. A successful anesthetic depends on many factors. First is the adherence to the clinical principles of neurosurgical anesthesia. Next the anesthesiologist should have an appreciation of the clinical pharmacology involved with epilepsy. A patient's comorbidities must be addressed. Then the anesthetic itself must be tailored to the procedure and the requirements for patient safety and optimal operating conditions. The low incidence of surgical complications and the successful outcomes (69%, 81%, and 89% seizure free in three large series, and another with over 70% of patients with significant improvement in patients with severest forms of epilepsy [139–142]) make these surgical procedures likely to increase significantly in the future.

REFERENCES

1. Eadie MJ. Epilepsy—from the Sakikku to Hughlings Jackson. *J Clin Neurosci.* 1995;2:156–162.
2. Gross RA. A brief history of epilepsy and its therapy in the western hemisphere. *Epilepsy Res.* 1992;12:65–74.
3. Hanna NJ, Black M, Sander JW, et al. *The national sentinel audit of epilepsy related death.* London: The Stationary Office; 2002.
4. Matthews WS, Barabas G. Suicide and epilepsy: a review of the literature. *Psychosomatic.* 1981;22:515–524.
5. Sander JW. The epidemiology of epilepsy revisited. *Curr Opin Neurol.* 2003;16:165–170.
6. Sathyaprabha N, Satishchandra P, Netravathi K, et al. Cardiac autonomic dysfunctions in chronic refractory epilepsy. *Epilepsy Res.* 2006;72 49–56.
7. Devinsky O, Effects of seizures on autonomic and cardiovascular function. *Epilepsy Currents.* 2004;4:43–46.
8. Standridge SM, Holland KD, Horn PS. Cardiac arrhythmias and ictal events within an epilepsy monitoring unit. *Pediatr Neurol.* 2010;42:201–205.
9. Jehi L, Najm IM. Sudden unexpected death in epilepsy: impact, mechanisms, and prevention. *Cleve Clin J Med.* 2008;75:S66–S70.
10. Malow BA, Weatherwax KJ, Chervin RD, et al. Identification and treatment of obstructive sleep apnea in adults and children with epilepsy: a prospective pilot study. *Sleep Med.* 2003;4:509–515.
11. Kwan P, Brodie MJ. Early identification of refractory epilepsy. *N Engl J Med.* 2000;342:314–319.
12. Baker GA, Jacoby A, Buck D, et al. Quality in life in people with epilepsy: a European study. *Epilepsia.* 1997;38:353–362.
13. Elger CE, Schmidt D. Modern management of epilepsy. *Epilepsy Behav.* 2008;12:501–539.
14. Nguyen A, Pharm B, Ramzan I. Acute in vitro neuromuscular effects of carbamazepine and carbamazepine-IO,II-epoxide *Anesthesia Analgesia.* 1997;84:886–890.
15. LaRoche SM, Helmers Sl. The new antiepileptic drugs. *JAMA.* 2004;291:605–614.
16. Werhahn KJ. Epilepsy in the elderly. *Dtsch Arztebl Int.* 2009;106: 135–142.
17. Verma NP, Dan Haidukewych D. Differential but infrequent alterations of hepatic enzyme levels and thyroid hormone levels by anticonvulsant drugs. *Arch Neurol.* 1994;51:381–384.
18. Ruiz-Gimenez J, Sanchez-Alvarez JC, Canadillas-Hildago F, et al. Antiepileptic treatment in patients with epilepsy and other comorbidities. *Seizure: Eur J Epilepsy.* 2010;19:375–382.
19. Donovan PJ, Cline D. Phenytoin administration by constant intravenous infusion: selective rates of administration. *Ann Emerg Med.* 1991;20:139–142.
20. T′ellez-Zenteno JF, Matijevic S, Wiebe S. Somatic comorbidity of epilepsy in the general population in Canada. *Epilepsia.* 2005;46:1955–1962.
21. Prasad VN, Chawla HS, Goyal A, et al. Incidence of phenytoin induced gingival hyperplasia in epileptic children: a six month evaluation. *J Indian Soc Pedod Prev Dent.* 2002;20:73–80.
22. Lafzi A, Farahani RM, Shoja MA. Phenobarbital-induced gingival hyperplasia. *J Contemp Dent Prac.* 2007;1:50–56.
23. Kawaguchi M, Sakamoto T, Furuya H, et al. Pseudoankylosis of the mandible after supratentorial craniotomy. *Anesth Analg.* 1996;83:7314.
24. Kawaguchi M, Sakamoto T, Ohnishi H, et al. Airway management in a patient with pseudoankylosis of the mandible following fronto-temporal craniotomy. *J Anesth.* 1994;8:346–348.
25. Zafarulla M. Pseudoankylosis of the mandible following a fronto-temporal craniotomy. *J Neurol Neurosurg Psychiatry.* 1985;48:1069–1070.
26. Kang DH, Park JC, Kim SO, et al. Intubation difficulty in patient with pseudoankylosis of temporo-mandibular joint after pterional craniotomy. *J Kor Neurosurg Soc.* 2004;36:166–167.
27. Yoshii AT, Hamamoto Y, Muraoka S, et al. Pseudoankylosis of the mandible as a result of methyl methacrylate-induced inflammatory cicatricial contracture of the temporal muscle after cranioplasty. *Br J Oral Maxillofac Surg.* 2001;39:374–375.
28. Engel J. ILAE classification of epilepsy syndromes. *Epilepsy Res.* 2006;**70S**:S5–S10.
29. Rosenow F, Luders H. Presurgical evaluation of epilepsy. *Brain.* 2001;124:1683–1700.
30. Wada JA. A fateful encounter: sixty years later—reflections on the Wada test. *Epilepsia.* 2008;49:726–727.
31. Simkins-Bullock J. Beyond speech lateralization: a review of the variability, reliability, and validity of the intracarotid amobarbital procedure and its nonlanguage uses in epilepsy surgery candidates. *Neuropsychol Rev.* 2000;10:41–74.
32. Milner B, Branch C, Rasmussen T. Study of short-term memory after intracarotid injection of sodium amytal. *Trans Am Neurol Assoc.* 1962;87: 224–226.
33. Dodrill CB, Ojemann GA. An exploratory comparison of three methods of memory assessment with the intracarotid amobarbital procedure. *Brain Cogn.* 1997;33: 210–223.
34. Loddenkemper T, Morris HH, Möddel G. Complications during the Wada test. *Epilepsy Behav.* 2008;13:551–553.
35. English J, Davis B. Case report: death associated with stroke following intracarotid amobarbital testing. *Epilepsy Behav.* 2010;17: 283–284.
36. Ammerman JM, Caputy AJ, Potolicchio SJ. Endovascular ablation of a temporal lobe epileptogenic focus—a complication of Wada testing. *Acta Neurol Scand.* 2005;112:189–191.
37. Baxendale SA. The Wada test. *Curr Opin Neurol.* 2009: 22:185–189.
38. Abou-Khalil B An update on determination of language dominance in screening for epilepsy surgery: the Wada test and newer noninvasive alternatives. *Epilepsia.* 2007;48:442–455.
39. Gelžinienė G, Endzinienė M, Vaičienė N, et al. Presurgical evaluation of epilepsy patients. *Medicina (Kaunas).* 2008;44:585–592.
40. Milby AH, Halpern CH, Baltuch GH. Vagus nerve stimulation in the treatment of refractory epilepsy. *Neurotherapeutics.* 2009;6:228–237.
41. McLachlan RS. Vagus nerve stimulation for intractable epilepsy: a review. *J Clin Neurophysiol.* 1997;14:358–368.
42. Amar AP, Apuzzo MLJ, Liu CY. Vagus nerve stimulation therapy after failed cranial surgery for intractable epilepsy: results from the Vagus Nerve Stimulation Therapy Patient Outcome Registry. *Neurosurgery.* 2004;55:1086–1093.
43. Handforth A, DeGiorgio CM, Schachter SC, et al. Vagus nerve stimulation therapy for partial-onset seizures. A randomized active-control trial. *Neurology.* 1998;51:48–55.
44. Zanchetti A, Wang SC, Moruzzi G. The effect of vagal stimulation on the EEG pattern of the cat. *Electroencephalogr Clin Neurophysiol.* 1952;4:357–361.
45. Zabara J. Inhibition of experimental seizures in canines by repetitive vagal stimulation. *Epilepsia.* 1992;33:1005–1012.
46. Penry JK, Dean JC. Prevention of intractable partial seizures by intermittent vagal stimulation in humans: preliminary results. *Epilepsia.* 1990;31(Suppl. 2):S4O–S43.
47. Guberman A. Vagus nerve stimulation in the treatment of epilepsy. *Can Med Assoc J.* 2004;171:1165–1166.
48. Abubakr A, Wambacq I. Long-term outcome of vagus nerve stimulation therapy in patients with refractory epilepsy. *J Clin Neurosci.* 2008: 15:127–129.
49. Foley JO, DuBois FS. Quantitative studies of the vagus nerve in the cat. *J Comp Neurol.* 1937;67:49–67.
50. Sheth RD, Stafstrom CE, Hsu D. Nonpharmacological treatment options for epilepsy. *Semin Pediatr Neurol.* 2005;12:106–113.
51. George MS, Nahas Z, Bohning DE, et al. Mechanisms of action of vagus nerve stimulation (VNS). *Clin Neurosci Res.* 2004;4:71–79.
52. Marrosu F, Serra A, Maleci A, et al. Correlation between GABA$_A$ receptor density and vagus nerve stimulation in individuals with drug-resistant partial epilepsy. *Epilepsy Research.* 2003;55:59–70.

53. Ardell JL, Randall WC. Selective vagal innervation of sino-atrial and atrioventricular nodes in canine heart. *Am J Physiol.* 1986;251:764–773.

54. Ali II, Pirzada NA, Kanjwal Y, et al. Complete heart block with ventricular asystole during left vagus nerve stimulation for epilepsy. *Epilepsy Behav.* 2004;5:768–771.

55. Amark P, Stodberg T, Wallstedt L. Late onset bradyarrhythmia during vagus nerve stimulation. *Epilepsia.* 2007;48:1023–1025.

56. Hatton KW, McLarney JT, Pittman T, et al. Vagal nerve stimulation: overview and implications for anesthesiologists. *Anesth Analg.* 2006;103:1241–1249.

57. Bernard EJ, Passannante AN, Mann B, et al. Insertion of vagal nerve stimulator using local and regional anesthesia. *Surg Neurol.* 2002;57:94–98.

58. Anneggers JF, Coan SP, Hauser WA, et al. Epilepsy, vagal nerve stimulation by the NCP system, all-cause mortality, and sudden, unexpected, unexplained death. *Epilepsia.* 2000;41;549–553.

59. Tecoma ES, Iragui VJ. Vagus nerve stimulation use and effect in epilepsy: what have we learned? *Epilepsy Behav.* 2006;8:127–136.

60. Lega BC, Halpern CH, Jaggi JL, et al. Deep brain stimulation in the treatment of refractory epilepsy: update on current data and future directions. *Neurobiol Dis.* 2010;38:354–360.

61. Schulze-Bonhage A. Deep brain stimulation: a new approach to the treatment of epilepsy. *Dtsch Arztebl Int.* 2009;106:407–412.

62. Halpern CH, Samadani U, Litt B, et al. Deep brain stimulation for epilepsy. *Neurotherapeutics.* 2008;5:59–67.

63. Voges J, Waezeggers Y, Maarouf M, et al. Deep-brain stimulation long-term analysis of complications caused by hardware and surgery—experiences from a single centre. *J Neurol Neurosurg Psychiatry.* 2006;77:868–872.

64. Moitra V, Permut TA, Penn RM, et al. Venous air embolism in an awake patient undergoing placement of deep brain stimulators. *J Neurosurg Anesthesiol.* 2004;16:321.

65. Yang I, Barbaro NM. Advances in the radiosurgical treatment of epilepsy. *Epilepsy Curr.* 2007;7:31–35.

66. Peragut JC, Rey M, Samson Y, et al. First selective amygdalohippocampal radiosurgery for mesial temporal lobe epilepsy. *Stereotact Funct Neurosurg.* 1995;64(Suppl. 1):193–201.

67. Rheims S, Fischer C, Ryvlin P, et al. Long-term outcome of gamma-knife surgery in temporal lobe epilepsy. *Epilepsy Res.* 2008;80: 23–29.

68. McDonalda CR, Normana MA, Tecomab E, et al. Neuropsychological change following gamma knife surgery in patients with left temporal lobe epilepsy: a review of three cases. *Epilepsy Behav.* 2004;5:949–957.

69. Modica, PA, Tempelhoff R, White PF. Pro- and anticonvulsant effects of anesthetics (part I). *Anesth Analg.* 1990;70:303–315.

70. Voss LJ, Ludbrook G, Grant C, et al. Cerebral cortical effects of desflurane in sheep: comparison with isoflurane, sevoflurane and enflurane. *Acta Anaesthesiol Scand.* 2006;50:313–319.

71. Kurita N, Kawaguchi M, Hoshida T, et al. The effect of sevoflurane and hyperventilation on electrocorticogram spike activity in patients with refractory epilepsy. *Anesth Analg.* 2005;101:517–523.

72. Hosain S, Nagarajan L, Fraser R, et al. Effects of nitrous oxide on electrocorticography during epilepsy surgery. *Electroencephalogr Clin Neurophysiol.* 1996;102:340–342.

73. Endo T, Sato K, Shamoto H, et al. Effects of sevoflurane on electrocorticography in patients with intractable temporal lobe epilepsy. *J Neurosurg Anesthesiol.* 2002;14:59–62.

74. Kofke WA, Tempelhoff R, Dasheiff RM. Anesthetic implications of epilepsy, status epilepticus, and epilepsy surgery. *J Neurosurg Anesthesiol.* 1997;9:349–372.

75. Modica, PA, Tempelhoff R, White PF. Pro- and anticonvulsant effects of anesthetics (part II). *Anesth Analg.* 1990;70:433–444.

76. Ragazzo PC, Galanopoulou AS. Alfentanil-induced activation: a promising tool in the presurgical evaluation of temporal lobe epilepsy patients. *Brain Res Rev.* 2000;32:316–327.

77. Herrick IA, Craen RA, Blume WT, et al. Sedative doses of remifentanil have minimal effect on ECoG. *J Neurosurg Anesthesiol.* 2002;14:55–58.

78. Walder B, Tramèr MR, Seeck M. Seizure-like phenomena and propofol. *Neurology.* 2002;58:1327–1332.

79. Benish SM, Cascino GD, Warner ME, et al. Effect of general anesthesia in patients with epilepsy: a population-based study. *Epilepsy Behav.* 2010: 17:87–89.

80. Ross J, Kearse A, Barlow MK, et al. Alfentanil-induced epileptiform activity: a simultaneous surface and depth electroencephalographic study in complex partial epilepsy. *Epilepsia.* 2008;42:220–225.

81. McGuire G, El-Beheiry H, Manninen P, et al. Activation of electrocorticographic activity with remifentanil and alfentanil during neurosurgical excision of epileptogenic focus. *Br J Anaesth.* 2003;91:651–655.

82. Gancher S, Laxer KD, Krieger W. Activation of eliptogenic activity by etomidate. *Anesthesiology.* 1984;61:616–618.

83. Smith M, Smith SJ, Scott A, et al. Activation of the electrocorticogram by propofol during surgery for epilepsy. *Br J Anaesth.* 1996;76:499–502.

84. Bekker A, Sturaitis MK. Dexmedetomidine for neurological surgery. *Neurosurgery.* 2005;57(Suppl 1):1–10.

85. Talke P, Stapelfeldt C, Garcia P. Dexmedetomidine does not reduce epileptiform discharges in adults with epilepsy. *J Neurosurg Anesthesiol.* 2007;19:195–199.

86. Leonhardt G, de Greiff A, Marks S et al. Brain diffusion during hyperventilation: diffusion-weighted MR-monitoring in patients with temporal lobe epilepsy and in healthy volunteers. *Epilepsy Res.* 2002;51:269–278.

87. Pomfrett CJD. The EEG during anaesthesia. *Curr Anaesth Crit Care.* 1998;9:117–122.

88. Flemming DC, Fitzpatrick J, Fariello RG, et al. Diagnostic activation of epileptoenic Foci by enflurane. *Anesthesiology.* 1980: 52:431–433.

89. Voss LJ, Sleigh JW, Barnard JPM, et al. The howling cortex: seizures and general anesthetic drugs. *Anesth Analg.* 2008;107:1689–1703.

90. Sato K, Shamoto H, Kato M. Effect of sevoflurane on electrocorticogram in normal brain. *J Neurosurg Anesthesiol.* 2002;14:63–65.

91. Kurita N, Kawaguchi M, Hoshida T, et al. Effects of nitrous oxide on spike activity on electrocorticogram under sevoflurane anesthesia in epileptic patients. *J Neurosurg Anesthesiol.* 2005;17:199–202.

92. Ada Y, Tiroyama S, Tanaka K, et al. The effect of dexmedetomidine on electrocorticography in patients with temporal lobe epilepsy under sevoflurane anesthesia. *Anesth Analg.* 2007;105:1272–1277.

93. Kurita N, Kawaguchi M, Hoshida T, et al. The effects of sevoflurane and hyperventilation on electrocorticogram spike activity in patients with refractory epilepsy. *Anesth Analg.* 2005;101:517–523.

94. Balakrishnan G, Grover KM, Mason K, et al. A retrospective analysis of the effect of general anesthetics on the successful detection of interictal epileptiform activity in magnetoencephalography. *Anesth Analg.* 2007;104:1493–1497.

95. Schuh L, Drury I. Intraoperative electrocorticography and direct cortical stimulation. *Semin Anesth.* 1997;16:46–55.

96. Bulsara KR, Johnson J, Villavicencio AT. Improvements in brain tumor surgery: the modern history of awake craniotomies. *Neurosurg Focus.* 2005;18:1–3.

97. Morgan JP. The first reported case of electrical stimulation of the human brain. *J Hist Med.* 1982;37:51–64.

98. Hans P, Bonhomme V. Anesthetic management for neurosurgery in awake patients. *Minerva Anesthesiol.* 2007;73:507–512.

99. Frost EAM, Booij LHSJ. Anesthesia in the patient for awake craniotomy. *Curr Opin Anaesthesiol.* 2007;20:331–335.

100. Aglio LS, Laverne D, Gugino LD. conscious sedation for intraoperative neurosurgical procedures. *Techn Neurosurg.* 2001;7:52–60.

101. Erickson KM, Cole DJ. Anesthetic considerations for awake craniotomy for epilepsy. *Anesthesiol Clin.* 2007;25:535–555.

102. Khu KJ, Doglietto F, Radovanovic I, et al. Patients' perceptions of awake and outpatient craniotomy for brain tumor: a qualitative study. *J Neurosurg.* 2010;112:1056–1060.

103. Wilson M Artru AA. Anesthesia for awake craniotomy. *Semin Anesth Perioperat Med Pain*. 2004: 23:230–236.

104. Bilotta F, Rosa G. "Anesthesia" for awake neurosurgery. *Curr Opin Anaesthesiol*. 2009;22:560–565.

105. Mack PF, Perrine K, Schwartz TH, et al. Dexmedetomidine and neurocognitive testing in awake craniotomy. *J Neurosurg Anesthesiol*. 2004;16:20–25.

106. Moore TA II, Markert JM, Knowlton RC. Dexmedetomidine as rescue drug during awake craniotomy for cortical motor mapping and tumor resection. *Anesth Analg*. 2006;102:1556–1558.

107. Rozet I. Anesthesia for functional neurosurgery: the role of dexmedetomidine. *Curr Opin Anaesthesiol*. 2008;21:537–543.

108. Ard JL Jr, Bekker AY, Doyle WK. Dexmedetomidine in awake craniotomy: a technical note. *Surg Neurol*. 2005;63:114–117.

109. Bekker AY, Kaufman B, Hany Samir H, et al. The use of dexmedetomidine infusion for awake craniotomy. *Anesth Analg*. 2001;92:1251–1253.

110. Souter MJ, Rozet I, Ojemann JG, et al. Dexmedetomidine sedation during awake craniotomy for seizure resection: effects on electrocorticography. *J Neurosurg Anesthesiol*. 2007;19:38–44.

111. Lobo F, Beiras A. Propofol and remifentanil effect-site concentrations estimated by pharmacokinetic simulation and bispectral index monitoring during craniotomy with intraoperative awakening for brain tumor resection. *J Neurosurg Anesthesiol*. 2007;19:183–189.

112. Leslie K, Bjorksten AR, Ugoni A, et al. Mild core hypothermia and anesthetic requirement for loss of responsiveness during propofol anesthesia for craniotomy. *Anesth Analg*. 2002;94:1298–1303.

113. Herrick IA, Craen RA, Gelb AW, et al. Propofol sedation during awake craniotomy for seizures: patient-controlled administration versus neurolept analgesia. *Anesth Analg*. 1997;84:1285–1291.

114. Herrick IA, Craen RA, Gelb AW, et al. Propofol sedation during awake craniotomy for seizures: electrocorticographic and epileptogenic effects. *Anesth Analg*. 1997;84:1280–1284.

115. Berkenstadt H, Ram Z. Monitored anesthesia care in awake craniotomy for brain tumor surgery. *IMAJ*. 2001;3:297–300.

116. Blanshard HJ, Chung F, Manninen PH, et al. Awake craniotomy for removal of intracranial tumor: considerations for early discharge. *Anesth Analg*. 2001;92:89–94.

117. Piccioni F, Fanzio M. Management of anesthesia in awake craniotomy. *Minerva Anesthesiol*. 2008;74:393–408.

118. Manninen PH, Balki M, Lukitto K, et al. Patient satisfaction with awake craniotomy for tumor surgery: a comparison of remifentanil and fentanyl in conjunction with propofol. *Anesth Analg*. 2006;102:237–242.

119. Prabhu VC, Vargas C, Benedict WJ Jr, et al. Cortical mapping in the resection of gliomas. *Contemp Neurosurg*. 2007;29:1–8.

120. Archer D, McKenna JMA, Morin L. Conscious-sedation analgesia during craniotomy for intractable epilepsy: a review of 354 consecutive cases. *Can J Anaesth*. 1988: 35:338–344.

121. Sarang A, Dinsmore J. Anaesthesia for awake craniotomy—evolution of a technique that facilitates awake neurological testing. *Br J Anaesth*. 2003;90:161–165.

122. Skucas, AP, Artru AA. Anesthetic complications of awake craniotomies for epilepsy surgery. *Anesth Analg*. 2006;102:882–887.

123. Serletis D, Berstein M. Prospective study of awake craniotomy used routinely and nonselectively for supratentorial tumors. *J Neurosurg*. 2007;107:1–6.

124. Hol JW, Klimek M, van der Helde-Mulder M, et al. Awake craniotomy induces fewer changes in the plasma amino acid profile than craniotomy under general anesthesia. *J Neurosurg Anesthesiol*. 2009;21:98–107.

125. Conte V, Magni L, Songa V, et al. Analysis of propofol/remifentanil infusion protocol for tumor surgery with intraoperative brain mapping. *J Neurosurg Anesthesiol*. 2010;22:119–127.

126. Frost EAM, Booij LHSJ. Anesthesia in the patient for awake craniotomy. *Curr Opin Anaesthesiol*. 2007;20:331–335.

127. Artru AA, Wilson M. Anesthesia for awake craniotomy. *Semin Anesth Perioperat Med Pain*. 2004;23:230–236.

128. Bonhomme V, Collette Franssen C, Hans P. Awake craniotomy. *Eur J Anaesthesiol*. 2009;26:906–912.

129. Huncke T, Chan J, Doyle W, Kim J, Bekker A. The use of continuous positive airway pressure during an awake craniotomy in a patient with obstructive sleep apnea. *J Clin Anesth*. 2008;20:297–299.

130. Gonzales J, Lombard FW, Borel CO. Pressure support mode improves ventilation in "asleep–awake–asleep" craniotomy. *J Neurosurg Anesthesiol*. 2006;18:88.

131. Yamamoto F, Kato R, Sato J, et al. Anaesthesia for awake craniotomy with non-invasive positive pressure ventilation. *Br J Anaesth*. 2003;90:382–385.

132. Pemberton PL, Dinsmore J. Bispectral index monitoring during awake craniotomy surgery. *Anaesthesia*. 2002;57:1244–1245.

133. De Sloovere V, De Deyne C, Wuyts J, et al. Bispectral index monitoring during asleep–awake technique for craniotomy. *Eur J Anaesthesiol*. 2009;26:443–444.

134. Girvin JP. Neurosurgical considerations and general methods for craniotomy under local anesthesia. *Int Anesthesiol Clin*. 1986;24:89–114.

135. Costello TG, Cormack JR, Hoy C, et al. Plasma ropivacaine levels following scalp block for awake craniotomy. *J Neurosurg Anesthesiol*. 2004;16:147–150.

136. Osborn I, Sebeo J. "Scalp block" during craniotomy: a classic technique revisited. *J Neurosurg Anesthesiol*. 2010;22:187–194.

137. Costello TG, Cormack JR. Anaesthesia for awake craniotomy: a modern approach. *J Clin Neurosci*. 2004;11:16–19.

138. Gebhard RE, Berry J, Maggio WW, et al. The successful use of regional anesthesia to prevent involuntary movements in a patient undergoing awake craniotomy. *Anesth Analg*. 2009;91:1230–1231.

139. Tanriverdi T, Olivier A, Poulin N, et al. Long-term seizure outcome after corpus callosotomy: a retrospective analysis of 95 patients. *J Neurosurg*. 2009: 110:332–342.

140. Cohen-Gadol AA, Wilhelmi BG, Collignon F, et al. Long-term outcome of epilepsy surgery among 399 patients with nonlesional seizure foci including mesial temporal lobe sclerosis. *J Neurosurg*. 2006: 104:513–524.

141. Elsharkawy AE, Alabbasi AH, Pannek H, et al. Long-term outcome after temporal lobe epilepsy surgery in 434 consecutive adult patients. *J Neurosurg*. 2009;110:1135–1146.

142. Salanova V, Markland O, Worth R. Temporal lobe epilepsy surgery: outcome, complications and late mortality rate in 215 patients. *Epilepsia*. 2002;43:170–174.

19.

SEVERE TRAUMATIC BRAIN INJURY

Ramachandran Ramani

Severe traumatic brain injury (TBI) has an extremely high mortality (30% to 45%) [1] and is the leading cause of death in adults less than 45 years of age. Fifty percent of the patients who survive TBI live with moderate or severe disability. Maximizing the likelihood of a positive outcome in these patients is challenging and requires a thorough understanding of the pathophysiology of TBI. The goal of the anesthesiologist while managing these patients is to optimize systemic and cerebral hemodynamics while maintaining cerebral perfusion to prevent secondary injury to the brain and promote recovery.

Care of the patient with TBI begins in the field as soon as possible after the primary head injury and continues during transport to the hospital and after arrival in the emergency department. Management of TBI patient can therefore be broadly divided into prehospital care and intrahospital care. Anesthesiologists play a critical role in the initial management of these patients, from resuscitation of the patient on arrival in the emergency department, anesthesia or sedation for diagnostic imaging, intraoperative management during a surgical procedure (e.g., decompressive craniectomy or evacuation of a hematoma), and management in the intensive care. The Brain Trauma Foundation has (BTF) published guidelines for management of TBI in 1999. Subsequently these guidelines were revised in 2003 and 2007 [2]. This chapter covers the pathophysiology of TBI followed by management. Each section of the management in this chapter is followed by a brief summary of the relevant BTF guidelines.

PATHOPHYSIOLOGY

Neuronal injury is a process that begins at the time of impact and continues for days afterward [3, 4]. In order to better describe treatment strategies, however, this process is commonly defined as *primary injury* that is caused by the mechanical effects of the impact and *secondary injury*, which describes the delayed process of cerebral edema and neuronal death. The initial traumatic event can cause a skull fracture, brain contusion, laceration, vascular injury, intracerebral clot, and axonal injury. Two distinct types of force occur at impact: linear acceleration and rotational movement. Linear acceleration causes injury at or close to the site of impact. Rotational movement causes injury some distance from the site of impact resulting in axonal injury (white matter damage) and injury to deep-seated nuclei. Diffuse axonal injury is a major predictor of mortality and morbidity in TBI and determines the long-term outcome as evaluated by the Glasgow Outcome Score (GOS). Most patients who are in a comatosed or vegetative state following TBI or are unable to return to their pre-injury functional level have had some type of axonal injury. Secondary injury that occurs as a result of subsequent physiologic processes can also cause axonal injury.

Multiple processes occur in response to the initial injury which exacerbate the primary brain damage; this is commonly referred to as *secondary injury*. Although the precise mechanisms remain unclear, changes to the cerebral environment seem to involve a complex interaction between cellular and molecular processes. Glutamate-driven excitotoxic effects, oxidative stress, inflammation, ion imbalance, and metabolic disarray have all been implicated in secondary injury. The ultimate result is progressive neuronal loss through necrosis and apoptosis. At the same time, intracellular changes caused by the excessive influx of calcium, which affects mitochondrial integrity, depletes cells of energy. The resultant accumulation of lactate leads to cytotoxic swelling, which, together with the increased permeability of the cerebral vasculature, results in cerebral edema, intracranial hypertension, and reduced cerebral perfusion.

While primary injury causes cell death close to the site of trauma secondary injury can induce widespread damage to neurons, glia, and axons. Biochemical factors that have been implicated in secondary injury (the *ischemic cascade*) include excitatory amino acids (e.g., glutamate), free radicals, and nitric oxide. Excitatory amino acids are initially released in response to the TBI, causing calcium influx into the cells. Intracellular calcium promotes synthesis of free radicals, which in turn promotes nitric oxide and excitatory amino acid synthesis. The initial response to TBI and neuronal injury is wide spread depolarization of neurons, glia and vascular endothelial cells. Increased glutamate levels then induce depolarization of traumatized cells, making it both a cause as well as product of depolarization and a major contributor to cell death and dysfunction in TBI.

Although primary brain injury cannot be reversed, secondary injury to the brain is potentially preventable. The two factors that have been identified to be primarily responsible for secondary injury are hypotension (systolic BP less than 90 mm Hg) and hypoxia (SpO_2 less than 90 mm Hg). Hypotension and hypoxia are among the five significant predictors of mortality in TBI, and both factors are independent predictors of mortality. Prevention and treatment of hypotension and hypoxia are therefore the mainstay of initial resuscitation following TBI. Additional physiological factors responsible for secondary injury are hypo- and hyperglycemia, hypo- and hypercarbia, and intracranial hypertension. In addition, the inflammatory response to tissue injury, cerebral edema, and excitotoxic effects can aggravate the existing neuronal damage. Cerebral edema and the resultant intracranial hypertension can decrease cerebral perfusion pressure (CPP), further exacerbating cerebral ischemia. More than 90% of the patients who die following TBI have evidence of ischemic damage in the brain.

The management in TBI is primarily focused on prevention and treatment of the secondary injury related to physiological derangement. Several treatment protocols have been developed to minimize the biochemical cascade that perpetuates neuronal damage. Current research focuses on calcium and glutamate antagonists and free radical scavengers. While these therapeutic modalities have worked well in a laboratory model, none of them have been found to be effective in clinical trials and no agent has progressed beyond phase III studies. Several recent studies suggest that progesterone may have a beneficial effect in patients with TBI, and a recent Cochrane Database review of three small randomized controlled trials concluded that it may improve neurologic outcome but the available evidence was still insufficient.

PREHOSPITAL CARE

Anesthesiologists in North America rarely participate in the prehospital care of patients with TBI, but it is important to understand the prehospital management in TBI to continue the optimal care after a patient arrives at the hospital. Although hypotension and hypoxia are detrimental to any patient, the outcome is significantly worse in patients with TBI who have a moderate (Glasgow Coma Scale [GCS] score 8–13) or severe (GCS score <8) head injury. In a study covering 717 patients from the Trauma Coma Data Bank (TCDB), hypoxia and hypotension were found to be independent predictors of morbidity and mortality [5]. Two studies have reported that the incidence of hypotension and hypoxia in the field in patients with TBI is 16% and 19% respectively. One Italian study found that the incidence of hypoxia in the field was 55% [6]. Even a single episode of hypotension can, double mortality and increase the morbidity significantly in a severe head injury [5].

Hypotension and hypoxia have even been reported in seemingly stable patients during transport. After the patient reaches the hospital, hypotension and hypoxia can still influence morbidity and mortality. This underscores the importance of adequate perfusion and oxygenation from the time of resuscitation in the field to definitive care in the hospital. A prehospital systolic blood pressure (SBP) that is less than 90 mm Hg is considered as hypotension and should be treated. Similarly, a patient with SpO_2 less than 90% with oxygen supplementation is considered to be hypoxic. Blood pressure should be measured every 5 minutes and SpO_2 should be continuously monitored in every patient who has a suspected TBI. SBP is generally monitored because it is easier to measure in the field and because recording a single value saves time. Maintaining an adequate CPP usually requires a SBP greater than 90 mm Hg. It is possible that mean arterial pressure (MAP) may be more important than SBP, but the data on outcome currently available are based on SBP predominantly.

Currently the recommended treatment for hypotension in the prehospital setting is a rapid infusion of 2 L of isotonic saline. Other acceptable options include lactated Ringers solution, hypertonic saline (7.5%), and hemoglobin substitutes. Hypertonic saline requires a smaller volume for resuscitation and because it is hyperosmolar, it promotes diuresis and decreases ICP. Hypertonic saline therefore offers the dual advantages of increasing blood pressure while decreasing ICP. However data regarding long-term outcome in patients treated with hypertonic saline infusion is inconsistent and abrupt rise in blood pressure may worsen bleeding if a patient has other injuries. There is no hemoglobin substitute currently approved by the FDA for clinical use. However artificial blood substitutes like perfluorocarbons are approved by the FDA for clinical trials in trauma patients. Because of the medical emergency patient consent has been waived.

The criteria for airway management in the hypoxic patient are unambiguous. Endotracheal intubation and mechanical ventilation are indicated in patients with a GCS less than 9, patients who are unable to maintain a patent airway, and patients who are unable to maintain a SpO_2 of more than 90% with oxygen supplementation. Rapid sequence intubation is the preferred intubation technique in patients who do not have a difficult airway. Although esmolol, lidocaine, and fentanyl have been used to provide sedation and control the sympathetic response to intubation, there is no evidence of improved outcome associated with these drugs.

After the airway is secured, ventilator settings include a tidal volume of 6 to 7 mL/kg and a rate of 10 to 12 per minute, with the goal of an end-tidal CO_2 ($ETco_2$) of 35 mm Hg. Hyperventilation is not recommended in the first 24 hours following a head injury, but mild hyperventilation ($ETco_2$ 25 to 30 mm Hg) may be considered in patients with intracranial hypertension. (Signs of increased ICP include non-reacting or dilated pupils, decerebrate posturing, or an abrupt decrease in GCS of more than 2 points in a patient with GCS less than 9.) In such cases hyperventilation is used as a bridge to definitive treatment, and the recommended respiratory rate is 20 for adults, 25 for children (up to 10 years of age) and 30 for infants.

> **BTF Guidelines**
>
> - *There is level II evidence that BP should be monitored and hypotension (SBP less than 90 mm Hg) should be avoided.*
>
> - *There is level III evidence that oxygenation status should be monitored and hypoxia (Spo_2 less than 90%) should be avoided.*

CPP AND ICP

The primary goals of the anesthesiologist are to maintain cerebral perfusion and oxygenation while providing optimal surgical conditions. Some specific aspects of TBI management in the hospital relevant to anesthesiologists include management of intracranial pressure (ICP), maintaining CPP, and avoiding hypoxia. Novel treatments, including brain tissue oxygenation-guided therapy ($Pbto_2$), hypothermia and cerebral protective agents are currently under investigation.

A large body of literature, published since the 1970s, supports the value of intensive care management of patients with TBI [7, 8]. The core of intensive care in this patient population is ICP monitoring and maintenance of optimal cerebral perfusion (CPP). The main objective of ICU care is to maintain optimal cerebral perfusion to avoid secondary injury to the brain and to promote recovery of the injured brain. CPP can be determined with the formula:

$$CPP = MAP - ICP$$

CPP should be maintained between 50 mm Hg and 70 mm Hg to maintain perfusion. Decreasing the CPP to less than 50 mm Hg can cause ischemia since the autoregulatory response of the brain vasculature is insufficient to maintain optimum cerebral blood flow (CBF). In fact, microdialysis measurements of metabolic parameters in the brain also show evidence of cerebral ischemia at a CPP below 50 mm Hg [9]. Decreasing the CPP can also increase ICP because hypotension can cause cerebral vasodilation and rise in cerebral blood volume. Transcranial Doppler and jugular venous oxygen tension (Sjo_2) recordings at various levels of CPP show that CBF, flow velocity, and venous oxygen tension plateau when CPP reaches 60 to 70 mm Hg. This suggests that the lower limit of pressure autoregulation is 60 to 70 mm Hg [10, 11].

Because ICP is an important determinant of CPP, much of the management strategy in TBI is guided by the goal of maintaining a normal ICP. These strategies include early and effective resuscitation to stabilize the vital signs, transfer to a trauma care center, early diagnosis of a mass lesion followed by surgical decompression if required, and ICU management. Intracranial hypertension can significantly decrease CPP and worsen outcome. Intracranial hypertension and systemic hypotension are the leading cause of mortality and morbidity in patients with TBI [12]. Increase in ICP is an indicator of impending cerebral ischemia and warrants immediate intervention. ICP should be treated when it rises above 20 mm Hg, and should be manipulated in increments of 5 mm Hg. Once ICP has fallen below 20 mm Hg, MAP should be manipulated to maintain a CPP of 50 to 70 mm Hg to ensure adequate cerebral perfusion. In patients with an ICP monitor in place, a decrease in ICP in response to an increase in CPP over 70 mm Hg implies that cerebral vasoconstriction is occurring as a normal response to increase in CPP. This in turn suggests a good prognosis. If, however, the patient responds to an increase in CPP with an increase in ICP, the most likely cause is impaired autoregulation in which case CBF passively increases with CPP; this suggests a poor prognosis.

The two most common techniques for monitoring ICP are intraventricular catheter and intraparenchymal monitor. The intraventricular catheter route of monitoring ICP offers the most accurate recording of ICP, permits the display of pressure waveforms and permits CSF drainage as a means to treat the intracranial hypertension. The ICP monitoring range should be between 0 and 100 mm Hg with an accuracy of ±2 mm Hg and error of 10%.

In patients with an abnormal CT, the incidence of raised ICP is between 53% and 63% [13]. Moreover, 13% of patients who have a head injury but have a normal CT scan have increased ICP. Risk factors for intracranial hypertension after closed head injury include age over 40 years, abnormal posturing, and SBP less 90 mm Hg. If a patient with a normal CT has two of these three factors (age over 40 years, abnormal posturing, SBP less than 90 mm Hg), the risk of intracranial hypertension is the same as in those with abnormal CT scan. One third of patients with a normal CT scan ultimately develop abnormal findings over time. ICP monitoring is therefore frequently indicated in patients with head injury. Indications for ICP monitoring include:

1) Severe head injury (GCS score less than 8) with an abnormal CT scan (cerebral contusion, hematoma, brain swelling, compressed cisterns).

2) Severe head injury (GCS score less than 8) with a normal CT scan and any two of the three risk factors (age greater than 40 years, abnormal posturing, systolic BP less than 90 mm Hg)

The original BTF guidelines (1999) for severe head injury management recommended that CPP be maintained above 70 mm Hg. This was revised in 2003 to decrease the minimum acceptable CPP to 60 mm Hg. Some older, retrospective studies suggested that a CPP of greater than 70 or 80 mm Hg would improve cerebral perfusion and therefore positively affect outcome. In a patient with intact pressure autoregulation, increasing the CPP above 70 mm Hg will induce cerebral vasoconstriction with a concomitant decrease in cerebral blood volume (CBV) and ICP. If, however, autoregulation is impaired, increasing the CPP above 70 mm Hg can cause passive cerebral vasodilation, which then increases ICP. Thus, ICP responds unpredictably to an increase in CPP, and the actual response depends on the response of the cerebral vasculature to the change in CPP. In one study, patients with a CPP that was greater than 70 mm Hg were compared with those in whom ICP was less than 20 mm Hg and CPP was greater than 50 mm Hg. The group with the higher CPP was found to have an increased incidence of ARDS, require more treatments for intracranial hypertension, have a higher incidence of refractory intracranial hypertension, and have a poor outcome at 6 months [14]. Thus the critical threshold for cerebral ischemia seems to be a CPP between 50 and 60 mm Hg; the CPP should ideally be maintained at a level 10 mm Hg above the ischemic threshold. Both components of CPP (MAP and ICP) should be treated individually to maintain cerebral perfusion while minimizing end-organ damage.

BTF Guidelines (summary)

- *There is no level I recommendation for ICP and CPP threshold.*

- *There is level II evidence for maintaining ICP less than 20 mm Hg.*

- *There is level II evidence that CPP greater than 70 mm Hg should be avoided.*

  o *There is level III evidence to avoid a CPP less than 50 mm Hg.*
  o *There is level III evidence to maintain a CPP of 50 to 70 mm Hg.*
  o *Ancillary methods of monitoring CBF, oxygenation and metabolism facilitate CPP management.*

ICP and CPP are both surrogate measures of cerebral perfusion; they indicate that the perfusion pressure to the brain is optimal, but do not accurately reflect CBF, cerebral oxygen delivery, or the brain's metabolic status. Although CBF can be measured with positron emission tomography (PET), xenon CT, or transcranial Doppler (TCD), these are primarily research tools and are not routinely used in the clinical setting. Brain oxygenation can be measured by jugular venous oxygen saturation (Sjo_2) and brain tissue oxygen tension ($Pbto_2$), while its metabolic status can be measured with a microdialysis catheter. Sjo_2 is a global measure of the balance between oxygen supply and demand. A Sjo_2 greater than 50% indicates that the brain is being perfused with an adequate supply of oxygen [14], while a fall in Sjo_2 to below 50% is associated with a poor prognosis. Prognosis is worse as the number of episodes where Sjo_2 is less than 50% increases. Desaturation (indicted by a drop in Sjo_2 below 50%) in the first 48 hours after head injury is more ominous. Increase in Sjo_2 above 75% reflects either luxury perfusion to the brain or cerebral infarction with a resultant decrease in oxygen demand. This also frequently indicates a poor prognosis. Brain arterial-venous oxygen difference ($A-Vdo_2$) is another index of prognostic value: a higher cerebral $A-Vdo_2$ is correlated with a better prognosis.

NEW AND EVOLVING TREATMENT STRATEGIES

Current management of patients with TBI is primarily focused on the prevention of secondary injury to the brain that is caused by hypoxia, hypoperfusion, hypercarbia and related factors [2, 15]. Over the years alternative treatment strategies such as hypothermia, barbiturate therapy, and cerebral protection have been explored as potential treatments for TBI. The relationship between increase in ICP, low CPP and cerebral ischemia resulting in poor outcome is well established. ICP-guided therapy has decreased the mortality in TBI from 60% to between 25% and 30% [16, 17]. Cerebral infarction, however, is related to intracranial hypertension in only 50% of patients with TBI [18], and some patients develop cerebral infarction with a normal ICP and CPP. Thus, there are mechanisms other than increase in ICP that seem to contribute to cerebral infarction in patients with TBI. Moreover, there is evidence of cerebral hypoxia ($Pbto_2$ less than 10 mm Hg) in 30% of patients with TBI who were resuscitated successfully as per the BTF guidelines in the early hours following TBI [19]. There is a poor correlation between CPP and the lactate to pyruvate ratio in the brain as measured by microdialysis technique. These data offer possible explanations for the plateau in outcome in ICP /CPP based treatment in recent years. In patients who die of TBI, between 80% and 90% have evidence of cerebral hypoxia and ischemia. This implies that despite of ICP/CPP-directed therapy, cerebral ischemia still occurs in patients with TBI.

In order to improve the care in TBI a technique of measuring CBL ischemia which is more sensitive in comparison to ICP /CPP is required. $PbtO_2$ seems to be one such marker. And treatment strategy should be developed focusing on optimizing $PbtO_2$ (rather than ICP /CPP) as a way of preventing /minimizing CBL hypoxia. Brain tissue oxygen tension $(PbtO_2)$-directed therapy is a novel strategy that seems to offer promise in TBI management. $PbtO_2$ is measured with a probe located on the surface of the brain close to the area of cerebral contusion, and reflects the balance between brain oxygen supply and demand in the region being monitored. $PbtO_2$ is a physiological measure that is potentially more sensitive than ICP and CPP as a marker of cerebral ischemia. Normal $PbtO_2$ varies from 37 mm Hg to 48 mm Hg. A $PbtO_2$ of 10 mm Hg to 15 mm Hg appears to be the threshold for cerebral ischemia. There is emerging evidence that $PbtO_2$ less than 15 mm Hg is associated with poor outcome in TBI. The duration of drop in $PbtO_2$ also contributes to CBL ischemia. Low $PbtO_2$ is linked to biochemical evidence of brain ischemia and correcting the $PbtO_2$ is correlated with a decrease in brain damage in laboratory studies.

Clinical management is guided by the response of $PbtO_2$ to changes in FiO_2 $(PbtO_2$ reactivity) and the correlation of $PbtO_2$ with CPP. Two types of $PbtO_2$ monitors are available—Licox (GMS, Kiel Mulkendorf, Germany) which measures $PbtO_2$ and temperature, and the Neurotrend monitor (Codman, Raynham, MA) which measures $PbtO_2$, $PbtCO_2$, pH, brain temperature. Although the brain constitutes only 2% of total body weight, it receives 15% of cardiac output and consumes 20% of the oxygen used by the body, making it far more vulnerable to hypoxia and ischemia than other organs. The value of monitoring $PbtO_2$ in the management of TBI lies in the fact that it may be more sensitive to compromised cerebral perfusion than CPP, allowing earlier and more definitive therapeutic intervention. The ideal ICP and CPP in patients with TBI seems to be constantly evolving, and $PbtO_2$-directed therapy offers specific advantages: ICP/CPP guided therapy is associated with side effects like fluid and electrolyte imbalances, pulmonary edema, and ARDS. $PbtO_2$ directed therapy might allow a higher ICP to be tolerated in some patients provided that there is no objective evidence of ischemia. Moreover, there have been several reports in which $PbtO_2$ monitoring enabled early identification of extracerebral complications.

Spiotta et al. compared $PbtO_2$-directed therapy with conventional ICP-directed therapy in patients with TBI [20]. Patients with TBI with a GCS score of 8 or less and Injury Severity Score greater than 16 with CT scan evidence of head injury were included in the study. The $PbtO_2$ monitoring probe was inserted on the abnormal side of the brain close to the site of primary injury over the normal white matter. The position was confirmed by increase in $PbtO_2$ with increase in FiO_2 for 5 minutes. In the control group standard stair case approach was followed for treating the ICP (target ICP less than 20 mm Hg) and maintaining CPP greater than 60 mm Hg. In the $PbtO_2$-directed therapy group standard ICP, CPP-guided therapy was followed and in addition goal was to maintain the $PbtO_2$ over 20 mm Hg. Despite the treatment if $PbtO_2$ was below 20 mm Hg for more than 15 minutes' decompressive craniotomy was carried out. There were 70 patients in the treatment group and 53 patients in the control group (where ICP guided therapy as per BTF guidelines was followed). Outcome was measured in terms of GOS at the end of 6 months. More patients in the treatment group required decompressive craniotomy and the duration of treatment also was longer (average of 4.7 days). In the treatment group 64.3% had a good outcome compared with 39.6% in the control group. Mortality was 25.7% versus 45.3%. The mean $PbtO_2$ in the treatment group was 36.5 ± 17 mm Hg. In patients who died $PbtO_2$ was significantly lower.

In another study by Narotham et al. five-year experience with $PbtO_2$-directed (139 patients) therapy was compared with the cohort of 41 patients managed as per conventional ICP/CPP-directed therapy [21]. The target $PbtO_2$ in the treatment group was 20 mm Hg. Outcome as per GOS was measured at the end of 6 months. In the treatment group 65% had a good outcome (GOS 1 or 2) compared with 44% in the control group. There was no correlation between ICP and $PbtO_2$. Patients with good outcome responded within 2 hours to $PbtO_2$-directed protocol. Predictors of good outcome were CPP over 75 mm Hg, with $PbtO_2$ over 25 mm Hg and ICP less than 15 mm Hg. All patients in the vegetative state had a $PbtO_2$ of less than 10 mm Hg for more than 2 hours. Failure to respond to $PbtO_2$ guided treatment was associated with 11 to 17 times odds ratio of death. In a literature review seven studies were identified where $PbtO_2$-guided treatment was compared with conventional ICP/CPP-guided treatment (491 patients) [22]. In the $PbtO_2$ group 61% had a favorable outcome compared with 41% in the standard treatment group.

> **BTF Guidelines**
>
> - **Both BTF as well as EBIC (European Brain Injury Consortium) guidelines emphasize on ICP/CPP-directed management in TBI.**
>
> - **Brain tissue oxygen monitoring is recommended in the guidelines.**

Hopefully the integration of $PbtO_2$ and ICP will allow an ideal ICP and CPP value to be identified that can predict cerebral ischemia facilitating early therapeutic intervention.

HYPOTHERMIA

The role of therapeutic hypothermia in the management of patients with TBI is controversial. At the present time, over 40 laboratory studies have concluded that mild to moderate hypothermia is protective, but clinical studies have failed to replicate its therapeutic efficacy. As of now therapeutic hypothermia is indicated and improves neurological outcome only in adult cardiac arrest survivors and neonatal hypoxia [23]. Multiple studies on hypothermia, including a major multi-institutional study, have not, however, found a beneficial effect in patients with TBI. Twenty-nine clinical studies on therapeutic hypothermia in TBI have been published so far, and although there is some suggestion that hypothermia is beneficial there is no clear evidence of improvement in outcome [24]. One proposed reason for this is that patients who suffer a cardiac arrest or neonatal hypoxia are treated immediately after a well-defined event, while cerebral ischemia after TBI is multifactorial. Several meta-analyses on this subject do suggest that hypothermia improves the outcome in patients with TBI [25, 26]. Despite so much of conflicting data the reason for pursuing this line of treatment in TBI is the convincing laboratory studies, which show that hypothermia has beneficial effect in TBI and the clinical evidence in cardiac arrest survivors and neonatal hypoxia. Besides most pharmacological treatment measures (e.g., calcium antagonists, glutamate antagonists, free radical scavengers) have not progressed beyond phase III trial, thus imploding us to look for nonpharmacological therapeutic measures.

In the failed hypothermia clinical trials several important observations have been reported which if addressed are likely to be of benefit in future studies [27, 28]. These are:

i) **Control of ICP with hypothermia:** In 18 studies (2096 patients) where mild hypothermia was used for treating TBI patient with refractory intra cranial hypertension, there was evidence of decrease in ICP in all of them. In 13 of these studies there was improvement in outcome with hypothermia. Even 2°C drop in temperature causes a significant decrease in ICP.

ii) **Hypothermia titrated to control the ICP:** Studies where hypothermia was titrated to control the ICP were associated with an improvement in outcome, compared with studies where hypothermia was maintained for a fixed period of time.

iii) **Duration of hypothermia:** It has been observed that if cooling is done for a minimum of 48 hours followed by gradual rewarming (0.25°C /6 hours) outcome is better.

iv) **Early cooling:** The window of opportunity for instituting hypothermia seems to be narrow. Preferably hypothermia should be induced within 2 hours of TBI. In one of the hypothermia studies it took as much as 8 hours to start inducing hypothermia. In Clifton's study it took 4.3 ± 1.1 hours to start cooling and 8.4 ± 3 hours to reach the target temperature.

v) **Cooling Techniques:** Techniques used for cooling determine how quickly and effectively the target temperature is achieved. In most of the older studies surface cooling has been used. Surface cooling takes a longer time to cool the patient. Intravascular cooling has been found to be very effective, predictable drop in temperature can be achieved and complications related to intravascular cooling technique are minimal. Polderman reported that with 1.5 L of cold normal saline (at 4 °C) infused over 30 minutes temperature drops from 36.9 °C to 34.6 °C within 30 minutes and to 32.9 °C in 60 minutes. Once the desired temperature is achieved temperature can be maintained by surface cooling.

vi) **Complications related to hypothermia:** In most studies done in the past several complications related to cooling have been reported like hypotension, immune suppression, bronchopneumonia, electrolyte imbalance etc.

vii) Hypothermia was beneficial only in patients who did not get barbiturate therapy as a part of the treatment.

Considering the various shortcomings of hypothermia studies in the past recently two new studies have been initiated—the NABISH II trial by Guy Clifton from Texas and one in Europe called the Eurothermia 3235 trial.

NABISH TRIAL II (NORTH AMERICAN BRAIN INJURY STUDY: HYPOTHERMIA IIR TRIAL)

Salient observations in the NABISH I trial were [29, 30]:

i) There was a delay in inducing hypothermia in the treatment group (4.3 hours) and cooling technique was slow (it took 8 hours to reach the target temperature).

ii) Patients who were less than 45 years old, hypothermic on admission (< 35 °C) and randomized to the hypothermia group had a better outcome at 6 months (52% versus 76% poor outcome).

iii) There was a decrease in ICP with hypothermia.

vi) Incidence of complications like hypotension was high in the hypothermia group.

In NABISH II trial early cooling and prevention of hypotension was the goal. Salient features of the NABISH II trial, which was started in 2005, are:

i) Subjects: Nonpenetrating TBI patients in the age group of 16 to 45 years, GCS score of 3 to 8 and identified within 2.5 hours of the injury.

ii) Initially cooling to 35 °C was instituted as soon as the patients were identified in the field, as quickly as possible (using an Arctic sun device—surface cooling) and, if need be, intravenous cooling with ice-cold saline was supplemented.

iii) Patients were be triaged in the hospital—cooling continued to 33 °C if subjects fulfilled inclusion criteria.

iv) ICP of less than 20 mm Hg, CPP of 60 to 70 mm Hg, MAP of greater than 70 mm Hg was maintained.

v) Cooling maintained for 48 hours followed by slow rewarming.

This study was started in 2005—original plan was to recruit 240 patients with TBI. However after 97 subjects were recruited an interim analysis was carried out and the study was prematurely discontinued, as there was no evidence of benefit with early hypothermia. The mortality in the hypothermia group was 60% compared with 56% in the normothermia despite instituting hypothermia within 1.6 hours of TBI. The investigators have concluded that there is no evidence at this point to institute early hypothermia in TBI. They have suggested that future trials should explore continuing hypothermia till ICP is controlled as is being studied in the Eurothermia trial.

Eurothermia 3235 trial [31]: The Eurothermia trial is focused on patients with TBI—adults up to 65 years of age, admitted within 72 hours after a head injury and with ICP over 20 mm Hg for 5 minutes after stage I and II treatment for ICP control (as per the Brain Trauma Foundation and European Brain Injury Consortium guidelines). Brief study protocol is included in the appendix at the end of the chapter.

The study will recruit 1800 subjects (900 in each group) over 41 months. Study group patients will be treated with hypothermia to control ICP below 20 mm Hg. Rest of the management protocol will be the same in both groups. In the TBI trials done in the past studies were powered to detect a 10% difference in outcome between the treatment group and control group. The Eurothermia study is powered to detect a 7% difference between the two groups (since 10% is considered to be very over ambitious goal). Outcome will be measured in GOS at the end of 3, 6 and 12 months.

BTF Guidelines

- *There is no level I or level II evidence to support the use of prophylactic hypothermia in TBI.*

- *There is no level III evidence that hypothermia decreases the mortality in TBI. However pooled data suggests that there is a decrease in mortality if hypothermia is maintained for more than 48 hours.*

ANESTHETIC MANAGEMENT

Patients with TBI may require anesthetic management for craniotomy, sedation for diagnostic procedures or sedation and analgesia in the ICU. Anesthetic agents have a variety of effects on the systemic and cerebral hemodynamics, and may therefore influence the outcome following TBI. There is a paucity of data on how the choice of a specific anesthetic agent affects long-term outcome in patients with TBI. One retrospective study [32] of 252 patients with TBI compared the effect of total intravenous anesthesia (TIVA) with volatile anesthetic agents. The TIVA group were anesthetized with propofol 75 to 150 µg/kg/min infusion with narcotic and some also received ketamine. The unadjusted outcome was better in the TIVA group—75% good outcome compared with 54% in the volatile anesthetic group (GOS). However, when the results were adjusted for Injury Severity Score, craniotomy versus craniectomy, and other confounding factors there was no difference in outcome between the two groups. Interestingly, mortality after TBI incurred during wartime has been decreasing over the last 40 years, independent of the choice of a specific anesthetic technique (19% in Lebanon, 16% in Vietnam, and 11% in Iraq) [32]. Another study that compared propofol with morphine for sedation in the ICU found no difference in outcome [33]. In a retrospective study in patients with TBI, 7 of 277 patients who were administered propofol infusion died of propofol infusion syndrome (presents with rhabdomyolysis, lactic acidosis, cardiac and renal failure) [34, 35]. Patients who were administered greater than 5 mg/kg/h of propofol for 48 hours or more are prone for propofol infusion syndrome. In the absence of outcome studies the choice of an anesthetic technique is determined by its effects upon intracranial and systemic hemodynamics [33].

Animal and human studies have demonstrated that the effects of propofol on cerebral hemodynamics and oxygen demand are superior to those of volatile anesthetics. Propofol decreases CMR_{O_2} by 50% to 68%, CBF by 53% to 70%, and CBV by 25%; this decrease in CBV reduces ICP. When given in high doses, however, propofol decreases MAP, which then decreases CPP and negates the beneficial effects on ICP. Propofol also decreases JV_{O_2} by up to 50%. When combined with hyperventilation, starting a propofol infusion can cause JV_{O_2} to drop below 50%, which is consistent with cerebral ischemia. Another study found that ICP was lower and CPP was higher in patients who received propofol as opposed to isoflurane or sevoflurane anesthesia [36, 37]. Starting hyperventilation decreased ICP in the isoflurane and sevoflurane groups but not in the propofol group. Sevoflurane decreases CMR_{O_2} to the same extent as does propofol, but has minimal effects on CBF and CBV [38]. Of the three commonly used volatile anesthetic agents sevoflurane has the least effect on cerebral vasculature. Hyperventilation can decrease CBF and CBV in patients who receive sevoflurane. There is conflicting data regarding the hemodynamic effect of sevoflurane and propofol. Target controlled infusion of propofol does not cause hypotension, but propofol does cause hypotension when given as a standard infusion. Sevoflurane combined with remifentanil is associated with a higher incidence of hypotension compared with propofol remifentanil combination. Some studies have shown EEG evidence of seizure activity in patients who receive high doses of sevoflurane. However in a study carried out in patients with temporal lobe epilepsy patients there was no evidence of seizure activity when they were anesthetized with either sevoflurane or propofol (up to 1.5 MAC).

Barbiturate therapy: Prophylactic administration of barbiturates is not indicated in patients with TBI. Barbiturates were associated with a poorer outcome and a higher mortality in comparison to mannitol when used to control ICP. The mortality was worse in the diffuse head injury group compared with those with focal injury. In patients with TBI who have refractory intracranial hypertension (i.e., no response to conventional measures for reducing ICP) barbiturates can be used to control ICP, but are frequently associated with hypotension (25% incidence of hypotension) that negates any benefit from ICP control. In a Cochrane review based on three randomized control trials in patients with TBI, the relative risk for poor outcome associated with barbiturate therapy was 1.15 though the RR for refractory ICP was 0.81 [39].

> **BTF Guidelines**
>
> - *Prophylactic administration of barbiturates for burst suppression is not recommended*
>
> - *Barbiturate therapy is recommended for controlling ICP refractory to standard medical and surgical therapy. Hemodynamic stability is essential before and during barbiturate therapy.*
>
> - *Propofol infusion can be used for ICP control. High dose propofol is associated with significant morbidity.*

Hyperventilation: More than 40% of patients with TBI have intracranial hypertension, which is the most common cause of death and disability in this population. Hyperventilation has been used as a treatment for intracranial hypertension for more than 20 years. In a survey, 83% of the trauma centers in the United States were using hyperventilation to decrease ICP in patients with TBI. Although hyperventilation does decrease ICP, it has numerous adverse effects. During the first few days after TBI, cerebral blood flow is 50% lower than the CBF in normal individuals (18 mL/100 g/min and 27 mL/100 g/min in two different studies). Moreover, CBF is lower in the contused area and CO_2 reactivity in the surrounding region is altered. Hyperventilation and hypocarbia on day one of head injury

induce cerebral vasoconstriction, profound decrease in CBF, resulting in a poor outcome at 3 and 6 months.

> **BTF Guidelines**
>
> - *Prophylactic hyperventilation is not recommended in TBI.*
>
> - *No hyperventilation is recommended in the first 24 hours following TBI.*
>
> - *After the first day if hyperventilation is required for controlling ICP, Sjo_2 or $Pbto_2$ should be monitored to ensure improvement in oxygen delivery to the brain tissues.*

CONCLUSIONS

In the management of the patient with TBI, the primary goal is early effective resuscitation of the patient to optimize the physiological parameters. Subsequently cerebral perfusion has to be optimized and maintained at optimal level to promote recovery of the injured brain. However, with this mode of therapy, outcome seems to have plateaued over the past 10 to 20 years. Therapeutic agents focused on neutralizing the ischemic cascade have not been effective in clinical trials. Another treatment strategy being followed is monitoring of brain tissue oxygenation ($Pbto_2$) and treatment focused on optimizing brain tissue oxygenation status. This seems to be a more effective method of monitoring and treating CBL ischemia in TBI. Hypothermia continues to hold promise. Based on the negative clinical trial with hypothermia in TBI patients the reasons for failure in the past seems to have been identified and also the possible approach likely to work in future trials. These are being addressed and a new trial following the treatment strategy likely to work is in progress in Europe.

APPENDIX

Salient features of the Eurothermia study protocol are:

i) The threshold for ICP control as per the BTF guideline is 20mm Hg. Treatment is focused on controlling the ICP with hypothermia and titrating hypothermia to an ICP of 20 mm Hg, because several studies in the past have established the efficacy of hypothermia when it is titrated to a physiological end point like ICP. (Figure 19.1)

ii) Early cooling is not a goal in this study. Early cooling is beneficial only in patients with a high ICP. This study will recruit a wider group of patients (injury within 72 hours with ICP greater than 20mm Hg) who are already receiving the standard treatment

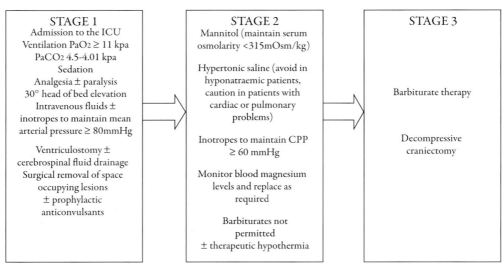

STAGE 1	STAGE 2	STAGE 3
Admission to the ICU Ventilation PaO2 ≥ 11 kpa PaCO2 4.5-4.01 kpa Sedation Analgesia ± paralysis 30° head of bed elevation Intravenous fluids ± inotropes to maintain mean arterial pressure ≥ 80mmHg Ventriculostomy ± cerebrospinal fluid drainage Surgical removal of space occupying lesions ± prophylactic anticonvulsants	Mannitol (maintain serum osmolarity <315mOsm/kg) Hypertonic saline (avoid in hyponatraemic patients, caution in patients with cardiac or pulmonary problems) Inotropes to maintain CPP ≥ 60 mmHg Monitor blood magnesium levels and replace as required Barbiturates not permitted ± therapeutic hypothermia	Barbiturate therapy Decompressive craniectomy

Figure 19.1 Management protocol Eurothermia 3235 *trial.*

measures for TBI. The delay in cooling is offset by the more aggressive cooling technique described below.

iii) Patients who are on barbiturate therapy will be excluded—a meta-analysis found that hypothermia is effective only inpatients that did not get barbiturate therapy.

iv) Cooling technique: Patients will be cooled with ice cold saline 20 ml to 30 ml /kg (up to 1.5 L infused over 30 minutes). Intravenous cooling has been found to be more effective than surface cooling. Temperature will be maintained with surface cooling.

v) The temperature range will be 32 °C to 35 °C. Hypothermia will be titrated to threshold ICP level (20 mm Hg). Minimum duration of hypothermia will be 48 hours while there will be no limit to maximum duration of hypothermia (cooling will be maintained as long as it is required to control the ICP).

vi) Rewarming will be slow—0.25 °C /every 6 hours to prevent rebound rise in ICP during rewarming.

vii) If ICP does not respond to cooling stage III treatment for ICP control will be instituted (decompressive craniotomy) and hypothermia will be discontinued.

The study will recruit 1800 subjects (900 in each group) over 41 months. Study group patients will be treated with hypothermia to control ICP below 20 mm Hg. Rest of the management protocol will be the same in both groups. In the TBI trials done in the past studies were powered to detect a 10% difference in outcome between the treatment group and control group. The Eurothermia study is powered to detect a 7% difference between the two groups (since 10% is considered to be very over ambitious goal). Outcome will be GOS measured at the end of 3, 6, and 12 months.

REFERENCES

1. Alkhoury F, Courtney J. Outcomes after severe head injury, a National Trauma Data Bank-based comparison of Level I and Level II trauma centers. *Am Surg.* 2011;77:277–280.
2. Bullock MR, Povlishock JT. Guidelines for the management of severe traumatic brain injury. Editor's Commentary. *J Neurotrauma.* 2007;24(Suppl 1).
3. Sharma D, Vavilala MS. Perioperative management of adult traumatic brain injury. *Anesthesiol Clin.* 2012;30:333–346.
4. Greve MW, Zink BJ. Pathophysiology of traumatic brain injury. *Mt Sinai J Med N Y.* 2009;76:97–104.
5. Chesnut RM, Marshall LF, Klauber MR, et al. The role of secondary brain injury in determining outcome from severe head injury. *J Trauma.* 1993;34:216–222.
6. Stocchetti N, Furlan A, Volta F. Hypoxemia and arterial hypotension at the accident scene in head injury. *J Trauma.* 1996;40:764–767.
7. Patel HC, Menon DK, Tebbs S, et al. Specialist neurocritical care and outcome from head injury. *Intens Care Med.* 2002;28:547–553.
8. Miller JD, Butterworth JF, Gudeman SK, et al. Further experience in the management of severe head injury. *J Neurosurg.* 1981;54:289–299.
9. Nordstrom CH, Reinstrup P, Xu W, et al. Assessment of the lower limit for cerebral perfusion pressure in severe head injuries by bedside monitoring of regional energy metabolism. *Anesthesiology.* 2003;98:809–814.
10. Chan KH, Miller JD, Dearden NM, et al. The effect of changes in cerebral perfusion pressure upon middle cerebral artery blood flow velocity and jugular bulb venous oxygen saturation after severe brain injury. *J Neurosurg.* 1992;77:55–61.
11. Chan KH, Dearden NM, Miller JD, et al. Multimodality monitoring as a guide to treatment of intracranial hypertension after severe brain injury. *Neurosurgery.* 1993;32:547–552; discussion 552–543.
12. McHugh GS, Engel DC, Butcher I, et al. Prognostic value of secondary insults in traumatic brain injury. results from the IMPACT study. *J Neurotrauma.* 2007;24:287–293.
13. Narayan RK, Kishore PR, Becker DP, et al. Intracranial pressure. to monitor or not to monitor? A review of our experience with severe head injury. *J Neurosurg.* 1982;56:650–659.
14. Robertson CS, Valadka AB, Hannay HJ, et al. Prevention of secondary ischemic insults after severe head injury. *Crit Care Med.* 1999;27:2086–2095.
15. Maas AI, Dearden M, Teasdale GM, et al. EBIC-guidelines for management of severe head injury in adults. European Brain Injury Consortium. *Acta Neurochir.* 1997;139:286–294.

16. Patel HC, Bouamra O, Woodford M, et al. Trends in head injury outcome from. 1989 to. 2003 and the effect of neurosurgical care. an observational study. *Lancet*. 2005;366:1538–1544.

17. Huang SJ, Hong WC, Han YY, et al. Clinical outcome of severe head injury using three different ICP and CPP protocol-driven therapies. *J Clin Neurosci* 2006;13:818–822.

18. Stein SC, Graham DI, Chen XH, et al. Association between intravascular microthrombosis and cerebral ischemia in traumatic brain injury. *Neurosurgery*. 2004;54:687–691; discussion 691.

19. Stiefel MF, Udoetuk JD, Spiotta AM, et al. Conventional neurocritical care and cerebral oxygenation after traumatic brain injury. *J Neurosurg*. 2006;105:568–575.

20. Spiotta AM, Stiefel MF, Gracias VH, et al. Brain tissue oxygen-directed management and outcome in patients with severe traumatic brain injury. *J Neurosurg*. 2010;113:571–580.

21. Narotam PK, Morrison JF, Nathoo N. Brain tissue oxygen monitoring in traumatic brain injury and major trauma. outcome analysis of a brain tissue oxygen-directed therapy. *J Neurosurg*. 2009;111:672–682.

22. Nangunoori R, Maloney-Wilensky E, Stiefel M, et al. Brain tissue oxygen-based therapy and outcome after severe traumatic brain injury. a systematic literature review. *Neurocrit Care*. 2012;17:131–138.

23. Marion D, Bullock MR. Current and future role of therapeutic hypothermia. *J Neurotrauma*. 2009;26:455–467.

24. Polderman KH. Induced hypothermia and fever control for prevention and treatment of neurological injuries. *Lancet*. 2008;371:1955–1969.

25. Sydenham E, Roberts I, Alderson P. Hypothermia for traumatic head injury. *Cochrane Database Syst Rev*. 2009 Apr 15;(2):CD001048.

26. Peterson K, Carson S, Carney N. Hypothermia treatment for traumatic brain injury. a systematic review and meta-analysis. *J Neurotrauma*. 2008;25:62–71.

27. Jiang JY. Clinical study of mild hypothermia treatment for severe traumatic brain injury. *J Neurotrauma*. 2009;26:399–406.

28. Polderman KH, Ely EW, Badr AE, et al. Induced hypothermia in traumatic brain injury. considering the conflicting results of meta-analyses and moving forward. *Intens Care Med*. 2004;30:1860–1864.

29. Clifton GL, Miller ER, Choi SC, et al. Lack of effect of induction of hypothermia after acute brain injury. *N Engl J Med*. 2001;344:556–563.

30. Clifton GL, Valadka A, Zygun D, et al. Very early hypothermia induction in patients with severe brain injury (the National Acute Brain Injury Study. Hypothermia II). a randomised trial. *Lancet Neurol*. 2011;10:131–139.

31. Andrews PJ, Sinclair HL, Battison CG, et al. European society of intensive care medicine study of therapeutic hypothermia (32-35 degrees C) for intracranial pressure reduction after traumatic brain injury (the Eurotherm 3235 Trial). *Trials*. 2011;12:8.

32. Grathwohl KW, Black IH, Spinella PC, et al. Total intravenous anesthesia including ketamine versus volatile gas anesthesia for combat-related operative traumatic brain injury. *Anesthesiology*. 2008;109:44–53.

33. Cole CD, Gottfried ON, Gupta DK, et al. Total intravenous anesthesia. advantages for intracranial surgery. *Neurosurgery*. 2007;61:369–377; discussion 377–368.

34. Otterspoor LC, Kalkman CJ, Cremer OL. Update on the propofol infusion syndrome in ICU management of patients with head injury. *Curr Opin Anaesthesiol*. 2008;21:544–551.

35. Cremer OL, Moons KG, Bouman EA, et al. Long-term propofol infusion and cardiac failure in adult head-injured patients. *Lancet*. 2001;357:117–118.

36. Petersen KD, Landsfeldt U, Cold GE, et al. ICP is lower during propofol anaesthesia compared with isoflurane and sevoflurane. *Acta Neurochir Suppl*. 2002;81:89–91.

37. Petersen KD, Landsfeldt U, Cold GE, et al. Intracranial pressure and cerebral hemodynamic in patients with cerebral tumors. a randomized prospective study of patients subjected to craniotomy in propofol-fentanyl, isoflurane-fentanyl, or sevoflurane-fentanyl anesthesia. *Anesthesiology*. 2003;98:329–336.

38. Engelhard K, Werner C. Inhalational or intravenous anesthetics for craniotomies? Pro inhalational. *Curr Opin Anaesthesiol*. 2006;19:504–508.

39. Roberts I, Sydenham E. Barbiturates for acute traumatic brain injury. *Cochrane Database Syst Rev*. 2012;12:CD000033.

20.

SPINAL SURGERY

Maria Bustillo

ANATOMY

The anatomy of the spine can be divided into the vertebral column and the spinal cord. The two structures are intimately related and surgery on one will affect the other.

VERTEBRAL COLUMN

The vertebral column is a bony structure composed of 33 vertebrae whose function is to protect the spinal cord. The presacral vertebrae consist of 7 cervical, 12 thoracic, and 5 lumbar bones. The 5 sacral and 4 coccygeal vertebrae fuse early in development. In adults, therefore, the spine is functionally reduced to 24 presacral vertebrae, one sacrum and one coccyx. The vertebral column normally exhibits four curves in the anteroposterior plane: Two forward curves, or lordoses are in the cervical and lumbar areas, and the two posterior curves or kyphoses, are in the thoracic and sacral areas.

The individual vertebrae that make-up the vertebral column are each a single bony structure consisting of a large body, bilateral pedicles, bilateral lamina, bilateral transverse processes, a spinous process, and four articular processes. The two pedicle laterally, the two lamina posteriorly, and the body anteriorly together form the anterior canal in which lies the spinal cord. The segmental nerves exit between the vertebrae through the intervertebral foramen. The four articular processes mate with corresponding processes on the vertebrae above and below to form the facet joints. The facet joint articulations provide posterior stability, and the body articulations provide anterior and vertical stability to the spinal column as a unit. In addition the facet joints provide flexion, extension and lateral rotation to the spine.

The anterior longitudinal ligament and the posterior longitudinal ligament are located anterior to and posterior to the vertebral column, respectively. They extend from the base of the skull and the atlas to the sacrum. The anterior ligament is attached to the anterior surface of the vertebrae and intervertebral discs. The posterior ligament is attached to the posterior surface of the vertebrae and the intervertebral discs and lies within the vertebral canal. These two ligaments provide stability in flexion and extension to the vertebral column. The posterior elements of the bony spine are joined by several lesser ligaments: The supraspinal and interspinal ligaments unite the spinous processes at each level, providing additional stability in flexion. The ligamentum flavum connects the vertebral laminae at each level and forms part of the posterior border of the intervertebral foramen.

The intervertebral discs are fibrocartilaginous joints composed of an interior nucleus pulposus surrounded and encapsulated by a tough annulus fibrosus. These two components provide a strong attachment between vertebrae, in addition the discs act as a very effective shock absorber during movement and activity. The facet joints are synovial joints between adjacent vertebrae posterior to the vertebrae canal. These joints are paired at each level, one on each side of the spine. As posterior elements the facet joints allow flexion of the spine. The facet joints at the cervical region are less rigid, thus allowing greater flexion of the neck.

SPINAL CORD

The spinal cord carries information to and from the brain and the rest of the body below the cranium and is contained within the vertebral canal. It is contiguous with the brain stem and the foramen magnum, and in the adult extends to the conus medullaris at about the level of the first or second lumbar vertebrae. The filum terminale attaches the end of the conus to the first coccygeal segment of the bony spine. The segmental spinal nerves enter and exit the cord on either side. Approximately 30 segments are involved. These are made up of 8 cervical, 12 thoracic, 5 lumbar, 5 sacral and a variable number of coccygeal segments. The cord exhibits two prominent bulges in the cervical and the lumbar areas, which corresponds to the origins of the nerves of the upper and lower extremities, respectively.

A cross section of the spinal cord reveals a mixture of white and grey matter. The grey matter is in the shape of an H surrounding the central canal and contains the cell bodies of the spinal neurons. The dorsal columns (most posterior) transmit sensory information including pain, position sense, touch and temperature. The ventral horn contains neurons associated with motor function and spinal reflexes. The surrounding white matter contains myelinated and unmyelinated fibers that communicate with higher and lower centers, including the brainstem and the cerebral cortex. The descending motor pathways travel in the white matter of the cord in the lateral and ventral areas. The corticospinal tract conducts primary motor impulses and the vestibulospinal and the rubrospinal tracts also participate in motor function. The dorsal areas of the white matter contain the dorsal column tracts, the spinothalamic tracts, and the spinoreticular tracts, which transmit sensory information to higher cord centers and the brain.

The dorsal roots conduct sensory information, including pain. All nerve cell bodies of afferent axons are located in the dorsal root ganglion. The ventral roots conduct primarily motor and afferent information from the cord to the periphery. The two roots combine in the spinal nerve as they traverse the vertebral foramen. The nerves then divides into three rami: dorsal, ventral and communicating. The ventral ramus continues as the primary spinal nerve, the dorsal ramus innervated the paraspinous muscles of the back and the facet joints at each level, and the communicating ramus provides segmental neuronal connections to the sympathetic chains.

The sympathetic nervous system is also segmental and traverses the length of the vertebral column in two chains anterior to the bony spine. Segmental communication is accomplished at each spinal segment via the communicating ramus of each segmental spinal nerve. The segmental spinal nerves are made up of the confluence of the dorsal root and a ventral root at each level. The spinal nerves exit the vertebral canal via the intervertebral foramina. These foramina are formed by the juxtaposition of adjoining vertebrae in the spinal column [1].

BLOOD SUPPLY

The blood supply to the spinal cord comes from the aorta via the vertebral and segmental or radicular arteries. The primary blood supply comes from the single anterior spinal artery in the anterior or ventral median sulcus and two posterior spinal arteries located in the area of the dorsal nerve rootlets. These three arteries arise as branches of the vertebral arteries at the base of the brainstem and traverse the entire length of the cord. The blood flow is augmented by multiple segmental radicular and medullary arteries that enter the intervertebral foramen. The arterial network of the three main blood vessels supplies blood to the interior of the cord through an extensive network of arterioles and capillaries. The density of the capillary bed reflects the metabolic demands of the different areas of the cord.

The anterior spinal artery supplies the anterior two thirds of the cord, and the posterior spinal arteries supply the posterior one third. Below the level of the cervical cord segments additional blood supply is provided by segmental or radicular arteries that arises as branches of the aorta and enter the cord arterial system. The most consistent of these arteries is the artery of Adamkiewicz, which is the largest segmental feeder in the thoracolumbar region of the cord. It usually enters as a single vessel between the ninth and the eleventh thoracic level. This vessel is thought to be the principal contributor to the arterial blood supply anterior thoracic and lumbar cord. Loss of this artery due to surgery or trauma may produce paraplegia below the thoracic region.

Venous drainage of the spinal cord is through radial veins serving the parenchyma. These veins feed into the coronal venous plexus or longitudinal veins in the surface of the cord, which in turn drain into medullary veins that penetrate the dura adjacent to the nerve roots to join the epidural venous plexus. The epidural or internal vertebral venous system drains into the external vertebral venous system, which in turn communicates with the azygous veins and vena cava. The veins in the epidural system are valveless and may therefore become engorged in conditions such as pregnancy and obesity [2, 3].

TYPES OF SPINAL SURGERY

TUMOR RESECTION

The clinical presentation of patients with spinal cord tumors includes pain, a neurological deficit, a progressive spinal deformity, or some combination of these symptoms. The surgical approach to tumors in this region is guided by the particular location and size of the tumor, the involvement of adjacent structures and the stability of the spine. Tumor resection is usually undertaken to relieve pressure on the spinal cord or to provide stability to the bony spine.

Spinal tumors are divided into four classifications: extradural, intradural, extramedullary, and intramedullary. *Extradural* tumors usually originate in the vertebral body or the epidural space. Primary tumors of this area include sarcomas, osteochondromas, chordomas, osteomas, multiple myelomas, and osteosarcomas. The majority of the extradural tumors are malignant, representing metastatic disease from lung, breast, prostate, hematopoietic, or lymphoid tissue. In the majority of patients, spinal metastasis involves the vertebral body and occurs through hematopoietic seeding or direct extension of a paravertebral tumor. The thoracic spine is the most common location of spinal metastasis, and pain caused by vertebral body involvement, mass effect on surrounding tissue, or nerve root compression is the most common presenting symptom. Neurological symptoms may vary from radiculopathy to cord dysfunction. Indications for surgical treatment include the presence of a progressive neurological deficit, severe pain unresponsive to medical treatment, progressive spinal instability, a radioresistant tumor, or an unknown primary tumor for which biopsy is otherwise impossible.

Intradural extramedullary tumors are located within the dura but outside of the substance of the spinal cord and may involve the arachnoid tissue, circulating CSF, nerve sheaths, dentate ligaments, filum terminale and vascular structures. Tumors that arise from this space are usually either nerve sheaths tumors or meningiomas and are histologically benign. The clinical presentation of an intradural extramedullary tumor usually includes a radiculopathy or myelopathy. Surgery is warranted for the treatment of benign intradural extramedullary tumors in order to treat the neurological deficit or prevent the deficit from worsening.

Intramedullary tumors are located within the substance of the spinal cord. Approximately 80% of these tumors in adults are astrocytomas and ependymomas. The typical clinical presentation consists of a myelopathy and sensory disturbance below the level of the spinal tumor. The primary treatment of an intramedullary tumor is laminectomy and surgical resection.

ARTERIOVENOUS MALFORMATIONS

Arteriovenous malformations (AVMs) are typically congenital and present with intermittent neurological findings that may resemble multiple sclerosis. These lesions produce a neurological deficit by causing thrombosis of vessels, resulting in spinal cord ischemia. They may also bleed into and around the spinal cord, compressing neural structures. AVMs of the spine are classified as either intradural or dural and subclassified as juvenile, glomus, or a direct arteriovenous fistula. The majority of the spinal AVMs are intradural. Intradural AVMs generally occur in young patients, have an acute onset, present with a subarachnoid hemorrhage or a bruit, and primarily involve the cervical and thoracic cord.

Dural arteriovenous fistulas make up the minority of spinal AVMs. These may be acquired lesions since they tend to occur in older patients with gradual onset and progressive worsening of symptoms and they tend to occur in the lower half of the spinal cord, commonly affecting the legs. The pathology of dural AVMs is related to venous hypertension. No valves exist in the intrathecal venous system. Retrograde flow from the dural arteriovenous fistula combined with anterograde flow from an intradural AVM produce venous hypertension that reduces cord blood flow and produces ischemic symptoms.

DISC HERNIATION

Intervertebral discs are composed of a well-hydrated central nucleus pulposus surrounded by an outer annulus fibrosus.

Disks deteriorate as part of the aging process, and may ultimately herniate if the annulus fibrosus breaks, opens or cracks allowing the nucleus pulposus to extrude. One of the most common indications for surgery of the spine is discectomy and removal of herniated nucleus pulposus material to treat a radiculopathy.

The most common location of disc herniation in the cervical spine is at C5-C6, and -C7 is the next most common. Herniation is most common in individuals older than 40 years. Symptoms include neck pain and radicular symptoms consisting of shoulder, arm and hand paresthesias, pain, or weakness in a nerve root distribution. Patients may also present with symptoms of cervical myelopathy if the herniated disc compresses the spinal cord. Herniated cervical discs may initially be managed conservatively, with physical therapy, nonsteroidal anti-inflammatory drugs, steroids, and physical therapy. Surgical management is indicated if conservative therapy fails or the patient develops progressive neurological symptoms surgical therapy is selected. An anterior cervical discectomy and fusion with or without anterior cervical plating is the most commonly performed procedure [4].

Symptomatic thoracic disc herniations are rare, but occur most commonly between levels T8 and T12. Peak incidence is in adults between the ages of 40 and 60 years. The majority are located centrally and cause a variety of symptoms including pain, myelopathy, and bladder dysfunction. The majority of patients with thoracic disc herniations are effectively managed with medical treatment. Indications for surgical intervention include failure of medical therapy after 4 to 6 weeks, progressive neurological deficits, or persistent radicular pain [5].

Lumbar disc herniation is very common, with an incidence of 1–3%. It is most common in people between the ages of 30 and 50 years old, and occurs twice as often in men as in women. Sciatica caused by a herniated lumbar disc is the most common cause of leg pain in the adult working population. The majority of lumbar herniations occur at the level of L4-L5 or L5-S1, and are most commonly located posterolateraly. The majority of patients with lumbar disc herniations are treated medically. Indications for surgery include significant motor deficits, severe pain unresponsive to medical treatment, or a large extruded disc fragment. A large, centrally located disc herniation may produce a *cauda equina syndrome*. Symptoms may include bowel or bladder dysfunction, saddle paresthesias, or acute or chronic radiating back pain. Muscle weakness or reflex abnormalities may be noted on physical examination. The presence of cauda equina syndrome warrants urgent medical attention and is an indication for surgical intervention [6].

SPINAL STENOSIS

Lumbar spinal stenosis may be of congenital or acquired origin or a combination of both. A patient with congenitally short pedicles has a shallow spinal canal that predisposes to spinal stenosis. Lumbar stenosis most commonly occurs at the L4-L5 level; next most common is the L3-L4 level. Clinical symptoms of lumber spinal stenosis include the gradual onset of leg and buttock pain combined with lower extremity sensorineural deficits. These symptoms progress over a period of months. Conservative management, including weight loss, physical therapy, nonsteroidal anti-inflammatory drugs, and epidural steroid injections is usually the first step in the management of patients with spinal stenosis. Laminectomy and decompression is indicated when is associated with pain and neurological findings and conservative treatment has failed [7].

SPONDYLOSIS

Lumbar spondylosis consists of nonspecific degenerative changes in the vertebral joint characterized by progressive degeneration of the intervertebral disc, with subsequent changes in the bone and the soft tissue [8]. One theory is that disc dehydration causes a loss of disc height, which is then responsible for bulging of the annulus fibrosus and ligamentum flavum into the spinal canal. Subsequent changes in loading of the facet joints cause arthrosis and osteophyte formation. The clinical spectrum of spondylosis includes spinal instability, spinal stenosis, and degenerative spondylolisthesis. Spinal stenosis is the most common of the spondylitic disorders. Cervical radiculopathy is defined as a neurological condition characterized by dysfunction of a cervical spine nerve, nerve root or both, and is the most common symptom of cervical degenerative disease. It is most commonly caused by lateral disc herniation, with narrowing of the lateral foramen or cervical spine instability cause by subluxation of the cervical vertebrae. Degenerative cervical disc disease is generally treated medically for a period of 4–6 weeks. Surgery is indicated if symptoms persist after 6 weeks of medical treatment.

SCOLIOSIS

Adult scoliosis is defined as any curvature in the spine greater than 10 degrees in a person whose spine is fully developed. Adult scoliosis is divided in two groups: *Idiopathic scoliosis* describes a curve that develops during adolescence but is treated during adulthood. *De novo scoliosis* describes a curve that appears after skeletal maturity. Degenerative disease is the most common cause of de novo scoliosis, although scoliosis may occur after previous spinal surgery or in patients with osteoporosis. Degenerative lumbar scoliosis occurs as part of the normal aging process and may lead to wedging of the vertebral bodies and discs with progressive spinal rotation and translation.

One of the most common indications for spinal surgery in the younger patient is correction of progressive scoliosis. The cause of scoliosis in this population may be either idiopathic or secondary to a disability such as paraplegia. Management depends on the degree of curvature of the spine and whether or not the disease is progressing. Abnormal geometry of the rib cage caused by thoracic scoliosis may produce restrictive pulmonary disease, impairing ventilation [8]. Patients with thoracic scoliosis may also present with arterial hypoxemia that is most likely caused by ventilation/perfusion abnormalities [9, 10]. They may also exhibit significantly decreased ventilatory capacity and reduced exercise tolerance and oxygen consumption despite normal pulmonary function testing at rest. Thoracic scoliosis may cause elevated pulmonary vascular resistance [11]. This condition may lead to pulmonary hypertension, right ventricular hypertrophy and eventually right ventricular failure. Pulmonary function testing should be performed preoperatively in patients with respiratory symptoms or decreased exercise tolerance [6].

Some conditions that are associated with scoliosis also affect the cardiovascular system. The most abnormality seen is mitral valve prolapse. Individuals with Duchenne's muscular dystrophy develop a cardiomyopathy in the second decade of life. The electrocardiogram in these patients may reveal prolonged PR and QRS intervals, ST abnormalities, bundle branch block, Q waves in the left precordial leads, and tall R waves in the right precordial leads. Ejection fraction may be decreased. Patients with Marfan's syndrome may have mitral and aortic insufficiency, aneurysm of the proximal ascending aorta, and abnormalities of the conduction system [7].

Most patients whose symptoms are limited to back pain are treated conservatively, most commonly with braces and exercise. Indications for surgical intervention include persistent pain not controlled with medical therapy, progressive neurological symptoms, worsening of respiratory function and postural imbalance. The goal of surgery is stabilization of the spine or correction of the deformity.

When correction is attempted, traction on the spinal cord during distraction of the vertebral bodies may cause neurological dysfunction thought to be caused by spinal cord ischemia. Intraoperative neurological monitoring with motor evoked potentials (MEPs) and somatosensory evoked potentials (SSEPs) of the spinal cord and of the effect of distraction is recommended. Management of the patient undergoing neurophysiological monitoring and its anesthetic implications are discussed in greater detail in Chapter 4. Other complications associated with this operation are large blood loss caused by exposure required for the surgery and post-operative respiratory complication.

TRAUMA

The most common causes of spine trauma are motor vehicle accidents, falls, violence, and sport-vehicle injuries. Spinal injuries tend to occur most commonly the more mobile areas of the spine, which includes the cervical spine and the thoracolumbar junction, with as many as one fifth of the injuries occurring at multiple levels. Damage to the spinal column may occur without injury to the cord or it can cause spinal cord injury (SCI) through various mechanisms, including compression, hemorrhage, and vasospasm, all of which result in cord ischemia and infarction. The nature of the bony injury is important, as it will guide further management of the patient irrespective of the SCI. The purpose of the spinal column is to provide support while protecting the spinal cord and nerve roots. An unstable injury puts the spinal cord at risk, and may require urgent surgical intervention to provide stability.

SCI frequently occurs in conjunction with other injuries. Cervical spine trauma is associated with blunt cerebrovascular injury, TBI, and facial fractures. Thoracic trauma is also associated with vascular injury in addition, one must consider the possibility of pneumothorax, myocardial contusion, pulmonary contusion. Lumbar spine fractures may be associated with bowel and solid viscous injury.

Surgical intervention for traumatic injury of the spine typically includes removal of foreign bodies, decompression of the spinal cord, stabilization of the bony spine to minimize further injury to the surrounding structures, particularly the spinal cord. Of primary concern, particularly in the preoperative period, is the prevention of further injury until surgical stability can be obtained. This concern particularly applies to the cases of cervical instability.

After initial resuscitation and evaluation, a detailed neurological evaluation is performed to detect the presence of neurological deficits. Traumatic injury of the spinal cord may result in systemic vasomotor and respiratory compromise. SCI is analogous to traumatic brain injury (TBI) in that there is both a primary and a secondary component. The initial injury typically involves damage to the bones and ligament s of the spinal column. Secondary injury to the spinal cord is mediated through a cascade of deleterious events similar to that seen in TBI, including induction of nitric oxide synthase, release of excitotoxic amino acids, cellular influx of calcium, oxidative stress, and lipid peroxidation. Secondary injury may be exacerbated by hypotension due to hemorrhage or neurogenic shock. Although SCI can occur without radiographic abnormalities, this phenomenon is more common in children than adults.

SPINAL CORD PROTECTION

Minimizing the extent of SCI is one of the most important aspects of patient management following any injury to the spinal cord. Early institution of pharmacological therapy combined with surgical decompression and stabilization of the spine improve the chances of a good neurological outcome. Mechanical compression that decreases blood supply to the cord leads to gradual, intermittent microinfarction. It is therefore important to pay close attention to

the maintenance of adequate blood pressure during surgery. This begins with invasive blood pressure monitoring using an intraarterial catheter so that transient reductions in perfusion can be identified and treated. The blood pressure should be maintained at or slightly above the patient's baseline [12]. Hypotension can be prevented with proper volume resuscitation, and in some cases pressors such as dopamine or phenylephrine will be necessary.

Unfortunately, studies of pharmacological therapy have yet been shown to significantly reduce spinal cord damage following traumatic injury [11]. Corticosteroid therapy and hypothermia remain an option but are not considered standard therapy. Administration of high-dose steroids for acute trauma or in patients with severe cervical myelopathy is controversial. Administration of high-dose steroids may result in delayed wound healing, hyperglycemia, gastrointestinal hemorrhage, sepsis, and infection. As a result, there is substantial variation in the application of an SCI protocol [13].

Hypertension has been suggested as a means to improve perfusion in the post-traumatic patient in whom the cord may be hypoperfused. One of the pathophysiological causes of chronic SCI in spondylitic myelopathy relates to poor neural perfusion. Although definitive data are lacking, early and aggressive intervention to maintain a mean arterial blood pressure above 85 mmHg for the first seven days after injury is recommended because autoregulation is impaired [14].

PREOPERATIVE EVALUATION AND PREPARATION

Patients presenting for surgery of the spine have a high incidence of cardiac, pulmonary and rheumatological disease. The preoperative evaluation should concentrate on the patient's neurological status as well as other comorbidities. Patients presenting for spine surgery may have significant pulmonary disease related to the specific spine abnormalities or to other risk factors like obesity, smoking, asthma, or COPD. Moreover, patients undergoing a thoracic spine procedure may have impaired pulmonary function in the postoperative period. Patients with scoliosis may have a significant component of restrictive lung disease. A chest radiograph and pulmonary function tests are therefore indicated for any patient undergoing thoracotomy for spine. Pulmonary function should be optimized prior to surgical correction of scoliosis. Documentation of the patient's baseline blood pressure will help to ensure that intraoperative blood pressure is maintained at a level sufficient to perfuse the spinal cord.

Patients may have neurological symptoms such as peripheral neuropathy or paraplegia that indicate spinal instability. Moreover, patients with history of rheumatoid arthritis may have poor jaw and neck mobility combined with cervical spine instability. A brief neurological evaluation of patients will uncover deficits that exist before the surgery. If the patient has evidence of cervical spine instability, the anesthesiologist should determine whether the patient can flex or extend the neck without symptoms. This maneuver, which should be part of the airway evaluation, may help to determine whether awake intubation with a fiberoptic bronchoscope is necessary. Imaging studies should also be reviewed as part of the routine preoperative evaluation.

The surgeon and the anesthesiologist should formulate a comprehensive anesthetic plan well in advance of the planned procedure. This plan should address the need for intraoperative neurophysiological monitoring and or invasive hemodynamic monitoring, patient positioning, fluid requirements and timing of extubation. A detailed explanation to the patient should include the risks of anesthesia and surgery, including intraoperative awareness (if neurophysiological monitoring is anticipated) and postoperative vision loss (if the procedure is planned in the prone position). Patients in whom an awake intubation may be indicated should be made aware of this possibility in order to ensure that they can understand and tolerate the procedure.

POSITIONING

Patients undergoing spine surgery may be placed in the supine, prone, or lateral decubitus position depending on the location of the surgical site. When the patient will be in any position other than supine, general anesthesia is induced and the airway is secured while the patient is in the supine position. The endotracheal tube must be secured to prevent dislodgment during positioning, and appropriate rescue devices (*e.g.*, laryngeal mask airways) should be immediately available in case the airway is lost. Whenever possible, intravascular access should obtained before the patient is positioned. The patient can then turned into the operating position while keeping the neck in line with the spine during the move. The anesthesiologist is ultimately responsible for coordinating the move and for positioning of the head, with the exception of patients with cervical instability, for whom neurosurgeon is responsible for the applying the headholder and positioning the neck. The position of the endotracheal tube is verified and the ability to ventilate the patient is reassessed immediately after positioning. Physiological monitors should be reconnected as soon as possible after positioning. In patients with severe myelopathy, the surgeon may wish to record baseline electrophysiological data before positioning the patient.

The prone position is used primarily for surgical access to the posterior fossa of the skull or the posterior spine. If the legs are at the level of the heart, hemodynamic reserve is maintained. Pulmonary function may be superior to the supine or lateral decubitus positions if there is no significant abdominal pressure and the patient is properly positioned.

The head may be supported face down with its weight borne by the bony structures or turned to the side. The patient's head should be kept in a neutral position using a surgical pillow, horseshoe headrest, Mayfield head pins, or other positioning device. Commercially available surgical pillows help to support the forehead, malar regions and the chin, and are usually designed to include a cutout for the eyes, nose and mouth.

The horseshoe head holder supports the forehead and the malar regions, gives excellent access to the airway but is more rigid and can cause ocular injury if the head moves. The Mayfield head pins support the head without any direct pressure to the face, may allow access to the airway, and keep the head firmly in one position. This device is primarily used for procedures involving the cervical spine. The neck is typically placed in a slightly flexed or neutral position in patients with spondylotic myelopathy or slightly extended for patients with atlantoaxial subluxation so as to maximize the diameter of the spinal canal.

Depending on the location of the surgery, the arms may be positioned at the patient's side and tucked in neutral position or abducted and placed on arm boards. Abduction should be limited to less than 90 degrees at the level of the shoulders and elbows to prevent excessive stretching of the brachial plexus. The elbows should be padded to avoid compression of the ulnar nerve, while padding under the axillary area helps to avoid compression injuries caused by a Wilson frame or Jackson. The legs should be padded and flexed slightly at the knees and hips. Venous compression devices should be applied to the lower extremities to minimize the risk of thromboembolism.

Regardless of the technique used to support the patient's the head, the eyes, face and airway should be checked at regular and frequent intervals. The patient's weight should be evenly distributed and supported by bony structures. There should be no pressure on the face, eyes, breasts, or genitals. The patient's position should be recorded in the anesthetic record, along with periodic checks. A plan should be established for rapid transition to the supine position if airway or cardiopulmonary complications occur.

The lateral position is used for lateral approaches to the cervical spine, anterior approaches to the upper thoracic spine and retroperitoneal approaches to the thoracolumbar junction and lumbar spine. In the lateral position, particular care must be directed to the position of the dependent arm to prevent brachial plexus injury and vascular compression; the use of an axillary roll is recommended for must procedures in the lateral position. The non-dependent arm is usually outstretched in front of the patient and should be supported on a pillow or padded armrest. The head should be supported in a neutral position to avoid extension or flexion of the cervical spine and endotracheal tube obstruction. It should be supported with a pillow or padded headrest. As in the supine position eyes should be free of pressure.

ANESTHETIC MANAGEMENT

INDUCTION

Induction of general anesthesia in patients with cervical spine injury requires careful planning. During induction of general anesthesia, spinal cord has not yet been mechanically decompressed, the neck musculature is unable to provide protective stabilization, hemodynamic variations may occur, and it is impossible to assess the patient's neurological status. Movement of the neck during airway management can cause compression of the spinal cord. In patients with subaxial spondylotic myelopathy, neck extension may cause narrowing of the spinal canal. Patients with rheumatoid arthritis or Down's syndrome may have atlantoaxial subluxation, and flexion of the neck may increase the atlantodental interval, narrowing the spinal canal.

If a patient with SCI did not require endotracheal intubation in the ER, definitive airway management will be required in the operating room. If the patient's cervical spine has been radiographically and clinically cleared prior to arrival, then the technique for induction of anesthesia and intubation should be determined by the patient's other co-morbidities, injuries and airway examination.

A rapid sequence induction with inline stabilization may be necessary in an uncooperative patient. Ideally, three people are necessary for this technique. One person manually stabilizes the patient's head positioning one hand on each side of the skull to hold the neck and head in neutral position. Another administers sedatives, muscle relaxants and applies cricoid pressure so that the third person can ventilate the patient during induction (if a rapid-sequence induction is not being performed) and perform direct laryngoscopy and intubation. Although it is commonly used in the emergency room, there is a slight risk of exacerbating the spine injury if the external immobilization is not performed properly. Moreover, axial stabilization implies that the head and neck are not in an ideal position for visualization of the vocal cords, and intubation may be difficult. For these reasons, a backup visualization technique such as a Glidescope should be immediately available or the anesthesiologist should be prepared to awaken the patient if the airway cannot be secured.

The most conservative airway management technique is an awake fiberoptic endotracheal intubation. This technique requires thorough administration of sprays and topical anesthesia with lidocaine to the nose, pharynx, larynx and proximal trachea. This is accomplished under light sedation with the patient spontaneously breathing. When properly performed there is minimal risk of neck motion and the patient remains responsive enough to allow assessment of neurological function after intubation.

MONITORING

Monitoring for spine surgery should include ASA standard monitors (noninvasive blood pressure, electrocardiogram, pulse oximetry, end-tidal CO_2, and core temperature). Complex spine and trauma surgery carries a risk of significant blood loss. A radial artery catheter is therefore essential for continuous monitoring of blood pressure and the ability to draw frequent sample for arterial blood gas analysis and measurement of hemoglobin concentration. The respiratory variation on arterial blood pressure (inspiratory increase in arterial blood pressure followed by a decrease on expiration) during mechanical ventilation (Pulse Pressure Variation, PPV) is not an indicator of blood volume but a predictor of fluid responsiveness [15]. In the operating room a goal-directed fluid therapy based on PPV monitoring has the potential to improved the outcome of patients undergoing high-risk surgery [16]. At least two large bore intravenous catheters should be inserted to facilitate fluid and blood product administration if extensive bleeding is anticipated. All patients undergoing extensive spine procedures should have a urinary catheter to measure urine output during and after the surgical procedure. Central venous pressure monitoring may be indicated if expected blood loss is large or if the patient has history of cardiovascular disease. A pulmonary artery catheter may be useful in patients with cardiomyopathy from Duchenne's muscular dystrophy or in the patient with pulmonary hypertension and right ventricular failure [6].

Intraoperative neurophysiological monitoring (IONM) is commonly used to minimize the risk of SCI in during many neurosurgical procedures. The use of IONM has substantially decreased the rate of paralysis after surgery for spinal deformity, and its use has been validated in cervical spinal surgery, and thoracic and lumbar laminectomy. The monitoring techniques most commonly used in the operating room include SSEPs, MEPs, and electromyography (EMG). Each technique examines a functionally separate area of the spinal cord, so the test that is chosen depends on the location of the surgery and the patient's preexisting injuries and deficits.

SSEPs are used to assess the functional integrity of the sensory pathways, which are comprised of the posterior columns of the spinal cord. This technique involves applying repeated electrical stimuli to a peripheral nerve while measuring the evoked response over the subcortical regions or the cerebral cortex and. As these evoked potentials are of very low amplitude, a computer averages the response to each stimulus in order to distinguish signals from background noise and the patients EEG. The time interval between the peripheral nerve stimulation and the recording of the evoked response in the cortex is defined as *latency*, while the size of the response is called the *amplitude*. In general, an increase in latency of 10% to 15% or more or a decrease in amplitude of 50% or more should be cause of concern. Increased latency (slower conduction), decreased amplitude, or a complete loss of the evoked potential indicates surgical injury or ischemia until proven otherwise.

MEPs assess the integrity of the spinal motor pathways (anterior columns). MEPs are elicited by transosseous electrical stimulation of the motor cortex using scalp electrodes. Conduction of these stimuli through the motor pathways is monitored as peripheral nerve impulses, electromyographic signals, or actual limb movements. Any response is considered to be positive, *i.e.*, it is characterized as "all or none." MEPs are considered to be the gold standard for monitoring the motor pathways. Injury to the central nervous system can occur at multiple levels and may involve multiple pathways. Because different arterial supplies serve the motor and sensory pathways, it is possible to injure to the motor tracts despite recording adequate signals if SSEPs alone are used, but it is unusual for the motor tracts to be significantly injured when SSEPs remain unchanged. To access central nervous system integrity more completely, both SSEPs and MEPs are monitored together [17].

The correct anesthetic technique is critical for successful intraoperative recording of cortical SSEPs or myogenic MEPs. The anesthetic technique is chosen to minimize effects on intraoperative neurophysiological monitoring. Potent volatile anesthetics produce a dose-dependent increase in latency and decrease in amplitude of cortically recorded SSEPs. MEPs recorded in muscle (myogenic) are severely attenuated or abolished by potent volatile anesthetics. There is no ideal anesthetic regimen for patients undergoing surgery with intraoperative monitoring. The management of the patient's physiological milieu is also important because central nervous system blood flow, temperature, and arterial carbon dioxide tension produce alterations in the responses consistent with neural functioning. Last, the management of pharmacological neuromuscular blockade is critical to myogenic MEP recording in which some muscle relaxation may be desirable for surgery but excessive blockade may eliminate responses. A close working relationship between the neuromonitoring team, anesthesiologist and surgeon is key to ensure successful monitoring and interpretation on IONM as well as patient safety during and after surgery [12, 18].

FLUID MANAGEMENT

Fluid management in the patient undergoing spinal surgery requires a balance between maintaining vascular volume to ensure an adequate blood pressure while avoiding venous congestion, which may be caused by fluid overload. The nature of the surgery to be performed influences the approach to fluid replacement. Surgery involving extensive surgery of the spine with denudement of the bone, such as scoliosis repair and extensive spinal fusion, may be associated with significant blood loss [19]. Patients undergoing such procedures typically receive large amounts of crystalloids and colloid plasma expanders in addition to blood products. This may result in admission to the intensive care unit. Patients who have received large amounts of fluids or blood products may have a significant amount of tissue edema, including airway edema. It is important to avoid glucose-containing solutions in patients undergoing spine surgery because hyperglycemia may exacerbate neurological injury [20]. The safety of postoperative extubation should be considered before the endotracheal tube is removed.

When appropriate, use of autologous blood and hemodilution may be used to minimize the need for banked blood should be considered. Autologous blood may be through preoperative donation, acute intraoperative removal with isovolemic hemodilution, or using blood salvage techniques. The only contraindication on autologous blood donors is the presence of bacteremia or tumor cell contamination. Intraoperative blood salvage may also reduce the need of homologous transfusion.

Acute normovolemic hemodilution (ANH) involves collection of whole blood from a patient. Surgery is then performed with a reduced red blood cell mass but a normal vascular volume immediately before surgery and replacement with crystalloid or colloid to maintain euvolemia. The blood is stored in the operating room at ambient temperature in a bag containing an anticoagulant until is re-infused if transfusion is indicated or after the majority of the blood loss has occurred. The goal of ANH is to reduce the hematocrit to 30% prior the beginning of surgery. This technique is well tolerated in most patients because the reduced oxygen-carrying capacity of blood is compensated for by an increase in cardiac output and enhanced venous return caused by a reduction in viscosity. Before using ANH, the anesthesiologist should consider the patient's underlying medical condition before the technique is implemented. Patients should have a hemoglobin concentration greater than 12gm/dl, and should not have significant coronary, pulmonary, renal or liver disease; severe hypertension; or infection and the risk of bacteremia.

POSTOPERATIVE CARE

EXTUBATION

The majority of patients can be extubated in the operating room if criteria for extubation have been met. Some patients may require postoperative intubation if ventilation is impaired due to high cervical or thoracic lesions, preoperative pulmonary impairment, metabolic derangement, or persistent muscle weakness. If the surgery was prolonged (i.e., length greater than 6 hours) or if the patient has significant facial edema, it may be safer to leave the patient intubated. Raising the head of the bed at least 45 degrees for several hours prior to extubation will allow the edema

POSTOPERATIVE PAIN CONTROL

Effective pain management facilitates early mobility, reduces postoperative pulmonary complications, may shorten length of stay in the hospital, and enhances patient satisfaction. In general, cervical spine surgery is associated with the least amount of postoperative pain, whereas spinal fusion and instrumentation procedures involving the thoracic and lumbar spine are associated with the most significant postoperative pain. Many patients with chronic back pain have been treated with opioids, and have developed tolerance. These patients may require several modalities, including intravenous or intrathecal medication as well as regional blockade and adjuvant medications. A comprehensive pain management strategy includes intermittent intramuscular and intravenous opioids used, continuous intravenous infusions of opioids, patient controlled analgesia (PCA), intrathecal opioids, intercostal blocks, paravertebral blocks, and continuous local anesthetic infusion via local placed catheters.

COMPLICATIONS

POSTOPERATIVE VISUAL LOSS

Postoperative vision loss (POVL) is rare but devastating complication of spine surgery that may result in permanent visual loss. Most of the cases of POVL involve ischemic optic neuropathy (ION) (89%), other causes include central retinal artery occlusion and ischemic lesion of the cerebral cortex. The incidence is less than 1:1000 and the pathophysiology of ischemic optic neuropathy is poorly understood. It is notable that ION almost always occurs without any accompanying evidence of vascular injury in other critical organs like the heart or the brain. This is true even in patients with preexisting coronary atherosclerosis, diabetes, or hypertension. This observation suggests that the optic nerve vasculature may be uniquely vulnerable to hemodynamic perturbations in the prone position in some patients.

More than two thirds of the cases of the ASA POVL Registry were related to spine surgery in the prone position. Most of the affected patients were relatively healthy and the lowest hematocrits and blood pressures varies widely; this may reflect a multifactorial etiology [12]. Risk factors associated with ION after spinal fusion are: obesity, male sex, use of Wilson frame, longer anesthetic duration, greater estimated blood loss and decrease percent colloid administration [25]. For patients undergoing lengthy spine surgery in the prone position, the risk of visual loss should be included while discussing perioperative risks with the patient [21]. The quality of evidence for preventive measures for postoperative ION after spinal surgery is very low, but it has been proposed that efforts aimed at reducing the duration or severity of venous congestion in the head may be beneficial [22–25].

RECURRENT LARYNGEAL NERVE INJURY

Neuropraxia of the recurrent laryngeal nerve is the most common complication after anterior cervical spine surgery. Although direct injury can occur at the time of the neck dissection, the nerve itself is rarely seen during the procedure. The precise cause of this complication remains unclear. Endotracheal balloon insufflation pressure and surgical retraction placement can be causative, and this phenomenon has been observed anatomically in cadaveric investigations. In one clinical study, releasing the air from the endotracheal cuff and reinflating after retractor blade placement decreased the rate of temporary vocal cord paralysis from 6.4% to 1.69% [26].

REFERENCES

1. Parsa AT, Miller JI. Neurological diseases of the spine and cord: surgical considerations. In Cottrell JE, Smith DS, eds. Anesthesia and Neurosurgery. 4th ed 4. St Louis, MO: Mosby; 2001:531–555.
2. Moore KL, Dalley AF II. Clinically Oriented Anatomy. Philadelphia, PA: Lippincott Williams & Wilkins; 2006:477–531.
3. Stier GR, Gabriel CL, Cole DJ. Neurosurgical diseases and trauma of the spine and the spinal cord: anesthetic considerations. In Cottrell JE, Young WL, eds. Neuroanesthesia. 5th ed. Philadelphia, PA: Mosby; 2010:343–389.
4. Kincaid MS, Lam MA. Anesthesia for neurosurgery. In Barash PG, Cullen BF, Stoelting RK, et al, eds. Clinical Anesthesia. 6th ed. Philadelphia, PA: Lippincott Williams & Wilkins; 2009:1005–1031.
5. Miller RD. Miller's Anesthesia. 7th ed. New York, NY: Churchill Livingston Elsevier; 2010:1160–1162
6. Kafer ER. Respiratory and cardiovascular functions in scoliosis and the principles of anesthetic management. *Anesthesiology.* 1980;32:339–351.
7. Weber W, Smith JP, Bricoe WA, et al. Pulmonary function in asymptomatic adolescents with idiopathic scoliosis. *Am Rev Respir Dis.* 1975; 111:389–397.
8. Bradford DS, LonsteinJE, Ogilvie JW, et al. Moe's Textbook of Scoliosis and Other Spinal Deformities. Philadelphia, PA: WB Saunders; 1987:41–45.
9. Barois A. Respiratory problems in severe scoliosis. *Bull Acad Natl Med.* 1999;183:721–730.
10. Ascani E, Bartolozzi P, Logroscino CA, et al. Natural history of untreated idiopathic scoliosis after skeletal maturity. *Spine.* 1986;11:784–789.
11. Sayer FT, Kronvall E, Nilson OG. Methylprednisolone treatment in acute spinal cord injury: the myth challenged through a structure analysis of published literature. *Spine J.* 2006;6:335–343.
12. Wang MY, Green BA. Operative nuances: open-door cervical expansile laminoplasty. *Neurosurgery.* 2004;54:119–124.
13. Kim KA, Wang MY. Anesthetic considerations in the treatment of cervical myelopathy. *Spine J.* 2006;6:207S–211S.
14. Hadley MN. Management of acute central cervical spine cord injuries, *Neurosurgery.* 2002;50(Suppl):S166–S172.
15. Michard F. Changes in Arterial Pressure During Mechanical Ventilation. Anesthesiology 2005;103:419–428.

16. Michard F, Lopes MR, Auler JO. Pulse Pressure Variation: Beyond the Fluid Management of Patients with Shock. *Critical Care* 2007;11:131–133.
17. Nuwer MR, Dawson EG, Carlson LG, et al. Somatosensory evoked potential spinal cord monitoring reduces neurologic deficits after scoliosis surgery. Results of large multicenter survey. *Electroencephalogr Clin Neurophysiol*. 1995;96:6–11.
18. Sloan TB, Heyer EJ. Anesthesia for intraoperative neurophysiologic monitoring of the spinal cord. *J Clin Neurophysiol*. 2002;19:430–443.
19. Nahtomi-Schick O, Kostvik JP, Winter BD, et al. Does intraoperative fluid management in spine surgery predict intensive care unit length of stay? *J Clin Anesth*. 2001;13:208–212.
20. Drummond J, Moore S. The influence of dextrose administration on neurologic outcome after temporary spinal cord ischemia in the rabbit. *Anesthesiology*. 1989;70:64–70.
21. Diener S. Highlights of anesthetic considerations for intraoperative monitoring, *Semin Cardiothorac Vasc Anesth*. 2010;14:51–53.
22. Lee LA, Roth S, et al. The American Society of Anesthesiology, postoperative visual loss registry. *Anesthesiology*. 2006;105:652–659.
23. Lee LA, Newman NJ, Wagner TA, et al. Postoperative ischemic optic neuropathy. *Spine (Phila Pa 1976)*. 2010;35:S105–S116.
24. Warner MA, Arens JF, Connis RT, Domino KB, Lee LA, Miller N, et al. Practice Advisory for Perioperative Visual Loss Associated with Spine Surgery: A report of the American Society of Anesthesiology Task Force on Perioperative Blindness. *Anesthesiology*. 2006;104:1319–1328.
25. Lee LA, Roth S, Todd MM, Posner KL, Polissar KL, Neradilek MB, Newman NJ, et al. (Postoperative Vision Group Loss) Risk factors associated with ischemic optic neuropathy after spinal fusion surgery. *Anesthesiology*. 2012;116(1)15–24.
26. Apfelbaum RI, Kriskovich MD, Haller JR. On the incidence, cause, and prevention of recurrent laryngeal nerve palsies during anterior cervical spine surgery. *Spine*. 2000;25:2906–2912.

21.

INTERVENTIONAL NEUROVASCULAR SURGERY

Ketan R. Bulsara and Keith J. Ruskin

INTRODUCTION

Interventional neurovascular surgery involves treatment of both hemorrhagic and ischemic stroke. Within the last decade, neurovascular surgery has undergone transformational changes. Recent developments in both microsurgery and endovascular treatment for neurovascular pathologies have improved outcomes by individualizing treatment decisions to the patient's clinical condition and comorbidities. It has never been more important to have a multidisciplinary team to address complex neurovascular pathologies, and optimal patient care requires collaboration between the anesthesiologist and the neurointerventional surgeon.

Although the specific technique used will vary with the vascular pathology, interventional neurovascular procedures generally begin with gaining access the femoral artery. Subsequently, through a series of catheters, a microcatheter is advanced into the target lesion for treatment. The specifics of each treatment are detailed here, but two overriding factors are that patient immobility and hemodynamic stability are critical to the success of the procedure. The lesions are often very small, and even a small movement on the part of the patient can result in disastrous consequences. In addition, the anesthesiologist may be required to manage unexpected issues (e.g., hemorrhage or unintentional vascular occlusion) during the course of the procedure. This requires that the anesthesiologist have a fundamental understanding of the pathophysiology of neurovascular disease as well as the interventional procedure.

HEMORRHAGIC STROKE

Cerebral aneurysms and arteriovenous malformations (AVMs), though rare, represent the more common causes of hemorrhagic stroke treated by interventional neurovascular surgeons. These lesions commonly present with seizures, intraparenchymal hemorrhages, or subarachnoid hemorrhage.

ANEURYSMS

Subarachnoid hemorrhage (Figure 21.1) is a life-threatening complication of an intracranial aneurysm that carries a significant morbidity even in patients who survive the initial event. In general, one third of patients who present with a ruptured aneurysm die before reaching the hospital and one third survive initial treatment but leave the hospital with a significant neurologic deficit. Only one third of patients survive the initial event with a good neurologic outcome. The best predictor we have of an aneurysm's risk of rupture is size. Both the International Study of Unruptured Aneurysms and the Unruptured Intracranial aneurysm study support the finding that aneurysms less than 1 cm in size have a less than 1% annual risk of rupture [1, 2]. This progressively increases with giant aneurysms (>2.5 cm) in the posterior circulation having an annual rupture rate of 10% a year.

A ruptured aneurysm is an unstable lesion with a significant risk of rehemorrhage. The cumulative risk of re-hemorrhage is as high as 26.5% within the first 2 weeks if the ruptured aneurysm is not treated [3]. In the immediate period, blood pressure management is critical in minimizing this. The International Subarachnoid Aneurysm Trial (ISAT) revealed decreased morbidity and mortality in patients who underwent endovascular treatment compared with microsurgical treatment. The long-term follow-up of these patients with a mean of 6 years still supported this advantage [4, 5]. These findings were reconfirmed in the Barrow Ruptured Aneurysm Trial [6]. The endovascular treated group had an extremely low but higher rate of re-rupture compared with the microsurgical group in the ISAT group [5]. Endovascular treatment of aneurysms has emerged as the first line treatment for ruptured aneurysms. The data on unruptured aneurysms are not as clearcut; however, the International Study of Unruptured Intracranial Aneurysms (ISUIA) prospectively evaluated 1692 patients who underwent microsurgical clipping or endovascular treatment of their aneurysms. The results of the prospective

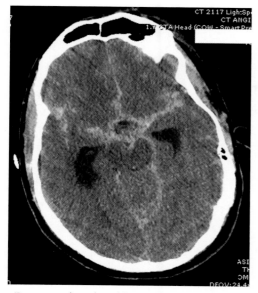

Figure 21.1 Extensive subarachnoid hemorrhage and hydrocephalus as manifested by increased size of temporal horns of the ventricular system.

ISUIA study favor a better outcome associated with coiled aneurysms [4, 5] (Figures 21.2 and 21.3).

A unique feature of subarachnoid hemorrhage is the development of delayed ischemia, also known as vasospasm. For an unclear reason, starting around day 3 after the hemorrhage, blood vessels begin to undergo vasoconstriction. Part of the treatment for this is elevating blood pressure. This phenomenon can persist for up to 21 days. In those patients who have clinical symptoms despite optimizing medical management neurointerventional surgery may be beneficial. This entails either superselective catheterization of intracranial vessels or mechanical angioplasty. These can both result in some decrease in systolic blood pressures: therefore it is essential that the anesthesia team work with the surgical team to ensure that the blood pressure stays within the needed range.

ARTERIOVENOUS MALFORMATIONS

An *AVM* is defined as an abnormal connection between arteries and veins without an intervening capillary network. The risk of hemorrhage annually is 2% to 4%. With a hemorrhage, there is 10% to 30% chance of death and a 30% to 50% change of permanent neurological deficits [7]. Increased rates of rupture have been associated with prior rupture, small lesion size, deep venous drainage, venous stenosis, single venous drainage, and large feeding artery aneurysms [8]. Interventional AVM treatment ranges from attempted cure, reduction of the nidus size in anticipation for radiosurgery or microsurgery, or treatment of high-risk features. There is a wide range of techniques in the embolization of AVMs including polyvinyl alcohol particles, fibers, microcoils, microballoons, cyanoacrylate monomers, ethanol, and ethylene vinyl alcohol [9]. Ethylene vinyl alcohol may have the most durable result (Figure 21.4).

Cyanoacrylate monomers have been associated with decreased obliteration rates, especially with radiosurgery [10].

ISCHEMIC STROKE

The only current FDA-approved treatment for ischemic stroke remains intravenous tPA within a 3-hour window that has now commonly been extended to 4.5 hours [11]. Most patients, however, cannot get to a treatment center before the 4.5-hour mark. It is precisely for this reason that intra-arterial therapy with lytic agents was attempted in the PROACT II trial [12]. This trial showed a trend toward improved recanalization if intra-arterial thrombolytic (prourokinase) was administered within 6 hours of stroke onset. Subsequently, series of mechanical thrombectomy devices have been developed that extend this time window to less than 8 hours after onset in the anterior circulation and 24 hours in the posterior circulation (MERCI, Penumbra, Solitaire, Trevo) (Figure 21.5). The latter two devices fall into the category of stent-retrievers,

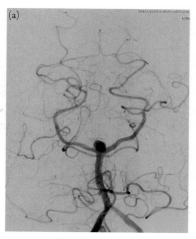
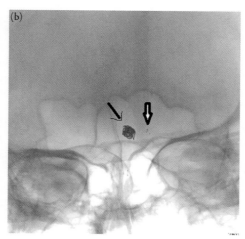
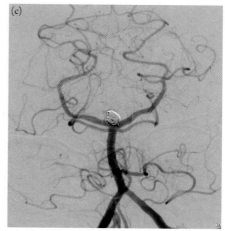

Figure 21.2 (a) Right vertebral angiogram showing complex unruptured basilar apex aneurysm. (b) Skull radiograph showing the distal tynes of the stent (open arrow) and the coil mass (closed arrow). (c) Right vertebral angiogram following stent-assisted coiling of complex unruptured basilar apex aneurysm.

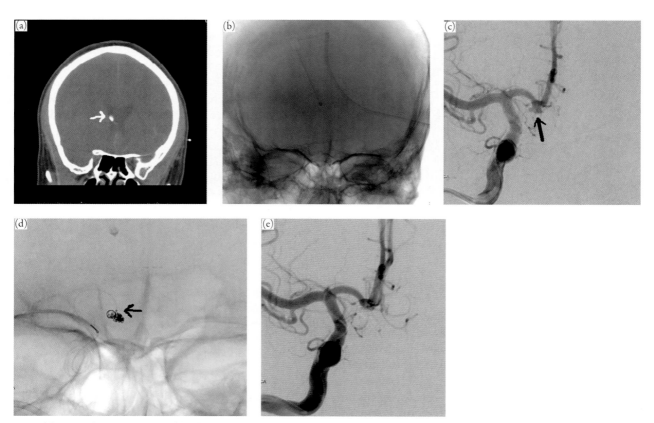

Figure 21.3   (a) Coronal reconstruction of head CT in patient with ventriculostomy following subarachnoid hemorrhage. (b) AP radiograph showing the ventriculostomy. (c) Ruptured 2.9-mm anterior communicating artery aneurysm (arrow). (d) Microcatheter (arrow) in ruptured aneurysm with adjacent coil mass. (e) Status post-coiling of ruptured anterior communicating artery aneurysm.

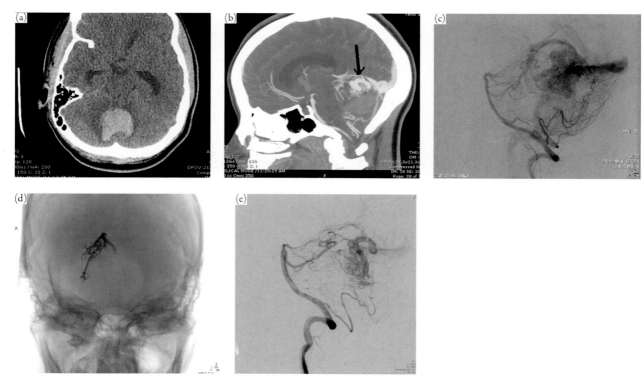

Figure 21.4   (a) Cerebellar hemorrhage. (b) Sagittal CTA showing AVM associated with hemorrhage (arrow). (c) Sagittal digital subtraction angiogram showing the arteriovenous malformation (arrow). (d) Ethylene vinyl alcohol embolization (ONYX) for size reduction. (e) Digital subtraction angiogram after ONYX embolization.

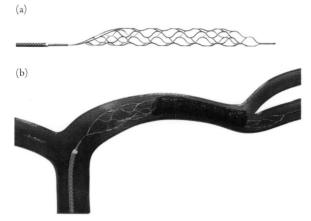

Figure 21.5 (a) Concept of a stent retriever: "stent on a stick." (b) Stent retriever expanding within a clot. Once the clot is attached to the stent retriever, the stent is withdrawn with the clot to recanalize the vessel.

which have demonstrated some of the highest recanalization rates [13, 14].

RADIATION PROTECTION

All personnel working in an interventional procedure suite should be familiar with radiation safety. Two imaging modes are used in the interventional suite: fluoroscopy and digital subtraction angiography (DiSA). DiSA requires a higher dose of radiation than fluoroscopy. When DiSA is being used, the interventional team usually moves away from the patient, and the anesthesiologist should stand well away from the tube and ideally behind a portable shield. There are three sources of radiation: Direct exposure to the X-ray beam that is emitted from the tube, scattered radiation that is reflected from the patient or other objects in the path of the primary beam, and radiation that leaks through the collimator. Three factors determine the radiation dose to which personnel are exposed: time, distance, and shielding. The anesthesiologist is rarely in control of the duration of fluoroscopy; this is dictated by the needs of the proceduralist. The amount of radiation decreases in proportion to the square of the distance from the source, such as doubling the distance from the tube decreases the amount of radiation by a factor of four. The anesthesia team should therefore be located as far away from the tube as is feasible and as permits appropriate patient care. The last element is shielding; all personnel should wear lead aprons that cover both the front and back of their bodies. Thyroid collars should also be worn. A recent study demonstrated that anesthesiologists' eyes receive a high dose of radiation during interventional procedures, so appropriate eye protection should be considered [15]. Dosimeter badges should be worn by personnel who work regularly in the interventional radiology suite to monitor radiation exposure [16].

ANESTHETIC MANAGEMENT

Management of the patient undergoing an interventional neurovascular procedure is a collaborative effort between the anesthesiologist and the treating physician. The anesthesiologist must also be protected from the radiation that will be used during the procedure, and must frequently work in a darkened room. Patients are frequently hemodynamically unstable and may have multiple comorbidities. Complications of the procedure (e.g., intracranial hemorrhage or vascular occlusion) may be rapid and life threatening, leaving only a brief window for effective treatment. Maintenance of patient immobility is a primary concern during these procedures, because sudden movement during a critical phase of the procedure may be cause significant injury. In many cases, the patient should be awake and able to cooperate with a neurologic examination as quickly as possible after surgery.

The anesthesiologist is usually tasked with managing the anticoagulation during the procedure, which involves monitoring activated clotting time (or other laboratory values) and administration of heparin or other drugs. One of the biggest risks during interventional neurovascular treatment is thromboembolic events. Anticoagulation can help decrease this risk, however, in the setting of a ruptured intracranial aneurysm, its use should be weighed carefully prior to at least partial securing of the aneurysm. The decision to initiate anticoagulation for ruptured and unruptured aneurysm is made by the treating physician. It is essential that the anesthesiologist clearly establish these parameters prior to case initiation. If heparin cannot be used (e.g., in a patient with heparin-induced thrombocytopenia), the hematology service should be consulted to determine the best anticoagulation regimen for the procedure. Given patient positioning, it is essential that comfortable access to the patient be established prior to the initiation of the procedure.

Preoperative evaluation involves a discussion of the planned procedure with the surgeon, a history and physical examination with particular attention to neurologic findings, and a review of laboratory and imaging studies. The patient's baseline blood pressure and cardiovascular reserve should be carefully evaluated for several reasons: The limits of autoregulation in an individual patient are dependent upon that specific patient's baseline blood pressure, and autoregulation may be impaired by factors such as subarachnoid hemorrhage. At some point during the procedure, manipulation of the patient's systemic blood pressure will probably be required (e.g., to slow blood flow through an AVM that is being embolized). Moreover, the patient might have received calcium channel blockers to treat vasospasm in the perioperative period. In addition to those monitors specified by the American Society of Anesthesiologists' Standards for Basic Intraoperative Monitoring, an intra-arterial catheter is usually inserted for continuous blood pressure monitoring.

GENERAL ANESTHESIA

Most patients receive general endotracheal anesthesia for complex neurointerventional procedures, especially those of long duration. The advantages of general anesthesia include a secure airway and an immobile patient. In a recent survey of active members of the Society of Vascular and Interventional Neurology, the majority of respondents indicated that they preferred general anesthesia, citing the risk of patient movement as the reason for this choice. The primary disadvantages of general anesthesia were reported to include loss of the neurologic examination, delays, and possible propagation of an ischemic insult due to hypotensive episodes. Nearly half stated that they would like the patient to be extubated at the end of the procedure if possible [17].

Airway management is dictated by the patient's status and preferences of the anesthesiologist. An endotracheal tube offers the advantages of a secure airway and facilitates interventions such as hyperventilation. There is, however, a report of three cases in which a laryngeal mask airway (LMA) was used in lieu of an endotracheal tube during coiling of an unruptured aneurysm [18]. The advantages of a supraglottic airway include minimizing the hemodynamic response to airway management and decreased coughing on emergence from anesthesia. The disadvantages of this technique include limited access to the airway and the potential need to secure the airway with an endotracheal tube should a catastrophic event occur during the procedure. Blood pressure should be monitored carefully while the airway is being secured, and laryngoscopy should be discontinued if the patient becomes hypertensive. In the absence of intracranial hypertension, normocapnia is usually desirable. Patients who are undergoing an interventional neurovascular procedure are most commonly hyperventilated as a treatment for intracranial hypertension after subarachnoid hemorrhage. Although hyperventilation is effective, it decreases intracranial pressure by causing cerebral vasoconstriction, which in turn decreases cerebral perfusion. It is therefore used as a bridge to the definitive management of intracranial hypertension (e.g., insertion of an intraventricular catheter).

No single anesthetic agent has been shown to be superior to any others, so the choice of the anesthetic is dictated by patient characteristics and the preferences of the anesthesiologist. A total intravenous anesthetic like remifentanil, possibly in combination with a low concentration of a potent volatile anesthetic, offers the advantages of a smooth, rapid awakening at the end of the procedure. Many anesthesiologists avoid the use of nitrous oxide because there are reports that it worsens outcome after neurosurgery, but the data remain equivocal [19, 20].

INTRAVENOUS SEDATION

The primary advantage of intravenous sedation and monitored anesthetic care is that this technique allows continuous monitoring of the patient. One recent study suggests that patients who receive general anesthesia for endovascular treatment of acute ischemic stroke are less likely to have a good outcome. The proposed mechanism is hypotension, although this may be due to preintervention risk factors that were not included in the stroke severity measures [21]. The goal of the anesthesiologist is to provide a comfortable patient who is able to cooperate with the procedure and with a neurologic examination. If intravenous sedation is chosen, the drugs used and level of sedation should be carefully chosen so as to minimize the possibility of airway obstruction because it will be difficult to access the patient's airway once the procedure has started. The use of a nasopharyngeal airway should be avoided in patients who have received anticoagulants because of the risk of profuse bleeding. Dexmedetomidine is a potent, highly selective α_2 agonist that is delivered as an intravenous infusion. It has sedative, analgesic, and anxiolytic properties, and it does not depress respiration. The effects of dexmedetomidine on cerebral metabolism remain unclear [22], but one small study in six patients receiving the drug in the neurocritical care unit found a statistical, but not clinically significant, effect on patient hemodynamics [23]. Dexmedetomidine may produce hypotension into the postanesthesia period, so patients receiving the drug should be closely monitored throughout the perioperative period, and the drug should be used in caution in patients who are dependent upon a normal blood pressure to maintain cerebral blood flow.

Patients who have had a neurologic injury and who receive sedation may develop a transient recurrence of a neurologic deficit from which they have previously recovered. Although there is no clear explanation for this phenomenon, the proposed mechanism is that compensatory remodeling occurs in response to the injury [24], and anesthetic agents may temporally disrupt the new connections. This effect has recently been shown to occur with GABAergic, but not anticholinergic, agents [25]. Although no specific recommendations can be made regarding the choice of a sedative, all team members should be aware that previously resolved focal deficits might reappear if GABAergic sedatives (e.g., midazolam, propofol) are used. Use of these agents may complicate intraprocedural neurologic monitoring, especially if a technique such as temporary balloon occlusion is attempted before permanently closing a vessel.

BLOOD PRESSURE

Blood pressure is managed in cooperation with the surgeon so as to maintain adequate end-organ perfusion while providing optimum procedural conditions and minimizing the risk of bleeding. In general, the systemic blood pressure should be kept within 20% of the patient's baseline blood pressure or a value that has previously been agreed upon by the surgeon and anesthesiologist and is dictated by the clinical situation. In patients with hemorrhagic stroke, for example, there is no definitive study on a specific blood pressure that will cause rehemorrhage, however, the consensus is that significant hypotension and systolic blood pressure greater than 160 mm Hg can adversely influence outcomes [26]. Many neurosurgeons generally try to keep the SBP between 100 and 140 mm Hg. In patients with ischemic stroke, however, maintaining relative hypertension (typically 30% to 40% above the patient's baseline) is essential to maintaining perfusion in ischemic brain. An intravenous phenylephrine infusion can be used to induce hypertension. If deliberate hypertension is being induced, the electrocardiogram should be monitored for signs of myocardial ischemia [27]. In patients who have received intravenous tPA, the systolic blood pressure should be kept less than 180 mm Hg to prevent hemorrhage into ischemic brain regions.

Intracranial Pressure

The anesthesiologist is frequently asked to manage ICP during neurointerventional procedures. If a ventriculostomy or other CSF diversion method is being used, the anesthesiologist should be familiar with its function before the start of the procedure. The transducer should be placed at the level of the mastoid process, and the various stopcocks and tubing should be routed so as to be accessible during the procedure. Most CSF drainage systems are designed to automatically close to prevent backflow of nonsterile CSF back into the ventricle; under no circumstances should the drainage system be inverted. In the case of the need for emergency placement of a ventriculostomy, access to the patient's head will be shared, requiring coordination between the anesthesia team and the neurointerventional team.

Anticoagulation

Anticoagulation is almost always used during neurointerventional procedures to minimize the risk of thromboembolic events, but there is no clear consensus on the ideal regimen. Most often, heparin is used and the treating physician determines the PTT or ACT to which therapy should be titrated. The anesthesiologist should readily have available the means to reverse heparin with protamine and furthermore ensure that adequate blood products are readily available. In general, a baseline activated clotting time (ACT) is obtained, after which an initial dose of intravenous heparin (70 units/kg) is administered; heparin is usually titrated to a target prolongation of approximately 2 to 3 times the baseline value. Heparin is then administered either continuously or as an intermittent bolus with hourly monitoring of ACT.

CATASTROPHIC COMPLICATIONS

A well thought-out plan, an understanding of the underlying physiology, and close communication between all team members are essential to a good outcome if a catastrophic complication occurs during the procedure. The primary responsibilities of the anesthesia team are to secure the airway and maintain oxygenation and perfusion. Simultaneously, the interventional team must determine whether the lesion is due to bleeding or to vascular occlusion and clearly communicate this to the anesthesia team because it influences anesthetic management.

In the case of aneurysmal rupture during the procedure, the rapid and effective collaboration between the anesthesiologist and the treating physician can minimize the potential disastrous outcome. If the patient is acutely bleeding, antihypertensives (e.g., labetalol, hydralazine, or a nicardipine infusion) should be used to decrease the blood pressure. The goal is to decrease blood flow through the lesion, with the specific blood pressure selected by the proceduralist and the anesthesiologist to facilitate management of the lesion while maintaining end-organ perfusion. If heparin was administered, it should be reversed with protamine (1 mg for each 100 U of heparin intravenously, usually not to exceed 50 mg). If the patient bleeds, he or she should be presumed to have intracranial hypertension, and steps should be taken to control ICP, including administration of mannitol, diversion of CSF through an intraventricular catheter, and hyperventilation.

If a vascular occlusion has occurred, the goal is to restore perfusion through a combination of induced hypertension and/or thrombolysis. If a decision is made to induce hypertension, the goal is usually to perfuse the ischemic brain through collateral blood vessels. The target blood pressure is generally determined by the anesthesiologists and the proceduralist. It is usually preferable to induce hypertension with a vasopressor (e.g., phenylephrine infusion) rather than reducing the depth of anesthesia.

CONCLUSIONS

Interventional neurovascular surgery has been shown to a safe and effective means of treating intracranial vascular lesions, and may in some cases be associated with a better outcome than intracranial surgery. The best chance of a good neurologic outcome depends upon a multidisciplinary team that includes the anesthesiologist and the neurointerventional surgeon. Patient immobility and hemodynamic stability are important, but ultimately the success of the procedure requires a fundamental understanding of the pathophysiology of neurovascular disease and interventional procedure.

REFERENCES

1. Morita A, Kirino T, Hashi K, et al. The natural course of unruptured cerebral aneurysms in a Japanese cohort. *N Engl J Med.* 2012;366:2474–2482.

2. Wiebers DO, Whisnant JP, Huston J 3rd, et al. Unruptured intracranial aneurysms: natural history, clinical outcome, and risks of surgical and endovascular treatment. *Lancet.* 2003;362:103–110.

3. Kassell NF, Torner JC. Aneurysmal rebleeding: a preliminary report from the Cooperative Aneurysm Study. *Neurosurgery.* 1983;13:479–481.

4. Molyneux A, Kerr R, Stratton I, et al. International Subarachnoid Aneurysm Trial (ISAT) of neurosurgical clipping versus endovascular coiling in 2143 patients with ruptured intracranial aneurysms: a randomised trial. *Lancet.* 2002;360:1267–1274.

5. Molyneux AJ, Kerr RS, Birks J, et al. Risk of recurrent subarachnoid haemorrhage, death, or dependence and standardised mortality ratios after clipping or coiling of an intracranial aneurysm in the International Subarachnoid Aneurysm Trial (ISAT): long-term follow-up. *Lancet Neurol.* 2009;8:427–433.

6. McDougall CG, Spetzler RF, Zabramski JM, et al. The Barrow Ruptured Aneurysm Trial. *J Neurosurg.* 2012;116:135–144.

7. Aoun SG, Bendok BR, Batjer HH. Acute management of ruptured arteriovenous malformations and dural arteriovenous fistulas. *Neurosurg Clin N Am.* 2012;23:87–103.

8. Stapf C, Mast H, Sciacca RR, et al. Predictors of hemorrhage in patients with untreated brain arteriovenous malformation. *Neurology.* 2006;66:1350–1355.

9. Zacharia BE, Vaughan KA, Jacoby A, et al. Management of ruptured brain arteriovenous malformations. *Curr Atheroscler Rep.* 2012;14:335–342.

10. Schwyzer L, Yen CP, Evans A, Zavoian S, Steiner L. Long-term results of gamma knife surgery for partially embolized arteriovenous malformations. *Neurosurgery.* 2012;71:1139–1148.

11. Hacke W, Kaste M, Bluhmki E, et al. Thrombolysis with alteplase 3 to 4.5 hours after acute ischemic stroke. *N Engl J Med.* 2008;359:1317–1329.

12. Furlan A, Higashida R, Wechsler L, et al. Intra-arterial prourokinase for acute ischemic stroke. The PROACT II study: a randomized controlled trial. Prolyse in Acute Cerebral Thromboembolism. *JAMA.* 1999;282:2003–2011.

13. Nogueira RG, Lutsep HL, Gupta R, et al. Trevo versus Merci retrievers for thrombectomy revascularisation of large vessel occlusions in acute ischaemic stroke (TREVO 2): a randomised trial. *Lancet.* 2012;380:1231–1240.

14. Saver JL, Jahan R, Levy EI, et al. Solitaire flow restoration device versus the Merci Retriever in patients with acute ischaemic stroke (SWIFT): a randomised, parallel-group, non-inferiority trial. *Lancet.* 2012;380:1241–1249.

15. Anastasian ZH, Strozyk D, Meyers PM, et al. Radiation exposure of the anesthesiologist in the neurointerventional suite. *Anesthesiology.* 2011;114:512–520.

16. Cousins C, Sharp C. Medical interventional procedures-reducing the radiation risks. *Clin Radiol.* 2004;59:468–473.

17. McDonagh DL, Olson DM, Kalia JS, et al. Anesthesia and sedation practices among neurointerventionalists during acute ischemic stroke endovascular therapy. *Front Neurol.* 2010;1:118.

18. Golshevsky J, Cormack J. Laryngeal mask airway device during coiling of unruptured cerebral aneurysms. *J Clin Neurosci.* 2009;16:104–105.

19. McGregor DG, Lanier WL, Pasternak JJ, et al. Effect of nitrous oxide on neurologic and neuropsychological function after intracranial aneurysm surgery. *Anesthesiology.* 2008;108:568–579.

20. Pasternak JJ, McGregor DG, Lanier WL, et al. Effect of nitrous oxide use on long-term neurologic and neuropsychological outcome in patients who received temporary proximal artery occlusion during cerebral aneurysm clipping surgery. *Anesthesiology.* 2009;110:563–573.

21. Davis MJ, Menon BK, Baghirzada LB, et al. Anesthetic management and outcome in patients during endovascular therapy for acute stroke. *Anesthesiology.* 2012;116:396–405.

22. Prielipp RC, Wall MH, Tobin JR, et al. Dexmedetomidine-induced sedation in volunteers decreases regional and global cerebral blood flow. *Anesth Analg.* 2002;95:1052–1059, table of contents.

23. Grof TM, Bledsoe KA. Evaluating the use of dexmedetomidine in neurocritical care patients. *Neurocrit Care.* 2010;12:356–361.

24. Chollet F, DiPiero V, Wise RJ, et al. The functional anatomy of motor recovery after stroke in humans: a study with positron emission tomography. *Ann Neurol.* 1991;29:63–71.

25. Lazar RM, Berman MF, Festa JR, et al. GABAergic but not anti-cholinergic agents re-induce clinical deficits after stroke. *J Neurol Sci.* 2010;292:72–76.

26. Diringer MN, Bleck TP, Claude Hemphill J 3rd, et al. Critical care management of patients following aneurysmal subarachnoid hemorrhage: recommendations from the Neurocritical Care Society's Multidisciplinary Consensus Conference. *Neurocrit Care.* 2011;15:211–240.

27. Lee CZ, Young WL. Anesthesia for endovascular neurosurgery and interventional neuroradiology. *Anesthesiol Clin.* 2012;30:127–147.

22.

CAROTID ENDARTERECTOMY AND CAROTID ARTERY BYPASS

Colleen M. Moran and Christoph N. Seubert

INTRODUCTION

The goal of carotid endarterectomy and carotid artery bypass is to prevent cerebral ischemia and ultimately strokes. Although neither procedure has changed much in the past 50 years, their prevalence as a treatment for cerebrovascular disease has varied markedly. Carotid endarterectomy (CEA) first gained widespread acceptance in the 1980's when routine carotid artery bypass was found to increase the risk of stroke in patients with symptomatic extracranial cerebrovascular disease [1]. Carotid artery bypass (extracranial/intracranial bypass; EC/IC bypass) has since been reserved for special indications that will be discussed in the last section of this chapter. Subsequent studies raised concerns with perioperative stroke rates of CEA, and ultimately two landmark studies at the turn of the century defined indications for CEA in symptomatic [2, 3] and asymptomatic patients [4] with significant carotid artery stenosis. CEA provides a durable mild reduction in stroke risk in both patient groups, provided perioperative morbidity is sufficiently low (Table 22.1). These changes in use of CEA and EC/IC bypass parallel our growing understanding of the pathophysiology of stroke, emphasizing the importance of plaque biology and embolic material over simple global or regional misery perfusion. Misery perfusion is defined as a state where cerebral blood flow is insufficient to match cerebral metabolic demand. Such a mismatch may be evident by a neurologic deficit at rest or may become evident only during tasks that increase metabolic requirements. Prolonged misery perfusion can result in a permanent neurologic deficit.

In recent years, carotid stenting in the interventional radiology suite has challenged the role of CEA. Early experience with carotid stents has shown that perioperative morbidity may be less than that of CEA, but that the risk of perioperative stroke remains higher than that of CEA [5]. Today many questions about the role of carotid artery stenting cannot yet be answered definitively [6, 7], but

new developments, including novel delivery systems, distal embolic protection, and proximal embolic protection [8], suggest that stenting may find a place in the treatment of cerebrovascular occlusive disease in the future.

SURGICAL CONSIDERATIONS

Surgical considerations for CEA center on the different phases of the operation and include brief interruption of blood flow through the blood vessel, the possibility of embolization, and hemodynamic changes in a patient with atherosclerotic disease (Figure 22.1). Exposure of the carotid artery requires manipulation of an atherosclerotic vessel with the attendant risk of dislodging embolic material from the carotid plaque. The endarterectomy itself requires the obligatory interruption of cerebral inflow on the operative side, even if only for the time it takes to place a shunt, which places the patient at risk for cerebral hypoperfusion. Reperfusion poses the risk of an embolic event. The newly increased blood flow may lead to normal perfusion pressure breakthrough. This occurs in vascular territories in which autoregulation has become impaired because of chronic hypoperfusion through a tight carotid stenosis. Finally, in the short term, CEA exchanges the thrombogenic situation of an ulcerated plaque with the thrombogenic situation of an exposed media layer of the vessel to which the endarterectomy is carried down. The transition areas to normal endothelial lining at the proximal and distal ends of the endarterectomy site are also possible sites for thrombogenesis and subsequent cerebral emboli.

MANIPULATION OF AN ATHEROSCLEROTIC VESSEL

Features of the carotid atherosclerotic plaque itself may cause atheroembolic material to break off and cause transient

Table 22.1 INDICATIONS AND "ACCEPTABLE" COMPLICATION RATES FOR CEA

PATIENT STATUS	DEGREE OF STENOSIS	PERIOPERATIVE COMPLICATIONS
Symptomatic	≥50–70%	<6%
Asymptomatic	≥60%	<3%

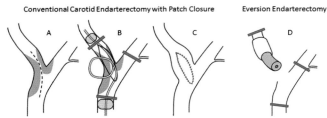

Conventional Carotid Endarterectomy with Patch Closure   Eversion Endarterectomy

Figure 22.1   Technique of carotid endarterectomy. The three panels on the left show the most frequent technique for carotid endarterectomy (A) The carotid is freed from surrounding tissue. The arterotomy is indicated by a dashed line (B) Cross clamps are applied in sequence to internal, common, and external carotid arteries. A shunt placed beyond the clamps can provide blood supply to the brain during the endarterectomy. (C) The arterotomy is closed with a patch, widening the bifurcation and decreasing turbulence to blood flow after unclamping (D) An alternative approach to the endarterectomy is the eversion of the internal carotid artery after transsection at the bifurcation. In this case closure of the arterotomy is by a circumferential suture line.

ischemic attacks or strokes. Plaque features such as intima/media thickness, erosion/ulceration, and thrombus or hemorrhage indicate a fragile plaque [9]. Anticoagulation and lipid-lowering therapy are complementary therapeutic approaches to decrease the risk of emboli, and thus are the cornerstone of medical therapy of cerebrovascular occlusive disease.

Antiplatelet agents such as aspirin and clopidogrel are the most common drugs used to inhibit thrombosis. CEA under dual antiplatelet therapy has been performed without an increased incidence of hemorrhagic complications [10]. Discontinuing anti-platelet medication in the perioperative period nearly doubles perioperative stroke risk [11], so at least one of these agents should be continued throughout the perioperative period [12]. Before clamping the carotid artery, an intravenous dose of heparin is typically administered to further decrease clot formation.

Lipid-lowering therapy with statins may cause regression of carotid artery stenosis (as measured by intima/media thickness) that is proportional to its effect on low-density lipoprotein cholesterol [13]. In addition to reducing lipid content in atheroma, statins also have anti-inflammatory properties that induce histologic changes in carotid plaque consistent with improved plaque stability [14].

Dissection of the carotid artery should be done gently to minimize mechanical disruption of the carotid plaque and dislodgement of emboli. Monitoring blood flow in the ipsilateral middle cerebral artery with transcranial Doppler,

discussed in greater detail below, can provide auditory warning of embolic events associated with manipulation of the vessel. Emboli stand out against the background sound of the Doppler signal as "high intensity transient" sounds ("HITs") also described as chirps.

CAROTID OCCLUSION

CEA involves dissection of plaque from within the vessel. This requires clamping the internal carotid artery distal to the stenosis, the common carotid artery proximal to the stenosis, and the external carotid artery distal to the carotid bifurcation (Figure 22.1), after which the artery is opened and the plaque removed. Temporary interruption of blood flow through the artery may be well tolerated if perfusion through collateral blood vessels is adequate. Sources of collateral perfusion include the circle of Willis, external-internal carotid collaterals such as the facial and ophthalmic arteries and leptomeningeal collaterals. The circle of Willis is incomplete in approximately half of the population, which may impair collateral perfusion [15]. Moreover, blood vessels supplying collateral blood flow may also have atherosclerotic disease, further impairing cerebral blood flow. In the absence of preoperative studies of cerebrovascular reactivity or blood flow, an individual patient's tolerance of carotid occlusion is difficult to predict. Even though patients with contralateral carotid occlusion require a shunt more frequently than patients in whom contralateral stenosis does not limit flow, many tolerate the cross-clamp without evidence of ischemia [16, 17]. The potential for inadequate cerebral blood flow during carotid occlusion has led to a variety of surgical practice patterns, where shunting is performed routinely, selectively based on evidence of ischemia or (now rarely) not at all. No studies clearly support the superiority of either routine or selective shunting [18]. In any event, patients should be monitored for evidence of hypoperfusion (see later).

REPERFUSION

Unclamping of the carotid artery may cause air, thrombo-emboli, or debris from the dissection to embolize. Debris from the endarterectomy or more likely air bubbles from the irrigation fluid may still reside in the arterotomy site. Careful irrigation before closure of the arterotomy and unclamping the internal carotid artery last minimizes the risk of embolic injury. A second and much more important source of emboli results from newly formed clot on the thrombogenic surface of the endarterectomy or from bleeding through the vasa vasorum [19]. New clot formation can be exacerbated by turbulent blood flow resulting from a technically imperfect repair. Technically inadequate endarterectomies may lead to an increase in the rate of emboli over the course of a few hours before complete thrombosis of the carotid occurs. Transcranial Doppler (TCD) can detect these emboli but does not help in distinguishing the type of embolic material.

Unclamping the carotid may also produce a significant and abrupt increase in cerebral blood flow. Before unclamping, blood flow may be reduced by removal of the shunt during final closure of the arteriotomy. The resulting normalization of cerebral blood flow may be problematic in patients with longstanding disease because autoregulation may be impaired distal to the lesion and resistance arterioles may not be able to constrict sufficiently to protect their distal vascular bed. This is termed *normal perfusion pressure breakthrough* and may be documented by TCD. Normal perfusion pressure breakthrough is diagnosed by a sustained increase in flow velocity to supranormal levels and manifests as a spectrum of symptoms ranging from headache to cerebral edema to frank intracerebral hemorrhage. Careful control of systemic blood pressure during and after unclamping minimizes the risk of this complication.

MEDICAL CONSIDERATIONS

Patients who are undergoing an elective carotid endarterectomy may have a variety of comorbidities and should undergo a comprehensive preoperative evaluation and medical optimization. Significant comorbidities are a common finding among patients with carotid artery disease. There has been considerable interest among practitioners as to whether assessment of preoperative patient characteristics can be correlated with postoperative morbidity and mortality. Some studies have suggested that age greater than 80, severe chronic obstructive pulmonary disease, severe congestive heart failure, renal failure, emergency surgery, and certain anatomical factors are risk factors for poor outcomes [20–22]. However, other recent large studies have demonstrated that there is little if any increased risk in the "high-risk" patient [23, 24]. It is unclear at this time if certain patients should be considered too high risk for a carotid endarterectomy. As the techniques for carotid stenting continue to evolve, avoidance of general or regional anesthesia may reduce morbidity and mortality for some patients.

The American Heart Association/American College of Cardiology (AHA/ACC) considers carotid endarterectomy an intermediate risk procedure. AHA/ACC guidelines recommend that heart rate control should be considered in patients with a poor functional status who have at least one of the following risk factors: diabetes mellitus, renal insufficiency, or a history of ischemic heart disease, heart failure, or cerebrovascular disease. Known severe cardiac disease or unstable angina warrants additional noninvasive testing such as an exercise stress test, dobutamine stress echocardiogram, or thallium scans after dipyridamole or adenosine administration [25]. It is important to note that preoperative studies, particularly those that are invasive, should only be performed if they will cause a change in patient management. The AHA/ACC does not recommend noninvasive cardiac testing beyond a resting electrocardiogram in asymptomatic patients who have good functional status (i.e., who are able to work at greater than or equal to 4 metabolic equivalents of activity). ECG should still be considered for patients with known coronary artery disease although the utility and most useful timing for ECG remains undefined. Coronary revascularization has historically been performed before vascular surgical procedures in an attempt to optimize cardiac perfusion, but a randomized controlled trial of patients without unstable angina or active myocardial infarction failed to demonstrate any benefit [26].

Medical optimization of patients for carotid endarterectomy may include drug therapy, including beta-blockers and anticoagulation. Beta blockers have been demonstrated to reduce the incidence of myocardial infarction and mortality in some patients undergoing non-cardiac surgery [27–29], but administering high doses of these drugs in naïve patients can increase the risk of stroke and death [30]. The AHA/ACC currently recommends that beta-blockers should be continued throughout the perioperative period and that they should be given to patients in whom myocardial ischemia is discovered on preoperative testing [25]. Beta blockers are probably helpful for patients undergoing vascular surgery who have more than one risk factor as listed previously, but additional randomized controlled studies are needed to help identify the patients who would most benefit from beta-blocker therapy.

Statins and antiplatelet agents may also reduce cardiovascular risk. Statins reduce the lipid content of the plaque and decrease inflammation within the plaque [31]. Both effects stabilize the plaque and reduce the risk of arterioarterial embolism. Large retrospective studies of patients who underwent carotid endarterectomy have correlated perioperative statin use with decreased risk of stroke or death [32, 33]. Aspirin has been studied extensively for use in CEA patients. In one large randomized trial, low-dose aspirin (81 mg or 325 mg daily) was more likely to prevent stroke, death, or myocardial infarction than higher doses [34]. Furthermore, a Cochrane review of six randomized controlled trials concluded that antiplatelet agents lowered the risk of stroke but did not affect mortality [35]. Dual antiplatelet therapy with aspirin and clopidogrel has been demonstrated in some trials to significantly reduce postoperative cerebral emboli without increasing bleeding complications [36, 37].

ANESTHETIC MANAGEMENT

Carotid endarterectomy can be performed under either regional or general anesthesia. Each option has several advantages as well as important limitations. The decision to pursue a particular anesthetic plan depends on the preferences and technical skills of both the surgeon and anesthetist. Although certain patients and practitioners may express a strong preference towards one type of anesthesia, it is important to understand the complexities of regional and general anesthetic approaches in order to provide the best care for each patient.

Regional anesthesia offers several important benefits for patients undergoing carotid endarterectomy. Most importantly, the patient's neurologic status can be continually assessed. If the patient's mental status deteriorates during the procedure, the surgeon can immediately insert a shunt. It is also possible to perform a reliable postoperative neurologic examination because the patient will not have any lingering effects of general anesthesia. Unfortunately, use of supplemental narcotics or sedation during the procedure will negatively affect the ability to assess the patient. The most convincing argument for a regional technique may be that it eliminates the need for expensive and complex neurologic monitoring, especially in resource poor settings [38, 39]. Another benefit of regional anesthesia may be a more stable intraoperative hemodynamic course [40], reflected in less use of vasopressors and less hypotension.

The choice to proceed with regional anesthesia also depends on the ability of the patient to cooperate during the block and subsequent operation. Once the procedure begins, it is difficult or impossible to secure the airway should the patient become neurologically compromised or hemodynamically unstable. Such a situation may occur if clamping the carotid artery results in a new neurologic deficit that does not reverse with placement of a shunt or unclamping of the artery. A recent large study concluded that overall perioperative conversion to general anesthesia either at the request of the patient or due to surgical and anesthestic complications was only 3.9% (69 of 1771 patients) [40].

Regional anesthesia for a carotid endarterectomy consists of a block of the cervical plexus. This can be performed as a superficial cervical plexus block by itself or combined with a deep cervical plexus block. Both typically require that the surgeon provide additional local anesthetic during the procedure, typically upon entering the carotid sheath. The superficial cervical plexus block uses as its entry point the midpoint of the posterior border of the sternocleidomastoid muscle, which frequently coincides with the crossing of the external jugular vein (Figure 22.2). From this entry point 10 to 12 mL of local anesthetic is injected along the posterior edge of the sternocleidomastoid muscle in a cranial and caudal direction while avoiding the external jugular vein. The deep cervical plexus block is performed either as a single injection at C3 or as three separate injections at C2, C3 and C4. At the cervical level contact is made between the needle and the lateral edge of the transverse process. The needle is then walked off the transverse process in a caudal direction so that its tip just lies above the spinal nerve root within the sulcus of the transverse process. Local anesthetic

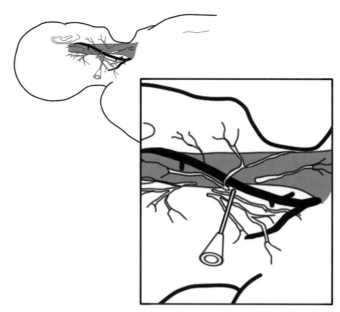

Figure 22.2   Superficial cervical plexus block for carotid endarterectomy. Terminal branches of the superficial cervical plexus come to the body surface near the midpoint of the posterior border of the sternocleidomastoid (SCM) muscle and provide sensory innervation of the neck. The anatomic landmark and entry point for regional anesthesia of the superficial cervical plexus is the midpoint of the posterior border of the SCM muscle, which corresponds in many patients to the point where the external jugular vein crosses the SCM muscle in its course from the angle of the jaw towards the middle of the clavicle. Local anesthetic is deposited in a cranial and caudal direction from the point of needle entry along the posterior border of the SCM muscle.

is injected either as a single fractionated 15-mL injection or as three separate 5-mL injections. Given this needle trajectory, it is possible to inject local anesthetic into the epidural or subarachnoid spaces during placement of a deep cervical plexus block. Injury to the ipsilateral vertebral artery, which may be an important source of collateral perfusion to the brain, or intra-arterial injection of local anesthetic resulting in a seizure are also possible complications of the deep cervical plexus block [41]. Addition of a deep cervical plexus block provides more rapid onset of anesthesia but does not improve significantly the quality of the anesthesia beyond that of a superficial cervical plexus block [42]. Patients can be lightly sedated with a benzodiazepine or an intermediate acting narcotic before the placement of the nerve block. Additional sedation and/or analgesics may be given to treat pain at the surgical site or inability to tolerate the surgical position.

General anesthesia offers a number of benefits for the patient undergoing carotid endarterectomy. The primary benefit of general anesthesia is that the airway is secure throughout the procedure. Many patients prefer to be asleep, because of the discomfort associated with the procedure. In addition, some patients may become claustrophobic because of the position of the drapes required for surgery on the neck. General anesthesia may also be beneficial for patients who have difficulty tolerating the surgical position because of respiratory disease, back pain, or other pathologies. Relative contraindications to regional anesthesia include morbid obesity, prior neck surgery or radiation, and inability to tolerate phrenic nerve paralysis. Surrogate measures of brain hypoperfusion (e.g., EEG, evoked potentials, or carotid stump pressure) allow the patient care team to monitor the patient during the procedure.

Numerous clinical trials have been undertaken in an attempt to determine the ideal anesthetic technique for the carotid endarterectomy. The largest randomized trial is the general anesthesia versus local anesthesia for carotid surgery (GALA), a multicenter, randomized controlled trial [40]. The primary outcomes studied were myocardial infarction, stroke, and death within randomization and 30 days of surgery. In this group of 3526 patients, there was no difference between regional and general anesthesia with regard to the primary outcome. Several subset analyses have also been completed with the goal of finding additional distinctions between these groups. There was limited evidence that regional anesthesia was more cost effective and resulted in less early neurocognitive dysfunction [39, 43]. Despite the very different anesthetic approaches that can be utilized for the carotid endarterectomy, it appears that the best decision is a shared one between the surgeon, anesthetist, and patient. The risks and benefits must be carefully weighed based on the individual patient as well as preferences of the physicians involved. Ultimately, both general and regional anesthesia appear to be equally safe in large population studies.

NEUROPHYSIOLOGIC MONITORING

A patient who is awake can be constantly assessed for a deteriorating neurologic status, but in patients who receive general anesthesia, monitoring neurologic function and blood supply may help to detect cerebral ischemia. Changes in cortical function may alert the anesthesiologist to increase blood pressure in order to maintain perfusion or serve as an indication for shunt placement. In patients who are unconscious, brain function can only be monitored indirectly with EEG and SEPs. Both of these techniques are relatively expensive, require equipment and time in the operating room, and rely on the presence of a skilled technician and/or neurologist for interpretation. Despite these limitations, however, EEGs and SEPs are commonly measured intraoperative parameters as they provide generally accurate information about a patient's neurological function.

The most common technique for monitoring brain function during a carotid endarterectomy is the EEG. EEG provides continuous information about cortical function but requires a tradeoff between spatial resolution (i.e., the number of EEG channels) and the amount of information to be interpreted. Bilateral placement of EEG allows

the clinician to identify both focal ipsilateral changes as well as contralateral ischemia secondary to incomplete collateral flow. A minimum of two leads over each cortex may discover the majority of changes related to inadequate blood flow, if placed over the watershed between anterior, middle, and posterior cerebral arteries in frontotemporal and frontoparietal positions. Changes in the EEG such as decreased amplitude and frequency may indicate intraoperative ischemia as result of carotid clamping, embolic events or hypotension (Figure 22.3). Hypothermia and changes in anesthetic depth can mimic ischemic changes but are typically symmetrical. Processed EEG simplifies the interpretation of the EEG (Figure 22.3) and identification of ischemic changes although the best diagnostic criteria remain controversial [44]. EEG may not detect all ischemia; false positive results range from 0% to as high as 4.5% in some studies [45]. Despite these limitations, EEG provides an excellent measure of global cortical function during carotid surgery.

Somatosensory potentials or SEPs can also be used to monitor brain function during carotid endarterectomy. Stimulation of the median nerve activates cortical territory perfused by the middle cerebral artery and boundary zone of the anterior and middle cerebral arteries (Figure 22.4). This allows the practitioner to selectively monitor one of the areas at greatest risk for ischemia. One advantage of SEPs is that this technique monitors subcortical pathways not captured on EEG. Monitoring SEPs does, however, require a slightly more involved setup and the intraoperative measurements are not as rapid as those of the EEG. The best measurements of function occur when both hemispheres are monitored. Their ability to detect ischemia is nearly as accurate as the EEG [44].

Cerebral blood supply can also be measured either directly or indirectly to help diagnose cerebral ischemia in patients who are receiving general anesthesia. TCD ultrasonography, stump pressures, and near-infrared spectroscopy are some of the techniques that may be used for this purpose.

TCD provides an approximation of cerebral blood flow by measuring the velocity of blood in the middle cerebral artery through a "window" in the temporal bone. Although it may be useful in many patients, it is technically impossible to perform in approximately 10% to 13% of patients, because the bone window prevents adequate visualization of the middle cerebral artery [46, 47]. Nevertheless, in patients with favorable anatomy the velocity can be constantly measured. A reduction in flow velocity of 60% at the time the carotid artery is occluded typically indicates cerebral hypoperfusion and requires placement of a shunt. TCD is unique in that it provides continuous assessment of embolic phenomena, which stand out against the background flow noise as musical chirps. As discussed earlier, emboli are the most frequent cause of new neurologic deficits in CEA. TCD is also the only technique that provides positive proof of normal perfusion pressure breakthrough after reperfusion. Blood pressure should be decreased in patients

Four Channels of Raw Electroencephalogram

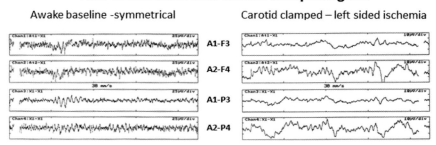

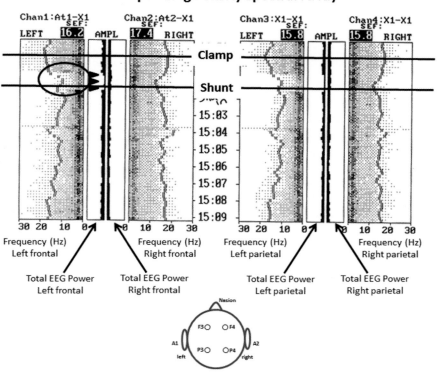

Figure 22.3 Monitoring for cerebral ischemia by electroencephalography (EEG). An example of cerebral ischemia upon clamping of the left carotid artery is presented. The top panel shows data from 4 channels of raw EEG. The montage is shown in the pictogram at the bottom of the figure. The awake baseline EEG is symmetrical and contains fast frequencies from muscle activity. After cross-clamping there is marked slowing and loss in amplitude in the left-sided EEG channels (A1-F3 and A1-P3). The bottom panel shows the processed EEG from the same 4 EEG channels in the same patient. The power present in different EEG frequencies is presented as the density of the printout over time in a density spectral array (DSA). Time indicated in the middle of the figure progresses from the top of the figure to the bottom. The spectral edge frequency, i.e. the frequency below which 95% of the EEG power resides, is depicted as a continuous line in the DSA displays of each EEG channel. Clamping of the internal carotid ("Clamp") results in a loss of fast frequencies in both left-sided channels as indicated by a black circle in the left frontal DSA display. Note also the loss of EEG power in both left-sided EEG channels indicated by black arrow heads in the left frontal EEG Power display. Insertion of a shunt ("Shunt") restores EEG symmetry.

in whom flow velocity is doubled after the cross-clamp is removed.

Measurement of stump pressure (the retrograde filling pressure of the operative blood vessel) is another method for assessing the adequacy of cerebral blood flow during carotid occlusion. A needle connected to a transducer is inserted into the internal carotid artery distal to the cross-clamp and the stump pressure is compared with the mean arterial pressure (Figure 22.5). Although higher pressures are generally suggestive of adequate collateral cerebral circulation, there has been considerable controversy about acceptable values.

Some studies found that patients with stump pressures ranging from 25 mm Hg to over 50 mm Hg had no neurologic changes [45, 48]. These findings underscore the limitation of this indirect one-time assessment.

Cerebral oximetry using near-infared spectroscopy is yet another method of assessing the adequacy of cerebral perfusion. A sensor is placed on the ipsilateral or bilateral frontal region. The device measures reflected light from both the brain and the intervening tissues, and a mathematical algorithm is used to calculate venous oxygenation at a particular location. It has been generalized to represent impaired cerebral

Somatosensory Evoked Potentials

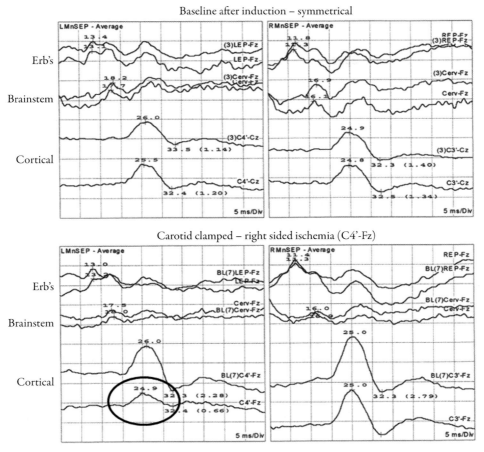

Figure 22.4 Somatosensory Evoked Potential (SSEP) Monitoring during CEA. Shown is data from a patient undergoing right CEA monitored with somatosensory evoked potentials. Potentials were recorded in response to median nerve stimulation over Erb's Point, the brainstem, and the contralateral somatosensory cortex. Baseline responses are reproducible and symmetrical. The response recorded after clamping the carotid artery shows a marked loss in amplitude in the right cortical signal as indicated by a black circle. Factors that suggest an SSEP change caused by ischemia are that peripheral and brainstem potentials from the same side are unchanged making technical problems with stimulation or recording unlikely and that the EPs from the contralateral side are unaffected suggesting no changes in global perfusion or anesthesia.

oxygenation with values less than 50% for single hemispheric changes or a 20% to 25% decrease from baseline. There is, however, no consensus about the usefulness of these values. Some studies have found an inverse relationship between cerebral oximetry values and ischemia during cross-clamping but others demonstrated a poor correlation [46, 47, 49].

Every technique for monitoring cerebral function or blood supply has several important advantages and disadvantages, and there is no definitive advantage of one method over another [50]. It will remain the judgment of the surgeon and anesthesiologist to determine the ideal monitor, if any, for a given patient.

PERIOPERATIVE COMPLICATIONS

Carotid endarterectomy carries the risk of worsening neurologic function due to a perioperative stroke or TIA,

myocardial ischemia, cranial nerve injury, or a postoperative wound hematoma.

The risk of myocardial infarction is a closely monitored outcome. The reported risk is low at approximately 1% [20, 51]. Since cardiac disease can certainly contribute to the cause of death, the occurrence of cardiac complications may be higher than reported. In fact, many of the large population studies on carotid endarterectomy report composite primary outcomes which include stroke, myocardial infarction, and death. As discussed previously, appropriate administration of beta-blockers, statins, and antiplatelet agents may help reduce the risk.

The reported incidence of stroke varies widely among different studies for several reasons including the indication for the procedure, clinical, and/or radiologic criteria for diagnosis, cohort size, experience of the surgeon(s), and numerous others. Some large recent studies found a rate of stroke of 1.31% to 6.5% [51–54]. The variables that were associated with an increased risk of stroke were not

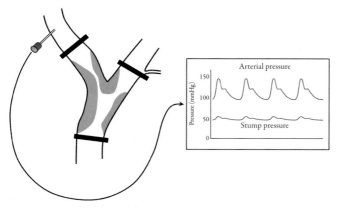

Measurement of the stump pressure. A needle connected via a fluid filled pressure line to a transduced is inserted into the distal internal carotid artery after cross-clamping. The measured "stump pressure" is compared with the invasively measured aterial pressure.

uniform among these studies. The NASCET group found that in symptomatic patients, hemispheric TIAs, left-sided procedures, contralateral carotid occlusion, and ipsilateral ischemia or an irregular plaque put patients at higher risk. Another large study in northern New England identified emergency surgery, contralateral carotid occlusion, congestive heart failure, preoperative stroke, and age greater than 70 correlated with increased risk in a cohort of symptomatic or asymptomatic patients [51]. The New York Carotid Artery Surgery study found that the presence of cranial nerve palsies, hematoma, and cardiac complications was associated with a higher rate of stroke [53]. From these studies, a conclusion can be drawn that numerous patient-, surgery-, or anesthetic-related factors can increase the risk of stroke, TIAs, and myocardial infarctions.

A wound hematoma is a potentially life-threatening complication of carotid endarterectomy. Arterial or venous bleeding can rapidly produce a significant airway obstruction. Depending on the size, location, and rate of expansion of the hematoma, immediate surgical intervention may be necessary. Urgent reexploration of a carotid endarterectomy is best managed under general endotracheal anesthesia because of the risk for tracheal compression and subsequent airway compromise [55]. Mask ventilation and intubation may be extremely difficult or even impossible with severe tissue edema and ongoing bleeding. In one study, 40% of patients that were initially deemed an "easy" intubation had a difficult airway when presenting for a hematoma evacuation [57]. The safest option for managing the airway may be an awake intubation while maintaining spontaneous ventilation. Conditions sometimes improve when the incision is opened and the pressure from the hematoma is released. If the patient appears to be in distress, the neck wound should be opened as quickly as possible, possibly even before the patient is transferred to the operating room for definitive management. If mask ventilation and intubation prove impossible, an immediate cricothyroidomy or tracheostomy may be required. Even after a endotracheal intubation,

tissue edema may persist or even worsen after reexploration, so postoperative intubation and mechanical ventilation should be considered.

Several nerves are at risk for injury during carotid endarterectomy either due to their anatomical position in the area of interest or from retractors placed to aid surgical visualization. Since identification of nerve injury is complicated by other factors such as postoperative swelling, difficulties with intubation or residual general anesthesia, it can be difficult to identify the affected nerve without a formal evaluation. Cranial nerve injury is relatively common after CEA, with an incidence of 5.5% to 10.6% but most patients make a full recovery [51, 54, 56]. The recurrent laryngeal nerve is a branch of the vagus nerve; injury to this nerve can cause unilateral vocal cord paralysis. The superior laryngeal nerve divides into the internal and external branches, which innervate the larynx and cricopharyngeal muscles, respectively. Damage to either branch can cause hoarseness. Hoarseness can also be caused by postoperative swelling or a hematoma [57]. Facial nerve injury, specifically to the marginal mandibular branch, may cause an asymmetric smile and drooling. Hypoglossal nerve injury produces tongue deviation to the injured side. Glossopharyngeal nerve damage can cause a globus sensation (a persistent feeling of having an obstruction in the throat) or difficulty swallowing. The accessory nerve innervates the trapezius and sternocleidomastoid muscles; injury may cause difficulty in turning the head and lifting the shoulder. One study noted that cranial nerves XII, X, and VII were most likely to be affected [56]. A careful postoperative neurologic examination should be performed to document the presence of any potential nerve injury.

CONSIDERATIONS FOR EXTRACRANIAL/ INTRACRANIAL BYPASS

GENERAL CONSIDERATIONS

EC/IC bypass is used to augment cerebral blood flow for several indications. This procedure will ensure distal perfusion if it is necessary to occlude a major intracranial artery (e.g., trapping of a complex aneurysm). EC/IC bypass will also mitigate cerebral hypoperfusion in the setting of a carotid occlusion caused, for example, by Moya-moya disease or atherosclerosis. Recent trials in patients with occlusive carotid disease support the ability of EC/IC bypass to normalize misery perfusion [58]. Whether this normalization translates to meaningful improvement in clinical outcomes remains to be determined [59, 60].

The most frequently performed anastomosis is from the superficial temporal artery to a branch of the middle cerebral artery [61]. This approach limits the number of anastomoses and uses only arterial conduit. Anesthetic management is focused on minimizing likelihood of arterial spasm or low flow, which might cause thrombosis at the anastomosis site. Adequate cerebral perfusion can be maintained by keeping the patient euvolemic and avoiding bolus administration of vasopressors and calcium as well as hyperventilation. The advent of indocyanine green fluorescence angiography has significantly improved the surgeons' ability to assess the quality of the anastomosis, which may help to improve patient outcome. Because cerebral inflow is occluded at the level of the distal middle cerebral artery, concerns about hemispheric hypoperfusion are less than for CEA, but because EC/IC bypass is performed under general anesthesia, the use of some type of monitoring for cerebral ischemia is recommended.

MOYA-MOYA DISEASE

Moya-moya disease is an inflammatory process that involves the terminal internal carotid artery, causes progressive restriction of cerebral inflow and ultimately results in cerebral hypoperfusoin and stroke. Moya-moya disease was originally described in Japan and describes its angiographic appearance, where continuation of flow from the distal internal carotid artery does not show the normal anatomy of discrete cerebral vessels such as middle and anterior cerebral arteries, but rather a network of neovascular collaterals, which give the appearance of the contrast media dissipating in a "puff of smoke." Patients with moya-moya disease benefit from surgery aimed at providing additional blood flow to the brain [62]. Approaches may be in the form of EC/IC bypass or by bringing vascular tissue in direct contact with the brain to allow formation of neovascular collaterals, a procedure called synangiosis. Vascular tissue may be in the form of the superficial temporal artery, dura or muscle. Anesthetic management is similar to that of EC/IC bypass [63].

CONCLUSIONS

Carotid surgery challenges anesthesiologists in many ways. From the preoperative medical optimization through the intraoperative integration of surgical approach, anesthetic choice and neurphysiologic monitoring to the management of postoperative complications, care for patients with carotid disease can be difficult. Safe care for appropriately selected patients can be achieved through different approaches provided the overall rate of complications remains low. On the one hand anti-platelet agents and statins have established a firm role. On the other hand operative technique, anesthetic approach and neuromonitoring vary dramatically between institutions. Nonetheless 50 years of research and practice provide sufficient information to design a rational approach to care that integrates patient preferences, surgical approach

and anesthetic management in a way that allows patients to realize the benefit of a reduced risk of stroke.

REFERENCES

1. EC/IC Bypass Study Group. Failure of extracranial-intracranial arterial bypass to reduce the risk of ischemic stroke. Results of an international randomized trial. *N Engl J Med*. 1985;313:1191–1200.
2. North American Symptomatic Carotid Endarterectomy Trial Collaborators. Beneficial effect of carotid endarterectomy in symptomatic patients with high-grade carotid stenosis. N Engl J Med. 1991;325:445–453.
3. European Carotid Surgery Trialists' Collaborative Group. MRC European Carotid Surgery Trial: interim results for symptomatic patients with severe (70-99%) or with mild (0-29%) carotid stenosis. *Lancet*. 1991;337:1235–1243.
4. Executive Committee for the Asymptomatic Carotid Atherosclerosis Study. Endarterectomy for asymptomatic carotid artery stenosis. *JAMA*. 1995;273:1421–1428.
5. Ederle J, Featherstone RL, Brown MM. Randomized controlled trials comparing endarterectomy and endovascular treatment for carotid artery stenosis: a Cochrane Systematic Review. *Stroke*. 2009;40:1373–1380.
6. Ederle J, Dobson J, Featherstone RL, et al; International Carotid Stenting Study Investigators. Carotid artery stenting compared with endarterectomy in patients with symptomatic carotid stenosis (International Carotid Stenting Study): an interim analysis of a randomised controlled trial. *Lancet*. 2010;375:985–997.
7. Brott TG, Hobson RW 2nd, Howard G, et al; CREST Investigators. Stenting versus endarterectomy for treatment of carotid-artery stenosis. *N Engl J Med*. 2010;363:11–23.
8. Stabile E, Salemme L, Sorrropago G, et al. Proximal endovascular occlusion for carotid artery stenting: results from a prospective registry of 1,300 patients. *J Am Coll Cardiol*. 2010;55:1661–1667.
9. Dempsey RJ, Vemuganti R, Varghese T, et al. A review of carotid atherosclerosis and vascular cognitive decline: a new understanding of the keys to symptomology. *Neurosurgery*. 2010;67:484–494; discussion 493–494.
10. Payne DA, Jones CI, Hayes PD, et al. Beneficial effects of clopidogrel combined with aspirin in reducing cerebral emboli in patients undergoing carotid endarterectomy, *Circulation*. 2004;109:1476–1481.
11. Goodney PP, Likosky DS, Cronenwett JL; Vascular Study Group of Northern New England. Factors associated with stroke or death after carotid endarterectomy in Northern New England. *J Vasc Surg*. 2008;48:1139–1145.
12. Engelter S, Lyrer P: Antiplatelet therapy for preventing stroke and other vascular events after carotid endarterectomy. *Cochrane Database Syst Rev*. 2003;(3):CD001458.
13. Yamada K, Yoshimura S, Kawasaki M, et al. Effects of atorvastatin on carotid atherosclerotic plaques: a randomized trial for quantitative tissue characterization of carotid atherosclerotic plaques with integrated backscatter ultrasound. *Cerebrovasc Dis* 2009;28:417–424.
14. Kunte H, Amberger N, Busch MA, et al. Markers of instability in high-risk carotid plaques are reduced by statins. *J Vasc Surg*. 2008;47:513–522.
15. Cho L, Mukherjee D. Basic cerebral anatomy for the carotid interventionalist: the intracranial and extracranial vessels. *Cathet Cardiovasc Interv* 2006;68:104–111.
16. Karmeli R, Lubezky N, Halak M, et al. Carotid endarterectomy in awake patients with contralateral carotid artery occlusion. *Cardiovasc Surg* 2001;9:334–338.
17. Tan TW, Garcia-Toca M, Marcaccio EJ Jr, et al. Predictors of shunt during carotid endarterectomy with routine electroencephalography monitoring. *J Vasc Surg*. 2009;49:1374–1378.
18. Rerkasem K, Rothwell PM: Routine or selective carotid artery shunting for carotid endarterectomy (and different methods of

monitoring in selective shunting). Cochrane *Database Syst Rev* 2009;:CD000190.

19. Naylor AR, Hayes PD, Allroggen H, et al. Reducing the risk of carotid surgery: a 7-year audit of the role of monitoring and quality control assessment. *J Vasc Surg.* 2000;32:750–759.

20. Ouriel K, Hertzer NR, Beven EG, et al. Preprocedural risk stratification: identifying an appropriate population for carotid stenting. *J Vasc Surg.* 2001;33:728–732.

21. Hsia DC, Moscoe LM, Krushat WM. Epidemiology of carotid endarterectomy among Medicare beneficiaries: 1985-1996 update. *Stroke.* 1998;29:346–350.

22. Goodney PP, Likosky DS, Cronenwett JL; Vascular Study Group of Northern New England. Factors associated with stroke or death after carotid endarterectomy in Northern New England. *J Vasc Surg* 2008;48:1139–1145.

23. Miller MT, Comerota AJ, Tzilinis A, et al. Carotid endarterectomy in octogenarians: does increased age indicate "high risk"? *J Vasc Surg.* 2005;41:231–237.

24. Flanigan DP, Flanigan ME, Dorne AL, et al. Long-term results of 442 consecutive, standardized carotid endarterectomy procedures in standard-risk and high-risk patients. *J Vasc Surg.* 2007;46:876–882.

25. Fleisher LA, Beckman JA, Brown KA, et al; American College of Cardiology Foundation/American Heart Association Task Force on Practice Guidelines; American Society of Echocardiography; American Society of Nuclear Cardiology;Heart Rhythm Society; Society of Cardiovascular Anesthesiologists; Society for Cardiovascular Angiography and Interventions; Society for Vascular Medicine; Society for Vascular Surgery. 2009 ACCF/AHA focused update on perioperative beta-blockade incorporated into the ACC/AHA. 2007 guidelines on perioperative cardiovascular evaluation and care for noncardiac surgery. *J Am Coll Cardiol.* 2009;54:e13–e118.

26. McFalls EO, Ward HB, Moritz TE, et al. Coronary-artery revascularization before elective major vascular surgery. *N Engl J Med* 2004;351:2795–2804.

27. Lindenauer PK, Pekow P, Wang K, et al. Perioperative beta-blocker therapy and mortality after major noncardiac surgery. *N Engl J Med.* 2005;353:349–361.

28. Poldermans D, Boersma E, Bax JJ, et al. The effect of bisoprolol on perioperative mortality and myocardial infarction in high-risk patients undergoing vascular surgery. Dutch Echocardiographic Cardiac Risk Evaluation Applying Stress Echocardiography Study Group. *N Engl J Med* 1999;341:1789–1794.

29. Mangano DT, Layug EL, Wallace A, et al. Effect of atenolol on mortality and cardiovascular morbidity after noncardiac surgery. Multicenter Study of Perioperative Ischemia Research Group. *N Engl J Med* 1996;335:1713–1720.

30. POISE Study Group, Devereaux PJ, Yang H, Yusuf S, et al. Effects of extended-release metoprolol succinate in patients undergoing non-cardiac surgery (POISE trial): a randomised controlled trial. *Lancet* 2008;371:1839–1847.

31. van der Most PJ, Dolga AM, Nijholt IM, et al. Statins: Mechanisms of neuroprotection. *Prog Neurobiol.* 2009;88:64–75.

32. McGirt MJ, Perler BA, Brooke BS, et al. 3-Hydroxy-3-methylglutaryl coenzyme A reductase inhibitors reduce the risk of perioperative stroke and mortality after carotid endarterectomy. *J Vasc Surg* 2005;42:829–836.

33. Stoner MC, Defreitas DJ. Process of care for carotid endarterectomy: perioperative medical management. *J Vasc Surg.* 2010;52:223–231.

34. Taylor DW, Barnett HJ, Haynes RB, et al. Low-dose and high-dose acetylsalicylic acid for patients undergoing carotid endarterectomy: a randomised controlled trial. ASA and Carotid Endarterectomy (ACE) Trial Collaborators. *Lancet.* 1999;353:2179–2184.

35. Engelter S, Lyrer P. Antiplatelet therapy for preventing stroke and other vascular events after carotid endarterectomy *Stroke* 2004;35:1227–1228.

36. Payne DA, Jones CI, Hayes PD, et al. Beneficial effects of clopidogrel combined with aspirin in reducing cerebral emboli in patients undergoing carotid endarterectomy. *Circulation.* 2004;109:1476–1481.

37. Sharpe RY, Dennis MJ, Nasim A, et al. Dual antiplatelet therapy before carotid endarterectomy reduces post-operative embolisation and thromboembolic events: post-operative transcranial Doppler monitoring is now unnecessary. *Eur J Vasc Endovasc Surg.* 2010;40:162–167.

38. Hariharan S, Naraynsingh V, Esack A, et al. Perioperative outcome of carotid endarterectomy with regional anesthesia: two decades of experience from the Caribbean. *J Clin Anesth* 2010;22:169–173.

39. Gomes M, Soares MO, Dumville JC, et al.; GALA Collaborative Group. Cost-effectiveness analysis of general anaesthesia versus local anaesthesia for carotid surgery (GALA Trial). *Br J Surg.* 2010;97:1218–1225.

40. GALA Trial Collaborative Group, Lewis SC, Warlow CP, Bodenham AR, et al.. General anaesthesia versus local anaesthesia for carotid surgery (GALA): a multicentre, randomised controlled trial. *Lancet.* 2008;372:2132–2142.

41. Pandit JJ, Satya-Krishna R, Gration P. Superficial or deep cervical plexus block for carotid endarterectomy: a systematic review of complications. *Br J Anaesth.* 2007;99:159–169.

42. Guay J. Regional anesthesia for carotid surgery. *Curr Opin Anaesthesiol.* 2008;21:638–644.

43. Weber CF, Friedl H, Hueppe M, et al. Impact of general versus local anesthesia on early postoperative cognitive dysfunction following carotid endarterectomy: GALA Study Subgroup Analysis. *World J Surg* 2009;33:1526–1532.

44. Florence G, Guerit JM, Gueguen B. Electroencephalography (EEG) and somatosensory evoked potentials (SEP) to prevent cerebral ischaemia in the operating room. *Neurophysiol Clin.* 2004;34:17–32.

45. Calligaro KD, Dougherty MJ. Correlation of carotid artery stump pressure and neurologic changes during 474 carotid endarterectomies performed in awake patients. *J Vasc Surg.* 2005;42:684–689.

46. Guarracino F. Cerebral monitoring during cardiovascular surgery. *Curr Opin Anaesthesiol.* 2008;21:50–54.

47. Moritz S, Kasprzak P, Arlt M, et al. Accuracy of cerebral monitoring in detecting cerebral ischemia during carotid endarterectomy: a comparison of transcranial Doppler sonography, near-infrared spectroscopy, stump pressure, and somatosensory evoked potentials. *Anesthesiology.* 2007;107:563–569.

48. Hans SS, Jareunpoon O. Prospective evaluation of electroencephalography, carotid artery stump pressure, and neurologic changes during 314 consecutive carotid endarterectomies performed in awake patients. *J Vasc Surg.* 2007;45:511–515.

49. Friedell ML, Clark JM, Graham DA, et al. Cerebral oximetry does not correlate with electroencephalography and somatosensory evoked potentials in determining the need for shunting during carotid endarterectomy. *J Vasc Surg.* 2008;48:601–606.

50. Bond R, Rerkasem K, Counsell C, et al. Routine or selective carotid artery shunting for carotid endarterectomy (and different methods of monitoring in selective shunting). *Cochrane Database Syst Rev.* 2002;(2):CD000190.

51. Goodney PP, Likosky DS, Cronenwett JL; Vascular Study Group of Northern New England. Factors associated with stroke or death after carotid endarterectomy in Northern New England. *J Vasc Surg.* 2008;48:1139–1145.

52. Chiesa R, Melissano G, Castellano R, et al. Carotid endarterectomy: experience in 5425 cases. *Ann Vasc Surg.* 2004;18:527–534.

53. Greenstein AJ, Chassin MR, Wang J, et al. Association between minor and major surgical complications after carotid endarterectomy: results of the New York Carotid Artery Surgery study. *J Vasc Surg.* 2007;46:1138–1144; discussion 1145–1146.

54. Ferguson GG, Eliasziw M, Barr HW, et al; The North American Symptomatic Carotid Endarterectomy Trial. Surgical results in 1415 patients. *Stroke.* 1999;30:1751–1758.

55. Shakespeare WA, Lanier WL, Perkins WJ, et al. Airway management in patients who develop neck hematomas after carotid endarterectomy. *Anesth Analg* 2010;110:588–593.

56. Sajid MS, Vijaynagar B, Singh P, et al. Literature review of cranial nerve injuries during carotid endarterectomy. *Acta Chir Belg* 2007;107:25–28.

57. Assadian A, Senekowitsch C, Pfaffelmeyer N, et al. Incidence of cranial nerve injuries after carotid eversion endarterectomy with a transverse skin incision under regional anaesthesia. *Eur J Vasc Endovasc Surg* 2004;28:421–424.

58. Yonas H, Przybylski GJ, Webster MW, et al. Diagnosis and treatment of high-risk patients from symptomatic carotid occlusive disease with STA-MCA bypass. *Acta Neurol Scand Suppl* 1996;166:114.

59. Jeffree RL, Stoodley MA. STA-MCA bypass for symptomatic carotid occlusion and haemodynamic impairment. *J Clin Neurosci.* 2009;16:226–235.

60. Grubb RL Jr, Powers WJ, Derdeyn CP, et al. The Carotid Occlusion Surgery Study. *Neurosurg Focus.* 2003;14(3):1–7.

61. Baaj AA, Agazzi S, van Loveren H. Graft selection in cerebral revascularization. *Neurosurg Focus.* 2009;26:E18.

62. Scott RM, Smith J, Robertson RL, et al. Long-term outcome in children with moyamoya syndrome after cranial revascularization by plial synangiosis. *J Neurosurg.* 2004;100:142–149.

63. Parray T, Martin TW, Siddiqui S. Moyamoya disease: a review of the disease and anesthetic management. *J Neurosurg Anesthesiol* 2011;23:100–109.

23.

POSITIONING FOR NEUROSURGERY

Richard B. Silverman

GENERAL PRINCIPLES

Most surgical procedures are performed with the patient in the supine position and with little consultation between the surgeon and anesthesiologist. In the neurosurgical operating room, however, patient positioning must be a collaborative effort that includes the anesthesiologist, neurosurgeon, and nursing staff because the patient must frequently be positioned in ways that entail significant physiologic and pathologic consequences [1]. Surgeons and anesthesiologists have devised several standard positions for a range of procedures that provide the surgeon with an optimal field while minimizing nonanatomic patient positioning. Although poor positioning may be tolerated with little sequelae in a patient undergoing a brief surgical procedure, an overlooked detail may result in long-term or permanent injury and disability after a long neurosurgical procedure [26]. The length and complexity of neurosurgery significantly increase the risks of malpositioning [25]. Understanding which procedures will require a specific position and the risks that are entailed allows the anesthesiologist to manage the relevant physiologic and anatomic issues.

PATIENT PREPARATION

The first step in patient positioning is to ascertain the security of the airway, monitors, intravenous access, and other invasive devices. Access will probably be restricted during most of the procedure, and unintentional dislodgement may create a life-threatening situation.

The first priority is to secure the airway. Procedures during which the patient will be awake with supplemental oxygen are perhaps the most complex. Patient movement may dislodge the nasal cannula and, with it, side stream end-tidal capnography. If the patient's head is under sterile drapes or out of the direct line of sight of the anesthesiologist, it is best to secure the O_2 and end-tidal CO_2 ($ETco_2$) tubing with tape or clear plastic dressings. If the patient's head will

be covered with drapes, a method to remove "tented" CO_2 should be provided. One possible technique is to secure suction tubing under the drapes. This will remove exhaled gas while drawing in fresh air. Before the surgery begins, the anesthesiologists and surgeons should agree on a plan in case it is necessary to convert to general anesthesia during the procedure.

In addition to ASA standard monitors, the use of invasive monitors such as an intra-arterial catheter should be considered carefully before surgery begins because access to the patient will be impaired when he or she is in the final surgical position. Intravenous and intra-arterial catheters should be tested and adequate function confirmed after positioning and before turning the patient over to the neurosurgeons. An intravenous catheter that no longer free-flows should not be pressurized unless the anesthesiologist has access to ensure that it has not become infiltrated, because this may quickly lead to a compartment syndrome.

In many cases, the head and face of the neurosurgical patient are out of direct view. If the patient is intubated, a straight, bent, or flexible connector should be chosen so as to minimize stress on the endotracheal tube. The breathing circuit should be positioned so that endotracheal tube and the capnography tubing are kinked and there is no force on the endotracheal tube.

During most surgical procedures, rotation of the table to the surgical position and patient positioning will require periods during which intravenous and intra-arterial catheters are capped, patient monitors are disconnected, and the breathing circuit and capnograph are disconnected from the patient. The amount of time that the patient is unmonitored should be minimized, and the monitors and breathing circuit should be briefly reconnected if extra time is needed. If at all possible, the pulse oximeter should remain connected throughout this period because the information it provides allows early detection of serious problems (e.g., hypoxemia or a dysrhythmia). During most procedures, some part of the patient will be available to the anesthesiologist. During spine procedures, this may be one or both arms, while the lower extremities may be the only accessible to the anesthesiologist. Additional intravenous access can be obtained from the saphenous veins and, if necessary, arterial lines placed in dorsalis pedis artery.

PADDING AND PRESSURE POINTS

Data from the Closed Claims Study suggest that positioning injuries are not uncommon and suggest that the anesthesiologist should pay special attention to the use of appropriate padding [9]. In the supine patient, the ulnar nerve should be padded and knees should be elevated with pillows to relieve pressure under the lower back. Should there be any conceivable risk to pressure on the eyes, the use of padded goggles should be considered, and in any event the eyes should periodically be checked to be sure that a small change in position has not created a pressure point. In the prone patient, the arms will either be tucked at the sides or extended over the head. In this case, susceptible areas include the ulnar nerve, the chest (including breasts in women), and the iliac crests. All areas that may come into contact with posts or other support structures should be carefully padded. If the patient's head will not be secured in a Mayfield head holder, a foam prone positioning pillow with cutouts for nose, airway, and eyes should be used to protect the face.

POSITIONING COMPLICATIONS

Prolonged surgical procedures have significant physiologic implications, particularly when the patient will not be in a normal anatomic position. Stasis, decreased venous return, and deep vein thrombosis may occur in any patient, but patients in the "park bench" and sitting positions are especially susceptible to these complications [9]. Elastic stockings or sequential compression devices should use whenever feasible and should be applied when the patient is brought into the operating room. Pharmacologic interventions such as low molecular weight heparin are not usually an option in most patients undergoing a neurosurgical procedure. Transition to the sitting position can cause a significant decrease in diastolic and mean arterial pressures that is caused by a shift in circulating blood volume to the lower extremities in a vasodilated, anesthetized patient [4, 5]. One study recommends administration of a volume load of 10 mL/kg of 6% hetastarch before positioning [27]. The noninvasive blood pressure cuff should periodically be moved in order to avoid injury, particularly if the procedure is lengthy and it will be used to measure blood pressure frequently. When patients are placed in the lateral position, lung areas 18 cm above the bed are not well perfused but receive the greatest inspired volumes during positive pressure ventilation. This leads to a significant ventilation-perfusion mismatch

[6–8]. In the prone position, however, intra-abdominal pressure rises. If the patient is not positioned appropriately, with bolsters to remove pressure from the abdomen, venous return will decrease in combination with an increase in SVR and PVR.

Although this chapter is focused on the neurosurgical patient, the principles of head, neck, and spine positioning transcend this particular area. The most basic caveat is to avoid extreme positioning, compression of neurovascular structures, or pressure on bony prominences and soft tissue. There is a wide range of flexion in the cervical spine, most of which occurs in the atlanto-occipital and mid cervical areas (C4-C5). Flexion causes the interspinous ligaments to stretch. Extreme flexion causes the posterior wall of the cervical canal to elongate more than the anterior wall. The spinal cord is tethered by the nerve roots, so positioning the neck in extreme flexion pulls the nerve roots cephalad against the undersurface of the foramina. This may cause injury, particularly when the foramina are narrowed or calcified. Extreme flexion may also cause ischemia at the C4-C5 level with resultant quadriplegia.

SPECIAL CONSIDERATIONS FOR ADVANCED MONITORING

Electrodes for neurophysiologic monitors should be coiled and taped to the patient, and then unwrapped and connected to monitoring equipment only after the patient is fully positioned. This will minimize the possibility that the cables are inadvertently disconnected or trapped between the patient and the table, which may cause an injury. If a precordial Doppler monitor will be used, it should be applied after the patient in order to maximize the possibility of maintaining a good signal throughout the procedure. Poor positioning of an intraventricular catheter or its associated transducer can cause false indications or impair drainage of cerebrospinal fluid, increasing ICP. The ICP monitor should be carefully monitored to prevent this from happening. Poor positioning of jugular bulb catheters or intra-arterial catheters will also cause false readings and may impair sampling during the procedure.

POSITIONING EQUIPMENT

HORSESHOE HEADREST

The horseshoe headrest may be used for patients who are in either the supine or prone position. It is usually attached to a Mayfield apparatus and secured to the table. The patient's head rests on a gel pillow that is wrapped with gauze. If the patient is in the prone position, there should be no pressure on orbits or mucous membranes, and these areas should be periodically checked throughout the surgical procedure. In the supine position, the headrest should be adjusted so that it conforms to the patient's head and stabilizes the cranium. Pressure necrosis and pressure-related hair loss can occur after long procedures, even if appropriate precautions are taken [23].

MAYFIELD APPARATUS

Perhaps the most widely used system for head fixation in cranial and cervical spine surgery is the Mayfield pins, clamp, and holder, collectively known as the *Mayfield skeletal fixation apparatus*. The clamp is firmly attached to the head using pins that penetrate into the skull. It is then rigidly affixed to the table using the holder. The advantage of this device is that it immobilizes the patient's head and neck while providing superior access to the surgical field.

Application of the Mayfield clamp is as painful as surgical skin incision. Coordination with the surgeon is therefore essential to prevent patient movement or a hemodynamic response. Additional narcotics or hypnotics should be administered, or the concentration of a potent volatile anesthetic should be increased prior to application of the head-holder. The patient should be monitored carefully as the device is applied, and the surgeon instructed to stop should additional anesthesia be required. Prior to applying Mayfield pins, the patient's head should be cleaned with chlorhexidine scrub and bacitracin ointment should be applied to the pins for both infection reduction and to decrease risk of embolism for pins sites. A strain gauge on the clamp allows the surgeon to choose the amount of force used; the clamp is typically applied with 60 to 80 pounds of force.

The Mayfield system is associated with several complications. Use of excessive force may cause a depressed skull fracture in children or patients with thin skulls. The device should also be used with caution in patients with severe head trauma in which a skull fracture is known or suspected. Unexpected patient movement after the device is applied can result in injury to the cervical spine or severe lacerations if the head is forcibly pulled out of the clamp. After the removal of the device at the end of the case, bleeding from pin sites is not uncommon. This can usually be managed with simple compression with gauze pads and by using a pressure dressing. If this is not sufficient to control bleeding, the holes can be sutured closed or surgical skin staples can be used to close the holes.

PRONE POSITIONING PILLOW

The prone positioning pillow can sometimes serve as an alternative to head fixation in pins for a patient who is in the prone position for a surgical procedure in the thoracic or lumbar areas. This device is rarely suitable for intracranial surgery or surgery on the cervical spine. It is made of two types of foam with different densities that have been formed into a block with hollow invaginations or holes for the endotracheal tube, eyes, and nose. The pillow comes in one standard height. The head and neck of a smaller patient may therefore be hyperextended with this pillow.

GARDNER-WELLS TONGS

The Gardner-Wells tongs are used in the patient needing anterior cervical disc distraction. This is a simple C-shaped piece of metal that uses pins similar to those in the Mayfield device to hold the patient's head. A rope is tied to the tongs and a weigh is cantilevered over the edge of the bed to apply traction to the head and neck. If the surgeon needs additional distraction, he or she may request the anesthesiologist to apply additional force to the rope. The surgeon will ask for the weights to be removed when distraction is no longer needed. The technique for applying and removing the device is similar to that for the Mayfield skeletal fixation device noted earlier.

FRAMES AND TABLES

A variety of tables are currently being used for the patient undergoing spine surgery. Each has its advantages and disadvantages, with the choice of the device often being dictated by the surgical procedure and by preference of the surgeon. Frames that support the patient with the hips and knees flexed at least 90 degrees, such as the Andrews' table and Hastings frame, offer wide exposure of the lumbar disks, and are designed to remove pressure from the abdomen, which decreases venous bleeding. Spinal fusion procedures with instrumentation or fixation require that the curvature of the spine is kept as close as possible to the normal lordotic curve of in the standing position. The Jackson table, a four-post frame like the Relton-Hall, or other frame systems that support the patient with 60 degrees or less flexion of the hips are better suited for these procedures. Some studies, however, suggest that the four-post frames are less effective at stabilizing the natural curvature of the spine than are chest rolls [24]. Spinal instrumentation procedures almost always require intraoperative C-arm fluoroscopy or x-ray imaging to ensure proper alignment of the vertebrae. A third consideration is cost: Surgical tables with hydraulic equipment that have been designed primarily for spine surgery in the prone position are more expensive and less compact and portable than are frames designed to be placed on top of a conventional operating table.

JACKSON TABLE

Spine surgery involving fusion and instrumentation often require specialized tables that optimize the surgical field while permitting the position of the vertebrae to be

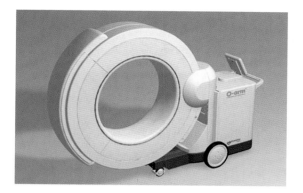

Figure 23.1   O-Arm, circumferential CT imaging.

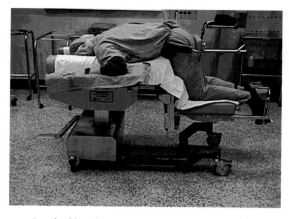

Figure 23.3   Standard kneeling position with hip stabilizer for lumbar surgery patient positioned.

manipulated. The Jackson table was patented in 1992, by to R. P. Jackson, and is also known as an *OSI table*, after the first company to market it (Mizohu OSI, Union City, CA), and it usually supports the patient with the hips flexed about 30 degrees. The Jackson Spinal table has several advantages, which include ease in positioning patients, particularly obese patients where the abdomen can hang free without being compressed. The patient can be tilted as needed for instrumentation, but there have been reports of failure during which a patient was accidently rotated too far and fell from the table [15].

This table offers the ability for rapid reconfiguration for intraoperative x-ray or CT imaging, which is particularly helpful during spine procedures (Figure 23.1). Figure 23.2 shows a model with her face resting in prone positioning pillow, but the head can just as easily be secured in a Mayfield pin apparatus for surgery on the cervical spine. In addition to its advantages for imaging, the table can be raised or lowered on either end and rotated as needed for spinal alignment. It also has a pair of hydraulic lifts that allow the table to be moved into Trendelenberg and reverse Trendelenberg positions.

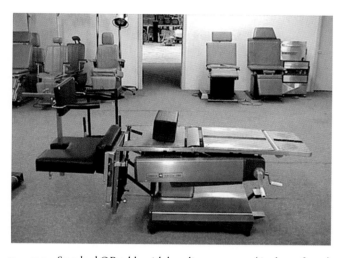

Figure 23.4   Standard OR table with kneeling apparatus (Andrews frame) and hip stabilizer.

ANDREWS FRAME

The Andrews Frame attaches to a conventional operating room table and supports a patient in the kneeling position (Figures 23.3, 23.4, and 23.5). It is designed to support the

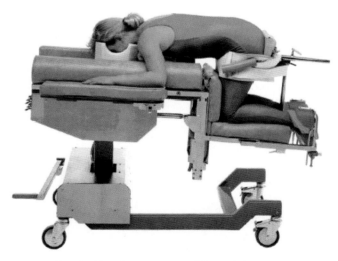

Figure 23.5   Standard kneeling position with hip stabilizer for lumbar surgery patient positioned.

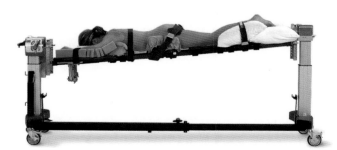

Figure 23.2   Jackson table.

chest and allowing the abdomen to hang free. This improves ventilation and decreases intra-abdominal pressure, which decreases venous pressure and bleeding. Until the patient is secured with thigh support bolsters, there is a significant amount of freedom, which places the patient at risk of sliding from the table during positioning. The pelvis is partially supported and the legs are positioned below the level of the heart, which increases venous stasis. The Andrews Frame does not offer any specific advantage over other positioning devices, and its selection is based on the surgeon's preference.

RELTON-HALL FRAME

The Relton-Hall frame is placed on top of a conventional operating table. It has a generally rectangular base frame, with four vertical posts that are clamped onto the frame and adjustable longitudinally and laterally. Its pads have a 45-degree inward tilt at the top of the vertical posts [24]. The pads are positioned under the anterolateral aspects of the pelvic girdle and under the lateral aspects of the upper thoracic cage as close to the midline as possible. The hips may be flexed up to 60 degrees. Intraoperative x-ray imaging is complicated by the orientation of the metal frame. Although lateral x-rays can be obtained, it is impossible to produce images in the anteroposterior orientation.

WILSON FRAME

The Wilson frame is commonly used to position patients for surgery of the thoracic and lumbar spine. Some studies have found that the Wilson frame is particularly useful for minimally invasive trasnforaminal lumbar interbody fusion (TLIF) procedures because it provides a satisfactory kyphosis and optimizes exposure. Some surgeons believe that it may be essential in these procedures [12] (Figures 23.6 and 23.7).

The Wilson frame has recently been associated with postoperative vision loss. The Postoperative Visual Loss Study Group found that there was a statistically significant increase in the incidence of ischemic optic neuropathy compared with other positioning devices [32]. However in the conclusions it was postulated that the reason the Wilson frame was associated with this increase in morbidity was

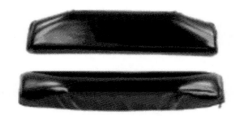

Figure 23.7   Wilson frame without patient.

that the positioning of the head was commonly below the level of the heart, leading to venous congestion. There was no available comparison or mention about repositioning (i.e., reverse Trandelenberg) to compensate for this. In light of this finding, it might be wise to check that patients on the Wilson frame do indeed have the level of the head at or above the level of their heart in insure good drainage.

FOUR-POST FRAME

Four padded bolsters on a Velcro board combined with "egg crate foam" is another option for positioning patients for spine surgery (Figure 23.8). The bolsters can easily be moved around on the Velcro board to accommodate patients with widely varying body habitus and a variety of surgical exposures. This system provides chest and pelvis support while also positioning the patient with good lordosis. It also allows for fluoroscopic examination, decreases abdominal pressure, and is easy to prepare. Two of the bolsters are specifically marked as "chest" and two are marked for "hips"; the chest bolsters are lower and flatter.

POSITIONING FOR SURGERY

SURGERY IN THE SUPINE POSITION

The supine position is the easiest for the anesthesiologists because the need to move the patient, catheters,

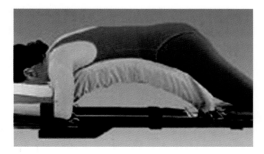

Figure 23.6   Wilson frame with patient positioned.

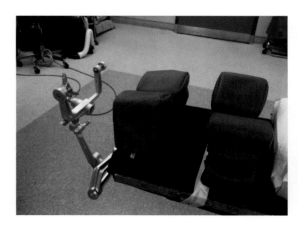

Figure 23.8   Mayfield frame.

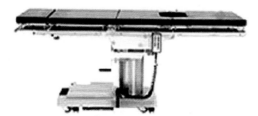

Figure 23.9   SKYTRON 6001 operating room table.

and monitors is minimized. Because anesthesia is usually induced in the supine position, the patient is awake during transfer. There are, however, important safety concerns.

The bed must be locked and capable of supporting the patient irrespective of how the base is positioned (Figure 23.9).

If the patient is not able to position him or herself (e.g., due to frailty, injury, pain, or paralysis), then assistance should be obtained from the nursing and surgical teams. Particularly for obese patients or those who are at risk for a spine injury, the use of a log roll with a roller board should be considered. If the cervical spine is unstable, then, the neurosurgeon may wish to control the neck. Patients with an unstable thoracic or lumbar spine should be transferred slow, gentle, and coordinated movements to minimize the risk of injury. If the patient is intubated, it is usually safest to disconnect the circuit before moving to minimize the risk of inadvertent extubation. Nearly all operating room tables and arm boards are built with foam padding over radiolucent risers. No additional cushioning is required for the supine patient except for a pillow under the head. For long procedures, pillows should be placed under the knees to slightly flex them, and heel pads should be considered.

When surgical procedure is near the face (e.g., for anterior cervical surgery) the patient's eyes may require additional protection with goggles or by placing a Mayo stand over the face.

Patients who are in the supine position are at high risk of injury to the arms leading to a malpractice lawsuit. Arms positioned at patient's side should be padded with foam around the ulnar prominence to protect the ulnar nerve. Poles rising from clamps on the bed rails should be positioned so that they are not pressing against any limb, and padding should be placed between such supports and the patient if there is any chance of movement during the procedure (e.g., pressure on the humerus can injure the radial nerve) (Figure 23.10). Sheets used to tuck the arms at the side should be secure so that the arm does not fall during the procedure. The draw sheet should also not be so tight as to inhibit venous return and flow through intravenous tubing, which can cause infiltration or venous congestion. Positioning the arms of obese patients may require a "sled" (Wells Arm Protector) board to minimize the risk of movement (see Figure 23.11).

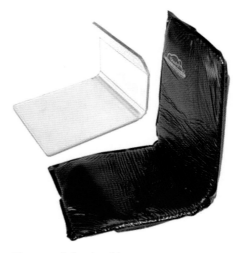

Figure 23.10   Plexi-arm sled and padding.

If the arms will be positioned away from the body, rotation should not exceed 90 degrees, particularly if the head is turned in the opposite direction. Overextending the arms may cause stretch injury of the brachial plexus. Hands resting on arm boards should be in neutral position or pronation whenever feasible.

The patient should also be positioned so as to support the natural lumbosacral curve. Placing a pillow under the knees will place the lumbar spine in a relatively neutral position. The patient's legs or ankles should not be crossed because this can cause venous compression and may cause pressure necrosis in a prolonged procedure. Legs should be protected with heel pads and sequential compression devices if they are not contraindicated.

The most common procedures performed on patients in the supine position anterior cervical spine surgery, subdural hematoma drainage, and transphenoidal pituitary resection. If the head can be turned, surgical procedures may include a transoral or retropharyngeal approach, suboccipital craniectomy, and intracranial surgery. For these procedures, however, the head is usually supported with a horseshoe head rest, the Mayfield pins, or Gardner-Wells tongs (Figure 23.12).

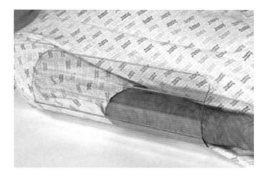

Figure 23.11   Plexi arm sled in position.

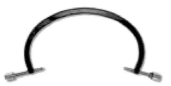

Figure 23.12   Gardner-Wells tongs.

Although the majority of these devices are applied after the induction of anesthesia, patients with an unstable spine require special consideration.

SURGERY IN THE PRONE POSITION

Many neurosurgical procedures require that the patient be placed in the prone position. Although the specific technique and apparatus varies with institutional preference, proper planning is essential to avoid unnecessary complications. Most patients are positioned using some type of frame or padded bolsters with the patient's arms placed above the head or at the sides.

Patients who will be in the prone position for surgery should be induced on a stretcher and positioned only after the endotracheal tube, intravenous catheters, and intra-arterial catheters are secured. Additional intravenous access beyond that which was required for induction should be considered to assure adequate access even if one catheter is lost during or after positioning. The decision to obtain additional access should take into account that it might be impossible after patient is positioned and draped.

Airway management presents additional concerns in patients who will be prone. The patient's head should be kept in a neutral position, avoiding extremes of extension, flexion, and rotation. The endotracheal tube should be positioned so that it will not migrate into a bronchus during flexion and will not move out of the trachea during extension. Most importantly, the endotracheal tube must be painstakingly secured so that it will not fall out during surgery. This can usually be accomplished with plastic tape and an adhesive such as Mastisol or benzoin. The tape should be protected while the surgeons are scrubbing the head and neck to prevent prep solution from wetting the tape. In general, applying tape circumferentially around the neck is not acceptable. It may be difficult to tape the endotracheal tube in a patient with a bushy beard, so the possibility of partially shaving the beard should be discussed with the patient before surgery.

After the airway and vascular access have been secured, the next step is to attach electrodes for neuromuscular (SSEP or motors) monitoring if appropriate. If motor evoked potentials are planned, a bite block consisting of a soft, rolled up 4 × 4 gauze pad should be placed into the mouth before positioning, taking care to make sure the tongue cannot be bitten when the jaw is stimulated.

The head holder should be attached while the patient is monitored and only after adequate anesthesia has been assured.

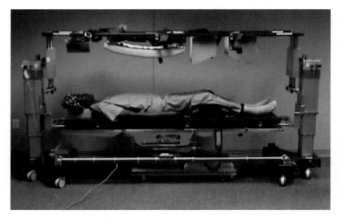

Figure 23.13   The Revolution System. In step 1, the patient is supine on the operating room table.

If a pillow is used to support the patient's face, hard goggles should be used or the eyes should be checked frequently during the procedure. If a prone positioning pillow is to be used, the anesthesiologist should check the face for pressure points and verify that the eyes are free; no additional eye protection is necessary aside from customary tape if the head is secured in a Mayfield frame. Before moving the patient, the operating room table should be at its lowest position and locked in order to minimize the risk of injury to staff and to prevent the table from moving during positioning. The stretcher should be positioned slightly above the table so that the patient is going downhill. Support apparatus, if used, should be securely attached to the table. Neurophysiologic monitoring electrodes should be disconnected and the wires gathered and secured to patient to prevent them from being pulled out. Intravenous tubing should also be disconnected, capped, and taped to the patients so they can be easily found and accessed after positioning the patient.

Several commercial devices can be used mechanically place the patient into the prone position. One such device is "The Revolution" system by Patient Safety Transport Systems, LLC [28]. However, most institutions still use manual techniques (Figures 23.13, 23.14, 23.15, 23.16, 23.17, and 23.18).

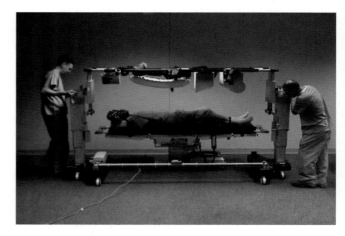

Figure 23.14   The Revolution System. In step 2, the device is lined up above the patient and lowered down onto him.

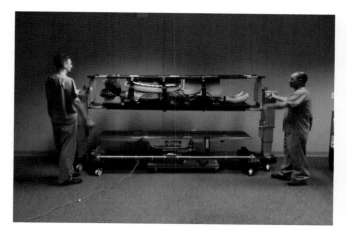

Figure 23.15   The Revolution System. In step 3, the upper and lower portions are secured and the patient is elevated above the operating room table.

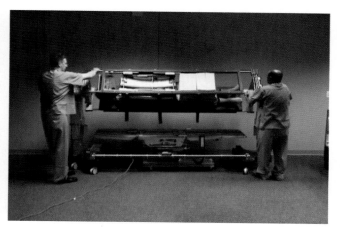

Figure 23.18   The Revolution System® the patient is lowered on the operating room table, the straps are released, the arms are positioned and the apparatus is raised up and removed.

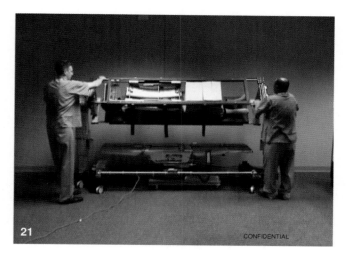

Figure 23.16   The Revolution System. In step 4, the patient is rotated.

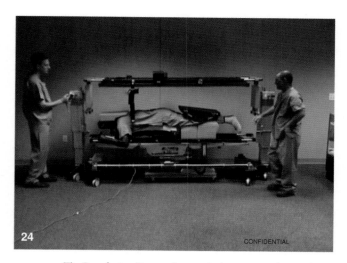

Figure 23.17   The Revolution System. In step 5, the patient is lowered onto the operating room table, the straps are released, the arms are positioned, and the apparatus is raised up and removed.

An organized group approach with an adequate number of assistants is essential to insure safety for the patient and the operating room team. There should be two or three assistants on the side of the table who are ready to receive the patient, two assistants on the side of the stretcher to roll the patient over to the receivers, and one person to guide the legs.

The breathing circuit should be disconnected from the endotracheal tube when the patient is ready for transfer. The anesthesiologist or neurosurgeon should be holding the head, directing the team, and counting so that the patient is moved smoothly. After the patient has been turned and is being held by the receivers, the endotracheal tube can be reconnected. After the position of the tube is confirmed by auscultation and capnography, the stretcher can be moved away from the table. The patient can now be placed in the final surgical position. The patient is adjusted under the collaborative direction of the neurosurgeon and anesthesiologist. The stretcher should remain either in the operating room or in the hallway but should be readily accessible so that in the patient can be turned to the supine position in an emergency.

The arms can be positioned either at the patient's sides or extended above the head. In general, the patient's arms are positioned in the extended position above the head for surgical procedures involving the lumbar or sacral levels of the spinal cord. The arms are usually positioned at the patient's sides for surgical procedures that involve the head or upper thoracic or cervical spine. The arms should not be allowed to fall from the table at any time as this may lead to brachial plexus injury. If the arms are to be placed on arm boards, they should be placed at the sides first, and then gently rotated onto the arm boards. The arms should be positioned in gentle abduction and extension of the upper arm with flexion of the elbow. The arms should not be positioned in extreme lateral hyper abduction; this will injure the capsule of the shoulder joint. The shoulder girdle should feel loose and never so taut as to appear to be stretching to reach 90 degrees. In that patient with a "frozen shoulder" caused by arthritis or previous surgery, it is best to leave the arms tucked at the side rather than trying to position them upward. Arms should be positioned slightly ventral in order to avoid traction on the brachial plexus. This may require that some padding be removed from the arm boards. If the arms are to be positioned at the patient's side, padding should be placed around bony prominences, especially at the elbow. If there is a need for iliac access, the arms can be tucked at the sides with a sheet, pillowcase, or surgical towel. Otherwise, one sheet can be drawn across the patient's back and the ends brought under the arms and back to midline. This will securely cradle the arms in a slightly ventral position.

After the airway and extremities have been secured, the chest and hips should be checked for pressure points and adequate support. The abdomen should be free, especially in overweight patients who have a pannus. This will ensure adequate ventilation and minimize venous bleeding. Male genitalia should be free of pressure points. Nipples and female breasts should be tucked between supports while trying to avoid direct pressure. In those who have had breast enhancement surgery, chest supports are ideally placed laterally and superior to the implants, but extended periods of pressure may still cause injury. The Concorde modification of the prone positioning is used primarily for intracranial surgery. The head is flexed and higher than the heart with arms positioned at the sides.

Some neurosurgeons may request that the airway be secured before induction in a patient who is undergoing surgery in the prone position and who has an unstable spine. The patient may then be asked assist with positioning, turning him- or herself prone and then testing to verify that the patient is neurologically intact before anesthesia is induced. This may also be an alternative in the obese patient for whom positioning under anesthesia could be challenging; one study has found it to be safe with a low risk of morbidity [11].

The knee-chest (kneeling) position is still occasionally used, but it is falling out of favor for several reasons. Although the patient is in a stable position, excessive pressure on the patient's knees may cause injury. This position also seems to produce a restrictive respiratory pattern (despite the fact that there is no pressure on the abdomen) that has caused many care teams to select alternative positions [14, 29].

The Concorde position involves placing the patient into the prone position while elevating the head. This position is commonly used for procedures on the cervical and upper thoracic spine because it permits good surgical access while also allowing venous drainage. The patient typically lies on chest rolls with the head secured in Mayfield pins. A restraining strap is secured under the buttocks and anchored to the table in a cephalad direction in order to keep the patient from sliding downward [25].

The lateral position is used for temporal craniotomy and sometimes for thoracic spine procedures, but only in patients who do not have an unstable spine. A *bean bag positioner* is a soft airtight bag filled with small plastic beads that becomes rigid when evacuated and is frequently placed on the operating room. table before the patient is moved on to it. A gel pad may also be placed on top of the beanbag for added padding. The head can be secured with a Mayfield apparatus, a padded horseshoe support, or with a foam pillow. The head should be positioned in a neutral position, facing in the anterior direction or slightly turned. The neck should be supple and in a neutral position. Excessive flexion can cause brachial plexus injury, particularly if there is any traction on the superior shoulder to aid surgical exposure. If a pillow or foam head rest is used, there should be no direct pressure on the ear because pressure necrosis may occur during prolonged surgery.

Turning the patient to the lateral position is a cooperative effort that involves the anesthesia, surgical, and nursing staff. The patient should be positioned only after the airway and intravenous and arterial catheters have been inserted and secured. The patient is typically turned by lifting the draw sheet. The patient is moved laterally to the side of the table corresponding to the side that will eventually be up, and then rolled over into position. is the person responsible for the movement and safety of the patients head (either the anesthesiologist or the neurosurgeon) should be directing the move. Once the patient is in the lateral position, his or her head, shoulders and upper thorax should be lifted an "axillary roll" should be placed several fingerbreadths below the axilla. This will protect the brachial plexus and the deltoid muscle. The upper arm can be supported with an armrest, a padded Mayo stand, or a pillow. The lower arm is typically placed on a padded arm board. The legs should be in a neutral position, slightly flexed, and well padded with foam or pillows. The common peroneal nerve is especially susceptible to injury because it lies at the neck of the fibula. In general, the lower leg is bent and the upper is straight to provide greater stability and prevent the patient from rocking from side to side. After positioning is satisfactory and all pressure points are padded, suction is applied to the bean bag, which forms a rigid cast to hold the patient in place. Lastly, the patient should be secured with straps or wide tape.

THE SITTING POSITION

The sitting, "park bench," and "lawn chair" positions are no longer frequently used but may be appropriate for surgery on the occipital area, the most posterior part of the cerebral hemisphere or of the posterior cranial fossa. Besides offering superior surgical exposure, the advantages of the sitting position include decreased venous pressure, which decreases bleeding, better decompression of the brain, improved drainage of CSF from and surgical site, and better ventilation. The sitting position offers unique challenges, including fatigue (because the surgeon must keep his or her hands elevated throughout the case), increased risk of postoperative hematomas, and mid-cervical quadriplegia from sitting and hypotension. This position carries the risk of causing significant complications and patient injury.

Patients undergoing surgery in the sitting position are usually receiving general endotracheal anesthesia. The primary advantage of this position for the anesthesiologist is that patients usually have lower airway pressure because there is less pressure on the diaphragm from abdominal contents. Because access to the airway during the procedure is extremely limited, repositioning or replacement of the endotracheal tube will be difficult or impossible. The tube should be well secured to the patient, and the breathing circuit should be supported so that there are no external forces on the tube.

The sitting position may cause hypotension and cardiovascular instability, and significant postural hypotension may occur, especially while the patient is being positioned. Even when sequential compression devices or surgical stockings are used, blood will pool in the lower extremities, which can reduce systemic arterial blood pressure and cerebral perfusion. Moreover, the sitting position is associated with an increase in the pulmonary and systemic vascular resistance [2, 3]. Surgical manipulation of the cranial nerves or brainstem can induce sudden changes in heart rate, including bradycardia or asystole, dysrhythmias, or arterial hypotension or hypertension.

After the patient has been placed in the sitting position, special attention should be placed on protecting and padding the boney prominences; particularly before a prolonged surgical procedure. The arms should be supported in order to prevent the brachial plexus from injury due to stretch. The ulnar nerve should be padded to prevent compression. The knees should also be slightly flexed to prevent excessive stretching of the sciatic nerve. The arms or knees should not be allowed to rest against the head-holding frame, and the feet should be in medium dorsiflexion.

Monitoring the patient in sitting position poses unique challenges. The transducer attached to the intra-arterial catheter is typically placed at the level of the right atrium in the supine patient. In the sitting patient, however, the transducer should be placed at the external auditory meatus so that it accurately reflects the pressure at the circle of Willis and provides the best indication of cerebral perfusion pressure. If the blood pressure is measured with a cuff, a correction factor of 7.7 mm Hg should be subtracted for every 10 cm of vertical distance between the external auditory meatus and the cuff. Management of blood pressure when the head is located a significant distance above the heart is critical because cerebral oxygenation in the beach-chair position has been show to be significantly reduced as compared with the lateral or supine positions [30]. Although there are no evidence-based guidelines, a panel of experts has recently recommended that mean arterial pressure be maintained in the range of 80 mm for these patients [13].

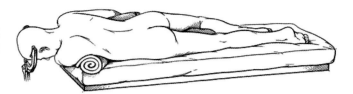

Figure 23.19   Three-quarters prone.

Venous air embolism (VAE) can occur during any surgical procedure in which the operative site is located above the heart, and patients in the sitting position are particularly susceptible to this complication. The key to managing VAE is to maintain a high suspicion, vigilant monitoring, and rapid intervention. This complication is discussed in depth later in this chapter.

The three-quarters prone or semiprone, lateral prone, or posttonsillectomy position is commonly used for posteriolateral cranial surgical approaches, and many of the issues surrounding this position combine those of the prone, lateral, and supine positions (Figure 23.19).

The patient can be induced in the supine position on a stretcher. A standard operating room table is used for the surgery, and positioning is usually facilitated with a beanbag patient positioner and a gel pad. After the airway, intravenous catheters, and all monitors have been secured, the head is placed into the headholder (frequently the Mayfield system). The head of the table is removed to accommodate the Mayfield apparatus. A draw sheet is then used to slide the patient to the right or left edge of the table, after which the patient is turned semiprone An arm board can be secured on top of the Mayfield support rods so as to support the downward arm. The head is secured in position with the Mayfield headholder. The hips should be slightly twisted so that the downward leg is straight and the upward leg is bent and padded to rest on a cushioned operating room table. The patient is stabilized with the beanbag and with tape and surgical towels to prevent movement. All pressure points, particularly the lower iliac crest, can then be padded. Depending on the patient's body habitus, there may or may not be a need for an axillary roll as the downward arm being is being cradled in a transom and might not be pressing against the brachial plexus. As with other positioning techniques, a plan should be made to access the airway and intravenous catheters if necessary and to intervene in an emergency. Intravenous access is usually not problematic as the upper arm is readily accessible.

COMPLICATIONS

SOFT TISSUE INJURIES

Although pressure injury may occur any time a patient is immobilized for a prolonged period, the length of cranial and neurospine procedures increases the risk of pressure necrosis. Repositioning is not feasible during these procedures, so the best way to decrease the risk of soft tissue injury is to adequately pad the patient and to distribute the patient's weight evenly. As has already been discussed, using a gel pad under the patient can help to cushion and distribute weight. Patients should be examined before positioning, and any skin breaks or soft tissue injury should be noted ahead of time. This is particularly important in elderly patients, those on chronic steroids, and those who have lost a significant amount of weight, leaving integument support structure more susceptible to trauma.

The endotracheal tube should not be pulled to the corner of the mouth, because this may cause pressure necrosis of the lips. A soft gauze pad may be rolled and placed between jaws to protect the patient against lip injury and from biting on endotracheal tube, tongue, or cheek during motor stimulation. Nasogastric and feeding tubes should also not be affixed tightly to the mucosa because this may also impair circulation and cause injury.

NEUROPATHY

Poor positioning of the upper extremities is associated with brachial plexus injury and also ulnar, median, and radial nerve injury. The American Society of Anesthesiologists' Closed Claims Study found 670 cases of 4183 claims (16%) of anesthesia-related nerve injury. Of those, ulnar nerve injury occurred in 28%, brachial plexus injury occurred in 20%, lumbrosacral nerve root occurred in 16%, and the spinal cord was injured in 13%. Of the ulnar nerve injuries, the majority (85%) was associated with general anesthesia. Although these data were not gathered in neurosurgical patients, it does highlight the need to carefully position the extremities [1].

The brachial plexus can easily be stretched to the point of injury in the anesthetized patient. Inadvertently dropping an arm in any position can cause permanent damage as can turning the head in the opposite direction while the patient is supine or dropping the head downward in the lateral position. This is exacerbated by applying downward traction to the arm and shoulder. In the lateral position, a roll should be placed under the axilla to relieve pressure from adjacent structures.

Some data suggests that monitoring the ulnar nerve with SSEPs may help to identify and avoid upper extremity nerve injuries when a patient is in the prone position [18]. In the prone patient, the arm should not be abducted more that 90 degrees and the elbows should be bent. In the supine patient arms should be at least 6 inches above the table. The use of clear drapes and frequent examination and repositioning (if feasible) is recommended to avoid injury [19].

The ulnar nerve can be damaged or sustain injury in the prone patient if the arms are raised above the head or if the elbows are allowed to rest on the edge of the mattress. The ulnar nerve can also be injured in the supine patient if the elbows or the lower humeral head are allowed to rest against the edge of the mattress.

The radial nerve travels in a spiral rotation around the humerus. If the humerus of a supine patient is pressed against an anesthesia screen, nerve injury could result in paresthesias.

Pressure against the inside of the tibial tuberosity can compress the saphenous nerve, while pressure on the outside of the tibial tuberosity will cause damage to the common peroneal nerve. The legs should not be crossed as this can cause long-term peroneal nerve damage, nor should legs be rotated or stretched as this can cause sciatic nerve damage. Last, padding of heels is recommended even in relatively short cases as break can easily occur.

EYE INJURIES

The unique positioning requirements and length of neurosurgical cases increase the risk of eye injury and postoperative visual loss. The patient's eyes should be closed and secured as soon as feasible after induction of anesthesia. (Some neurovascular surgeons routinely check the pupils after the patient is positioned.) The eye can be injured during airway management, placement of neurophysiologic monitors, and positioning. Skin preparation solutions can flow into the eyes, causing a chemical burn. If the patient will be in the supine position (e.g., for a procedure involving the anterior cervical spine) protective hard goggles can be used to protect the eyes against instruments that are placed on drapes that cover the face.

In the prone position, no pressure should be placed on the globes. Whenever feasible, the patient's head should be checked during the procedure in case the head or a positioning device has shifted. One way to ensure that there is no pressure on the eyes is to use a Mayfield positioning system. Although the risk of infection at the pin sites is exceedingly low, bleeding and cosmetically undesirable scars are not uncommon. Moreover, pins can slip or the device can fail, causing abrupt and possibly life-threatening head movement.

If a positioning pillow will be used, it should be placed over the patient while supine, so that the openings can be properly aligned and the endotracheal tube placed into its own opening before the patient is turned. There are several devices that offer a padded surface that position the patient's head above a mirror. This allows the face to be seen throughout the procedure, the anesthesiologist can then verify that the airway is secure and that there is no pressure on the globes. No single method has been found to be significantly better than the other, so to the positioning technique is usually driven by local practice, but vigilance is important, as is the understanding that no method is totally without its risks.

Ischemic optic neuritis (fully discussed in Chapter 20) is a rare but devastating complication that may involve one or both eyes and may result in partial or complete blindness.

The etiology of postoperative blindness in nonocular surgery is still not totally clear. The incidence is reported to be 0.0008% but it rises to 0.11% after cardiac surgery and 0.08% after spine surgery. In 26 cases of ischemic optic neuritis following spine surgery a MEDLINE search revealed most of the cases involved the posterior ION (PION) ($n = 17$) and remainder were anterior (AION, $n = 5$) [10, 17]. Although the precise etiology remains unclear, a combination of prolonged surgery, perioperative anemia, fluid resuscitation with large amounts of intravenous crystalloid, arterial hypotension and decreased intraocular perfusion pressure, preexisting arteriosclerosis, and prone positioning were potential factors of postoperative vision loss [16].

VENOUS AIR EMBOLISM

VAE occurs when air enters the circulation through open bridging veins in the cranium and through large venous sinuses when venous pressure is lower than atmospheric pressure. The air then travels through the venous system the heart, where it can continue to the pulmonary arteries or create an "air-lock" in the right ventricle. Right heart strain may cause arrhythmias and massive ventricular dilatation. Because the lungs are not perfused, dead space is dramatically increased, which results in profound hypoxia. Cardiac output is decreased, causing systemic hypotension that may progress to cardiovascular collapse. Paradoxical air embolism can produce bubbles that lodge in the cerebral blood vessels (causing a stroke) or in the coronary arteries (causing myocardial ischemia). Additional complications of VAE include thrombocytopenia [31].

Although patients undergoing surgery in the sitting position are at increased risk for venous air embolism, VAE can occur whenever the operative site is above the level of the heart. The likelihood of VAE is higher during neurosurgical procedures because of open venous channels such as those in the skull. VAE can occur during application of the Mayfield pins because the holes that they produce in the bony cortex can provide an opportunity for air entrainment. For this reason, antibiotic ointment is usually placed onto the skull pins so as to create an airtight seal.

Air entrainment can be slow and insidious or rapid. A small, continuous stream of air bubbles may enter the venous system and become distributed throughout the lung, causing an inflammatory response while increasing dead space and causing hypoxia. Air may also cross into the systemic circulation through a patent foramen ovale or through the pulmonary vasculature, causing micro inflammation and ischemia. As more air is entrained, pulmonary hypertension, hypoxemia, and impaired gas exchange eventually result. Rapid air entrainment can rapidly lead to cardiovascular collapse via two mechanisms. An air lock in the right atrium will cause right atrial pressure to rise and left atrial pressure to fall. Air can also to migrate into the arterial circulation. In those patients who entrain air and have a patent foramen ovale or VSD, air can enter the systemic circulation, resulting in ischemia in the heart or brain.

The patient is at risk for VAE any time the surgical incision will be located above the heart or any time surgery involves a venous complex. The anesthesiologist should have a high index of suspicion for VAE and should formulate a plan for diagnosis and management. Transesophageal echocardiography has the highest sensitivity for detection of VAE because it will show even tiny bubbles. It is not feasible, however, to insert a TEE in most neurosurgical patients. Moreover, the display must be monitored continuously. Precordial Doppler monitoring is a sensitive technique for the detection of VAE. Moreover, it is noninvasive and does not require continuous observation. The Doppler probe is placed over the right border at the third or fourth intercostal space. When the probe is positioned correctly, blood flow through the heart will be heard on the loudspeaker. Partially filling a syringe with sterile saline solution, shaking it to create microscopic bubbles, and then rapidly injecting it into an intravenous catheter will simulate a VAE. A characteristic murmur or distinct change in tones is an indication that air bubbles are being entrained. The least sensitive monitor is end tidal nitrogen in a patient who is breathing only oxygen or nitrous oxide. The presence of end tidal nitrogen then indicates room air entrainment. This technique is rarely feasible, however, because it requires that a mass spectrometer be used to analyze the respiratory gases; few commercially available monitors offer this option. If no specific monitoring is being used, a sudden, rapid drop in $ETco_2$, combined with hypotension and an elevated $Paco_2$ is consistent with VAE.

If VAE is suspected, the first response should be to alert the surgeons and ask them to flood the field with saline, which should always be available. If large areas of cranium are exposed, bone wax should be applied to all open bone edges. The operative site should be covered with wet sponges and the operating room table should be positioned in Trendelenberg to increase venous pressure relative to atmosphere. If at all possible patient should be positioned with left side down (closest to the operating room pads). This will help to prevent air in the right side of the heart to eject out the pulmonary arteries. If a central venous catheter is present, it should be vigorously aspirated for air and continue to do so until no further air can be obtained. Depending on the volume of air entrained, systemic pressures can fall due to an air lock. Aggressive fluid resuscitation is recommended as well as increasing the Fio_2 to 100% to help oxygenation with increased dead space. In the most catastrophic scenarios, cardiopulmonary bypass may be considered. However, the time to arrange such treatment of such physiologic derangement would probably be too late. Although personal experience suggests that conservative management with repositioning and aspiration has been sufficient, there is no way to immediately assess the magnitude of the embolus and therefore it is recommended to have all modalities available.

SPECIAL ISSUES

OBESITY

Obese patients are difficult to position correctly, may have increased operative time, and are more likely to experience complications related to positioning. Obese patients may also have a variety of comorbidities that are exacerbated by positioning and by the neurosurgical procedure itself. Common concerns include diabetes, which can cause skin breakdown, pulmonary insufficiency, and sleep apnea. The obese patient will be difficult to move and position and safely (for both patient and staff), and heavy extremities may fall unobserved while positioning the patient or during the procedure [11].

Sedation should be used sparingly if at all so that the patient can assist with transfer if necessary. Correct positioning during anesthetic induction and airway management is critical. When the obese or nonobese patient is supine, there can be as much as a 10% to 40% decreases in FRC; FRC in the obese patient may already be below the closing capacity.

Positioning of the head is guided by nonmobile structures such as the ears. If the patient will be supine, a gel pad under the head, particularly during long procedure, may minimize the risk of pressure alopecia. If the head will be secured to the table, the angle of the neck should be compared with bony structures because in-line or neutral positioning may otherwise not be obvious. If patient is supine, generous padding is recommended, particularly under bony prominences. Should the patient be lateral position, an axillary roll of sufficient size should be placed to reduce weight on shoulder and brachial plexus [20].

If the patient will be in the prone position, accommodation must be made to allow the abdomen to hang free. This will allow displacement of abdomen during inspiration and also keep pressure off of the vena cava and aorta. Ventilation and cardiovascular function is usually well preserved in the obese, prone patient so long as the upper chest and pelvis are well supported and the abdomen is unloaded [21, 22]. If a patient is on egg crate foam padding a hole should be made underneath the abdomen. In the prone position, alignment of the head neck and spine is best done with bony structures. The anterior aspects of thighs of patients in the prone position must also be padded. If a Jackson table will be used, the thigh rests and anterior tibial rests must be in correctly positioned. Transposing them will put all the support on the anterior thighs, which could lead to severe pressure necrosis.

BREAST IMPLANTS

Proper positioning of the patient with either breast implants or breast reconstruction after mastectomy is essential to avoid disfiguring injury. Although a variety of procedures and materials are in current use, the principles are constant; less pressure directly on the implants (or natural breasts) is better. Bolsters should be placed under the clavicle and lateral to the breasts. The breasts should be tucked inward (medially) and cephalad with as little direct contact as possible. Although some older publications suggest that breasts be positioned outward, this causes direct pressure and stretching that can cause tearing, ecchymosis, and postoperative pain. In all circumstances (both male and female), the nipples should be free from direct pressure, because this can also lead to necrosis.

THE PATIENT WITH AN UNSTABLE CERVICAL SPINE

Maintaining alignment of the cervical spine is absolutely critical in the presence of a fracture, ligamentous injury, or other reason to suspect instability. If the patient must be turned to the prone position, the movement should be as smooth as possible. If the patient arrives in the operating room with a cervical collar in place, he or she should be assumed to have an unstable cervical spine. Multiple assistants are essential in order to move the patient's head and body as a single unit, and the turn is directed by the physician who is controlling the head and neck should direct the turn. If possible, the collar should be replaced after airway management is complete and removed only after the patient is in the final surgical position. Leaving the collar in place during surgery can lead to a surgical site infection, skin injury due to pressure or a chemical burn (inform pooled prep solution), venous congestion and inability to assess if neck is properly positioned through out the procedure. At the end of the procedure, the decision as to whether to replace the collar usually rests with the surgeon.

PATIENTS WITH INTRAVASCULAR COOLING DEVICES (COOLGUARD)

Intravascular cooling devices are used both for prevention and as treatment of brain ischemia. This device is inserted in the femoral vein as is a central line and directly cools the circulating blood. If a patient with this catheter must be placed in the prone position, the line should be adjusted so that there is no kinking and the cooled fluid can flow freely through the catheter. If the patient is positioned on bolsters, they should be checked to make sure they are on the anterior iliac crest and not compressing the insertion site of the cooling line.

CONCLUSIONS

Surgery for neurological procedures tends to require positions other than the straight-forward supine position.

Anatomical and physiological considerations must be carefully assessed as they can easily render a successful operation a disaster riddled with complications. The time length of neurosurgical procedures and the fact most of the patient is covered in drapes makes the initial plan and survey even more paramount. Even with the best of forethought periodic evaluation is mandatory and as feasible re-positioning encourage.

REFERENCES

1. Cheney FW, et al. Nerve Injury associated with anesthesia: a closed clams analysis. *Anethesiology*. 1999;90:1062–1069.
2. Dutton A, The effects of posture during anesthesia *J Calif West Med*. 1933;37:145–150.
3. Backofen JE, Schauble JF. Hemodynamic changes with prone positioning during general anesthesia. *Anesth Analg*. 1995;64:194.
4. Wadsworth R, et al. The effect of four different surgical positions on cardiovascular parameters in healthy volunteers. *Anaesthesia*. 1966;51:819–822.
5. Sudheer PS, et al. Hemodynamic effects of the prone position: a comparison of proprofol total intravenous and inhalation anesthesia. *Anaesthesia*. 2006;61:138–141.
6. Pelosi P, et al. Prone positioning improves pulmonary function in obese patients during general anesthesia. *Anesth Analg*. 1996;83:578–583.
7. Nyren S, et al. Pulmonary perfusion is more uniform in the prone than in the supine position; scintigraphy in healthy humans. *J Appl Physiol*. 1999;86:1135–1141.
8. Dharmavaram S, et al. Effect of prone positioning systems on hemodynamic and cardiac function during lumbar spine surgery: an echocardiographic study. *Spine*. 2006;31:1388–1393
9. American Society of Anesthesiologists Task Force on Perioperative Blindness. Practice advisory for perioperative visual loss associated with spine surgery: American Society of Anesthesiologists, Chicago, Ill. 1997.
10. Baig MN, et al. Vision loss after spine surgery; review of the literature and recommendations. *Neurosurg Focus*. 2007;23:E1.
11. Wu SD, Yilmaz M, et al. Awake endotracheal intubation and prone patient self-positioning; anesthetic and positioning considerations during percutaneous nephrolithotomy in obese patients. *J Endourol*. 2009;23:1599–1602.
12. Cardoso MJ, Rosner MK. Does the Wilson frame assist with optimizating surgical exposure for minimally invasive lumbar fusion? *Neurosurg Focus*. 2010;28:E20.
13. Lee L, Caplan R. APSF Workshop: Cerebral perfusion experts share views on management of head-up cases. *Newsl Anesth Patient Safety Found*. 1997;24:45–68.
14. Yilmaz C, Buyrukcu SO, et al. Lumbar microdiscectomy with spinal anesthesia; comparison of prone and knee-chest positions in means of hemodynamic and respiratory function. *Spine*. 2010;35:1176–1184
15. Dauber MH, Roth S. Case report: Operating table failure; another hazard of spine surgery. *Anesth Analg*. 2009;108:904–905.
16. Ho VTG, Newman NJ, et al. Ischemic optic neuropathy following spine surgery. *J Neurosurg Anesthesiol*. 2005;17:38–44.
17. Shen Y, Drum M, Roth S. The prevalence of perioperative visual loss in the United States: A 10-year study from 1996 to 2005 of spinal, orthopedic, cardiac, and general surgery. *Anesth Analg*. 2009;109:1534–1545.
18. Schwartz DM, Drummond DS, Hahn M, et al. Prevention of positional brachial plexopathy during surgical correction of scoliosis. *J Spinal Disord*. 2000;13:178–182.
19. Uribe JS, Kolla J, Omar H, et al. Brachial plexus injury following spinal surgery: A review. *J Neurosurg Spine*. 2010;13:552–558.
20. Brodsky JB. Positioning the morbidly obese patient for anesthesia: A review. *Obes Surg*. 2002;12:751–758.
21. Mure M, Domino KB, Lindhahl SG, at al. Regional ventilation-perfusion distribution is more uniform in the prone position. *J Appl Physiol*. 2000;88:1076–1083.
22. Pelosi P. Corri M. Calappi E, et al. The prone position during general anesthesia minimally affects reparatory mechanics while improving functional residual capacity and increasing oxygen tension. *Anesh Analg*. 1995;80:955–960.
23. Matsushita K, Inoue N, et al. Postoperative pressure-induced alopecia after segmental osteotomy at the upper and lower frontal edentulous areas from distraction osteogenesis. *Oral Maxillofac Surg*. 2010 May 9. [Epub ahead of print]
24. Guanciale C, et al. Chest rolls for positioning in spinal surgery. *Spine*. 1996;21:964.
25. Anderton JM, Keen RI, Neave R. *Positioning the surgical patient*. New York: Butterworths; 1988.
26. Martin JT, Warner MA. *Positioning in anesthesia and surgery* (3rd ed.). Philadelphia: WB Saunders; 1997.
27. Akavipat P, Mett P. Does reploading with colloids prevent hemodynamic changes when neurosurgical patients are subsequently changed to the seated position? *J Med Assoc Thai*. 2005;88:247–251.
28. Personal communications and photos provided by operating room Safety Inc., d/b/a The Revolution. Sales and support information, Berwyn, Pa.
29. Rigamonti A, Gemma M, Rocca A, et al. Prone versus knee-chest position for microdiscectomy; a prospective randomized study of intra-abdominal pressure and intraoperative bleeding. *Spine*. 2005;30:1918–1923.
30. Murphy GS, Szokol JW, Marymount JH, et al. Cerebral oxygen desaturation events assessed by near-infrared spectroscopy during shoulder arthroscopy in the beach chair and lateral decubitus positions. *Anesth Analg*. 2010;111:496–505.
31. Schafer St, Sandalcioglu IE, et al. Venous air embolism during semi-sitting craniotomy evokes thrombocytopenia. *Anaesthesia*. 2011;66:25–30.
32. Lee LA, Roth S, et al. The Postoperative Visual Loss Study Group. *Anesthesiology*, 2012;116.

24.

AIRWAY MANAGEMENT FOR THE PATIENT WITH AN UNSTABLE CERVICAL SPINE

Eric A. Harris

INTRODUCTION

Cervical spine injury (CSI) continues to be a leading cause of morbidity and mortality in the developed world. Recent epidemiological studies indicate that cervical spine injuries accompany 1.8% [1] to 4% [2] of blunt trauma injuries and cause an estimated 6000 deaths and 5000 new cases of quadriplegia per year [3]. The incidence of CSI increases to 7.3% when the patient presents with a Glasgow Coma Scale (GCS) score of less than 8 [4]; 80% of the cases occur in patients between the ages of 18 and 24 (predominantly automobile, diving, and contact sports related injuries) and men present with CSI four times more frequently than women. Nearly half of the patients with significant CSI die at the scene of the injury [5], while 50% of motor vehicle patients with CSI and 90% of sport injury patients with CSI will become quadriplegic [6]. It is encouraging to note that less than 5% of severe CSIs secondary to automobile accidents occur in patients restrained with safety belts [7], but the continued lack of motorcycle and bicyclist helmet laws in many states ensures a steady stream of patients with CSI (currently only 20 states and the District of Columbia require all motorcyclists to wear a helmet [8]. Between 10% [9] and 32.3% [10] of these patients require endotracheal intubation within 30 minutes of arrival to the emergency department. It is therefore critical that anesthesiologists, who are often one of the primary care providers for these patients, can manage an airway that may exist in delicate balance with a cervical spine lesion.

Airway management in this patient population requires an understanding of the anatomy of the cervical spine and the underlying injury to develop a strategy for securing the airway. The once-reliable combination of sandbags and tape or the rigid cervical collar have (in many locales) been replaced by more sophisticated devices aimed at providing enhanced cervical immobility. This equipment may need to be removed to adequately access the airway, and then replaced after manipulation is complete. Furthermore, the radiographic three-view series traditionally used to assess the integrity of the cervical spine may be supplemented with more sensitive technology such as high-resolution computed tomography (CT) and magnetic resonance imaging (MRI) scans. These imaging techniques generally require more time to complete and often require that the patient be transferred from the emergency department or trauma center to a specialized imaging area. It may be prudent to secure the airway before moving the patient.

If the CSI is accompanied by damage to the spinal cord, the anesthesia team may be forced to manage the airway in a hemodynamically unstable patient. Centrally mediated bradycardia (caused by interruption of the T1-T4 cardio-accelerator fibers) and significant hypotension (secondary to a lack of vasoconstriction below the level of the lesion) add a sense of urgency to the immediate establishment of a secure airway. Other considerations such as head injury with increased ICP, skull fracture, facial trauma, the likelihood of a full stomach, and compression of the airway by cervical hematoma [11] further complicate the scenario. Conscious patients who are aggressive or uncooperative may be especially challenging.

There is that there is no single standard of care for management of the airway in a patient with suspected CSI, as outcome data have failed to find a single best course of action [12], but many different approaches to these patients have a high success rates with concurrent low morbidity. Of course, individual institutions and communities may endorse specific standards of care.

ANATOMY OF THE CERVICAL SPINE

The upper cervical spine, defined as the upper two cervical vertebrae, allows for normal flexion/extension of 24 degrees at both the atlanto-occipital and atlantoaxial junctions [13]. The transverse, apical, and alar ligaments maintain

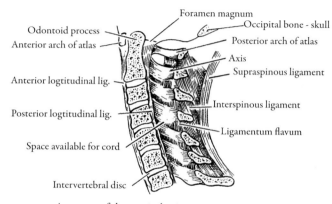

Figure 24.1 Anatomy of the cervical spine. (From Crosby ET. Airway management in adults after cervical spine trauma. *Anesthesia*. 2006;104:1293–1318.)

Labels in figure:
Odontoid process
Anterior arch of atlas
Anterior logtitudinal lig.
Posterior logtitudinal lig.
Space available for cord
Intervertebral disc
Foramen magnum
Occipital bone - skull
Posterior arch of atlas
Axis
Supraspinous ligament
Interspinous ligament
Ligamentum flavum

stability of the cervical spine, with smaller contributions from the anterior and posterior longitudinal ligaments. The transverse ligament is clinically significant as it limits anteroposterior translation between the dens and the anterior arch of the atlas (the atlas–dens interval, noted on lateral neck radiographs) to 3 mm. Disruption of this ligament will allow translation up to 5 mm, and destruction of the other supporting ligaments will allow translation up to 10 mm. These ligaments also limit posterior displacement of the dens and inhibit encroachment into the space available for the cord (SAC). The SAC, defined as the diameter of the spinal canal measured in the anteroposterior plane at the C1 level excluding the odontoid process, typically measures 20 mm [14]. The odontoid process normally occupies one third of the C1 diameter, with the remaining two thirds (the SAC) divided equally between the spinal cord and the remaining space [15], which acts as a cushion to allow some degree of cord enlargement without compression and compromise. The ligaments, in addition to the intervertebral discs, the facet joints, the interspinous ligament, and the supraspinous ligaments, also offer support to the lower cervical spine (C5-C8), offering a further 66 degrees of flexion-extension at this level (Figure 24.1).

C2, C6, and C7 are especially vulnerable to CSI, with almost one third of injuries occurring at C2 and over one half at C6 or C7 [16]. Approximately 10% of patients with CSI have fractures at other levels of the spine [17].

ATLANTO-OCCIPITAL DISSOCIATION (AOD)

AOD deserves special mention because patients have a critically unstable cervical spine and are often in dire need of airway management. The condition is almost uniformly fatal, present in 6% [18] to 8% [19] of patients in fatal traffic accidents but only 0.6% of blunt trauma patients alive on admission to the emergency department [20]. It is more common in children due to the less stable anatomical configuration of their craniocervical junction [19]. The causes

of injury are multifactorial and include spinal cord transsection, subarachnoid hemorrhage [21], and vascular insufficiency to the brainstem and cord secondary to carotid and/or vertebral artery rupture [22], thrombosis [23, 24], or vasospasm [25]. Presentation is variable: in one series of 79 cases patients ran the gamut from asymptomatic (18%) to single cranial nerve deficits [most often cranial nerve VI] (10%), unilateral limb deficits (34%), and quadriparesis or quadriplegia [21]. Airway intervention is often necessary due to concurrent facial trauma, retropharyngeal swelling, and brainstem injury resulting in cardiorespiratory compromise [26].

RADIOGRAPHIC CONFIRMATION OF CERVICAL-SPINE INJURY

Plain radiographic imaging of the cervical spine is the standard first intervention undertaken to ascertain the presence or absence of injury, a necessary step before immobilization devices can be removed. Early recognition of CSI is vital: the incidence of secondary neurological deficits in patients not initially recognized as having a spinal injury is 10.5%, compared with 1.4% among patients who are correctly diagnosed on initial examination [27]. The cross-table lateral view (CTL), once considered sufficient to rule out CSI [28], has been shown to underestimate the true incidence by up to 67% [29]. The three-view series (CTL, open mouth, and anteroposterior) has a sensitivity between 64% [30] and 90% [31]; its deficiency, visualization of the cervicothoracic junction, is often corrected by the addition of a supplementary swimmer's view [32]. While many clinicians use the three-view series to guide patient management [33], others feel that a five-view series (the original three views, as well as right and left obliques) should be used to rule out CSI [34, 35]. Dynamic fluoroscopy has been shown to add little predictive value to plain radiographs [36]. CT is perhaps a better tool to detect occult injury; when combined with the three-view cervical series the negative predictive value is reported to be 99%, rising to 100% when sagittal reconstruction of the entire cervical spine is performed [37, 38]. Helical CT is perhaps the most sensitive imaging modality in high-risk patients [39, 40].

MRI is useful to diagnose ligament injuries but has not been shown to be superior to CT imaging studies and a normal neurological examination for clearing the cervical spine [41–43]. At present, MRI is typically reserved for patients with normal x-ray and CT imaging who present with persistent neurological deficits. Spinal cord injury without radiological abnormality (SCIWORA) is a recognized condition seen most often among the pediatric population [44, 45]. It typically presents in conjunction with central cord syndrome, diagnosed clinically by weakness in the limbs (upper extremities more affected than lower) and variable sensory loss below the level of the lesion. Fortunately most children with SCIWORA recover fully [46], often responding to a course of high-dose intravenous steroids [47].

Some clinicians question the need to perform any testing at all for the majority of victims presenting with blunt trauma. Citing the enormous financial and manpower cost, as well as the patients' exposure to radiation, they are studying whether radiographic examination is warranted in patients who have a low suspicion of CSI. The National Emergency X-Radiography Utilization Study (NEXUS) was conducted with the intention of developing a set of clinical criteria that would categorize the blunt trauma patient as being at low risk for CSI [48, 49]. To be classified as low risk, patients had to meet the following criteria:

1. No midline cervical tenderness

2. No focal neurological deficit

3. Normal level of alertness

4. No intoxication

5. No painful distracting injury (e.g., long bone fractures, visceral injuries, large lacerations, burns, degloving, or crush injuries)

These criteria were applied to a population of 34,069 blunt trauma victims; 33,251 were deemed to be low risk for CSI, out of which only 8 were found to have evidence of CSI and only 2 had a clinically significant injury. Thus this simple screening tool had a 99% sensitivity for the presence of probable CSI prior to radiographic confirmation.

The Canadian CT Head and Cervical Spine Study group studied 8924 victims of suspected CSI injury in an attempt to make the selection criteria even more straightforward

[50]. Patients were evaluated based on the following three questions:

1. Is there any high-risk factor present that suggests the need for radiographic studies?

2. Are there low risk factors that would allow a safe assessment of cervical range of motion?

3. Is the patient able to actively rotate the neck 45 degrees to the left and right?

These three criteria had a 100% sensitivity in identifying patients with CSI. A follow-up study comparing the Canadian criteria with NEXUS [51] proved that the former is both more sensitive (99.4% versus 90.7%) as well as more specific (45.1% versus 36.8%) at identifying CSI.

Many centers are now following guidelines endorsed by both the American Association of Neurologic Surgeons and the Congress of Neurologic Surgeons. These guidelines state that patients with low clinical risk for CSI may have immobilization devices removed without radiographic examination [52]. Patients must typically meet three criteria (summarized in Figure 24.2) to be considered low risk:

1. The patient must have no focal neurological deficits. Sensory deficits are associated with an 8.9% risk of CSI [53]; the risk rises to 54% with motor deficits and approaches 100% when respiratory compromise is also present [54].

2. The patient must have a clear sensorium and be free from distracting injuries. If these criteria are present in a patient with suspected CSI the incidence approaches 5% [55].

3. The patient must have no complaints of neck pain or tenderness. When the mechanism of injury suggests CSI, neck pain is present in 4% [53] of confirmed cases.

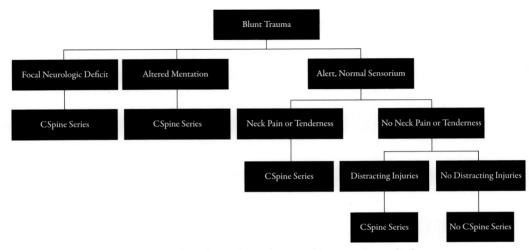

Figure 24.2   A proposed algorithm to evaluate the need for radiographic evaluation of the cervical spine [54].

Several series have confirmed that the incidence of CSI among patients who fulfill all three of the above criteria approaches zero [17, 56, 57]. Patients who are obtunded, intubated, or otherwise do not fulfill these criteria should have (at a minimum) a three-view cervical spine plain film series supplemented with a CT of the craniocervical junction and any other indicated exams [58].

CERVICAL SPINE MOTION DURING AIRWAY MANAGEMENT

Cervical spine movement is an inevitable consequence of airway manipulation [59]. Several series with cadavers [60, 61] (done with both normal and C1-C2 disrupted cervical spines) have illustrated cervical displacement, expansion of the disc space, and narrowing of the SAC during airway maneuvers both basic (mask ventilation, insertion of an oral airway) and advanced (orotracheal intubation with a laryngoscope, insertion of an esophageal obturator airway, blind nasal intubation). This movement occurred despite the presence of restraining devices such as rigid collars, sand bags, and tape. Surprisingly, preintubation maneuvers (mask ventilation, jaw thrust, and chin lift) were found to cause the greatest degree of cervical spine movement and SAC compromise [61]. Oral and nasal intubations in cadavers resulted in little cervical spine motion, and the difference between the two routes was statistically insignificant.

Studies of the effects of direct laryngoscopy have been performed on subjects who are awake (topically anesthetized) [62] and under general anesthesia [63]. Insertion of the blade causes clinically insignificant cervical displacement in both cohorts; elevation of the blade causes superior rotation of the occiput on C1 with mild inferior rotation of C3-C5. Insertion of the endotracheal tube slightly aggravates the occipital-C1 rotation. Removal of the laryngoscope blade resulted in a return of the cervical anatomy towards normal, although the exact previous anatomic position was not reached. Thus all significant movement seems focused upon the atlanto-occipital region with minimal disruption of the subaxial cervical segments [26]. All measurements fell within the normal range of motion of the cervical spine, although these patients' cervical spines were intact. Changes of this magnitude are not safe in a patient with an injured cervical spine or a reduced SAC.

There have been multiple attempts to find one blade that is superior to the others in this patient population. Several studies [64–67] have proved that there are no significant differences in the risk of cervical spine injury between the Macintosh, Miller, Belscope, or McCoy blades, although one study showed less axial distraction with the Miller blade [68]. The McCoy blade, with its flexible jointed tip, provides enhanced glottic exposure with less force [69] exerted and reduced physiological stress [70]; this may be

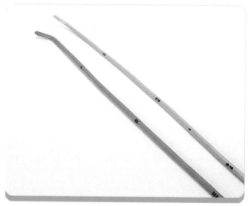

Figure 24.3 A gum elastic bougie [left] and a Frova intubating introducer [right].

significant in the patient with factors (e.g., spinal immobilization) that complicate laryngoscopy [64–71].

When visualization of the vocal cords is limited, a gum elastic bougie [72, 73] (Figure 24.3, left) or a Frova intubating introducer (Cook Critical Care, Bloomington, IN) (Figure 24.3, right) may be used as an aid to intubation. By accepting a view of only the arytenoid cartilages and using one of these devices, the anesthesiologist can successfully intubate the trachea, often in less than 25 seconds [74], while using less force to displace the glottis structures.

Rigid fiberoptic laryngoscopes may also be used to secure the airway in the patient with suspected cervical spine injury. The Bullard scope (Gyrus ACMI Corp., Norwalk, OH) (Figure 24.4) was compared with the Macintosh blade in a population of patients placed on rigid boards; half of the patients received MILI, the other half did not. Cervical spine extension was greatest in the Macintosh non-MILI group, reduced in the Macintosh-MILI group, but lowest among the patients intubated with the Bullard laryngoscope (with which MILI did not significantly reduce cervical spine movement [75]. Although time to intubation was prolonged in the Bullard-MILI cohort, all patients were intubated in less than 60 seconds. Similar results were obtained when the Bullard was compared with a Miller blade [66]. Furthermore, another study suggests that MILI has a significantly smaller chance of worsening the grade view

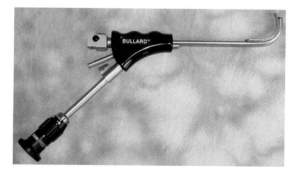

Figure 24.4 The Bullard scope.

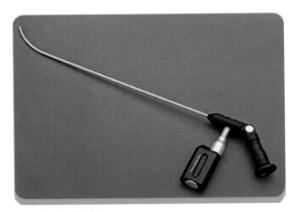

Figure 24.5   The Bonfils fiberscope.

of the larynx when used with a Bullard scope (as opposed to a Macintosh blade) [76]. The Bullard is also a promising alternative to flexible fiberoptic bronchoscopy: a small study (17 patients, all with cervical immobilization devices and/or MILI) comparing the Bullard scope with a flexible fiberoptic device showed no significant differences in success rates; all patient were intubated during the first attempt with either device [77]. In a larger study of 50 adults, time to intubation was significantly reduced when comparing the Bullard to a flexible fiberoptic bronchoscope, and the presence of cricoid pressure (which had no effect on the Bullard's success rate) resulted in a 56% failure rate among the flexible fiberoptic cohort [78]. The Bonfils fiberscope (Karl Storz Endoscopy, El Segundo CA) (Figure 24.5) provides an alternative to the Bullard, also significantly reducing cervical spine motion compared with the Macintosh blade [79]. The WuScope (Pentax Medical Co., Montvale NJ) (Figure 24.6) also has its proponents [80] despite limited penetration of the market.

The laryngeal mask airway has been extensively studied and found to exert little dynamic change to the cervical spine [81, 82]. Insertion and removal of an intubating laryngeal mask airway (ILMA) cause only 1 to 3 degrees of cervical spine *flexion* [83]; it is interesting to note the

contrast between the ILMA and the laryngoscope, which causes cervical spine *extension* [84]. The ILMA can also be easily inserted when the patient is immobilized in a rigid cervical collar [85–87] and/or MILI is being applied [88–90]. A cadaveric study suggested that standard and intubating laryngeal mask airways exert a high degree of pressure against C2 and C3 during insertion, cuff inflation, and while in situ; the authors of the study concluded that while this caused posterior displacement of the upper cervical spine (up to 2.8 mm at C3) it was impossible to determine whether there was any clinical significance [91, 92]. Case reports provide favorable anecdotal evidence for the use of both the classical [93] and the Fastrach ILMA (LMA North America Inc., La Jolla, CA) [94] used in conjunction with a flexible fiberoptic scope in patients with CSI. In the latter case the authors cite minimal cervical motion obtained at the expense of a prolonged intubation time (versus direct laryngoscopy), although the intubation times they cited (25 to 35 seconds for the ILMA/fiberoptic combination) were not excessive.

The C-Trach (LMA North America Inc., La Jolla, CA) (Figure 24.7) improves upon the design of the ILMA by adding an LCD screen and light source, thereby providing a continuous fiberoptic view of the glottis during airway manipulation. Clinical studies suggest that it is an excellent tool for performing an awake intubation on a patient with an unstable cervical spine [95]. Esophageal intubation is significantly reduced versus blind intubation via the ILMA [96] and intubation time is shorter than when a standard ILMA (versus direct laryngoscopy) is used [97, 98].

SPINAL IMMOBILIZATION

The significant decrease in mortality and morbidity secondary to CSI over the past half century has largely been attributed to the prevalence of spinal immobilization

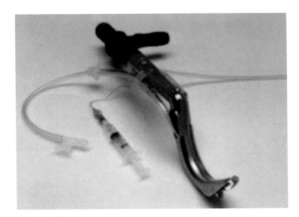

Figure 24.6   The WuScope.

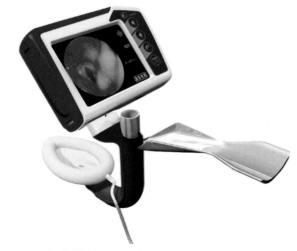

Figure 24.7   The C-Trach

techniques in blunt trauma victims [99, 100]. Although prospective randomized evidence linking cause and effect is lacking [101] and some question the need for immobilization of low-risk patients with CSI [102, 103], immobilization remains the standard of care in most facilities [104]. The precise characterization of immobilization is variable throughout the literature, with some authors referring to passive devices and others including hands-on techniques such as manual stabilization with or without traction [105].

The rigid cervical collar combined with a backboard seems to be the preferred method of spinal immobilization. A half-spine board or Kendrick Extrication Device (Ferno-Washington Inc., Wilmington OH) (Figure 24.8) are useful adjuncts in the pediatric population [106]. Hard foam or plastic collars are significantly more effective than soft foam, but alone are not sufficient to provide adequate immobility [107, 108]. Fresh cadavers with a C5-C6 injury and a Philadelphia collar in place showed more than 5 mm of cervical spine movement (typically extension) during basic airway maneuvers [109]. The addition of sand bags on either side of the head, with 3-inch tape or a strap holding the head in a midline position, provides a greater degree of immobilization (limiting the spine to 5% of its normal range of motion [110].

Side effects secondary to spinal immobilization result less from the decision to immobilize but rather the duration of immobilization [104, 111, 112]. It is universally accepted that the rapid clearance of the cervical spine and removal of immobilization devices, when clinically indicated, is of benefit [113]. Cutaneous pressure ulcers are the greatest culprit, most common when the immobilization device is present for greater than 2 days. These ulcers are a common source of sepsis and closure may require a split thickness skin graft [114]. Intracranial pressure (ICP) is elevated by the continuous presence of a rigid cervical collar [115, 116], which is especially undesirable in a patient who may already have an elevated ICP and poor intracranial compliance [117]. Access to the neck and mouth are limited, complicating

airway management and making central venous catheter placement more difficult. The presence of a rigid cervical collar has been shown to significantly reduce interincisor distance [118], thereby complicating laryngoscopy or LMA insertion. Most practitioners remove the anterior portion of the collar prior to manipulating the airway, maintaining manual in-line immobilization (MILI) until the airway is secured and the collar can be reattached.

Cadaveric studies to evaluate MILI have yielded mixed results, with some concluding it does not enhance cervical spine stability [119, 120] and others finding a small protective effect [84]. Yet, in vivo MILI has been clinically proved to reduce movement of the spinal column during laryngoscopy more effectively than the use of rigid collars alone [108–120]. It is equally effective when performed from the head of the bed (the provider grasps the mastoid processes and cradles the occiput) or from the patient's side (the provider grasps the occiput and cradles the mastoid processes). By design, MILI significantly reduces the ability to extend the patient's head (10 to 15 degrees in controls reduced to 4 to 5 degrees with MILI applied [121], thereby precluding an effective sniffing position for laryngoscopy. Nolan and Wilson revealed that this worsened the laryngoscopic view by one grade in 35.6% and by two grades in 9.5% of their study population (N = 157) [122]. Wood et al. [123] and Heath [124] reported similar results from smaller studies.

The acceptance of MILI in clinical practice is by no means universal. Some authors have suggested that the risk of hypoxia from a degraded laryngoscopic view may outweigh the benefit of immobilization, and MILI is therefore not an a priori requirement [125]. Others suggest that MILI may even increase the degree of subluxation of unstable cervical segments [120], possibly by limiting the rest of the cervical spine from accommodating the forces associated with direct laryngoscopy [84]. Yet despite the lack of a benefit borne out by randomized clinical trials [126], most clinicians believe that spinal immobilization is a necessary precaution. If cervical spine immobilization is desired, MILI has been shown to cause less airway distortion than cervical collars, tape, or sandbags in both human and cadaver models [68, 124]. The adverse effects of MILI may be minimized by the concurrent application of jaw thrust and/or cricoid/anterior laryngeal pressure; although this maneuver was once contraindicated in the patient with an unstable spine, recent clinical experience has proved that it is safe and effective [60, 109].

Cephalad traction, once an accepted component of MILI, is no longer recommended by most experts [127]. Several studies have demonstrated excessive distraction at the site of the CSI (up to 8 mm [128]) as well as posterior subluxation [84] and spinal cord stretching [129] when traction was applied. Despite the natural elasticity of both the dura mater and the cord itself, traction may aggravate the initial injury and result in secondary trauma to the injured cord [130, 131], possibly converting an incomplete

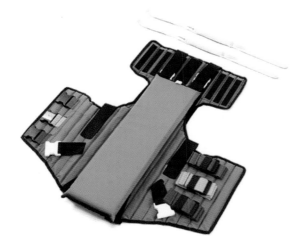

Figure 24.8   The Kendrick extrication device.

cord lesion into a complete transection. Brieg demonstrated that the application of 5 kg of traction to a partially severed cord resulted in separation of wound edges and a decreased neural conductivity in the cord [132]. Case reports support the supposition that axial traction results in morbidity and mortality following CSI [133].

In-line stabilization of the cervical spine may also be provided by external fixation devices (e.g., a halo vest fixation device,) seen most frequently when a patient presents for subsequent surgery after the initial injury. These pieces of equipment preclude practically any alignment of the oral, pharyngeal, and tracheal axes, making awake intubation the preferred choice [134], typically with the assistance of a fiberoptic scope [135], Bullard laryngoscope [136], or ILMA [137].

PRACTICE PREFENCES AMONG ANESTHESIOLOGISTS

Two important decisions must be made before attempting to secure the airway of a conscious patient with a compromised cervical spine. First, the physician must decide if the patient will be intubated awake or unconscious. Subsequently, the anesthesiologist must decide what tool(s) will be used to secure the airway. Several large studies have been conducted to gauge how anesthesiologists choose to answer these vital questions. One of the largest compared attending anesthesiologists in U.S. training programs to their surgical colleagues, all members of the Eastern Association for the Surgery of Trauma [138]. Patients were classified into one of the following groups: (1) elective (spontaneous ventilation, stable vital signs), (2) urgent (spontaneous ventilation, unstable vital signs), or (3) emergent (apneic, unstable vital signs). Both groups favored orotracheal intubation in all three categories, although anesthesiologists were more prone to use flexible fiberoptic bronchoscopy in all scenarios, including endotracheal tube replacement in patients with CSI [139]. Surgeons were statistically more likely to use a blind nasal intubation in the elective population, and more than twice as likely to perform a surgical airway in emergency patients (19% versus 7%).

Anesthesiologists tend to prefer awake intubations in most studies, often using a fiberoptic bronchoscope (FOB). One of the benefits to intubating the patient awake is that neurological status can be assessed immediately after intubation if excessive sedation was not administered. A study of American Society of Anesthesiologists members revealed that when faced with a cervical spine–injured patient, 78% of the respondents chose awake fiberoptic intubation as their preferred method to secure the airway. (The remaining 22% induced general anesthesia and intubated the patient with direct laryngoscopy [140].) A similar study conducted among members of the Canadian Anesthesiologists' Society showed similar results: 67% of physicians preferred an awake intubation, and 63% would use a flexible FOB [141]. A large study of 454 patients with confirmed CSI suggests awake fiberoptic intubation is indeed safe: 169 of the patients were intubated in this manner, while the remainder required no intubation. Among each group the incidence of sensory and/or motor deficits arising between hospital admission and discharge was identical at 2.4% [142], which is remarkable considering the greater degree of CSI that was likely sustained by the patients who required airway management.

If general anesthesia is induced before securing the airway, one small study of 16 patients with CSI suggests that the use of neuromuscular blocking agents does not affect outcome. There were no subsequent neurological complications among patients who did or did not receive neuromuscular blocking agents [143].

A study of physicians treating patients with cervical spine disease (e.g., cervical arthritis, ankylosing spondylitis) revealed that 75% of respondents listed fiberoptic bronchoscopy as their first choice, although only 59% admitted that they were comfortable (and felt adequately skilled) to successfully use the device [144]. This insecurity has been reflected in studies measuring the success of flexible fiberoptic intubations in patients with cervical pathology. One study conducted among patients with CSI cited a success rate of only 83.3% (95% CI 72%–94.6% [145]). Another large study examined 327 patients presenting for elective cervical spine surgery and found that 12% developed arterial oxygen desaturation (84% ± 4%) during awake fiberoptic examination [146]. Others authors have reported cases of complete airway obstruction during fiberoptic intubation attempts ultimately requiring surgical intervention to secure the airways [147].

The benefits of reduced cervical movement are eliminated when the fiberoptic intubation becomes difficult or if the operator is uncomfortable with the technique. Furthermore, in patients with brain injury accompanying CSI, fiberoptic bronchoscopy can significantly increase intracranial pressure; this increase is not reliably blunted by the administration of narcotics, benzodiazepines, or nebulized lidocaine [148]. Barbiturates will blunt this ICP response but may be dangerous in the face of hemodynamic instability [149].

Many clinicians find the GlideScope requires much less manual dexterity and training than the flexible FOB [150]. While visualization of the glottis is comparable to rigid or flexible FOB, the ease of use comes at the expense of greater cervical excursion (comparable to that seen with the use of a Macintosh blade [151]). This was proved in patients both with [152] and without [153] the use of cervical immobilization. In contrast, the AirWay Scope (Pentax Medical Co., Montvale NJ) (Figure 24.9) has been used successfully in patients with halo-vest fixation [154] and shown to cause less cervical spine motion compared with Macintosh laryngoscopy [155].

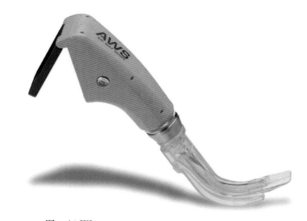

Figure 24.9   The AirWay scope.

THE CASE AGAINST DIRECT LARYNGOSCOPY

In 1987, an untested hypothesis was published in the emergency medicine literature asserting that direct laryngoscopy was an unsafe practice in a patient with cervical spine injury [156]. The author theorized that this technique of orotracheal intubation was directly responsible for excessive cervical movement and secondary spinal injury. Blind nasal intubation or cricothyrotomy were deemed to be the only appropriate airway management techniques in this population, and this (unproven) recommendation was incorporated into the then current Advanced Trauma Life Support protocol. A subsequent review article suggested that flexible fiberoptic bronchoscope was the only safe way to secure the airway in a CSI patient [157]. However, many medical centers remained skeptical about the purported dangers of direct laryngoscopy and continued to use this technique as their preferred method of airway control [142, 158, 159] despite a growing number of published case reports linking direct laryngoscopy with secondary spinal injury [160–167]. The risks of direct laryngoscopy may have been overstated, however. McLeod and Calder [168] reviewed all of the published case reports and concluded that none were able to draw a causal relationship between laryngoscopy and the worsening neurological condition; instead, the reports in aggregate describe patients with numerous confounding causes of possible injury including failure to immobilize the cervical spine after injury [161–165], failure to apply MILI [166], malpositioning during the operative procedure [164], and failure to recognize a congenital cervical spine deformity [162] or preexisting neurological disease [163]. Although individual case reports may suggest that direct laryngoscopy aggravates the neurological condition, it may also be true that a disproportionately large number of patients with significant CSI will require airway support, and the worsening neurological status will continue to develop and manifest after intubation by any technique.

Most clinicians now maintain that intubation via most methods is safe, provided proper cervical stabilization precautions are observed. Case series (ranging in size up to 335 patients [169] with suspected [158–170] or confirmed [138–171] CSI have reported no increased incidence of neurological damage after orotracheal intubation via direct laryngoscopy. Direct laryngoscopy was noted to be safe in both the awake [142–172] and anesthetized [173] patients, being no more risky than the previously touted blind nasal approach [174]. These results have also been published in the emergency medicine literature, including several successful case series of CSI intubations via direct laryngoscopy performed in the emergency department [175, 176].

While the size and volume of these case series lends more credence to the safety of direct laryngoscopy, there have yet to be large, controlled trials to conclusively prove that laryngoscopy is safe. Crosby concluded that the uncommon nature of progressive neurological injury in patients with CSI (approximately 2%) makes it extremely difficult to prove that direct laryngoscopy worsens cervical spine injury. A study designed to test whether direct laryngoscopy doubles this baseline incidence would require the participation of over 1800 patients [12]. Until such a study is performed, we can only speculate (based upon a plethora of anecdotal evidence) that direct laryngoscopy is safe and not contraindicated in the presence of CSI.

ALTERNATIVE INTUBATION TECHNIQUES

Direct laryngoscopy, fiberoptic intubation, or the use of some type of laryngeal mask airway seem to be the preferred tools for airway management of the patient with CSI, and a surgical airway may be necessary when other techniques have failed or immediate definitive airway access is required. In addition, a variety of airway management techniques are effective and cause little cervical spine movement when used properly.

Blind techniques, once considered the gold standard of CSI airway management, have fortunately been largely supplanted by these alternative methods. Blind tactile digital intubation is poorly tolerated by the conscious or semi-conscious patient and exposes the clinician to the risk of being bitten [177]. The Augustine guide (Augustine Medical Inc, Eden Prairie, MN) (Figure 24.10), a tool devised to facilitate blind orotracheal intubation, does improve the success rate and results in little cervical spine movement. However, this technique results in considerable laryngopharyngeal trauma in a significant majority of patients [178]. Blind oral intubation is facilitated via the placement of an intubating LMA [122], with success rates cited between 90% [179] and 95% [180]. As noted previously, insertion of the ILMA results in little cervical spine excursion.

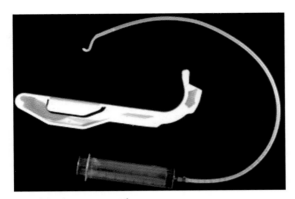

Figure 24.10 The Augustine guide.

The blind nasal approach is more challenging to perform than the oral approach and results in no less cervical spine motion [181]. While some studies suggest a success rate of over 90% [182, 183] (especially with the aid of ETT cuff inflation in the oropharynx [184, 185]), this is far from universal. One study comparing blind nasal to orotracheal intubation found the latter technique to be superior in terms of success rate (100% versus 65%), mean number of attempts (1.3 versus 3.7), and time to accomplish (64 versus 276 seconds) [186]. The nasal route may cause bleeding in the airway, making subsequent attempts at fiberoptic bronchoscopy more difficult. Blind nasal intubation also carries the risk of intracranial penetration [187]. In contrast, the use of a lighted stylet device significantly improves the success rate and decreases the complications of nasal intubations among this population. The StyletScope (Nihon Koden Corp., Tokyo, Japan) [188], the Trachlight (TL; Laerdal Medical, Wappinger Falls, NY), as well as other lighted stylet devices [189] have the versatility to be used for both oral and nasal approaches to the airway.

The TL is composed of three separate pieces: a reusable handle that contains three AAA batteries, a flexible wand (available in adult, pediatric, and infant sizes) and a stiff retractable wire stylet. For an oral intubation, the stylet is inserted into the flexible wand and the endotracheal tube is threaded over the wand and secured to the handle. The wand length can be adjusted with a control on the handle and should extend to the distal tip, but not beyond, the ETT. The wand/ETT complex is then bent at a 90-degree angle. A common mistake is to place a less exaggerated bend in the stylet, typical of intubation with a laryngoscope. However, the aim of this device is to focus the light against the anterior tracheal wall, where the anesthesiologist will be better able to see it. A 45-degree bend in the stylet will aim the light down the trachea, making successful intubation more difficult [190]. When the unit is turned on, a bright light at the end of the wand will illuminate; after 30 seconds the light will begin to blink, both to inform the operator of elapsed time and to minimize heat production. Localized tissue damage is unlikely if the light source is maintained inside the distal tip of the ETT [191].

The head may be left in a neutral position with MILI applied for intubation. After the patient is preoxygenated, the TL/ETT complex is inserted into the midline of the oropharynx and inserted posteriorly following the curvature of the tongue. A faint glow will be noted in the anterior neck as the device enters the vallecula (dimming of the room lights may be helpful [192]). The unit is advanced with a rocking motion, in the midline, until a bright, well-circumscribed red glow is seen inferior to the thyroid cartilage, indicating passage of the device into the glottic opening (Figure 24.11). A red glow on either side of the neck indicates placement of the device in the piriform sinus; the TL should be retracted several centimeters and re-advanced in the midline. Repositioning is also indicated if a diffuse glow is seen beneath the thyroid cartilage, indicating esophageal placement. Continued difficulty with positioning may be solved with the application of a jaw thrust maneuver which lifts the epiglottis off the posterior pharyngeal wall. The wire stylet is then withdrawn approximately 10 cm, allowing the tip of the ETT to curl anteriorly past the vocal cords, further enhancing the likelihood of endotracheal positioning. The unit is then advanced several centimeters more (into the trachea) and the ETT is unlocked from the TL, which is then removed from the airway.

Nasal intubation with the TL is also performed in the neutral position, and as with the oral TL route the application of MILI results in minimal cervical motion [193]. The wire stylet is removed from the TL to give the wand more flexibility so that it does not cause bleeding in the nasopharynx. The TL/ETT complex is inserted via either nare and inserted until the bright red glow is seen below the thyroid cartilage, as described earlier. Prior application of a vasoconstrictor to the nose, and the softening and/or lubrication of the ETT will facilitate insertion via this route.

Extraglottic devices are especially useful in the "can't intubate/can't ventilate" scenario; they are considered to be first-line devices in this limb of the ASA difficult airway algorithm. These devices can be inserted while the head and neck remain in a neutral position, making them ideal for the unanticipated difficult airway in the patient with CSI. The Combitube (CBT), once used solely for airway

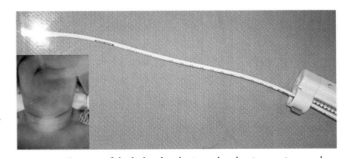

Figure 24.11 Passage of the lighted stylet into the glottic opening results in a well-circumscribed red glow on the anterior neck (inset).

management outside the hospital, is an easily inserted and is an effective rescue device in the operating or emergency departments [194] (Figure 24.12). The CBT is a dual-lumen tube with a single large distal opening and several smaller holes along the shaft. It is available in two sizes, as 37 Fr for use in adults 4 to 6 feet in height and a 41 Fr for adults over 6 feet tall. The device has two balloons, each with a separate inflation port. The larger balloon (85 cm² of volume in the small CBT, 100 cm² in the large) obstructs the posterior pharynx and prevents escape of oxygen out of the patient's nose and mouth. The smaller balloon (10 cm² of volume in both sizes) seals the esophagus, minimizing gastric distention. The tube is inserted blindly into the mouth and advanced along the curvature of the tongue. The head is left in the neutral position [195] to maximize the ease of insertion and minimize cervical motion. If resistance is met, a jaw thrust maneuver is helpful to elevate the soft tissue structures. Two black marks on the proximal portion of the tube indicate depth of advancement; the teeth (or alveolar ridge in edentulous patients) should rest between these markings. The CBT will enter the esophagus in over 95% of insertion attempts. After insertion of both balloons, ventilation through Port #1 will force oxygen through the lateral pharyngeal openings in the tube. Due to the esophageal and hypopharyngeal obstructions, the oxygen flows retrograde up the esophagus and into the trachea (the only unobstructed path it can take). If the trachea is intubated blindly, the pharyngeal cuff can be deflated and the patient can be ventilated through Port #2 (in which case the CBT functions like an ETT). Although the CBT (when placed in the esophagus) does not provide the same level of aspiration protection as a cuffed ETT, it is a useful device especially in an emergency to allow ventilation with minimal cervical movement until a more definitive airway can be obtained [196].

The King LT (Consort Medical, UK) is a similar supraglottic device (Figure 24.13). It is shorter than the CBT, has a single pilot balloon connected to both cuffs, and does not have a patent distal lumen. This property, as well as the shortened size, precludes direct ventilation of the trachea in contrast this to the CBT, with which endotracheal

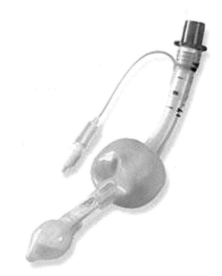

Figure 24.13   The King LT supraglottic device

insertion is unlikely but possible. It is available in six sizes (selected according to patient weight) and three different varieties (the standard disposable LT, as well as reusable and disposable versions with an accessory gastric suction channel [197]). As with the CBT the LT is inserted blindly with the head and neck in a neutral position, following the curvature of the hard palate. Markings on the tube align with the teeth to ensure proper depth of insertion. Inflation of the single pilot balloon inflates both the pharyngeal and esophageal balloons, allowing ventilation via side ports. Proper insertion is easily performed with minimal training [198], and insertion times are comparable to those of the LMA [199].

Retrograde intubation (RI) is a technique best suited for the elective management of a difficult airway; alternatively, it may be considered when intubation is problematic but ventilation proceeds without difficulty. It is not suitable for the "can't intubate/can't ventilate" scenario because it will require too much time even in skilled hands. Like the techniques discussed above it is very useful in the patient with CSI because it is performed with the head and neck in a neutral position. It is a blind technique that is not affected by maxillofacial trauma or the presence of blood in the airway. RI can be performed using a variety of common supplies, such as an epidural catheter [200] or a Fogarty balloon catheter. However, it is most easily accomplished with the use of a prefabricated RI kit containing all of the necessary supplies (except the ETT) such as the kit made by Cook Critical Care (Cook Medical, Bloomington, IN). This kit contains an 18-gauge needle that is used to puncture the cricothyroid membrane in the cephalad direction. If the patient is conscious, injecting 4 mL of 4% lidocaine through the needle should provide sufficient topical anesthesia. The J-wire is then inserted through the needle and threaded until it is visible in the oral cavity. Asking the

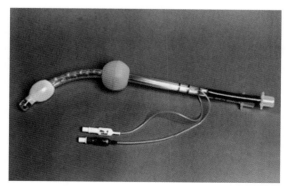

Figure 24.12   The Combitube.

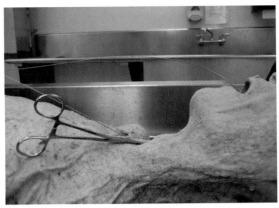

Figure 24.14   During a retrograde intubation, a clamp is used to secure the wire in place.

patient to protrude his/her tongue often causes the wire to spring out of the mouth; if the wire remains in the oropharynx, Magill forceps can be used to retrieve it. Alternatively, if a nasal intubation is preferred, forceps can be used to direct the wire posteriorly into the nasopharynx until it can be retrieved from one of the nares. In either case, the wire is advanced until the black positioning mark is flush with the neck, at which point the needle is removed and a clamp is applied to the wire to prevent additional movement (Figure 24.14). A tapered catheter is threaded onto the wire and advanced until resistance is felt (typically at about 20 cm) indicating it is abutting the posterior surface of the cricothyroid membrane. The wire is then removed and the tapered catheter is advanced several centimeters to ensure its placement below the vocal cords (Figure 24.15). An adapter can be placed at the proximal end of the catheter to permit positive pressure ventilation if needed. The endotracheal tube is then advanced over the tapered catheter into the trachea, and the catheter is then removed [201]. In one series of such patients Barriot reported successful RI times of less than 5 minutes [202].

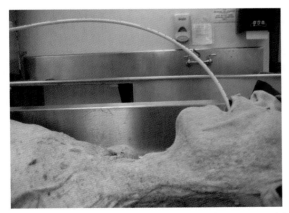

Figure 24.15   The tapered catheter allows for easier advancement of the endotracheal tube, and can also be used as a conduit for oxygenation.

SPECIAL CONSIDERATIONS FOR MOTORCYCLISTS

Few jurisdictions require that motorcyclists wear helmets, and only 53% of riders protect themselves with helmets when not required to do so [203]. The use of helmets significantly decreases the incidence of traumatic brain injury but does not reduce the occurrence of cervical or thoracic spine fractures [204, 205]. Paradoxically, the presence of a motorcycle helmet complicates airway management. Removal of the helmet almost certainly causes some degree of cervical spine movement [206, 207] even when performed under continuous fluoroscopy. As a result, the clinician must decide whether or not to leave the helmet in place during primary assessment. Open-face helmets offer protection to the forehead and cranium but do not cover the eyes, face, or jaw, or neck (in some cases a removable visor may add some protection). These helmets typically interfere the least with airway management and can often be left in place during bag-mask ventilation and laryngoscopy. Full-face helmets offer the most protection by completely obscuring the nose, mouth, and the upper portion of the neck, but access to the airway is practically impossible unless the helmet is removed. A third type of helmet, a modular type, functions as a full-face helmet with a removable face shield. Since airway access is unobstructed, these are considered to be the same class as open-face helmets.

Although there is currently no consensus on whether helmets should be routinely removed prior to airway management, most clinicians leave the helmet in place if the airway is reasonably accessible (i.e., open-face and modular helmets). If a full-face helmet prevents direct laryngoscopy (or any oral technique), then the clinician must weigh the possibility of success of a surgical or nasal airway (either blind nasal or TL-assisted [208] against the risks of carefully removing the helmet while maintaining cervical spine immobility. These alternative techniques may be the only option in a patient with a full-face helmet that cannot be removed (e.g., in the setting of penetrating trauma.)

Patients who present with CSI secondary to sports injuries may also present with a helmet in place. In general, these types of helmets do not obscure the airway to the same degree as motorcycle helmets, especially since the face-shield portion of a sports helmet is often removable with a screwdriver. Several studies have shown that removal of these helmets results in significant cervical spine movement [209, 210]. The airway is often unobstructed by these helmets and should almost always be left in place [211] until the cervical spine has been cleared radiographically.

CONCLUSION

Airway management for the patient with cervical spine injury or pathology is a challenging clinical problem. The absence of a single best strategy for managing these cases means that there are a variety of options and not one single, evidence-based practice mandate. The adoption of prehospital immobilization in the 1970s significantly reduced the incidence of secondary neurological injury, which before that time was estimated at 10% to 25% [212]. Studies of airway management have significantly changed the original Advanced Trauma Life Support (ATLS) guidelines [213] that required all patients to be managed with a surgical airway as well as the subsequent recommendation of nasotracheal intubation for unconscious, spontaneously breathing patients [214]. Oral intubation has been shown to be a safe alternative in this patient population [215], even with the use of cricoid pressure to overcome the deleterious effects of MILI upon laryngoscopic view. While bougies, lighted stylets, and other adjunct devices may assist the laryngoscopist who fails to obtain a clear view with MILI, their use does not guarantee a successful intubation of the difficult airway [216]. In these cases, it is permissible to relax or completely release MILI temporarily for the sake of obtaining a clearer view of the glottic opening; the potential harm to the cervical spine is outweighed by the benefit of a secure airway [85]. Despite anecdotal warnings about the potential deleterious effects of MILI [217], orotracheal intubation [218], or the induction of general anesthesia prior to intubation [142] (all of which have been theoretically linked to postintubation neurological deficits), the evidence points to a contrary conclusion. A 10-year retrospective study demonstrated no differences in neurological outcomes with intubation performed awake versus after the induction of general anesthesia, with orotracheal intubation via direct laryngoscopy versus airway access via other methods, or with MILI versus no MILI [219]. Attaining and maintaining a stable airway should be the primary concern for the anesthesia provider caring for a patient with CSI; the method chosen to attain this goal seems less important than its successful completion.

REFERENCES

1. Crosby ET, Lui A. The adult cervical spine: implications for airway management. *Can J Anaesth.* 1990;37:77–93.
2. Patterson H. Emergency department intubation of trauma patients with undiagnosed cervical spine injury. *Emerg Med J.* 2004;21:302–305.
3. Davenport M. Fracture, cervical spine. http://emedicine.medscape.com/article/824380-overview.
4. Hills MW, Deanne SA. Head injury and facial injury: is there an increased risk of cervical spine injury? *J Trauma.* 1993;34:549–554.
5. Mark NH. Guidelines for management of acute cervical spine injuries. *Neurosurgery.* 2002;50:1.
6. Ghafoor AU, Martin TW, Gopalakrishanan S, et al. Caring for the patients with cervical spine injuries: what have we learned? *J Clin Anesth.* 2005;17:640–649.
7. Huelke F, O'Day J, Mendelsohn RA. Cervical injuries suffered in automobile crashes. *J Neurosurg.* 1981;54:316–322.
8. Insurance Institute for Highway Safety. Current US motorcycle and bicycle helmet laws—February. 2010. http://www.iihs.org/laws/HelmetUseCurrent.aspx.

9. Criswell JC, Parr MJA, Nolan JP. Emergency airway management in patients with cervical spine injuries. *Anaesthesia.* 1994;49:900–903.
10. Jaberi M, Mitchell K, MacKenzie C. Cricothyroidotomy: good, bad, or ugly? *Trauma Care.* 2001;1:13.
11. Calder I, Koh K. Cervical haematoma and airway obstruction. *Br J Anaesth.* 1996;76:888–889.
12. Crosby ET. Airway management in adults after cervical spine trauma. *Anesthesia.* 2006;104:1293–1318.
13. Jofe MH, White AA, Panjabi MM. Clinically relevant kinematics of the cervical spine. *The Cervical Spine, 2nd Ed* Edited by the Cervical Spine Research Society. Philadelphia, PA: JB Lippincott; 1999:57–69.
14. Hensinger RN. Congenital anomalies of the atlantoaxial joint. *The Cervical Spine, 2nd Ed.* Edited by the Cervical Spine Research Society. Philadelphia, PA: JB Lippincott; 1989:236–243.
15. Steel HH. Anatomical and mechanical considerations of the atlanto-axial articulations. *J Bone Joint Surg.* 1968;50:1481–1490.
16. Davidson JSD, Birdsell DC. Cervical spine injury in patients with facial skeletal trauma. *J Trauma.* 1989;29:1276–1278.
17. Ringenberg BJ, Fisher AK, Urdaneta LF, et al. Rational ordering of cervical spine radiographs following trauma. *Ann Emerg Med.* 1988;17:792–796.
18. Alker GJ Jr, Oh YS, Leslie EV, et al. Postmortem radiology of head and neck injuries in fatal traffic accidents. *Radiology.* 1975;114:611–617.
19. Bucholz RW, Burkhead WZ, Graham W, et al. Occult cervical spine injuries in fatal traffic accidents. *J Trauma.* 1979;19:768–771.
20. Chiu WC, Haan JM, Cushing BM, et al. Ligamentous injuries of the cervical spine in unreliable blunt trauma patients: incidence, evaluation, and outcome. *J Trauma.* 2001;50:457–464.
21. Przybylski GJ, Clyde BL, Fitz CR. Craniocervical junction subarachnoid hemorrhage associated with atlanto-occipital dislocation. *Spine* 1996;21:1761–1768.
22. Lee C, Woodring JH, Walsh JW. Carotid and vertebral artery injury in survivors of atlanto-occipital dislocation: case reports and literature review. *J Trauma.* 1991;31:401–407.
23. Gabrielsen TO, Maxwell JA. Traumatic atlanto-occipital dislocation with case report of a patient who survived. *Radiology.* 1966;97:624–629.
24. Evarts CM. Traumatic occipito-atlantal dislocation. Report of a case with survival. *J Bone Joint Surg.* 1970;52-**A**:1653–1660.
25. Powers B, Miller MD, Dramer RS, et al. Traumatic anterior atlanto-occipital dislocation. *Neurosurg.* 1979;4:12–17.
26. Crosby E. Airway management after upper cervical spine injury: what have we learned? *Can J Anesth.* 2002;49:733–744.
27. Reid DC, Henderson R, Saboe L, et al. Etiology and clinical course of missed spine fractures. *J Trauma.* 1987;27:980–986.
28. Shaffer MA, Doris PE. Limitation of the cross table lateral view in detecting cervical spine injuries: a retrospective analysis. *Ann Emerg Med.* 1981;10:508–512.
29. Woodring JH, Lee C. Limitations of cervical radiography in the evaluation of acute cervical trauma. *J Trauma.* 1993;34:32–39.
30. Hashem R, Evans CC, Farrokhyar F, et al. Plain radiography does not add any clinically significant advantage to multidetector row computed tomography in diagnosing cervical spine injuries in blunt trauma patients. *J Trauma* 2007;66:423–428.
31. Grossman MD, Reilly PA, Gillett T, et al. National survey of the incidence of cervical spine injury and approach to cervical spine clearance in US trauma centers. *J Trauma.* 1999;47:684–690.
32. Ajani AE, Cooper DJ, Sceinkestel CD, et al. Optimal assessment of cervical spine trauma in severe nonpenetrating closed head injury: a prospective study. *Anaesth Intensive Care.* 1998;26:487–491.
33. Freemyer B, Knopp R, Piche J, et al. Comparison of five-view and three-view cervical spine series in the evaluation of patients with cervical trauma. *Ann Emerg Med.* 1989;18:818–821.
34. Krochmal P. Clinical criteria to rule out cervical-spine injury. *N Engl J Med* 2000;343:1338–1339.
35. Hoffman JR, Mower WR, Wolfson AB. Validity of a set of clinical criteria to rule out injury to the cervical spine in patients with blunt trauma. *N Engl J Med* 2000;343:94–99.

36. Davis JW, Kaups KL, Cunningham MA, et al. Routine evaluation of the cervical spine in head-injured patients with dynamic fluoroscopy: a reappraisal. *J Trauma.* 2001;50:1044–1047.

37. Hadley MN. Guidelines of the American Association of Neurologic Surgeons and the Congress of Neurologic Surgeons: radiographic spinal assessment in symptomatic trauma patients. *Neurosurgery.* 2002;50 (suppl):S36–S43.

38. Morris CGT, McCoy E. Clearing the cervical spine in unconscious polytrauma victims—balancing risk and effective screening. *Anaesthesia.* 2004;59:464–482.

39. Nunez DB, Ahmad AA, Coin CG, et al. Clearing the cervical spine in multiple trauma victims: a time effective protocol using helical computed tomography. *Emerg Radiol.* 1994;1:273–278.

40. Brohi K, Healy M, Fotheringham T, et al. Helical computed tomographic scanning for the evaluation of the cervical spine in the unconscious intubated trauma patient. *J Trauma.* 2005;58:897–901.

41. Shuster R, Waxman K, Sanchez B, et al. Magnetic resonance imaging is not needed to clear cervical spines in blunt trauma patients with normal computed tomographic results and no motor deficits. *Arch Surg.* 2005;140:762–766.

42. Hogan GJ, Mirvis SE, Shanmuganathan K, et al. Exclusion of unstable cervical spine injury in obtunded patients with blunt trauma: is MR imaging needed when multi-detector row CT findings are normal? *Radiology.* 2005;237:106–113.

43. Benzel EC, Hart BL, Ball PA, et al. Magnetic resonance imaging for the evaluation of patients with occult cervical spine injury. *J Neurosurg.* 1996;85:824–829.

44. Siddiqui A. Airway management for Cervical Injury. *Saudi Med J.* 2009;30:1133–1137.

45. Grabb PA, Pang D. Magnetic resonance imaging in the evaluation of spinal cord injury without radiographic abnormality in children. *Neurosurgery.* 1994;35:406–414.

46. Hadley MN, Zabramski JM, Browner CM, et al. Pediatric spinal trauma—review of 122 cases of spinal cord and vertebral column injuries. *J Neurosurg.* 1988;68:18–24.

47. Kriss VM, Kriss TC. SCIWORA (spinal cord injury without radiographic abnormality) in infants and children. *Clin Pediatr* 1996;35:119–124.

48. Hoffman JR, Mower WR, Pollack CV, et al. Validity of a set of clinical criteria to rule out injury to the cervical spine in patients with blunt trauma. *N Engl J Med.* 2000;343:94–99.

49. Mower WR, Hoffman JR, Pollack CV, et al. Use of plain radiography to screen for cervical spine injuries. *Ann Emerg Med.* 2001;38:1–7.

50. Stiell IG, Wells GA, Vandemheen KL, et al. The Canadian cervical spine rule for radiography in alert and stable trauma patients. *JAMA.* 2001;286:1841–1848.

51. Stiell IG, Clement CM, McKnight RD, et al. The Canadian cervical spine rule versus the NEXUS low-risk criteria in patients with trauma. *N Engl J Med.* 2003;349:2510–2518.

52. Hadley MN. Guidelines of the American Association of Neurologic Surgeons and the Congress of Neurologic Surgeons: radiographic spinal assessment in asymptomatic trauma patients. *Neurosurg.* 2002;50(Suppl):S30–S35.

53. Kreipke DL, Gillespie KR, McCarthy MC, et al. Reliability of and indication for cervical spine films in trauma patients. *J Trauma.* 1989;29:1438–1439.

54. Ivy ME, Cohn SM. Addressing the myths of cervical spine injury management. *Am J Emerg Med.* 1997;15:591–595.

55. Neifeld GL, Keene JG, Hevesy G, et al. Cervical injury in head trauma. *J Emerg Med.* 1988;6:203–207.

56. Roberge RJ, Wears RC, Kelly M. Selective application of cervical spine radiography in alert victims of blunt trauma: a prospective study. *J Trauma.* 1988;28:784–788.

57. Velmahos GC, Theodorou D, Tatevossian R, et al. Radiographic cervical spine evaluation in the alert asymptomatic blunt trauma victim: much ado about nothing? *J Trauma.* 1996;40:768–774.

58. Lockey AS, Handley R, Willett K. Clearance of cervical injury in the obtunded patient. *Injury.* 1998;29:493–497.

59. Crosby ET. Considerations for airway management for cervical spine surgery in adults. *Anesthes Clin.* 2007;25:511–533.

60. Donaldson WF III, Heil BV, Donaldson VP, et al. The effect of airway maneuvers on the unstable C1-C2 segment: a cadaver study. *Spine.* 1997;22:1215–1218.

61. Hauswald M, Sklar DP, Tandberg D, et al. Cervical spine movement during airway management: cinefluoroscopic appraisal in human cadavers. *Am J Emerg Med* 1991;9:535–538.

62. Jorton WA, Fahy L, Charters P. Disposition of the cervical vertebrae atlanto-axial joint, hyoid and mandible during x-ray laryngoscopy. *Br J Anaesth.* 1989;63:435–438.

63. Sawin PD, Todd MM, Traynelis VC, et al. Cervical spine motion with direct laryngoscopy and orotracheal intubation: an *in vivo* cinefluoroscopic study of subjects without cervical abnormality. *Anesthesia.* 1996;85:26–36.

64. Laurent SC, De Melo AE, Alexander-Wiliams JM. The use of the McCoy laryngoscope in patients with simulated cervical spine injuries. *Anaesthesia.* 1996;51:74–75.

65. MacIntyre PR, McLeod ADM, Hurley R, et al. Cervical spine movements during laryngoscopy: comparison of the Macintosh and McCoy laryngoscope blades. *Anaesthesia.* 1999;54:413–418.

66. Hastings RH, Vigil AC, Hanna R, et al. Cervical spine movement during laryngoscopy with the Bullard, Macintosh and Miller laryngoscopes. *Anaesthesia.* 1995;82:859–869.

67. Gajraj NM, Chason DP, Shearer VE. Cervical spine movement during orotracheal intubation: comparison of the Belscope and Macintosh blades. *Anaesthesia.* 1994;49:772–774.

68. Gerling MC, Davis DP, Hamilton RS, et al. Effects of cervical spine immobilization technique and laryngoscope blade selection on an unstable cervical spine in a cadaver model of intubation. *Ann Emerg Med* 2000;36:293–300.

69. McCoy EP, Mirakhur RK, Rafferty C, et al. A comparison of the forces exerted during laryngoscopy. The Macintosh versus the McCoy blade. *Anaesthesia.* 1996;51:912–915.

70. McCoy EP, Mirakhur RK, McCloskey BV. A comparison of the stress response to laryngoscopy. The Macintosh versus the McCoy blade. *Anaesthesia.* 1995;50:943–946.

71. Uchida T, Hikawa Y, Saito Y, et al. The McCoy levering laryngoscope in patients with limited neck extension. *Can J Anaesth.* 1997;44:674–676.

72. Nolan JP, Wilson ME. An evaluation of the gum elastic bougie. Intubation times and incidence of sore throat. *Anaesthesia.* 1992;47:878–881.

73. Nocera A. A flexible solution for emergency intubation difficulties. *Ann Emerg Med.* 1996;27:665–667.

74. Nolan JP, Wilson ME. Orotracheal intubation in patients with potential cervical spine injuries. An indication for the gum elastic bougie. *Anaesthesia.* 1993;48:630–633.

75. Watts ADJ, Gelb AW, Bach DB, et al. Comparison of Bullard and Macintosh laryngoscopes for endotracheal intubation of patients with a potential cervical spine injury. *Anaesthesia.* 1997;87:1335–1342.

76. Cooper SD, Benumof JL, Ozaki GT. Evaluation of the Bullard laryngoscope using the new intubating stylet: comparison with conventional laryngoscopy. *Anesth Analg.* 1994;79:965–970.

77. Cohn AL, Zornow MH. Awake endotracheal intubation in patients with cervical spine disease: a comparison of the Bullard laryngoscope and the fiberoptic bronchoscope. *Anesth Analg.* 1995;81:1283–1286.

78. Shulman GB, Connelly NR. A comparison of the Bullard laryngoscope versus the flexible fiberoptic bronchoscope during intubation on patients afforded inline stabilization. *J Clin Anesth.* 2001;13:182–185.

79. Rudolph C, Schneider JP, Wallenborn J, et al. Movement of the upper cervical spine during laryngoscopy: a comparison of the Bonfils intubation fiberscope and the Macintosh laryngoscope. *Anaesthesia.* 2005;60:668–672.

80. Smith CE, Pinchak AB, Sidhu RS, et al. Evaluation of tracheal intubation difficulty in patients with cervical spine immobilization. Fiberoptic (WuScope) versus conventional laryngoscopy. *Anesthesia.* 1999;91:1253–1259.

81. Nakazawa K, Tanaka N, Ishikawa S, et al. Using the intubating laryngeal mask airway (LMA-Fastrach) for blind endotracheal intubation in patients undergoing cervical spine operation. *Anesth Analg.* 1999;89:1319–1321.

82. Waltl B, Melischek M, Schuschnig C, et al. Tracheal intubation and cervical spine excursion: direct laryngoscopy versus intubating laryngeal mask. *Anaesthesia.* 2001;56:221–226.

83. Kihara S, Watanabe S, Brimacombe J, et al. Segmental cervical spine movement with the intubating laryngeal mask during manual in-line stabilization in patients with cervical pathology undergoing cervical spine surgery. *Anesth Analg.* 2000;91:195–200.

84. Lennarson PJ, Smith DW, Sawin PD, et al. Cervical spinal motion during intubation: efficacy of stabilization maneuvers in the setting of complete segmental instability. *J Neurosurg (Spine 2).* 2001;94:265–270.

85. Komatsu R, Nagata O, Katama K, et al. Intubating laryngeal mask airway allows tracheal intubation when the cervical spine is immobilized by a rigid collar. *Br J Anaesth.* 2004;93:655–659.

86. Asai T, Shingu K. Tracheal intubation through the intubating laryngeal mask in patients with unstable necks. *Acta Anaesth Scand.* 2001;45:818–822.

87. Moller F, Andres AH, Langenstein H. Intubating laryngeal mask airway (ILMA) seems to be ideal device for blind intubation in case immobile spine. *Br J Anaesth.* 2000;85:493–494.

88. Asai T, Murao K, Tsutsumi T, et al. Ease of tracheal intubation through the intubating laryngeal mask during manual in-line head and neck stabilisation. *Anaesthesia.* 2000;55:82–85.

89. Asai T, Wagle AU, Stacey M. Placement of the intubating laryngeal mask is easier than the laryngeal mask during manual in-line stabilisation. *Br J Anaesth.* 1999;82:712–714.

90. Komatsu R, Nagata O, Kamata K, et al. Comparison of the intubating laryngeal mask airway and laryngeal tube placement during manual in-line stabilisation of the neck. *Anaesthesia.* 2005;60:113–117.

91. Keller C, Brimacombe J, Keller K. Pressures exerted against the cervical vertebrae by the standard and intubating laryngeal mask airways: a randomized controlled cross-over study in fresh cadavers. *Anesth Analg.* 1999;89:1296–1300.

92. Todd MM, Traynelis VC. Experimental cervical spine injury and airway management methods. *Anesth Analg.* 2001;93 :799–800.

93. Asai T. Fiberoptic tracheal intubation through the laryngeal mask in an awake patient with cervical spine injury. *Anesth Analg.* 1993;77:404.

94. Schuschnig C, Waltl B, Erlacher W, et al. Intubating laryngeal mask and rapid sequence induction in patients with cervical spine injury. *Anaesthesia.* 1999;54:787–797.

95. Bilgin H, Yylmaz C. Awake intubation through C-Trach¨ in patients with unstable cervical spine. *Anaesthesia.* 2006;61:513–514.

96. Liu EHC, Goy RW, Chen FG. The LMA C-Trach¨, a new laryngeal mask airway for endotracheal intubation under vision: evaluation in 100 patients. *Br J Anaesth.* 2006;96:396–400.

97. Bilgin H, Bozkurt M. Tracheal intubation using the ILMA, C-Trach¨ or a McCoy laryngoscope in patients with simulated cervical spine injury. *Anaesthesia.* 2006;61:685–691.

98. Pandit JJ, MacLachlan K, Dravid RM, et al. Comparison of times to achieve tracheal intubation with three techniques using the laryngeal mask or intubating laryngeal mask airway. *Anaesthesia.* 2002;57:128–132.

99. DeVivo MJ, Krause JS, Lammertse DP. Recent trends in mortality and causes of death among persons with spinal cord injury. *Arch Phys Med Rehabil.* 1999;80:1411–1419.

100. DeLorenzo RA. A review of spinal immobilization techniques. *J Emerg Med.* 1996;14:603–613.

101. Kwan I, Bunn F, Roberts I; on behalf of the WHO Prehospital Trauma Care Steering Committee. Spinal immobilisation for trauma patients. *Cochrane Database Syst Rev.* 2001;2:CD002803.

102. Hauswald M, Braude D. Spinal immobilization in trauma patients: is it really necessary? *Curr Opin Crit Care.* 2002;8:566–570.

103. Kennedy FR, Gonzalez P, Beitler A, et al. Incidence of cervical spine injury in patients with gunshot wounds to the head. *Southern Med J.* 1994;87:621–623.

104. Hadley M. Guidelines of the American Association of Neurologic Surgeons and the Congress of Neurologic Surgeons: cervical spine immobilization before admission to hospital. *Neurosurgery.* 2002;50(Suppl):S7–S17.

105. Knopp RK. The safety of orotracheal intubation in patients with suspected cervical-spine injury. *Ann Emerg Med.* 1990;19:603–604.

106. Huerta C, Griffith R, Joyce SM. Cervical spine stabilization in pediatric patients: evaluation of current techniques. *Ann Emerg Med.* 1987;6:1121–1126.

107. Alberts LR, Mahoney CR, Neff JR. Comparison of the Nebraska collar, a new prototype cervical immobilization collar, with three standard models. *J Orthop Trauma.* 1998;12:425–430.

108. Majernick TG, Bieniek R, Houston JB, et al. Cervical spine movement during orotracheal intubation. *Ann Emerg Med.* 1986;15:417–420.

109. Aprahamian C, Thompson BM, Finger WA, et al. Experimental cervical spine injury model: evaluation of airway management and splinting techniques. *Ann Emerg Med* 1984;13:584–588.

110. Podolsky S, Baraff LJ, Simon RR, et al. Efficacy of cervical spine immobilization methods. *J Trauma.* 1983;23:461–465.

111. Morris CG, McCoy EP, Lavery GG. Spinal immobilisation for unconscious patients with multiple injuries. *Br Med J.* 2004;329:495–499.

112. Morris CG, McCoy EP. Cervical immobilization collars in the ICU: friend or foe? *Anaesthesia.* 2003;58:1051–1055.

113. Gupta KJ, Clancy M. Discontinuation of cervical spine immobilisation in unconscious patients with trauma in intensive care units—telephone survey of practice in the South and West region. *Br Med J.* 1997;314:1652–1655.

114. Morris CG, Mullan B. Clearing the cervical spine after polytrauma: implementing unified management for unconscious victims in the intensive care unit. *Anaesthesia* 2004;59:755–761.

115. Davies G, Dealin C, Wilson A. The effect of a rigid collar on intracranial pressure. *Injury.* 1996;27:647–649.

116. Kolb JC, Summers RI, Galli RL. Cervical collar-induced changes in intracranial pressure. *Am J Emerg Med.* 1999;17:135–137.

117. Hunt K, Hallworth S, Smith M. The effects of rigid collar placement on intracranial and cerebral perfusion pressures. *Anesthesia.* 2001;56:511–513.

118. Goutcher CM, Lochhead V. Reduction in mouth opening with semi-rigid cervical collars. *Br J Anaesth* 2005;95:344–348.

119. Lennarson PJ, Smith D, Todd MM, et al. Segmental cervical spine motion during orotracheal intubation of the intact and injured spine with and without external stabilization. *J Neurosurg (Spine 2)* 2000;92:201–206.

120. Brimacombe J, Keller C, Kunzei KH, et al. Cervical spine motion during airway management: a cinefluoroscopic study of the posteriorly destabilized third cervical vertebrae in human cadavers. *Anesth Analg.* 2000;91:1274–1278.

121. Hastings RH, Wood PR. Head extension and laryngeal view during laryngoscopy with cervical spine stabilization maneuvers. *Anesthesia.* 1994;80:825–831.

122. Nolan JP, Wilson ME. Orotracheal intubation in patients with potential cervical spine injuries. *Anaesthesia* 1993;48:630–633.

123. Wood PR, Dresner M, Hayden Smith J, et al. Direct laryngoscopy and cervical spine stabilization. *Anaesthesia.* 1994;49:77–78.

124. Heath KJ. The effect on laryngoscopy of different cervical spine immobilization techniques. *Anaesthesia.* 1994;49:843–845.

125. Manoach S, Paladino L. Manual in-line stabilization for acute airway management of suspected cervical spine injury: historical review and current questions. *Ann Emerg Med.* 2007;50 :236–245.

126. Kwan I, Bunn F, Roberts I. Spinal immobilisation for trauma patients. *Cochrane Database Syst Rev..* 2001;CD002803.

127. Bejjani GK, Rizkallah RG, Tzortidis F, et al. Cervical spinal cord injury during cerebral angiography with MRI confirmation: case report. *Neuroradiology*. 1998;40:51–53.

128. Bivins HG, Ford S, Bezmalinovic Z, et al. The effect of axial traction during orotracheal intubation of the trauma victim with an unstable cervical spine. *Ann Emerg Med*. 1988;17:25–29.

129. Kaufman JJ, Harris JH Jr, Spencer JA, et al. Danger of traction during radiography for cervical trauma (letter). *JAMA*. 1982;247:2369.

130. Bohlman J, Bahniuk E, Rashkulinecz G. Mechanical factors affecting recovery from incomplete cervical spinal cord injury. *Johns Hopkins Med J*. 1979;145:115–125.

131. Brieg A. Overstretching and circumscribed pathologic tension in the spinal cord. *J Biomech*. 1970;3:7–9.

132. Brieg A. *Adverse Mechanical Tension in the Central Nervous System*. Stockholm, Sweden: Almgvist & Wiskell; 1978.

133. Scher AT. Overdistraction of cervical spinal injuries. *S Afr Med J* 1981;59:639–641.

134. Kang M, Vives MJ, Vaccaro AR. The halo-vest: principles of application and management of complications. *J Spinal Cord Med*. 2003;26:186–192.

135. Canaioni D, Rodola F, Barbi S, et al. The use of the fibroscope for tracheal intubation in severe cervical instability with the Halo cranial traction system. *Minerva Anestesiol*. 1991;57:775–776.

136. Cohn AI, Lau M, Leonard J. Emergent airway management at a remote hospital location in a patient wearing a halo traction device. *Anesthesia*. 1998;89:545–546.

137. Sener EF, Sarihasan B, Ustun E, et al. Awake tracheal intubation through the intubating laryngeal mask airway in a patient with halo traction. *Can J Anaesth*. 2002;49:610–613.

138. Lord SA, Boswell WC, Williams JS, et al. Airway control in trauma patients with cervical spine fractures. *Prehosp Dis Med*. 1994;9:44–49.

139. Wright TM, Vinayakom K. Endotracheal tube replacement in patients with cervical spine injury. *Anesthesia*. 1995;82:1307–1308.

140. Rosenblatt WH, Wagner PJ, Ovassapian A, et al. Practice patterns in managing the difficult airway by anesthesiologists in the United States. *Anesth Analg*. 1998;87:153–157.

141. Jenkins K, Wong DT, Correa R. Management choices for the difficult airway by anesthesiologists in Canada. *Can J Anesth*. 2002;49:850–856.

142. Meschino A, Devitt JH, Koch JP, et al. The safety of awake tracheal intubation in cervical spine injury. *Can J Anesth*. 1992;39:114–117.

143. Chekan E, Weber S. Intubation with or without neuromuscular blockade in trauma patients with cervical spine injury. *Anesth Analg*. 1990;70:S54.

144. Ezri T, Szmuk P, Warters RD, et al. Difficult airway management practice patterns among anesthesiologists practicing in the United States: have we made any progress? *J Clin Anesth*. 2003;15:418–422.

145. Dunham CM, Barraco RD, Clark DE, et al. EAST Practice Management Guidelines Work Group: Guidelines for emergency tracheal intubation immediately after traumatic injury. *J Trauma*. 2003;55:162–179.

146. Fuchs G, Schwarz G, Baumgartner A, et al. Fiberoptic intubation in 32 patients with lesions of the cervical spine. *J Neurosurg Anesth*. 1999;11:11–16.

147. McGuire G, El-Beheiry H. Complete upper airway obstruction during awake fiberoptic intubation in patients with unstable cervical spine fractures. *Can J Anesth*. 1999;46:176–178.

148. Kerwin AJ, Croce MA, Timmons SD, et al. Effects of fiberoptic bronchoscopy on intracranial pressure in patients with brain injury: a prospective clinical study. *J Trauma*. 2000;48:878–883.

149. Schwartz ML, Tator CH, Rowed DW, et al. The University of Toronto head injury treatment study: a prospective randomized comparison of pentobarbital and mannitol. *Can J Neurolog Sci*. 1984;2:434–440.

150. Cooper RM. Use of a new videolaryngoscope (GlideScope) in the management of a difficult airway. *Can J Anesth*. 2003;50:611–613.

151. Turkstra TP, Craen RA, Pelz DM, et al. Cervical spine motion: a fluoroscopic comparison during intubation with lighted stylet, GlideScope, and Macintosh laryngoscope. *Anesth Analg*. 2005;101:910–915.

152. Robitaille A, Williams SR, Tremblay MH, et al. Cervical spine motion during tracheal intubation with manual in-line stabilization: direct laryngoscopy versus GlideScope® videolaryngoscopy. *Anesth Analg*. 2008;106:935–941.

153. Wong DM, Prabhu A, Chakraborty S, et al. Cervical spine motion during flexible bronchoscopy compared with the Lo-Pro GlideScope. *Br J Anaesth*. 2009;102:424–430.

154. Maruyama K, Yamada T, Hara K, et al. Tracheal intubation using an AirWay Scope in a patient with halo-vest fixation for upper cervical injury. *Br J Anaesth*. 2009;102:565–566.

155. Maruyama K, Yamada T, Kawakami R, et al. Randomized cross-over comparison of cervical spine motion with use of the AirWay Scope and Macintosh laryngoscope with in-line stabilization: a video-fluoroscopic study. *Br J Anaesth*. 2008;101:563–567.

156. Walls RM. Orotracheal intubation and potential cervical spine injury (letter). *Ann Emerg Med*. 1987;16:373.

157. Chestnut RM. Management of brain and spine injuries. *Crit Care Clin*. 2004;20:25–55.

158. Suderman VS, Crosby ET, Lui A. Elective oral tracheal intubation in cervical spine injured adults. *Can J Anesth*. 1991;38:785–789.

159. Grande CM, Barton CR, Stene JK. Appropriate techniques for airway management of emergency patients with suspected spinal cord injury. *Anesth Analg*. 1988;67:714–715.

160. Farmer J, Vaccaro A, Albert TJ, et al. Neurologic deterioration after cervical spinal cord injury. *J Spinal Disord*. 1998;11:192–196.

161. Muckart DJ, Bhagwanjee S, van der Merwe R. Spinal cord injury as a result of endotracheal intubation in patients with undiagnosed cervical spine fractures. *Anesthesia*. 1997;87:418–420.

162. Redl G. Massive pyramidal tract signs after endotracheal intubation: a case report of spondyloepiphyseal dysplasia congenital. *Anesthesia*. 1998;89:1262–1264.

163. Yan K, Diggan MF. A case of central cord syndrome caused by intubation: a case report. *J Spin Cord Med*. 1997;20:230–232.

164. Yaszemski MJ, Shepler TR. Sudden death from cord compression associated with atlanto-axial instability in rheumatoid arthritis. *Spine*. 1990;15:338–341.

165. Hastings RH, Kelley SD. Neurologic deterioration associated with airway management in a cervical spine-injured patient. *Anesth*. 1993;78:580–583.

166. Liang BA, Cheng MA, Tempelhoff R. Efforts at intubation—cervical injury in an emergency circumstance? *J Clin Anesth*. 1999;11:349–352.

167. Powell RM, Heath KJ. Quadriplegia in a patient with an undiagnosed odontoid peg fracture: the importance of cervical spine immobilization in patients with head injuries. *J R Army Med Corps*. 1996;142:79–81.

168. McLeod ADM, Calder I. Spinal cord injury and direct laryngoscopy: the legend lives on. *Br J Anaesth*. 2000;84:705–708.

169. Talucci RC, Shaikh KA, Schwab CW. Rapid sequence induction with oral endotracheal intubation in the multiply injured patient. *Am Surg* 1988;54:185–187.

170. Shatney CH, Brunner RD, Nguyen TQ. The safety of orotracheal intubation in patients with unstable cervical spine fracture or high spinal cord injury. *Am J Surg*. 1995;170:676–680.

171. Norwood S, Myers MB, Butler TJ. The safety of emergency neuromuscular blockade and orotracheal intubation in the acutely injured trauma patient. *J Am Coll Surg*. 1994;179:646–652.

172. McCrory C, Blunnie WP, Moriarity DC. Elective tracheal intubation in cervical spine injuries. *Irish Med J*. 1999;90:234–235.

173. Scanell G, Waxman K, Tommaga G, et al. Orotracheal intubation in trauma patients with cervical fractures. *Arch Surg*. 1993;128:903–906.

174. Holley J, Jordan R. Airway management in patients with unstable cervical spine fractures. *Ann Emerg Med*. 1989;10:1237–1239.

175. Rhee KJ, Green W. Holcroff JW, et al. Oral intubation in the multiply injured patient: the risk of exacerbating spinal cord damage. *Ann Emerg Med*. 1990;19:511–514.

176. Wright SW, Robinson GG, Wright MB. Cervical spine injuries in blunt trauma patients requiring emergent endotracheal intubation. *Am J Emerg Med*. 1992;10:104–109.

177. Stewart RD. Tactile orotracheal intubation. *Ann Emerg Med*. 1984;13:175–178.

178. Kautzky M, Granz P, Krafft P, et al. Traumatizing effects of blind oral intubation using the Augustine Guide. *J Oral Maxillofac Surg* 1996;54:156–161.

179. Heath ML, Allagain J. Intubation through the laryngeal mask. A technique for unexpected difficult intubation. *Anaesth*. 1991;46:545–548.

180. Kapila A, Addy EV, Verghese C, et al. The intubating laryngeal mask airway: an initial assessment of performance. *Brit J Anaesth*. 1997;79:710–713.

181. Langeron O, Birenbaum A, Amour J. Airway management in trauma. *Minerva Anestesiol*. 2009;75:307–311.

182. Danzl DF, Thomas DM. Nasotracheal intubation in the emergency department. *Crit Care Med*. 1980;8:677–682.

183. Iserson KV. Blind nasotracheal intubation. *Ann Emerg Med*. 1981;10:468–471.

184. Van Elstraete AC, Pennant JH, Gajraj NM, et al. Tracheal tube cuff inflation as an aid to blind nasotracheal intubation. *Br J Anaesth*. 1993;70:691–693.

185. Van Elstraete AC, Mamie JC, Mehdaoui H. Nasotracheal intubation in patients with immobilized cervical spine: a comparison of tracheal tube cuff inflation and fiberoptic bronchoscopy. *Anesth Analg*. 1998;87:400–402.

186. Dronen SC, Merigian KS, Hedges JR, et al. A comparison of blind nasotracheal and succinylcholine-assisted intubation in the poisoned patient. *Ann Emerg Med*. 1987;16:650–652.

187. Horellou MF, Mathe D, Feiss P. A hazard of naso-tracheal intubation. *Anaesth*. 1978;33:73–74.

188. Kihara S, Yaguchi Y, Taguchi N, et al. The StyletScope˜ is a better intubation tool than a conventional stylet during simulated cervical spine immobilization. *Can J Anesth*. 2005;52:105–110.

189. Verdile V, Heller M, Paris P, et al. Nasotracheal intubation in traumatic craniofacial dislocation: use of the lighted stylet. *Am J Emerg Med*. 1988;6:39–41.

190. Christodoulou CC, Hung OR. "Blind intubation techniques" in *Management of the Difficult and Failed Airway, 2nd Edition*. Hung OR, Murphy MF, eds. McGraw Hill Medical, Toronto CA; 2008:195–196.

191. Nishiyama T, Matsukawa T, Hanaoka K. Safety of a new lightwand device (Trachlight): temperature and histopathological study. *Anesth Analg*. 1998;87:717–718.

192. Hung OR, Pytka S, Morris I, et al. Clinical trial of a new lightwand (TL) to intubate the trachea. *Anesth*. 1995;83:509–514.

193. Inoue Y, Koga K, Shigematsu S. A comparison of two tracheal intubation techniques with Trachlight and Fastrach in patients with cervical spine disorders. *Anesth Analg*. 2002;94:667–671.

194. Agro F, Frass M, Benumoff JL, et al. Current status of the Combitube: a review of the literature. *J Clin Anesth*. 2002;14:307–314.

195. Urtubia R, Aguila C. Combitube: a study for proper use. *Anesth Analg*. 1999;89:803.

196. Deroy R, Ghoris M. The Combitube˙ Elective anesthetic airway management in a patient with cervical spine fracture. *Anesth Analg*. 1998;87:1441–1442.

197. Asai T, Shingu K. The laryngeal tube. *Br J Anaesth*. 2005;95:729–736.

198. Finteis T, Genzwuerker H, Blankenberg A, et al. Airway management by nonmedical personnel a prospective, randomized comparison of laryngeal masks, combitubes, and laryngeal tubes. (German) *Notfall Rettungsmed*. 2001;4:327–334.

199. Doerges V, Ocker H, Wenzel V, et al. The laryngeal tube: a new simple airway device. *Anesth Analg*. 2000;90:1220–1222.

200. Hung OR, Al-Qatari M. Light-guided retrograde intubation. *Can J Anaesth*. 1997;44:877–882.

201. Bhardwaj N, Yaddanapudi S, Makkar S. Retrograde tracheal intubation in a patient with a halo traction device. *Anesth Analg*. 2006;103:1628–1629.

202. Barriot P, Riou B. Retrograde technique for tracheal intubation in trauma patients. *Crit Care Med*. 1988;16:712–713.

203. Motorcycle helmets. http://www.saferoads.org/motorcycle-helmets, Jan. 2010.

204. Orsay EM, Muelleman RL, Peterson TD, et al. Motorcycle helmets and spinal injuries: dispelling the myth. *Ann Emerg Med*. 1994;23:802–806.

205. Goslar PW, Crawford NR, Petersen SR, et al. Helmet use and associated spinal fractures in motorcycle crash victims. *J Trauma*. 2008;64:190–196.

206. Kolman JM, Hung OR, Beauprie IG, et al. Evaluation of cervical spine movement during helmet removal. *Can J Anaesth*. 2003;50:A18.

207. Laun RA, Lignitz E, Haase N, et al. Mobility of unstable fractures of the odontoid during helmet removal. A biomechanical study. *Unfallchirurg*. 2002;105:1092–1096.

208. Vu M, Guzzo A, Hung OR, et al. A novel method for endotracheal intubation in patients wearing full-face helmets. *World Cong Anesth*. 2003:CD104.

209. Laprade RF, Schnetzler KA, Broxterman RJ, et al. Cervical spine alignment in the immobilized ice hockey player. A computed tomography analysis of the effect of helmet removal. *Am J Sport Med*. 2000;23:800–803.

210. Swenson TM, Lauerman WC, Blanc RO, et al. Cervical spine alignment in the immobilized football player. Radiographic analysis before and after helmet removal. *Am J Sport Med*. 1997;25:226–230.

211. Waninger KN. On-field management of potential cervical spine injury in helmeted football players: leave the helmet on! *Clin J Sport Med*. 1998;2:124–129.

212. Crosby ET. Tracheal intubation in the cervical spine-injured patient. *Can J Anaesth*. 1992;39:105–109.

213. Wood PR, Lawler PGP. Managing the airway in cervical spine injury. A review of the Advanced Trauma Life Support protocol. *Anaesthesia*. 1992;47:792–797.

214. McHale SP, Brydon CW, Wood MLB, et al. A survey of nasotracheal intubating skills among Advanced Trauma Life Support course graduates. *Br J Anaesth* 1994;72:195–197.

215. Dunham CM, Britt LD, Stene JK. Emergency tracheal intubation in the blunt injured patient. *Panamerican J Trauma*. 1989;1:9–12.

216. Levitan RM. Myths and realities: the "difficult airway" and alternative airway devices in the emergency setting. *Acad Emerg Med*. 2001;8:829–832.

217. Turner LM. Cervical spine immobilization with axial traction: a practice to be discouraged. *J Emerg Med* 1989;7:385–386.

218. Joyce SM. Cervical immobilization during orotracheal intubation in trauma victims. *Ann Emerg Med* 1988;17:88.

219. Suderman VS, Crosby ET. Elective oral tracheal intubation in cervical spine-injured adults. *Can J Anaesth*. 1991;38:785–789.

25.

NEUROSURGERY IN PEDIATRICS

Craig D. McClain and Sulpicio G. Soriano

Pediatric neuroanesthesiologists manage patients with a wide spectrum of neurosurgical lesions that are age specific. Pediatric patients present with pathology that includes congenital anomalies, neoplasms, epilepsy, cerebrovascular lesions, and traumatic brain injury and a variety of anatomic, physiologic, and pathologic factors affect the management pediatric patient from infancy to adolescence. This chapter reviews the salient features of each of these conditions as it relates to the developing central nervous system (CNS).

DEVELOPMENTAL CEREBROVASCULAR PHYSIOLOGY

The CNS undergoes significant changes that include growth of the cranial vault and age-related modifications in hemodynamics. The neonate has open fontanels and cranial sutures. Insidious increases in intracranial volume due to slow growing tumors are often masked by a compensatory separation of the cranial sutures and protrusion of the fontanels. A rapid increase in cranial volume caused by hemorrhage or obstructed CSF flow will frequently result in life-threatening intracranial hypertension. The posterior fontanelle is usually closed by 2 months of age and the anterior fontanelle is closed in 96% of infants by 2 years. After the fontanelles have closed, intracranial compliance is similar to that of an adult.

Cerebral blood flow (CBF) is coupled tightly to metabolic demand, and both increase proportionally immediately after birth, peak between 2 and 4 years of age, and stabilize at 7 to 8 years of age. These changes mirror the changes in neuroanatomical development. CBF in a conscious, healthy child is estimated to be 100 mL/100 g, and approaches that of an adult (50 mL/100 g) during the teenage years. The range of blood pressure that is autoregulated is narrow and lower in normal newborns (20 to 60 mmHg). This reflects the low cerebral metabolic requirements and blood pressure during the perinatal period. The slope of the autoregulatory curve drops rises significantly at the lower and upper limits of the curve, making neonates vulnerable to cerebral ischemia and intraventricular hemorrhage. There is a linear correlation between CBF and systemic blood pressure in premature neonates. Critically ill premature and term neonates do not have intact cerebral autoregulation, resulting in CBF that varies passively with cerebral perfusion pressure (CPP). The lower limit of cerebral autoregulation appears to be equivalent among older and younger children. Since children less than 2 years have lower baseline mean arterial pressures; they may have less autoregulatory reserve and can theoretically be at greater risk of cerebral ischemia. Since the head of the infant and child accounts for a large percentage of the body surface area and blood volume, a larger percentage of cardiac output is directed to the brain. Infants are therefore at increased risk for hemodynamic instability during neurosurgical procedures.

PREOPERATIVE EVALUATION

The initial evaluation of the pediatric neurosurgical patient should include a thorough interview of the patient's parent or care taker. Older children may be able to participate in their care and should be allowed to do so if appropriate. Perioperative anxiety is often minimized during the preoperative interview with by explaining what will happen to both child and parent in a reassuring manner. A thorough organ-based history and physical examination should focus on potential physiological derangements and coexisting disease states that may increase the risk of perioperative complications. In the pediatric population special emphasis should be placed on obtaining a history of congenital anomalies (e.g., heart, lung, and CNS), craniofacial syndromes, neuromuscular disease, and prematurity. Children who were born prematurely frequently present with underlying chronic pulmonary disease, postoperative apnea in infancy, and varying degrees of neurocognitive dysfunction. If the patient is a newborn who is scheduled for an emergency neurosurgical procedure, time may not permit a thorough preoperative evaluation. In this case, rapid measurement of oxygen saturation on room air and transthoracic echocardiogram (if clinically feasible) should rule out the presence of significant congenital cardiac defects that can cause rapid deterioration in the perioperative period.

Preoperative fasting guidelines have evolved and are frequently dictated by regional practices. The purpose of limiting oral intake is to minimize the risk of pulmonary aspiration of gastric contents on induction. Prolonged fasting periods and vomiting may, however, cause hypovolemia and hypoglycemia, which can exacerbate hemodynamic and metabolic instability under anesthesia. Therefore the general trend has been to allow oral consumption of clear liquids up to 2 hours before induction of anesthesia in infants. Obtunded patients and patients who are vomiting should be fasted before surgery and a rapid sequence induction may be required.

The need for specialized preoperative testing is guided by the nature of the neurosurgical lesion. Most patients with CNS tumors undergo extensive imaging studies as part of the neurosurgical evaluation. The anesthesiologist should review these studies before surgery to determine whether the patient has intracranial hypertension or is at risk for herniation. Resection of brain and spinal cord lesions may require intraoperative neurophysiologic monitoring; this should be discussed with the surgical team in advance of the procedure. Pituitary lesions are associated with endocrine derangements and these patients may require perioperative consultation with an endocrinologist.

INTRAOPERATIVE MANAGEMENT

PREMEDICATION

A smooth transition into the operating suite alleviates parental and patient distress and plays a significant role in the care of the pediatric neurosurgical patient. The choice of a specific technique is dependent on the level of anxiety and the cognitive development and age of the child. Parental presence during induction of anesthesia is common in pediatric operating rooms and should be an option for the parent if the surgical team is appropriately trained. Children are usually old enough to manifest separation anxiety between the ages of 9 to 12 months and 6 years. In this age group, an anxiolytic drug provides a smooth and stress-free separation from the parents for induction of anesthesia. The patient's ability to cooperate and his or her neurological and fasting status determine the level of sedation needed for parental separation. Oral midazolam (0.25–0.5 mg/kg) is particularly effective in relieving anxiety and producing amnesia in children without intravenous access. This technique may also decrease the possibility of recall if an

opioid-based anesthetic technique is used. Obtunded and lethargic patients do not require premedication with sedatives and should have an anesthetic induction performed in an expeditious manner.

INDUCTION TECHNIQUES AND POSITIONING

The specific technique used for induction of anesthesia is dictated by the patient's comorbidities and neurologic status. Anesthesia can be induced with sevoflurane, nitrous oxide, and oxygen by mask in a fasted, neurologically stable patient who does not have intravenous access. Sevoflurane has virtually replaced halothane as the principal anesthetic for induction of anesthesia in infants and children. Induction with sevoflurane is rapid and smooth, with minimal depression of the cardiovascular system. Intracranial hypertension is exacerbated by hypercarbia and hypoxia, which may occur if the airway becomes obstructed during induction. Therefore, the anesthesiologist should gradually take over respiration and gently hyperventilate to minimize the cerebrovascular effects. In patients with intravenous access, anesthesia can be induced with a rapid acting hypnotic drug (e.g., propofol). Neuromuscular blockade is established with a nondepolarizing muscle relaxant. If the patient is at risk for aspiration, a rapid-sequence induction with succinylcholine is acceptable. Contraindications to the use of succinylcholine include malignant hyperthermia susceptibility, muscular dystrophies, and recent denervation injuries. If succinylcholine cannot be used, rocuronium can produce ideal intubating conditions within 2 minutes but does not allow spontaneous ventilation to return quickly if the airway is lost.

The pins of the head holder are designed to penetrate the skull with a force of up to 36 kg. The level of surgical stimulation is comparable to that of a skin incision, so supplemental analgesia should be administered before application of the head holder. Local anesthesia (e.g., bupivacaine with epinephrine) can be injected into the scalp and periosteum to decrease blood loss and provide supplemental analgesia. The total dose of bupivacaine should not exceed 2.5 mg/kg or 1 mL/kg of 0.25% solution.

The head of the patient is typically elevated to improve exposure and enhance cerebrospinal fluid (CSF) and venous drainage. This increases the risk that air emboli will enter the venous system through open channels in bone and sinuses. Paradoxical air embolism may occur in patients with cardiac defects that produce a left to right shunt for example, in patients with a patent foramen ovale or ductus arteriosus. Most pediatric neurosurgeons place their patients in the prone position for posterior fossa craniotomy, but the sitting position is still occasionally used for children who are older than 3 years of age and who have midline lesions and particularly in patients with morbid obesity in whom ventilation may be compromised.

A nasotracheal tube may be less likely to be displaced and more easily secured, especially in patients in the prone position. Proper positioning of the endotracheal tube is essential because extremes of neck flexion or extension can cause endobronchial intubation or accidental extubation. Careful auscultation of breath sounds after positioning is mandatory, and adequate clearance between the patient's chin and sternum should be ensured. Before draping, it is important to pad all pressure points and be certain that the endotracheal tube and all intravascular catheters and tubing are secure and accessible.

VASCULAR ACCESS

Secure intravenous access is essential before the start of the neurosurgical procedure. The decision to use peripheral or central catheters and the size of the catheters used is determined by the anticipated blood loss and need to administer vasoactive drugs. Two large peripheral venous cannulae are usually sufficient for most craniotomies in infants and children. In some patients, however, peripheral intravenous access may be difficult to secure and central venous cannulation may be necessary. A central venous catheter may not be feasible in children because the smaller bore may hinder rapid infusion of fluids and blood products. Moreover, children may have an increased risk of a pneumothorax, especially in neonates and infants. Cannulation of the femoral vein avoids the risk of pneumothorax associated with subclavian catheters and does not interfere with cerebral venous return as may be the case with jugular catheters. Femoral catheters are also more easily accessible to the anesthesiologist.

Blood loss may be significant during a craniotomy, and hemodynamic instability can occur as a result of fluid shifts or as a response to surgical manipulation of the brain. An intra-arterial catheter provides continuous blood pressure monitoring and sampling for blood gas analysis. Although the radial artery is the most commonly cannulated vessel, the dorsalis pedis and posterior tibial arteries may also be used for this purpose in infants and children.

MAINTENANCE OF ANESTHESIA

The choice of anesthetic drugs for maintenance of has not been shown to affect the outcome in neurosurgery in adults and has not been examined in pediatric patients. The choice of a specific technique therefore depends on the patient's medical condition, the surgical procedure, and the preference of the individual anesthesiologist. The most frequently used technique during neurosurgery consists of an opioid (i.e., fentanyl, sufentanil or remifentanil) and low-dose (less than 0.5 MAC) isoflurane or sevoflurane. Dexmedetomidine is frequently used in combination with opioids and a potent volatile anesthetic to as an adjunct to general anesthesia. This anesthetic regimen offers several advantages: It does not significantly affect most intraoperative neurophysiologic monitoring. Dexmedetomidine improves perioperative hemodynamic stability while reducing in opioid requirements and decreasing the time required for emergence from general anesthesia. Rapid administration of a dexmedetomidine bolus may, however, induce bradycardia and hypertension in small infants and children. Awareness under anesthesia in children has been reported to be 0.8%, which is significantly higher than that reported for adults. The use of processed EEG has been advocated in order to better estimate the depth of anesthesia, but the utility of these monitors in children less than 3 years of age is still in question. Routine use of preoperative benzodiazepines should provide some degree of amnesia in addition to decreasing patient anxiety.

Because sudden movements during neurosurgery may be life threatening, deep neuromuscular blockade is usually maintained during most procedures. Patients on chronic anticonvulsant therapy usually require a larger dose of neuromuscular blocking agents and some narcotics because of induced enzymatic metabolism of these agents. The use of neuromuscular blocking agents should be discussed with the surgical and monitoring teams if assessment of motor function during seizure and spinal cord surgery is planned. In many cases, these drugs may be used to facilitate endotracheal intubation and then allowed to wear off before monitoring is required.

MANAGEMENT OF FLUIDS AND BLOOD LOSS

Meticulous fluid and blood administration is essential in order to minimize hemodynamic instability, especially in the pediatric patient. Stroke volume is relatively fixed in the neonate and infant, so the patient should be kept normovolemic throughout the intraoperative period. Normal saline is generally chosen because it is mildly hyperosmolar (308 mOsm/kg) and should minimize cerebral edema, but rapid infusion of more than 60 mL/kg of normal saline may cause hyperchloremic acidosis. The routine administration of glucose-containing solutions is generally avoided during neurosurgical procedures, except in patients who are at risk for hypoglycemia. Patients who might require glucose-containing intravenous fluids include those with diabetes mellitus, children who are receiving total parental alimentation, and premature and small newborn infants. When it is required, glucose should be delivered with an infusion pump while closely monitoring serum glucose levels.

Circulating blood volume depends on the age and size of the patient. Newborn premature infants have a circulating blood volume of approximately 100 mL/kg total body weight; full term newborns have a volume of 90 mL/kg; infants have a blood volume of 80 mL/kg. Maximal allowable blood loss (MABL) can be estimated using a simple formula:

MABL = ESTIMATED CIRCULATING BLOOD VOLUME * (STARTING HEMATOCRIT − MINIMUM ACCEPTABLE HEMATOCRIT)/ STARTING HEMATOCRIT

Transfusion of 10 mL/kg of packed red blood cells increases hemoglobin concentration by 2 g/dL. Pediatric patients are susceptible to dilutional trombocytopenia in the setting of massive blood loss and multiple red blood cell transfusions. Low platelet counts or in some cases, excessive bleeding in acute settings necessitate the administration of 5 to 10 mL/kg of platelets, which should increase the platelet count by 50,000 to 100,000/mm³.

1. Intraoperative blood loss due to microvascular bleeding can sometimes be decreased by administration of antifibrinolytic drugs. Tranexamic acid is a synthetic amino acid lysine analog that forms a reversible complex with both plasminogen and plasmin. It competitively blocks the conversion of plasminogen to plasmin, which is responsible for the degradation of fibrin. This stabilizes blood clots that have already formed and enhances hemostasis. The routine use of tranexemic acid in surgical procedures with excessive blood loss such as posterior spine fusions and craniosynotosis reconstructive procedures has been shown to decrease blood loss in pediatric patients.

PHYSIOLOGIC MONITORS

Routine monitors for all patients undergoing anesthesia for neurosurgical procedure include a stethoscope (precordial or esophageal), electrocardiograph, pulse oximeter, noninvasive blood pressure, respiratory gas analysis, and body temperature. An intra-arterial cannula is usually inserted for continuous blood pressure monitoring after induction of anesthesia. Arterial access also allows sampling of blood for blood gases analysis, electrolytes, hematocrit, and serum osmolality. Central venous pressure may not accurately reflect vascular volume, especially in a child in the prone position, and is usually not monitored.

SPECIFIC ISSUES

CONGENITAL DISORDERS

Myelomeningocele

Myelomeningocele occurs because the posterior neural tube fails to close, resulting in a malformation of the vertebral column and spinal cord and other CNS anomalies. The spinal defect can occur anywhere along the vertebral column,

although lumbar and low thoracic defects are most common. In the most severe forms (rachischisis), the neural plate is a raw, fleshy plaque that can be seen through a vertebral column defect (spina bifida) and the skin. A protruding membranous sac containing meninges, CSF, nerve roots, and a dysplastic spinal cord often protrudes through the defect in meningocele or myelomeningocele. Tracheal intubation of a neonate with a myelomeningocele can be challenging depending on the size and location of the defect. The supine patient may be elevated on rolled-up towels, taking care to create a port through which the myelomeningocele may protrude. The neonate can also be positioned in the right lateral decubitus position to allow an unimpeded arc from right to left for laryngoscopy and intubation. Blood and fluid loss depends on the size of the myelomeningocele and the amount of tissue dissection required to repair the defect. Hydrocephalus is present in 80% of neonates with myelomeningocele or encephalocele. A ventriculoperitoneal shunt may therefore be implanted immediately after the initial repair of the myelomeningocele or within several days after primary closure.

Hydrocephalus

Hydrocephalus is commonly seen in pediatric neurosurgical patients. It has a laundry list of etiologies that include intraventricular or subarachnoid hemorrhage, congenital anomalies (e.g., aqueductal stenosis) trauma, infection, and tumors. Hydrocephalus is ideally managed by treating the underlying problem. If this is not possible, however, surgical implantation of a drain or shunt may be necessary. The most common place to drain CSF through an implanted shunt is the peritoneal cavity, but the right atrium or pleural cavity may also be used. The anesthetic technique to be used depends on the patient's symptoms. In a patient with an intact mental status or one in whom intravenous access cannot be established, an inhalation induction with sevoflurane and gentle cricoid pressure may be used. If, however, the patient is obtunded, is at risk for herniation, or has a full stomach, intravenous access should be established in order to perform a rapid sequence induction with a sedative/hypnotic drug and succinylcholine followed by tracheal intubation. Although implantation of a ventriculoperitoneal shunt is relatively straightforward, patients may be at increased risk for aspiration of gastric contents caused by the combination of use an altered mental status and recent peritoneal. VAE may occur during placement of the distal end of a ventriculoatrial shunt if the operative site is above the heart. Acute obstruction of a ventricular shunt usually requires urgent treatment because an acute increase in intracranial pressure in the relatively small cranial vault of the infant and child can be life threatening.

Craniosynotosis

Craniosynostosis is a condition in which the fibrous sutures of the skull close prematurely. The resulting abnormal growth of the skull may cause abnormalities in skull shape and facial features that are cosmetically unappealing. If the skull cannot expand to accommodate the growing brain, the patient can develop increased intracranial pressure. Remodeling procedures are most likely to have a good result if they are done early in life. Patients may also present for reconstruction with craniofacial syndromes that include an abnormal airway. Intubation of the trachea in these patients requires specialized techniques that are beyond the scope of this chapter. This surgery entails the risk of significant blood loss, necessitating the replacement of an infant's circulating blood volume or more. Blood loss varies with individual patients but increases with the number of sutures are involved. Large-bore intravenous access and arterial blood pressure monitoring are therefore essential for these procedures. Venous air embolus commonly occurs during the surgery, but maintaining adequate intravascular blood volume decreases this risk. Early detection of a VAE with continuous precordial Doppler ultrasound may allow treatment to be instituted before large amounts of air are entrained. In the setting of a VAE large enough to produce hemodynamic instability, the operating table can be placed in the Trendelenburg position to improve cerebral perfusion and prevent further entrainment of intravascular air. Special risks exist in neonates and young infants since potential right-to-left cardiac mixing lesions can result in paradoxical emboli.

NEOPLASMS

Brain tumors are the most common solid tumors in children. Signs of an intracranial lesion may be difficult to assess in infants and preverbal children but may include vomiting, irritability, or lethargy. Cranial nerve palsies and ataxia are also common findings; respiratory and cardiac irregularities are usually seen in patients with large tumors that impinge on the brainstem or that cause intracranial hypertension. The introduction of image-guided surgery in the treatment of brain tumors, vascular lesions and seizure foci has surgical precision, making it possible to accurately localize a tumor and its margins. Frame-based and frameless navigation systems use images obtained preoperatively to create a three-dimensional representation of the brain. Intraoperative magnetic resonance imaging allows the surgical team to assess the extent of mass resection on an ongoing basis. This offers surgeons the ability to achieve total mass resection while limiting the amount of healthy tissue that is removed.

Posterior Fossa Tumors

Cerebellar astrocytomas and meduloblastomas are the most common tumors of the posterior fossa and account for almost half of all pediatric CNS tumors. Malignancies affecting the brainstem (astrocytoma and ganglioglioma) and fourth ventricle (ependymoma) are less common. These space-occupying lesions often obstruct CSF flow and cause intracranial hypertension. These tumors may impinge on brainstem structures vital to the control of respiration, heart rate, and blood pressure, complicating the intraoperative management of these patients. Vital structures such as nuclei of the cranial nerves and respiratory centers are located anterior to the floor of the fourth ventricle and can be irritated or injured during the procedure. Respiratory control centers can be damaged during surgical dissection. Stimulation of the nucleus of cranial nerve V can cause hypertension and tachycardia. Irritation of the nucleus of the vagus nerve may result in bradycardia or postoperative vocal cord paralysis. Continuous observation of the blood pressure and ECG are essential to detect encroachment on these vital structures and guide the surgical manipulation of this area. The surgeon may wish to position the patient with the operative site above the heart in order to reduce bleeding and brain swelling. This may, however, increase the propensity for air entrainment into venous and bony sinuses.

Supratentorial Tumors

Approximately 25% of intracranial tumors in children involve the cerebral hemispheres, and the most common tumor types are astrocytomas, oligodendrogliomas, ependymomas, and glioblastomas. These tumors typically present with a new-onset seizures or focal deficits. Choroid plexus papillomas usually arise from the choroid plexus of the lateral ventricle. They are rare and occur most often in children younger than 3 years of age. Patients with these tumors present with hydrocephalus that is caused by increased production of CSF combined with obstruction of CSF outflow. Hydrocephalus usually resolves with surgical resection. Succinylcholine should be avoided in patients with motor weakness because hyperkalemia may result from massive depolarization. Nondepolarizing muscle relaxants and narcotics may be metabolized more rapidly in patients who are taking anticonvulsant medications. Cortical stimulation may be used to help identify motor areas in patients with tumors that lie near the motor or sensory strips. Nondepolarizing neuromuscular blocking agents can usually be used during induction, but then should be discontinued until mapping is no longer required. Since potent volatile agents can depress the cortical stimulation and detection of ictal activity, nitrous oxide and narcotics are usually sufficient to prevent patient movement during these periods.

Tumors that occur in the midbrain include craniopharyngiomas, optic gliomas, pituitary adenomas, and hypothalamic tumors and account for approximately 15% of intracranial tumors. Hypothalamic tumors (hamartomas, gliomas, and teratomas) frequently present with precocious puberty in children who are large for their chronological age.

Craniopharyngiomas are the most common perisellar tumors in children and adolescents and may be associated with hypothalamic and pituitary dysfunction. Symptoms often include growth failure, visual impairment, and endocrine abnormalities. Signs and symptoms of hypothyroidism should be sought during the preoperative evaluation. Routine laboratory studies in these patients should include thyroid and pituitary function tests. Steroid replacement therapy with either dexamethasone or hydrocortisone is may be required because the integrity of the hypothalamic-pituitary-adrenal axis may be uncertain. Diabetes insipidus may be present before surgery and commonly occurs in the perioperative period. A careful history that includes questions about nocturnal drinking and enuresis may elicit the presence of diabetes insipidus. Abnormally high output of dilute urine in the face of hypernatremia and hyperosmolality is diagnostic of diabetes insipidus. Laboratory studies should therefore include serum electrolytes and osmolality, urine-specific gravity, and urine output. Postoperative diabetes insipidus is marked by a sudden large increase in dilute urine output associated with a rising serum sodium concentration and osmolality. If diabetes insipidus is not present before surgery, it probably will not occur until the postoperative period. There appears to be an adequate reserve of antidiuretic hormone in the posterior pituitary gland that is capable of providing normal homeostasis for many hours even if the hypothalamic-pituitary stalk is injured during surgery. Initial management consists of infusion of a dilute crystalloid solution to replace the urine output. Frequent measurement of serum electrolyteis essential. In the setting of prodigious urine output (which may be up to 1 L/hr in an adult), an infusion of aqueous vasopressin (1–10 mU/kg/hr) should be started along with fluid administration that matches urine output and estimated insensible losses.

In infants and young children, an approach through a frontal craniotomy between the frontal lobes provides the best access to the pituitary gland. Transsphenoidal surgery is generally reserved for adolescents and older children with pituitary adenomas. Patients with pituitary tumors should receive the same monitoring and vascular access as for other midbrain tumors. Patients are usually intubated orally to give the surgeon optimal access to the nasopharynx, and preparations for an emergent craniotomy should be anticipated in case unexpected massive bleeding develops. Since the surgical exposure is limited, closure of the access site occurs. Nasal packs are also inserted at the end of surgery so patients should be fully awake before extubation of the trachea.

EPILEPSY

Surgical treatment of epilepsy may be indicated in patients with medically intractable epilepsy. Patients may undergo a series of procedures, including implantation of electrodes with subsequent mapping of eloquent areas and seizure paths. Patients then return to the operating room for removal of the electrodes, and may return for a third time for excision of the seizure focus. Intraoperative neurophysiologic monitors sometimes guide resection of the epileptogenic focus, and

general anesthetics can compromise the sensitivity of these devices. Cortical stimulation is sometimes used to mimic the seizure pattern or identify areas on the motor strip, and these responses may be ablated if neuromuscular blockade is present during the surgery. Some epileptogenic foci are in close proximity to cortical areas controlling speech, memory, motor or sensory function, and monitoring of patient and electrophysiologic responses is required to minimize the risk of iatrogenic injury to these areas. Chronic administration of anticonvulsant drugs (e.g., phenytoin and carbamazepine) induces rapid metabolism and clearance of several classes of anesthetic agents that include many neuromuscular blocking agents and opioids. Patients may have abnormally high requirements for these drugs and close monitoring of their effect and frequent redosing may be required. If a second craniotomy is scheduled within 3 weeks of the primary procedure, nitrous oxide should be avoided until after the dura is opened. Intracranial air can persist for up to 3 weeks after a craniotomy and nitrous oxide can cause rapid expansion of air cavities, resulting in tension pneumocephalus. An elective repeat craniotomy is most commonly scheduled for removal of grids and strips used for invasive EEG monitoring and subsequent resection of the seizure focus.

A variety of techniques have been advocated to facilitate intraoperative assessment of motor-sensory function and speech, including surgery with local anesthesia and no sedation and an "asleep-awake-asleep" technique in which the general anesthesia is induced, after the patient is awakened for functional testing, and general anesthesia is again induced with patient cooperation is no longer needed. Propofol does not interfere with the ECoG if it is discontinued 20 minutes before monitoring in children undergoing an awake craniotomy. Remifentanil and dexmedetomidine have also been used successfully in this setting. It is, however, imperative that candidates for craniotomy under local anesthesia or sedation be mature and psychologically prepared to participate in this procedure.

The vagal nerve stimulator is another advance in the surgical treatment of epilepsy. Although its exact mechanism of action is not understood, it appears to inhibit seizure activity at brainstem or cortical levels. It has been shown to benefit many patients who are disabled by intractable seizures and has minimal side effects. Implantation of a vagal nerve stimulator is a relatively simple procedure that involves creation of a left subpectoral muscle pocket for the impulse generator and placement of the electrode on the left vagal nerve. The electrode is then passed through a subcutaneous tunnel to the generator. The anesthetic management of patients for implantation of vagal nerve stimulators is determined by the patient's comorbidities.

CEREBROVASCULAR DISEASE

Cerebrovascular lesions are rare in pediatric patients and commonly manifests as hemorrhagic or ischemic stroke.

These vascular anomalies are categorized as structural (i.e., aneurysms or arterial dissections), pathologic (i.e., arteriovenous malformations [AVMs], vein of Galen malformations, arteriovenous fistulas [AVFs] and cavernous malformations), and progressive arteriopathies (e.g., moya-moya syndrome or heritable arteriopathies). Recent advances in interventional radiology offer diagnostic as well as therapeutic options for the management of these lesions. In general, the primary goal of the anesthesiologist is to optimize cerebral perfusion while minimizing the risk of bleeding.

A surgical approach to a cerebrovascular lesion always entails the risk of massive blood loss that should be aggressively treated with blood replacement and vasopressor therapy. Transient hypotension can be treated with either repeated bolus doses or a vasopressor infusion (e.g., dopamine, epinephrine, norepinephrine) during fluid resuscitation. Cerebral ischemia can be caused by hypoperfusion due to blood loss or by inadvertent occlusion of parent arteries by the surgeon. A large AVM in neonates may be associated with high-output congestive heart failure and require vasoactive support. Initial treatment of a large AVMs often consists of staged intravascular embolization in the interventional radiology suite. A small number of patients with high-flow AVMs may develop intraparenchymal hematoma and cerebral edema in the postoperative period. This is caused by markedly increased blood flow in newly perfused cerebral vessels during hypertensive episodes after embolization or surgical resection of the AVM. This phenomenon should be anticipated after treatment of high-flow lesions and can sometimes be avoided through staged embolization before surgical resection and maintenance of normal to slightly low blood pressure postoperatively. Vasodilators such as labetalol or nitroprusside may be necessary to control a hypertensive crisis.

Moya-moya is a rare chronic vasoocclusive disorder of the internal carotid arteries that presents as transient ischemic attacks and/or recurrent strokes in childhood. Moya-moya *disease* is the idiopathic form of moyamoya, while moya-moya *syndrome* is defined as the arteriopathy found in association with another condition, such as prior radiotherapy to the head or neck for optic gliomas, craniopharyngiomas, and pituitary tumors; genetic disorders such as Down syndrome, neurofibromatosis type I, large facial hemangiomas, sickle cell anemia, and other hemoglobinopathies; autoimmune disorders such as Graves disease, congenital cardiac disease, or renal artery stenosis. The goal of anesthetic management is to optimize cerebral perfusion with aggressive preoperative hydration and maintaining normotension or mild hypertension during surgery and the postoperative period. Intraoperative normocapnia is essential, because both hypercapnia and hypocapnia can lead to steal phenomenon from the ischemic region and further aggravate cerebral ischemia. Intraoperative EEG monitoring may utilized during surgery to detect cerebral ischemia and the anesthetic drugs needs to be modified

by avoid high inspiratory concentrations of isoflurane. Optimization of cerebral perfusion should be extended into the postoperative period maintain euvolemia and using sedatives and opioids to prevent hyperventilation induced by pain and crying.

NEUROENDOSCOPY

Technological advances in endoscopic surgery have provided less invasive approaches to the surgical management of CNS lesions. Since neuroendoscopic techniques are designed to minimize surgical incision, dissection, and blood loss, less aggressive fluid replacement and invasive hemodynamic monitoring are becoming the norm. Endoscopic strip craniectomies are associated with decreased blood loss, decreased surgical time, and improved postoperative recovery time during endoscopic strip craniectomy in neonates and infants. Endoscopic third ventriculostomy is another approach for the treatment of obstructive hydrocephalus in infants and children. A flexible fiberoptic scope is inserted through a trocar and provides a working channel that allows the neurosurgeon to insert a ventricular catheter or make fenestrations'. Despite the relative safety of this procedure, hypertension, bradycardia, and other arrhythmias have been reported in conjunction with acute intracranial hypertension due to lack of egress of irrigation fluids and/or manipulation of the floor of the third ventricle.

TRAUMATIC BRAIN INJURY

Protecting the brain in the pediatric neurosurgical or trauma patient requires a multiorgan approach to minimizing morbidity and mortality. Brain injury is an evolving process that extends beyond the initial insult. Since second insults can progressively worsen outcome, basic life support algorithms should be immediately applied to ensure a patent airway, spontaneous respiration, and adequate circulation. Progression of the primary neuronal injury can be attenuated by preventing hypotension and hypoxia, which are consequences of trauma. Progression of the primary neuronal injury can be attenuated by elimination the inciting event and optimizing cerebral metabolic supply and demand. Rapid implementation of advanced life support algorithms is essential in the management of these patients.

Securing a patent airway and restoring oxygenation and ventilation (breathing) are paramount in advanced life support algorithms. Infants and young children who are trauma victims are predisposed to C1-C2 cervical disruptions, which may be difficult to diagnose in cervical spine radiographs. There should be minimal cervical spine manipulation during tracheal intubation of the head-injured infant. Hyperventilation has traditionally been utilized to acutely treat intracranial hypertension. However, it can increase the volume of severely hypoperfused tissue within the injured brain by acute CBF reduction and increase in $CMRo_2$.

Therefore, hyperventilation should only be used acutely and not sustained in order to exacerbate cerebral ischemia.

Age appropriate nomograms of blood pressure in pediatric patients should dictate the endpoints of resuscitation. Hypotension is associated with greater mortality in children than adults. Therefore, hypotension secondary to trauma and/or blood loss should be aggressively treated by securing large bore intravenous catheters and restoration of fluid deficits. Vasopressors such as dopamine, phenylepherine, norepinephrine, or epinephrine can be utilized to augment CPP. The use of intracranial pressure monitoring in infants and children with severe head injury with a Glasgow Coma Scale less than or equal to 8 is strongly supported by several clinical several clinical studies. However, age-specific differences in cerebral hemodynamics necessitate modifying these variables. Pronounced morbidity and mortality occur after the ICP is persistently elevated above 20 mm Hg. However, the value of "less than 20 mm Hg" was artificially set and lower increments were not fully tested in pediatric patients. Ventricular catheters should be inserted to monitor intracranial pressure measurements provide a conduit to withdraw CSF.

One of the most controversial topics in the management of brain-injured patients is the goal for CPP. Several pediatric studies demonstrate that lower CPP levels are associated with better outcome when compared to adult values. Maintaining the CPP above 40 mm Hg appears to be associated with the best outcome in pediatric patients. However, studies in infants need to be performed in order to assess the efficacy of even lower CPP.

Cooling

Induced hypothermia has been unequivocally shown to reduce neurological injury in preclinical studies. Its efficacy in the clinical setting has been controversial. Head cooling and mild hypothermia has been demonstrated to be protective in asphyxiated neonates. A phase II NIH Trial demonstrated that induced hypothermia can be a safe therapeutic option in children with TBI. However an international multicenter trial of induced hypothermia in pediatric patients reported that hypothermia did not improve the neurologic outcome and may increase mortality.

Drugs

Endotracheal intubation and mechanical ventilation mandate prolonged sedation and, in severe cases, neuromuscular blockade. Sedation with intermittent doses of midazolam, fentanyl or morphine is imperative to minimize discomfort and agitation. Prolonged propofol infusion has limited utility in pediatrics due to its association with a fatal syndrome of bradycardia, rhabdomyolysis, metabolic acidosis, and multiple organ failure (propofol infusion syndrome). Brain swelling can be initially managed by hyperventilation and elevating the head above the heart. Should these maneuvers fail, mannitol can be given at a dose of 0.25 to 1.0 g/kg intravenously. This will transiently alter cerebral hemodynamics and raise serum osmolality by 10 to 20 mOsm/kg. However, repeated dosing can lead to extreme hyperosmolality, renal failure and further brain edema. Furosemide is a useful adjunct to mannitol in decreasing acute cerebral edema and has been shown in vitro to prevent rebound swelling due to mannitol. All diuretics will interfere with the ability to utilize urine output as a guide to intravascular volume status. The use of hypertonic saline (3% NaCl) has been shown to decrease ICP and improve CPP in pediatric patients. High-dose barbiturate therapy produces a burst suppression pattern on the EEG and results in a reduction in cerebral metabolic rate. Refractory intracranial hypertension can be treated by thiopental infusions. However, myocardial depression and hypotension are unacceptable side effects of this therapy and can be minimized by increasing intravascular volume and providing ionotropic support.

Decompressive Craniotomy

Reduction of severe, refractory intracranial hypertension may require surgical decompression of hemorrhagic and edematous brain tissue. A significant decrease in ICP and improved 6-month outcome have been reported in the children undergoing the decompressive craniectomy. Bifrontal or frontotemporal decompressive craniotomy for management refractory intracranial hypertension due to "shaken baby syndrome" have been shown to significantly decrease mortality in the when compared to the medically managed children. Despite the severity of this surgical approach, studies in children and adults demonstrate the utility of this approach in reducing refractory intracranial hypertension and an improvement in outcome. Therefore, decompressive craniotomy has a role as a last attempt at managing moribund head injured infants and children.

SUMMARY

Pediatric neurosurgical patients provide a variety of conditions are unique to small infants and children. A basic understanding of age-dependent variables and the interaction of anesthetic and surgical procedures are essential in minimizing perioperative morbidity and mortality.

BIBLIOGRAPHY

McClain CD, Soriano SG, Rockoff MA. Chapter 24: Pediatric neuroanesthesia. In: Cote CJ, Lerman J, Anderson BJ (Eds.), *A practice of anesthesia for infants and children* (5th ed.). 2013. Philadelphia: Elsevier Saunders.

Kochanek PM, Carney N Adelson PD, et al. Guidelines for the acute medical management of severe traumatic brain injury in infants, children, and adolescents—second edition. *Pediatr Crit Care Med* 2012;13(Suppl 1):S1–S82.

26.

ACUTE CARE SURGERY IN THE CRITICALLY ILL NEUROSURGICAL PATIENT

Joss J. Thomas and Avinash B. Kumar

INTRODUCTION

Advances in anesthesiology, critical care, and the prehospital care of patients with neurologic injury have resulted in patients being brought to the operating room with multiple comorbidities. Patients who were once considered to be "too sick for anesthesia" are now routinely undergoing surgery. Anesthetic management of critically ill patients who require neurosurgery requires an understanding of the pathophysiology of both the underlying neurologic process and that of the other comorbidities.

Managing intensive care unit (ICU) patients in the operating room presents a unique set of challenges for the anesthesia provider. These patients are frequently dependent upon mechanical ventilation and may be on multiple medications, including vasoactive infusions. Therapeutic goals may be different than those for routine neurosurgery case. Cerebral injury has several etiologies but the pathophysiologic common pathway involves (either individually or in combination) the lack of oxygen, essential nutrients and glucose to the brain tissue. This chapter will discuss some of the cardinal elements in the operating room management of patients who present from the neurocritical care unit.

NEUROLOGIC INJURY AND MECHANICAL VENTILATION

In the operating room setting with an intubated patient, ventilation strategies to reduce further neurologic injury are primarily based on maintaining adequate brain oxygenation and ventilation, since both can affect intracranial pressure (ICP). While it may be intuitive to consider maximal oxygen therapy in the light of brain injury, no study has demonstrated any benefit from the use of high Fio_2 [1]. In fact, as long as oxygen saturation is considered adequate, increasing Fio_2 is not necessary [2]. In addition, the risk of mild

hypercapnia on worsening neurologic injury has not been substantiated [3].

Hyperventilation has been used in the acute setting to reduce ICP. The goal of hyperventilation would be to reduce $Paco_2$ from 40 to 60 mm Hg (normal range) to a reduced range of 25 to 35 mm Hg [4]. However, it is not recommended that it should be continued on a long-term basis because it is associated with increased morbidity and mortality [5].

NEUROLOGIC INJURY, FLUID AND GLUCOSE MANAGEMENT

Fluid restriction as a management strategy is not supported by the current traumatic brain injury guidelines but continues to be used widely mostly based on historic teaching [6]. The current evidence for a positive fluid balance versus a fluid restrictive management strategy and outcomes in brain-injured patients are controversial [7].

Conventional medical therapy for cerebral vasospasm following subarachnoid hemorrhage is "triple H" or hypertension, hypervolemia, and hemodilution therapy. Recent evidence looking into the most important "H" in the triple H therapy points toward hypertension (aided with or without vasoactive medications) as being the most important and with the least effective being hemodilution [8. 9]. Hemodilution from generous fluid prescription was also associated with more non-neurologic complications such as respiratory failure, pulmonary edema, and congestive heart failure [8].

The causes of hyperglycemia in brain injury patients are multifactorial, ranging from acute catecholamine release, activation of hypothalamic pituitary axis, release of inflammatory cytokines, to acquired insulin resistance and iatrogenic causes such as large volume dextrose containing fluid prescription and total parenteral nutrition [10].

Hyperglycemia has been associated with poorer outcomes in SAH, ischemic stroke, and traumatic brain-injured patients. It is not, however, clear if the hyperglycemia itself is the cause of poor outcomes or it is just a marker for an underlying problem [10]. Hyperglycemia and hyponatremia are common iatrogenic consequences following the infusion of large volumes of dextrose-containing solutions, so large volumes of dextrose-containing fluids should be avoided in neurocritical care patients.

The role of intensive insulin therapy has been controversial in neurologic injury patients. The original intensive care study on tight glucose control dictated a blood glucose goal of 80 to 110 mg/dL [11]. The optimal target blood glucose levels in the neurocritical patient are not established, but there is consensus about the need for careful monitoring of blood glucose in this patient population. The current recommendation in acute ischemic stroke and traumatic brain injury patients is to maintain the blood glucose in the range between 110 and 180 mg/d: [12]. Results of ongoing and future trials are awaited to better define an optimal target for glycemic control.

DIRECT THROMBIN INHIBITORS

In 2010, the U.S. Food and Drug Administration (FDA) approved the use of dabigatran for the prevention of stroke in view of its superiority to warfarin for stroke and systemic embolism rates, as shown in some large randomized clinical trials. Dabigatran is a synthetic oral anticoagulant that acts as a direct, competitive inhibitor. It binds directly to the clot-bound and free thrombin. It also and has the advantage over warfarin because it does not require routine lab monitoring of prothrombin times or international normalized ratios (INRs). However, there are no effective reversal agents in the event of a devastating intracranial bleed. A case of fatal intracranial hemorrhage was reported by Garber et al. [13]. In addition, the authors have indicated that usual reversal agents such as factor VIIa and fresh frozen plasma are ineffective since it acts at the very last steps of the coagulation cascade. In view of the fact that the drug is renally excreted, dialysis can remove up to 60% of the drug in 2 to 3 hours. Following the thrombin time as a way to assess the effects of dabigatran during catastrophic bleeding is essential.

INTRACRANIAL HEMORRHAGE

Intracranial hemorrhage is a potentially life-threatening medical emergency, especially if the hemorrhage is ongoing. If the hemorrhage is due to a coagulopathy, the underlying cause must be corrected in a timely manner so that the size of the hematoma does not increase and cause increased ICP. Coagulopathy can be caused by anticoagulants used to treat other medical conditions (e.g., chronic atrial fibrillation).

Patients who develop an intracranial hemorrhage while being treated with an anticoagulant are at an increased risk of mortality relative to patients not taking these agents [14]. The specific management of a coagulopathy depends on the type of anticoagulant that was administered. For example, warfarin and heparin impair the coagulation cascade in clot formation, whereas aspirin and clopidogrel inhibit platelet function.

WARFARIN-ASSOCIATED INTRACRANIAL HEMORRHAGE

Warfarin-associated intracranial hemorrhage (WICH) is defined as intracranial hemorrhage that is associated with an INR greater than 1.3 [15]. Warfarin is being increasingly used to prevent strokes because of strong evidence in favor of anticoagulation [16]. Because patients are surviving longer, the incidence of WICH is increasing [17]. The treatment of warfarin coagulopathy can be challenging since the reversal of effect is slow, but rapid resolution of Warfarin-induced coagulopathy is critical to decreasing hematoma progression and improving patient survival. Treatment in the setting of active bleeding is multimodal, and drugs such as intravenous vitamin K (10 mg intravenous) take at least 6 to 24 hours for full effect. Vitamin K is normally administered as 1 mg orally or 0.5 mg intravenously because higher doses may lead to overcorrection and subsequent resistance to warfarin when anticoagulation therapy is resumed. Administration of a higher dose of vitamin K will make it difficult to achieve a therapeutic INR when warfarin therapy is reinitiated. Fresh frozen plasma is therefore recommended in a patient who is going to the operating room for intracranial surgery to remove the clot. Fresh frozen plasma should be ordered in advance of the scheduled surgery because it must be thawed prior to use and may not be immediately available. Once it has been administered, its effects may last up to 12 to 32 hours. Transfusion-related circulatory overload and acute lung injury are associated with the use of fresh frozen plasma, so the amount necessary to reverse the warfarin effect should be calculated. Figure 26.1 shows the calculation of volume of plasma needed depending on current INR and target INR [18]. In view of this increased risk of overload and lung injury, a better alternative is the use of prothrombin complex concentrates. These are safer than plasma but have been associated with a thrombogenic effect [19].

The use of recombinant factor VII (rFVIIa) remains controversial, and this drug is currently not FDA approved for use in intracranial hemorrhage, although there are centers which use it for this purpose. The Factor Seven for Acute Hemorrhagic Stroke (FAST) trial failed to confirm that rFVIIa administered within 4 hours of onset improves survival or functional outcome [20]. However, its use in WICH has shown to be effective in reversing effects of bleeding

Step 1. Decide on Target INR.

Clinical Situation	Target INR
Moderate bleeding, high risk of thrombosis	2.0–2.1
Serious bleeding, moderate risk of thrombosis	1.5
Serious or life-threatening bleeding, low risk of thrombosis	1.0

Step 2. Convert INR to Prothrombin Complex (expressed as a percentage of normal plasma).

	INR	Approximate %
Overanticoagulation	>5	5
	4.0–4.9	10
Therapeutic range	2.6–3.2	15
	2.2–2.5	20
	1.9–2.1	25
Subtherapeutic range	1.7–1.8	30
	1.4–1.6	40
Complete reversal to normal	1.0	100

Step 3. Calculate the Dose.

Formula for calculating the dose:

(target level as a percentage– present level as a percentage)×
body weight in kg– ml of plasma or IU of prothrombin-complex concentrate

Example: a patient with pulmonary embolism 3 months ago now has major intestinal bleeding; present INR – 7.5, target INR – 1.5, body weight – 80 kg:

(40–5)×80 – dose of 2800 ml or IU

Figure 26.1   Calculation of volume of FFP based on INR levels.

induced by warfarin within 15 minutes after an intravenous bolus. The use of factor VIIa in patients on warfarin and with traumatic intracranial hemorrhage may decrease the amount of time required to normalize the INR but there is no difference in mortality [21]. A meta-analysis of the safety and efficacy of the drug did not show improvement in mortality.

INTRACRANIAL HYPERTENSION

Cerebral edema is an acute response of the brain parenchyma to an insult. In adults, the cranial fontanelles have closed and the cranium is essentially a rigid box containing the brain itself, cerebrospinal fluid, and blood [22]. The Monro–Kellie doctrine dictates that the volume within the cranium is fixed and the addition of any further volume is at the expense of components already present. Normal ICP ranges from 5 to 15 mm Hg. The major consequences of sustained intracranial hypertension are ischemia and, ultimately, physical displacement of brain parenchyma causing potentially life-threatening herniation syndromes.

Any primary cause of uncontrolled rise in ICP is associated with a poor prognosis. The association with poor prognosis following traumatic brain injury (TBI) is high, especially with rise in ICP in the first 24 hours post injury [23].

Some of the important causes of increased ICP are outlined in Table 26.1 [24]

Table 26.1   **CAUSES OF INCREASED ICP [1]**

- Cerebral edema (vasogenic or cytotoxic)
- Mass lesion (e.g., hemorrhagic contusion, subdural hemorrhage)
- Obstructive hydrocephalus
- Posttraumatic seizure active (subclinical status epilepticus)
- Venous sinus thrombosis
- Decreased sedation and analgesia when on mechanical ventilation

INDICATIONS FOR MONITORING ICP IN THE NEUROLOGIC ICU (TBI GUIDELINES)

The initial clinical presentation of intracranial hypertension can be variable, ranging from a headache to a severely depressed level of consciousness. An astute neurologic examination and the Glasgow Coma Scale (GCS) are the primary tools that are widely used at the bedside to determine the need for ICP monitoring. The GCS is also used to determine the need for mechanical ventilation in the neurologically compromised patient. A decreasing motor component of the GCS in the setting of TBI is an indication that ICP may be increased.

Some of the potential indications for ICP monitoring are listed in Table 26.2 (BT guidelines 2008).

Table 26.2 **INDICATIONS FOR MONITORING ICP (BT GUIDELINES 2008)**

- GCS score ≤8
- Presence of other major injuries and hemodynamic compromise that may necessitate endotracheal intubation
- Development of hydrocephalus in a patient following acute subarachnoid hemorrhage
- Abnormal noninvasive ICP monitor numbers (e.g., increased pulsatility and abnormal waveforms on transcranial Doppler measurements
- Need for inducing barbiturate coma or aggressive sedation following severe TBI
- Postoperatively following the removal of large intracranial mass lesion

Attempts to monitor ICP noninvasively have been largely unsatisfactory [25]. In patients who require ICP monitoring, a ventricular catheter connected to an external strain-gauge transducer is the most accurate and cost-effective method of monitoring ICP. Intraventricular catheters are preferable to other methods because they are accurate, they can be recalibrated, and they allow drainage of CSF [26].

Other classes of devices used to monitor ICP include the parenchymal catheters (e.g., Camino catheter; Integra, Inc., Plainsboro, NJ). The major disadvantages of intraparenchymal catheters are the inability to drain CSF and the inherent tendency for "electrical drift" artifact once the catheter has been in place for several days. Once this system is placed into a patient, it cannot be re-zeroed or corrected for drift. Other less commonly used devices include the subarachnoid bolt and the epidural device [27]. The subarachnoid bolt has a tendency to read lower values than a ventricular catheter and the question of accuracy has led to its decline in use [28]. Epidural or extradural devices have the advantage of avoiding penetration of the dura, but the inelasticity of the dura, together with the difficulty in making sure that the transducer lies flat or co-planar to the dura leads, can lead to recording of falsely higher pressures [29].

MANAGING ACUTE INTRACRANIAL HYPERTENSION IN THE ICU

Managing a patient with a rapidly deteriorating neurologic status is a challenge; especially when the patient also has an acute increase in ICP. Management strategies for an acute rise in ICP include both medical and surgical interventions.

MEDICAL INTERVENTIONS

1. Prophylactic hyperventilation
2. Patient positioning
3. Hyperosmolar therapy
4. Temperature control
5. Barbiturate coma

SURGICAL INTERVENTIONS

1. Placement of an external ventricular drainage device
2. Decompressive craniectomy

PROPHYLACTIC HYPERVENTILATION

Aggressive hyperventilation (arterial $PaCO_2$ ≤25 mm Hg) had previously been a cornerstone in the management of severe traumatic brain injury (TBI) because it rapidly decreases ICP (by causing cerebral vasoconstriction and decreasing cerebral blood flow [CBF] and cerebral blood volume) [30]. Surveys conducted in the 1990s and later found more than 80% of centers in the United States of America used prophylactic hyperventilation as a first-line measure in the management of intracranial hypertension. A growing body of evidence suggests that hyperventilation is detrimental, especially in the first 24 hours following TBI. Hyperventilation is, therefore, no longer recommended as a routine part of clinical practice at this time. The most recent edition of the Brain Trauma Guidelines reflects this change in approach to managing TBI [31].

PATIENT POSITIONING

Elevation of the head of the bed to 30 degrees is a simple bedside maneuver that can help decrease ICP, provided there are no contraindications to this position (e.g., spine precautions) [32]. This intervention is restricted to those patients in whom there is no significant compromise in cerebral perfusion when the head of the bed is raised [33, 34].

TEMPERATURE CONTROL

Fever is common following brain injury, and aggressive treatment of hyperthermia is an important part of the management of the brain-injured patient [35]. Fever has been associated with worse outcomes following subarachnoid hemorrhage, TBI, and acute ischemic strokes [36].

The benefits of actively cooling patients to mild hypothermia (33 °C) using external cooling devices, cold saline infusions, or intravenous cooling catheters are controversial. Multiple studies of therapeutic hypothermia in the management of ICP and TBI have had contradictory outcomes [37, 38]. Although some patients may benefit from therapeutic hypothermia, it is currently not possible to make a uniform recommendation for therapeutic hypothermia in all brain-injured patients.

HYPEROSMOLAR THERAPY

Mannitol and hypertonic saline are the mainstays of hyperosmolar therapy in the management of intracranial hypertension. The primary mechanism of action is to raise the serum osmolality, which creates an osmotic gradient and draws water from the interstitial compartment of the brain to the intravascular compartment. This effect is more pronounced in normal brain tissue compared with the injured areas of the brain [27]. Mannitol is filtered in the glomerulus and is not reabsorbed in the renal tubules, thus creating an osmotic gradient that enhance water loss through the kidneys.

Mannitol can cause significant alterations in electrolytes and osmolality. Rapid administration of mannitol can also cause in hypotension, especially in the fluid-restricted patient. Mannitol-induced fluid shifts and renal fluid losses can cause electrolyte derangements (particularly hypokalemia, hypomagnesemia, and hypophosphatemia). Overly aggressive use of mannitol can result in a form of acute kidney injury called osmotic nephrosis, which is characterized by proximal tubular vacuolization and swelling of the cells lining the renal tubules, thus decreasing the effective size of the lumen [39]. Plasma osmolarity should, therefore, be monitored in patients receiving multiple doses of mannitol and not allowed to increase beyond 320 mOsm/L (the traditionally defined safe threshold for renal tubular necrosis) [27].

Hypertonic saline (HS) is rapidly gaining acceptance in the United States. The encouraging results from prehospital administration of HS as part of the "small-volume resuscitation" approach in TBI patients has ultimately resulted in more widespread use in the ICU. HS produces an osmotic gradient, dehydrating brain tissue and reducing ICP while augmenting volume resuscitation and increasing circulating blood volume, mean arterial pressure (MAP), and cerebral profusion pressure (CCP). Concentrations ranging from 3% through 23.4% are used in small aliquots in the management of ICH [40]. When used in isovolemic concentrations in a recent prospective randomized trial, HS (7.5%) was found to be more effective than mannitol in reducing ICP. HS (7.5%) remains the most commonly used concentration of HS in the United States [41].

There are several potential and theoretical complications that have been associated with HS therapy, including phlebitis, exacerbation of heart failure, hyperchloremic metabolic acidosis, and myelinolysis. The use of HS has additional advantages in maintaining hemodynamics and reducing the inflammatory response and possibly reduce incidence of ARDS. However, two recent landmark clinical trials in which concentrated saline was used in TBI and hemorrhagic shock were halted by the National Heart, Lung, and Blood Institute because there was no survival benefit. However, the safety of using HS was not questioned and there was no evidence that HS solutions were harmful [42, 43]. HS is ideally administered through a central venous catheter to minimize the risk of phlebitis. The goal of HS therapy is an increase in serum sodium concentration to 145 to 155 mEq/L (and serum osmolality, approximately 300 to 320 mOsm/L). It is imperative to closely monitor serum sodium and osmolality to avoid severe hypernatremia (Na^+ >165 mEq/L). This is continued while HS therapy is discontinued in order to avoid rebound hypernatremia [40]. There are currently no large, randomized clinical trials comparing conventional osmotic agents with HS solution in equiosmolar and equivolumic concentrations and long-term functional outcomes in critically ill brain-injured patients. Osmotic agents such as mannitol seem to have stood the test of time and maintain a role in the treatment of cerebral edema and elevated ICP. Hypertonic saline has the added advantage of potentially improving hemodynamics and may be more useful in a patient who is already in shock or is hemodynamically unstable.

BARBITURATE THERAPY

High-dose barbiturate therapy may be used in patients who have failed conventional first-line therapies like hyperosmolar therapy. Pentobarbital has emerged as the preferred agent in high-dose barbiturate therapy because of its greater efficacy as compared to other barbiturates. Pentobarbital also has a shorter physiologic half-life when administered as repeated boluses or a continuous infusion. Pentobarbital is usually administered as a bolus of about 3 to 10 mg/kg given slowly (not to exceed 50 µg/min) followed by an infusion of 1 to 3 mg/kg/h [44], which is then titrated to produce burst suppression on the electroencephalogram (EEG). Pentobarbital coma (PBC) is maintained for 48 hours or until the underlying pathophysiologic mechanism has been reversed.

PBC probably works by decreasing the cerebral metabolic rate as evidenced by the decrease in CBF, cerebral oxygen consumption, and reduced arteriovenous oxygen difference. Barbiturate therapy also reduces intracellular acidosis (which is a significant contributor to secondary neuronal damage) through inhibition of phosphofructokinase, pyruvate, and lactate production. Barbiturates also decrease the release of the excitatory amino acids glutamate and aspartate and may blunt the "neuroexcitotoxicity" thought to occur in the patient with severe TBI [45].

Barbiturates produce a sustained decrease in the arterial blood pressure frequently necessitating vasoactive medications to maintain CPP. Other commonly recognized side effects of barbiturate therapy include hepatic and renal dysfunction, systemic hypothermia, immunosuppression, and a delayed return of consciousness. However, one of the less well-recognized complications is that of severe potassium disturbances. Prolonged sedation, even after the termination of the infusion, is another important drawback of this therapy [25].

DECOMPRESSIVE CRANIECTOMY

The modern proponents of decompressive craniectomy (DC) described the technique as early as 100 years ago. Although cranial decompression theoretically improves the pressure–volume relationship, its use in the management of refractory intracranial hypertension remains controversial. The term "decompressive craniectomy" encompasses a range of surgical techniques (scalp closure only, duraplasty with autologous or synthetic patch), location of decompression (frontal, temporal, etc.), and hemisphere (unilateral or bilateral) designed to achieve satisfactory cranial volume expansion [46].

There are no specific guidelines or protocols stating exactly when or in what circumstances DC is appropriate. DC has been used as a last resort for cases with refractory ICH. However, recently, the Brain Trauma Foundation suggested that the use of DC should be considered earlier as a therapeutic option given emerging evidence supporting its use for early ICP control [47].

The procedure itself (i.e., DC) and the second staged cranioplasty needed to replace the bone flap represent major surgery and carry significant risk. Some of the common complications following DC include subdural hygromas, secondary wound infection, extension of the hemorrhage/contusion, and the fascinating syndrome of the trephined: a late complication consisting of headaches, confusion, dizziness, memory difficulties, and mood disturbances. Motor disturbances, including progressive contralateral upper limb weakness in an area not previously affected by injury, may also occur. In a majority of the cases, this syndrome can be reversed with cranioplasty [46].

CONCLUSIONS

Maintaining CPP or managing ICP. What is more important? ICP is one determinant of CPP (CPP = [MAP – ICP]) and thus, is also an indirect determinant of CBF.

Cerebral injury has several etiologies, but the common pathophysiologic pathway involves (either individually or in combination) the lack of oxygen, essential nutrients, and glucose to the brain tissue. The overall management strategy is to optimize and balance these elements. These patients presents with some unique challenges for the operating room anesthesiologist. A careful evidence-based approach should be encouraged, with consideration given to the principles of effective mechanical ventilation, hemodynamics, fluid management, glycemic management, and ICP control.

REFERENCES

1. Stocchetti N, Maas AI, Chieregato A, et al. Hyperventilation in head injury: a review. *Chest.* 2005;127:1812–1827.
2. Reinert M, Barth A, Rothen HU, et al. Effects of cerebral perfusion pressure and increased fraction of inspired oxygen on brain tissue oxygen, lactate and glucose in patients with severe head injury. *Acta Neurochir (Wien).* 2003;145:341–349; discussion 349–350.
3. Lowe GJ, Ferguson ND. Lung-protective ventilation in neurosurgical patients. *Curr Opin Crit Care.* 2006;12:3–7.
4. Bratton SL, Chestnut RM, Ghajar J, et al. Guidelines for the management of severe traumatic brain injury. XIV. Hyperventilation. *J Neurotrauma.* 2007;24(Suppl 1):S87–S90.
5. Haitsma JJ. Physiology of mechanical ventilation. *Crit Care Clin.* 2007;23:117–134, vii.
6. Clifton GL, Miller ER, Choi SC, et al. Fluid thresholds and outcome from severe brain injury. *Crit Care Med.* 2002;30:739–745.
7. Fletcher JJ, Bergman K, Blostein PA, et al. Fluid balance, complications, and brain tissue oxygen tension monitoring following severe traumatic brain injury. *Neurocrit Care.* 2010 13:47–56.
8. Muench E, Horn P, Bauhuf C, et al. Effects of hypervolemia and hypertension on regional cerebral blood flow, intracranial pressure, and brain tissue oxygenation after subarachnoid hemorrhage. *Crit Care Med.* 2007;35:1844–1851; quiz 1852.
9. Treggiari MM, Deem S. Which H is the most important in triple-H therapy for cerebral vasospasm? *Curr Opin Crit Care.* 2009;15:83–86.
10. Godoy DA, Di Napoli M, Rabinstein AA. Treating hyperglycemia in neurocritical patients: benefits and perils. *Neurocrit Care.* 2010;13:425–438.
11. van den Berghe G, Wouters P, Weekers F, et al. Intensive insulin therapy in the critically ill patients. *N Engl J Med.* 2001;345:1359–1367.
12. Quinn TJ, Lees KR. Hyperglycaemia in acute stroke—to treat or not to treat. *Cerebrovasc Dis.* 2009;27(Suppl 1):148–155.
13. Garber ST, Sivakumar W, Schmidt RH. Neurosurgical complications of direct thrombin inhibitors—catastrophic hemorrhage after mild traumatic brain injury in a patient receiving dabigatran. *J Neurosurg.* 2012;116:1093–1096.
14. Toyoda K, Yasaka M, Nagata K, et al. Antithrombotic therapy influences location, enlargement, and mortality from intracerebral hemorrhage. The Bleeding with Antithrombotic Therapy (BAT) Retrospective Study. *Cerebrovasc Dis.* 2009;27:151–159.
15. Brody DL, Aiyagari V, Shackleford AM, et al. Use of recombinant factor VIIa in patients with warfarin-associated intracranial hemorrhage. *Neurocrit Care.* 2005;2:263–267.
16. Aguilar MI, Hart RG, Kase CS, et al. Treatment of warfarin-associated intracerebral hemorrhage: literature review and expert opinion. *Mayo Clin Proc.* 2007;82:82–92.
17. Flaherty ML, Haverbusch M, Sekar P, et al. Long-term mortality after intracerebral hemorrhage. *Neurology.* 2006;66:1182–1186.
18. Schulman S. Clinical practice. Care of patients receiving long-term anticoagulant therapy. *N Engl J Med.* 14 2003;349:675–683.
19. Makris M, Greaves M, Phillips WS, et al. Emergency oral anticoagulant reversal: the relative efficacy of infusions of fresh frozen plasma and clotting factor concentrate on correction of the coagulopathy. *Thromb Haemost.* 1997;77:477–480.
20. Mayer SA, Brun NC, Begtrup K, et al. Efficacy and safety of recombinant activated factor VII for acute intracerebral hemorrhage. *N Engl J Med.* 2008;358:2127–2137.

21. Nishijima DK, Dager WE, Schrot RJ, et al. The efficacy of factor VIIa in emergency department patients with warfarin use and traumatic intracranial hemorrhage. *Acad Emerg Med.* 2010;17:244–251.

22. Ganong W. *Review of medical physiology.* 17th ed. London: Prentice Hall International; 1995.

23. Miller JD, Butterworth JF, Gudeman SK, et al. Further experience in the management of severe head injury. *J Neurosurg.* 1981;54:289–299.

24. Rangel-Castilla L, Gopinath S, Robertson CS. Management of intracranial hypertension. *Neurol Clin.* 2008;26:521–541, x.

25. Perez-Barcena J, Llompart-Pou JA, Homar J, et al. Pentobarbital versus thiopental in the treatment of refractory intracranial hypertension in patients with traumatic brain injury: a randomized controlled trial. *Crit Care.* 2008;12:R112.

26. Maas AI, Stocchetti N, Bullock R. Moderate and severe traumatic brain injury in adults. *Lancet Neurol.* 2008;7:728–741.

27. Jantzen JP. Prevention and treatment of intracranial hypertension. *Best Pract Res Clin Anaesthesiol.* 2007;21:517–538.

28. Miller JD. ICP monitoring—current status and future directions. *Acta Neurochir (Wien).* 1987;85:80–86.

29. Dorsch NWC, Symon L. *The validity of extradural measurement of the intracranial pressure.* Berlin: Springer-Verlag; 1975.

30. Raichle ME, Plum F. Hyperventilation and cerebral blood flow. *Stroke.* 1972;3:566–575.

31. Brain Trauma Foundation. Guidelines for the management of severe traumatic brain injury. *Journal of Neurotrauma.* 2007;24(Suppl 1):S1–106.

32. Fan JY. Effect of backrest position on intracranial pressure and cerebral perfusion pressure in individuals with brain injury: a systematic review. *J Neurosci Nurs.* 2004;36:278–288.

33. Ng I, Lim J, Wong HB. Effects of head posture on cerebral hemodynamics: its influences on intracranial pressure, cerebral perfusion pressure, and cerebral oxygenation. *Neurosurgery.* 2004;54:593–597; discussion 598.

34. Schneider GH, von Helden GH, Franke R, et al. Influence of body position on jugular venous oxygen saturation, intracranial pressure and cerebral perfusion pressure. *Acta Neurochir Suppl (Wien).* 1993;59:107–112.

35. Wolfe TJ, Torbey MT. Management of intracranial pressure. *Curr Neurol Neurosci Rep.* 2009;9:477–485.

36. Polderman KH. Induced hypothermia and fever control for prevention and treatment of neurological injuries. *Lancet.* 2008;371:1955–1969.

37. Fox JL, Vu EN, Doyle-Waters M, et al. Prophylactic hypothermia for traumatic brain injury: a quantitative systematic review. *CJEM* 2010;12:355–364.

38. Badjatia N. Fever control in the neuro-ICU: why, who, and when? *Curr Opin Crit Care.* 2009;15:79–82.

39. Dickenmann M, Oettl T, Mihatsch MJ. Osmotic nephrosis: acute kidney injury with accumulation of proximal tubular lysosomes due to administration of exogenous solutes. *Am J Kidney Dis.* 2008;51:491–503.

40. Bhardwaj A, Ulatowski JA. Hypertonic saline solutions in brain injury. *Curr Opin Crit Care.* 2004;10:126–131.

41. Vialet R, Albanese J, Thomachot L, et al. Isovolume hypertonic solutes (sodium chloride or mannitol) in the treatment of refractory posttraumatic intracranial hypertension: 2 mL/kg 7.5% saline is more effective than 2 mL/kg 20% mannitol. *Crit Care Med.* 2003;31:1683–1687.

42. National Heart, Lung, and Blood Institute. NHLBI stops enrollment in study of concentrated saline for patients with traumatic brain injury. 2009. https://roc.uwctc.org/tiki/tiki-index.php

43. National Heart, Lung, and Blood Institute. The NHLBI halts study of concentrated saline for patients with shock due to lack of survival benefit. 2009. http://www.nhlbi.nih.gov/news/press-releases/2009/the-nhlbi-halts-study-of-concentrated-saline-for-patients-with-shock-due-to-lack-of-survival-benefit.html

44. Eisenberg HM, Frankowski RF, Contant CF, et al. High-dose barbiturate control of elevated intracranial pressure in patients with severe head injury. *J Neurosurg.* 1988;69:15–23.

45. Marshall GT, James RF, Landman MP, et al. Pentobarbital coma for refractory intra-cranial hypertension after severe traumatic brain injury: mortality predictions and one-year outcomes in 55 patients. *J Trauma.* 2010;69:275–283.

46. Li LM, Timofeev I, Czosnyka M, et al. Review article: the surgical approach to the management of increased intracranial pressure after traumatic brain injury. *Anesth Analg.* 2010;111:736–748.

47. Kakar V, Nagaria J, John Kirkpatrick P. The current status of decompressive craniectomy. *Br J Neurosurg.* 2009;23:147–157.

27.

OCCLUSIVE CEREBROVASCULAR DISEASE—PERIOPERATIVE MANAGEMENT

Ryan Hakimi, Jeremy S. Dority, and David L. McDonagh

Occlusive cerebrovascular disease is a common clinical entity that is managed with a variety of medical and surgical therapies. The intraoperative management of patients undergoing neurovascular procedures to treat this condition is perhaps the most challenging work of the neuroanesthesiologist. This chapter provides an overview of the various occlusive cerebrovascular disease states and the perioperative management of patients undergoing corrective procedures.

The most common cause of occlusive cerebrovascular disease is atherosclerosis, which can be divided into three main categories: conditions involving the extracranial carotid arteries, the intracranial cerebral arteries, and the vertebrobasilar arteries. Nonatherosclerotic causes of occlusive cerebrovascular disease are also addressed in this chapter.

OCCLUSIVE EXTRACRANIAL CAROTID DISEASE

Extracranial atherosclerosis accounts for 15% to 20% of all ischemic strokes [1, 2]. Occlusive extracranial carotid disease (Figure 27.1) has historically received the greatest attention because it is readily accessible and amenable to intervention and has the greatest body of literature supporting its treatment. Three prospective carotid endarterectomy (CEA) trials have demonstrated that symptomatic patients who have greater than 70% carotid stenosis benefit from CEA [North American Symptomatic Carotid Endarterectomy Trial (NASCET), European Carotid Surgery Trail (ECST), Veterans Affairs Cooperative Study (VA Coop Study)] [3–5]. CEA has also been shown to prevent ischemic strokes in asymptomatic patients younger than 75 years of age who have greater than 70% stenosis (Asymptomatic Carotid Surgery Trial] [6]. However, few medical treatment options were available at the time of these trials.

A randomized controlled trial [Carotid Revascularization Endarterectomy versus Stenting Trial (CREST)] of over 2500 patients compared carotid stenting using a distal protection device to open CEA in symptomatic and asymptomatic patients with carotid occlusive disease. No statistically significant difference was found in the primary composite endpoint of stroke, myocardial infarction (MI), or death in the periprocedural period, or ipsilateral stroke within 4 years after randomization [7]. In post-hoc analyses, acute MI was more prevalent in the CEA group (2.5% versus 1.1%, $p = .03$) while acute ischemic stroke was more prevalent in carotid stenting (CS) group (4.4% versus 2.3%, $p = .01$). Further analyses could not differentiate any significant treatment effect based on age, sex, or symptomatic (versus asymptomatic) status.

CEA and CS procedures that were performed in these large trials were done by very experienced surgeons and interventionalists, while physicians with equivalent levels of skill may not be available at all centers. The location and anatomy of the stenotic lesion also guide the decision to choose CEA or CS, as lesions cephalad to the mandible may not be accessible to CEA. Similarly, vessel accessibility (vascular tortuosity, obesity, etc.) may impact the ability to gain arterial access or deliver and deploy the carotid stent to its optimal position. Lastly, patients who are considered to be at too high of a risk for surgical CEA should be considered for CS at the current time.

The patient undergoing either CEA or CS is at risk for ischemic stroke and myocardial infarction during the periprocedural period. However, quality of life measures at one year amongst survivors demonstrate that ischemic stroke has a greater adverse effect than myocardial infarction across a wide range of health-status domains [7]. Individual patient characteristics also guide the treatment of extracranial carotid stenosis. Older age is associated with an increased risk for adverse events with CS [8–11]. These adverse events have been attributed to vessel tortuosity and calcification [12]. Younger patients have been shown to have better outcomes with CS, while older patients have had better outcomes with CEA [12]. The low absolute numbers of

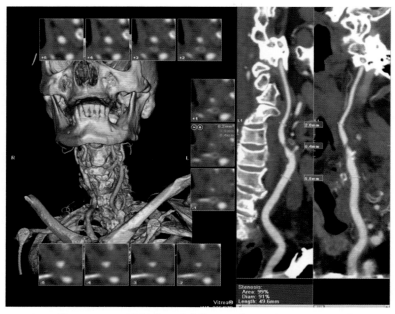

Figure 27.1   CTA image & reconstruction—72yo woman with high grade left internal carotid artery stenosis (approximately 90%).

postprocedural ischemic strokes and myocardial infarctions suggest that both procedures are safe for patients with extracranial carotid stenosis.

When there are no contraindications to revascularization in a patient with TIA or ischemic stroke, it is reasonable to perform the procedure within 2 weeks of the ischemic event [13]. Patients with a large hemispheric infarction are at a higher risk for reperfusion injury or hemorrhagic conversion, so carotid revascularization may be delayed for a period of 6 weeks or longer. Carotid revascularization is not indicated in patients with complete occlusion (i.e., 100% stenosis) of the symptomatic internal carotid artery or in patients who have severe debility such that revascularization would not be expected to improve [14].

OCCLUSIVE INTRACRANIAL CEREBRAL ARTERY DISEASE

Intracranial cerebral arterial stenosis can be attributed to wide variety of causes including, but not limited to, atherosclerosis, intimal fibroplasia, and vasculitis [14]. When extracranial carotid disease is not discovered in the diagnostic evaluation of a patient who has had a TIA or stroke, additional vascular imaging studies should be obtained to rule out intracranial cerebral artery disease [14]. It is estimated that intracranial atherosclerosis accounts for up to 10% of ischemic strokes and TIAs [15]. The Stenting & Aggressive Medical Management for Preventing Recurrent Stroke in Intracranial Stenosis (SAMMPRIS) Trial, randomized patients with symptomatic severe intracranial atherosclerosis to either angioplasty and stenting

with aggressive medical therapy or aggressive medical therapy alone. The study was stopped after the enrollment of 451 patients because the interventional arm had a high rate of stroke and death (14.7 versus 5.8%; $p = .002$) [16]. As such, medical management is currently the treatment of choice in patients with symptomatic intracranial atherosclerosis. Stenting of the intracranial vessel can be considered in symptomatic patients who fail aggressive medical therapy, if the patient is willing to enter a trial registry [17].

OCCLUSIVE VERTEBROBASILAR ARTERIAL DISEASE

Although patients with vertebral artery disease are at increased risk for stroke, MI, and death, the pathophysiology and management of occlusive vertebral artery disease is not as well understood as occlusive extracranial carotid disease (see Figure 27.2). The vertebral arteries are divided into four segments (V1-V4), the first three of which are extracranial. Atherosclerosis most commonly affects the proximal or V1 portion of the vertebral arteries. Lesions of the V2 and V3 portion may be caused by osteophytes on the transverse processes that interfere with blood flow through the artery when the patient turns his or her head [14]. Symptomatic intracranial vertebral artery stenosis has an associated annual 8% stroke rate, while basilar artery stenosis carries an 11% annual stroke rate [18–20]. Vertebrobasilar arterial stenosis has been associated with multiple ischemic episodes and places the patient at a higher risk of early recurrent ischemic stroke than does carotid stenosis [21].

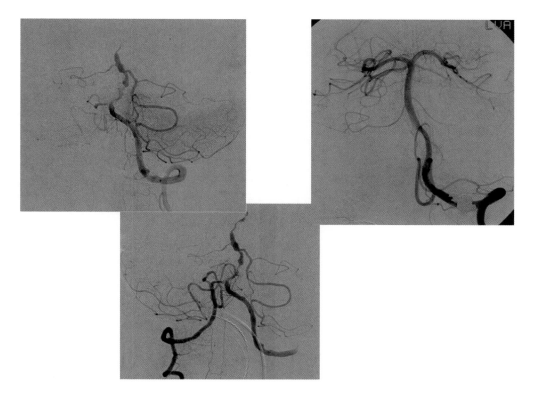

Figure 27.2 Conventional Angiography—70yo woman with severe basilar artery atherosclerotic disease (left: two images) compared with a normal basilar artery (right).

Initial evaluation of patients for whom vertebral artery revascularization is being considered usually begins with CT or MR angiography. Techniques used for noninvasive imaging typically do not allow adequate visualization of the vertebral artery origins, therefore conventional cerebral angiography is usually necessary as part of the evaluation [14].

At the present time, no specific medical, endovascular or surgical treatment for vertebrobasilar arterial stenosis has been studied in a randomized controlled trial. Most practitioners therefore follow the same medical recommendations as those for carotid atherosclerotic disease. Three months of anticoagulation is recommended [22–25] in patients with angiographic evidence of thrombus within an extracranial vertebral artery. In patients who have an ischemic stroke from intracranial vertebrobasilar atherosclerotic stenosis, aspirin is recommended for secondary stroke prevention [19, 26]. A randomized trial of Warfarin versus Aspirin for Symptomatic Intracranial Disease (WASID) concluded that warfarin anticoagulation offered no benefits over aspirin for secondary (recurrent) stroke prevention [19]. Endovascular stenting of atherosclerotic vertebrobasilar disease remains an option for patients who have failed medical therapy, and arterial bypass surgery is reserved for patients with medically intractable symptomatic vertebrobasilar stenosis that is not amenable to endovascular therapy.

SPECIAL POPULATIONS

Fibromuscular dysplasia (FMD) and cervical artery dissection are the most common nonatherosclerotic causes of occlusive cerebrovascular disease [14]. FMD is a noninflammatory, nonatherosclerotic stenosis of a vessel caused by thickening of the intimal, medial, and/or adventitial layers of the arterial wall [27–29]. It can affect any part of the cerebrovascular system, although bilateral internal carotid artery stenosis is most common. It most commonly affects middle-aged women who may be symptomatic or asymptomatic. Symptomatic presentations include ischemic stroke, TIA, Horner's Syndrome, dissection, and subarachnoid hemorrhage [27–29]. Medical treatment is most commonly with antiplatelet medications, while revascularization has been described on a limited basis [14].

Cervical arterial dissection involving the carotid or vertebral arteries may result from minor or major trauma, or with no apparent precipitant at all. CT angiography is typically used to screen for dissection following traumatic brain or neck injury. Subintimal dissection tends to cause stenosis, while subadventitial dissection leads to aneurysmal degeneration. Standard treatment consists of anticoagulation for a period of months, but this is not based on high-level evidence. Stenting of the vessel may be indicated in some patients.

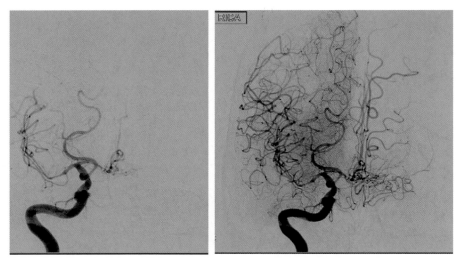

Figure 27.3   Conventional Angiography (early and late phase)—39yo woman with vasospasm due to subarachnoid hemorrhage. The M1 and A1 segments (1 segments of the MCA and ACA vessels) are severely narrowed. Endovascular therapy would entail angioplasty or intra-arterial vasodilators.

Vasospasm is a condition in which there is an imbalance between intrinsic vasodilators (e.g., nitric oxide) and vasoconstrictors (e.g., endothelins), which decreases the caliber of the intracranial vessels and increases the risk of ischemic stroke (see Figure 27.3). The pathophysiology of vasospasm is, however, highly complex and involves inflammatory cascades, histopathologic changes in the vessel wall, and neural-glial responses to injury [30]. Vasospasm is most commonly encountered in patients with aneurysmal subarachnoid hemorrhage, in whom the resulting ischemic strokes are referred to as "delayed ischemic deficits." It can, however, also be seen after traumatic brain injury and in vasculitides from a multitude of etiologies.

Moyamoya disease (see Figure 27.4) is a condition of unknown etiology in which there is progressive stenosis and occlusion of the intracranial carotid arteries and/or proximal vessels of the Circle of Willis [31]. Cerebral angiography has a characteristic "puff of smoke" appearance caused by tenuous cerebral perfusion through a multitude of small collateral vessels. Adult patients are at risk for both ischemic and hemorrhagic stroke. Medical therapy is limited and has been largely disappointing. Given that patients are at risk for both ischemic and hemorrhagic strokes, antithrombotic therapy poses the risk of exacerbating a hemorrhagic stroke. Individual patients may be managed with antiplatelet therapy or vasodilatory calcium channel blockers [31]. Indirect or direct surgical revascularization procedures (reviewed later) are used with success in many patients.

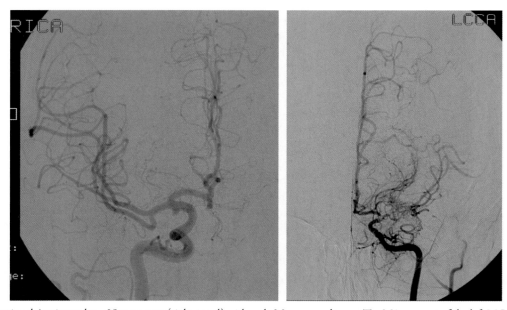

Figure 27.4   Conventional Angiography—28yo woman (right panel) with early Moyamoya disease. The M1 segment of the left MCA is occluded. A normal M1 vessel is shown (left panel).

BRAIN IMAGING

CT studies with intravenous contrast dye are usually the first step in the evaluation of patients with suspected cerebrovascular disease. Noncontrast CT imaging of the brain, although readily available, is of limited value in the assessment of patients with cerebrovascular disease given its poor visualization of the brainstem and posterior fossa, as well as insufficient information regarding the vasculature. MRI of the brain without gadolinium allows detailed evaluation of the brainstem and cerebellum while offering better visualization of small ischemic lesions, which may be isodense on brain CT. MRI imaging can be limited by its availability and its medical and surgical contraindications, which include incompatible implanted devices such as pacemakers and defibrillators, claustrophobia, and extreme obesity. MR angiography (MRA) with or without contrast is used to evaluate the cerebral vasculature.

CEREBROVASCULAR IMAGING

Every imaging technique has advantages and disadvantages. Because the quality of images produced by noninvasive imaging techniques, and neuroradiologic expertise in interpretation, may vary from one center to another, no single imaging modality can be universally recommended for all patients and all disease processes [14].

CONVENTIONAL CEREBRAL ANGIOGRAPHY

Conventional cerebral angiography is the gold standard for the evaluation of intracranial and extracranial arterial stenotic lesions. Factors limiting the use of conventional angiography include its cost and availability and the fact that it requires arteriotomy and the administration of iodinated IV contrast dye. When performed by experienced operators, conventional cerebral angiography carries a less than 1% risk for iatrogenic stroke [32, 33]. This technique is generally considered when evaluating intracranial or extracranial vascular disease for surgical intervention or when noninvasive vascular imaging is nondiagnostic, provides conflicting data, or is contraindicated [14]. In patients with renal dysfunction, conventional cerebral angiography may be a reasonable choice that limits the patient's exposure to iodinated contrast while providing definitive imaging of a single vascular territory [14]. Overall, few patients need conventional cerebral angiography for the evaluation of their cerebrovascular disease unless being evaluated for possible neurovascular surgery.

DUPLEX ULTRASONOGRAPHY

Duplex ultrasonography (DUS) is an inexpensive, readily available, and widely used technique [14]. DUS estimates the degree of arterial stenosis by measuring the peak systolic and diastolic Doppler velocities in the extracranial internal carotid artery and the ratio of the peak systolic velocity of the extracranial internal carotid artery to the ipsilateral common carotid artery. The use of *brightness mode* (B-mode) imaging permits the assessment of plaque morphology. Morphologic plaque features that have been associated with a greater risk for ischemic stroke include the presence of ulceration, echolucency, intraplaque hemorrhage, and high lipid content [34, 35]. Hypoechoic plaques are associated with embolic cortical and subcortical ischemic strokes [36]. DUS allows not only visualization of the extracranial internal and external carotid arteries but also a small portion of the cervical vertebral arteries. It provides information about the physiology of the vascular circulation, demonstrating variations in the normal direction of flow caused by conditions such as subclavian steal, or flow reversal through the external carotid artery to compensate for a highly stenotic internal carotid artery.

The utility of DUS is limited in patients with a short, thick neck, and variability in vascular anatomy from individual to individual may prevent adequate internal carotid artery assessment. Imaging is optimal in blood vessels located below the mandible. DUS may produce spurious results when performed by less experienced operators in unaccredited laboratories, leading to either underestimation or overestimation of the extent of stenosis. Visualization of the vertebral arteries is often inadequate and may be limited to determination of flow direction (antegrade or retrograde).

DUS is recommended as the first-line diagnostic test in the evaluation of asymptomatic patients with known or suspected carotid stenosis and permits determination of the hemodynamic significance of a stenotic lesion [14]. The presence of a carotid bruit in an asymptomatic patient is often a reason to obtain a DUS to rule out carotid stenosis, although the probability of detecting a carotid stenosis greater than 75% in a patient with a bruit is approximately 1.2% [37]. DUS may also be indicated in the presence of two or more risk factors for atherosclerosis in an asymptomatic patient, and intimal-medial thickness screening can be utilized in cerebrovascular risk assessment; although this remains controversial as various panels have conflicting recommendations for screening of this asymptomatic population [14]. Patients who are to undergo a revascularization procedure for extracranial carotid stenosis should also be evaluated by MRA, CTA, or conventional angiography to determine whether concomitant intracranial cerebral arterial disease is present [14]. DUS has additional indications including the follow-up evaluation post-carotid revascularization procedures and intra-operative assessment of a patient undergoing CEA or CS [38].

TRANSCRANIAL DOPPLER ULTRASONOGRAPHY

Transcranial Doppler ultrasonography (TCD) is a noninvasive modality that allows evaluation of intracranial cerebral blood flow velocity. TCD is performed by *insonating* the cerebral blood vessels with a 2-MHz probe through the temporal bone, the orbit, and the foramen magnum to measure flow through the anterior cerebral, middle cerebral, posterior cerebral, vertebral, and basilar arteries [39]. TCD is intrinsically limited by its "blind" insonation of the cerebral blood vessels through the cranium, but some systems use color Doppler imaging to directly visualize each vessel (transcranial color-coded duplex sonography) and allow some anatomic localization. Like DUS, TCD provides physiological information in that it can demonstrate flow reversal and/or collateral flow in vessels compensating for a stenotic or occluded vessel. TCD in combination with DUS is noninvasive and permits evaluation of the entire cerebrovascular system without the administration of contrast agents.

CTA

CTA provides rapid visualization of the intracranial and extracranial cerebrovascular anatomy and identifies stenoses, vascular malformations, and aneurysms. This technique has become more readily available as the resolution of CT scanners has improved. Unlike DUS or "time-of-flight" (noncontrast) MRA, CTA allows direct visualization of the vessel lumen. Its use is limited by the fact that it requires the administration of iodinated contrast dye, which carries risks that include iodine allergy, potential renal injury, and interactions with medications such as metformin. The utility of CTA is limited in patients with significant arterial calcification, dental implants, and surgical clips, all of which produce x-ray scatter and make the images difficult to interpret.

CTA should be considered as the next diagnostic step when evaluating patients with symptoms referable to the distributions of the internal carotid arteries and DUS is equivocal, nondiagnostic or suggests a complete occlusion of one or more internal carotid arteries [14]. CTA is preferred over DUS for imaging of the vertebrobasilar system, offering improved sensitivity [14]. CT perfusion is a developing imaging modality that permits evaluation of the hemodynamic significance of a stenotic or occluded artery (i.e., regional cerebral blood flow), but the literature supporting its use in daily clinical practice is limited at present.

MRA

MRA can be used to image the cerebral blood vessels either with or without gadolinium contrast. Intracranial imaging without gadolinium contrast relies on *time-of-flight imaging* which digitally subtracts the brain parenchyma from the image, allowing visualization of the intracranial vasculature. It is difficult to obtain satisfactory images of the extracranial cerebrovascular system without the administration of gadolinium (i.e., "contrast-MRA") because of artifact caused by the vertebral bodies.

MRA produces images of the vertebral arteries that are superior to CTA and DUS in some studies [40]. MRA, however, is prone to overestimation of the degree of carotid stenosis compared with conventional cerebral angiography [14]. MRA is also less sensitive than CTA or DUS to arterial calcification. Like DUS, MRA can provide information about plaque morphology [41] but MRA is far superior for imaging the vertebrobasilar system [14].

Although it provides superior images, gadolinium contrast dye is associated with nephrogenic systemic fibrosis (NSF), especially in patients with preexisting kidney disease (GFR less than 30 mL/min) [42]. Gadolinium should also be avoided in patients on dialysis [43]. Before obtaining an MRA of the blood vessels in the neck, the patient's glomerular filtration rate (GFR) should be determined and the potential risks of NSF should be considered if it is less than 30 mL/min. Newer, open MRI machines that use lower field strengths are rarely capable of producing high-quality MRA images, making this procedure more difficult to obtain in patients who are claustrophobic.

PREOPERATIVE EVALUATION

The preoperative evaluation begins with a thorough history and physical examination, including a basic neurological history and examination that establishes the patient's baseline deficits and level of functioning. Neurovascular imaging studies should be reviewed so that the neuroanesthesiologist understands the patient's anatomy, the planned procedure, and the risk of potential injury from hypo- or hypertension (i.e., cerebral hypo- or hyperperfusion). In cases where carotid revascularization is planned, the risk of ischemic stroke varies with the patient's preoperative clinical status. A patient with a symptomatic stenosis (i.e., stroke or transient ischemic attack referable to the vessel being revascularized) has a higher risk for subsequent ischemic stroke than would an asymptomatic patient. A patient with hemispheric ischemic symptoms (e.g., weakness or aphasia) has a higher risk for ischemic stroke than does one with amaurosis fugax (fleeting monocular blindness). Additional risk factors include the requirement for an urgent procedure and/or reoperation (as opposed to primary surgery) [44–46]. Patients with contralateral carotid occlusion, or restenosis after a previous CEA, face an even higher risk of perioperative stroke or death [47].

Management of hypertension is an important part of secondary stroke prevention in the outpatient setting. In general, medical management of hypertension after an acute ischemic stroke is important and backed by high level evidence, but specific universal blood pressure goals have not been established [48]. Blood pressure should be controlled if there is sufficient time before the planned cerebrovascular surgery. In the asymptomatic patient with extracranial carotid or vertebrobasilar disease, a systolic blood pressure of less than 140 mm Hg is recommended [48–50]. The neuroanesthesiologist should then use the patient's baseline blood pressure as a guide to intraoperative hemodynamic management.

Administration of statins to achieve an LDL less than 100 mg/dL is supported in all symptomatic or asymptomatic patients with carotid or vertebral atherosclerosis. Statin dose in patients who have had an ischemic stroke should be titrated to achieve a goal LDL of less than 70 mg/dL [48]. Statins should be continued perioperatively. The presence of diabetes increases a patient's risk for ischemic stroke by 2- to 5-fold [51]. Perioperative normoglycemia is the goal and the patient should have been screened for diabetes (or the efficacy of the current diabetic treatment regimen) in the workup of his/her cerebrovascular disease by obtaining a hemoglobin A1c level. The patient's smoking history is also valuable because the risk of carotid artery vasospasm, in addition to other smoking-related perioperative complications, during CS is greater in patients who are smokers and those with hypertension [52].

CARDIAC IMAGING: ECHOCARDIOGRAPHY

The preoperative cardiac evaluation is guided by the patient's age, medical history, comorbidities, and functional status. Patients with cerebrovascular atherosclerotic disease often have concomitant coronary atherosclerotic disease, and functional status may be difficult to assess because of either limited mobility or a sedentary lifestyle. In many cases, cerebrovascular surgery cannot be postponed while the patient undergoes an elective cardiac revascularization procedure. The purpose of the preoperative work-up is therefore to identify acutely decompensated cardiac conditions that may need short-term medical optimization or chronic conditions that are stable but may present problems during the perioperative period.

In general, the cardiac workup is designed to aid the neuroanesthesiologist with the patient's hemodynamic management during the perioperative period. At a minimum, most patients should receive a baseline electrocardiogram to identify asympomatic conduction abnormalities and to serve as a basis for comparison if cardiac abnormalities arise. Transthoracic echocardiography (TTE) may be considered to assess ventricular and valvular function in a patient with limited functional status but in whom functional cardiac studies (i.e., stress echocardiography or nuclear imaging) would not change management or lead to coronary revascularization procedures.

TTE should be performed as part of the routine evaluation of acute stroke patients to find an underlying cause

such as intracardiac thrombi, right to left intracardiac shunt, left atrial dilatation, valvular vegetations, or other structural abnormalities that could cause cardioembolic ischemic strokes [48]. When TTE results are nondiagnostic or equivocal, transesophageal echocardiography (TEE) may be indicated. TEE has a higher sensitivity than TTE in detecting right-to-left shunts as well as in evaluating the thoracic aorta, which may be worthwhile in certain patients undergoing carotid revascularization [14].

RECOMMENDATIONS FOR PREOPERATIVE MANAGEMENT OF PATIENTS UNDERGOING CEA

Aspirin (81 to 325 mg) should be started before surgery and continued indefinitely after the surgery [48, 53]. Various other antiplatelet medications may also be considered about four weeks after CEA for ongoing primary or secondary stroke prevention. Antihypertensives should be administered as needed to control the patient's blood pressure throughout the perioperative period, although a specific target is not recommended nor is a specific medication regimen. Periprocedural use of beta-blockers and angiotensin inhibitors has, however, been associated with better surgical outcomes in patients undergoing CEA [54, 55]. In one retrospective study, initiating statin therapy for at least one week before CEA was associated with a decreased length of stay and lower risk of periprocedural ischemic stroke, TIA, myocardial infarction, and death [56]. A multivariate analysis of the data, adjusting for demographics and comorbidities, suggests that antecedent statin use is associated with a 3-fold reduction in stroke and a 5-fold reduction in death following CEA.

RECOMMENDATIONS FOR PREOPERATIVE MANAGEMENT OF PATIENTS UNDERGOING CATHETER-BASED TREATMENTS

Preoperative management of the patient undergoing transluminal endovascular procedures is focused on managing hypertension and minimizing the risk of thromboembolic complications during and after the procedure. Most patients will be placed on dual antiplatelet therapy with aspirin (81 to 325 mg/day) and clopidogrel (75 mg/day) before CS or intracranial stenting, and this therapy will be continued for a minimum of 30 days after the procedure. Ticlopidine 250 mg twice daily may be substituted in patients who cannot tolerate clopidogrel [14]. The administration of antihypertensive medications is recommended before and after CS [14]. Patients should be evaluated for occlusive peripheral arterial disease that would preclude vascular access for the procedure. Since a large volume of contrast dye may be administered during the procedure, patients should be evaluated for baseline renal insufficiency.

INTRAOPERATIVE MANAGEMENT:

Arterial blood pressure is monitored invasively in nearly all patients undergoing neurovascular procedures under general anesthesia. When possible, the catheter should be inserted before induction to facilitate close monitoring of blood pressure during the induction of general anesthesia. Venous access should include large bore catheters for fluid administration. Central venous access may be required for safe delivery of vasopressors and hyperosmotic agents (e.g., mannitol and/or hypertonic saline).

Goals for management of systemic arterial pressure should be agreed on by the neuroanesthesiologist and neurosurgeon before starting the procedure, recognizing that the parameters should be individualized for the patient and the procedure. These parameters are inherently arbitrary and based on the opinions of the attending neurosurgeon and neuroanesthesiologist, which makes communication between the anesthesia and surgical teams all the more essential. Moreover, there is no evidence to suggest that using systolic blood pressure as opposed to mean blood pressure as a target offers improved outcome. One strategy is to target a systolic pressure on the assumptions that oligemic areas of brain parenchyma that are distal to the occlusive lesion may only be perfused during systole, and that systolic blood pressure is the main risk factor for hemorrhagic complications.

The ideal intraoperative monitor would provide continuous information about cerebral blood flow in the areas at risk of ischemia or hyperperfusion injury during cerebrovascular surgery. TCD and electrophysiologic monitoring techniques (EEG or evoked potentials) may be used to estimate the adequacy of cerebral perfusion. TCD is not feasible in the vast majority of patients, however, because the surgical site overlies the vessel of interest and it is difficult to access the head during the surgical procedure. TCD may be a more viable option for in patients undergoing endovascular procedures. Other monitoring techniques, such as EEG and near-infrared spectroscopy, have the same limitations in regards to intracranial vascular procedures but could be utilized for endovascular surgery or carotid revascularization because the entire scalp is accessible during the procedure. There is no standard of care for monitoring neurovascular surgery, so these various techniques should be used in cases where the neurovascular surgeon and neuroanesthesiologist believe that they will optimize care and outcome.

CAROTID REVASCULARIZATION

Open. The anesthetic management of patients undergoing open CEA has been extensively studied in large randomized trials such as the General Anaesthesia versus Local Anaesthesia for Carotid Surgery (GALA) trial [57, 58]. Regional (i.e., cervical plexus block) anesthesia in an awake patient and general anesthesia are both acceptable options.

The anesthetic technique varies based on surgeon preference, and neither approach has been shown to be superior to the other. Maintenance of adequate cerebral perfusion pressure is critical until the artery has been repaired and often requires the use of vasopressors. A temporary shunt may be used by some surgeons during carotid occlusion in order to maintain perfusion of the ipsilateral cerebral hemisphere; this carries a risk of neurologic complications most directly from embolic complications from shunt placement [59]. An alternate method of assessing cerebral perfusion is to monitor the neurologic status of an awake patient under regional anesthesia. Electroencephalographic, evoked potential, cerebral oximetry, or TCD can also detect cerebral hypoperfusion.

Despite lack of evidence for a clear clinical benefit, some surgeons request that propofol be administered during carotid cross-clamping to achieve pharmacologic burst suppression. If burst suppression is anticipated, EEG monitoring may be required, and can be performed with dedicated equipment and a neurophysiologist, or simply guided using a depth of anesthesia monitor such as the bispectral index. The typical dose required to achieve burst suppression is a 1- to 2-mg/kg bolus followed by an infusion at 150 to 200 µg/kg/min.

The carotid sinus reflex may cause an abrupt onset of hypotension and bradycardia during manipulation of the carotid artery or after reperfusion and should be anticipated by the anesthesiologist. Lidocaine injection in the surgical field can ameliorate this problem, although its use and effectiveness are debatable [60].

Endovascular. Endovascular stenting of the carotid artery may be performed under mild or moderate sedation with or without the presence of an anesthesia team. Like CEA, hypotension should be avoided in the period before the stenotic vessel is dilated, after which hypertension leading to hyperperfusion injury is the concern [61].

Patients undergoing either the open or endovascular procedure are at risk for post-operative cerebral hyperperfusion, so systemic hypertension should be treated promptly after blood flow through the internal carotid artery has been restored [62]. This can be accomplished with beta-blockers (e.g., metoprolol, labetalol, or esmolol infusions), dihydropyridine calcium channel blockers (e.g., nicardipine or clevidipine infusions), or nitrates (e.g., nitroglycerin or nitroprusside). Alternately, postoperative hypotension can occur, particularly after carotid stenting, and patients may require hemodynamic support with vasopressors for a brief period of time after the procedure.

INTRACRANIAL REVASCULARIZATION

Endovascular: Intracranial Angioplasty and Stenting

The primary goal of the anesthesiologist during intracranial endovascular procedures is to prevent patient movement during delicate and sometimes painful manipulation of intracranial vessel [62]. Simultaneously, tight hemodynamic control is essential to avoid injury due to hypoperfusion or hyperperfusion. It is important to communicate with the endovascular surgeon and to be aware of the stage of the procedure, which may not be intuitively obvious to the anesthesia team watching the angiographic images. There is very little pain during or after the procedure, except for vascular compression after the access port is withdrawn from the artery. Short-acting, potent analgesics like remifentanil are therefore particularly useful during maintenance anesthesia. Emergence hypertension is common and should be anticipated, particularly in this patient population (who often have baseline hypertension). High blood pressure can be safely treated with a variety of intravenous agents including beta-blockers and calcium channel blockers.

Open Vascular Bypass

EDAS. Encephaloduralarteriosynangiosis (EDAS) or encephalomyoarteriosynangiosis (EMAS) procedures are performed primarily in patients with moya-moya disease [31]. A vascular pedicle containing a branch of the temporal artery (with or without attached temporalis muscle) is mobilized and laid on the frontal lobe in the territory of the middle cerebral artery territory [63].

EDAS and EMAS are accomplished without the need to interrupt local or global cerebral blood flow, but patients with moya-moya disease have a very high risk of intraoperative ischemic injury because of the tenuous nature of their cerebral perfusion. It is therefore critical that the neuroanesthesiologist maintain cerebral perfusion pressure throughout the procedure. There is, however, no evidence base to further guide specific therapy [31]. One suggested practice is to begin administration of vasopressors before induction of anesthesia to prevent even brief episodes of relative hypotension, avoid significant changes in $PaCO_2$ (i.e., normocapnia) and continue vasopressors throughout the intraoperative period. Intracerebral steal is a theoretical concern with the halogenated anesthetic agents, so the use of a propofol intravenous anesthesia may be preferable. Our practice is to use high inspired oxygen concentrations (FIO_2 1.0) through most of the procedure, but any benefit remains speculative. The cerebral vasculature often contains microaneurysms and other fragile vessels that may be prone to bleeding. Patients with moya-moya disease are therefore also at risk for intracerebral hemorrhage if the blood pressure becomes too high.

VESSEL-TO-VESSEL BYPASS

Vascular bypass procedures are sometimes performed in patients with occlusive cerebrovascular disease refractory to medical management. The extracranial to intracranial arterial bypass study conducted 30 years ago found no benefit to surgical bypass for patients with internal carotid and middle cerebral artery occlusion [64]. These procedures are, however, still used occasionally for patients with occlusive cerebrovascular disease or to bypass giant intracranial aneurysms. A venous (e.g., saphenous vein) or arterial (e.g., temporal artery or free radial artery) graft is used to connect the extracranial carotid circulation to the middle or posterior cerebral arteries (or possibly other vessels). A "STAMCA" (Superficial Temporal Artery to Middle Cerebral Artery) bypass is commonly used for extracranial to intracranial vascular bypass in patients with moya-moya disease or to bypass an occluded middle cerebral artery.

These procedures involve temporary occlusion of the target vessel proximal to the site of anastomosis for an extended period of time (often longer than 30 minutes). Neuroprotective maneuvers are therefore commonly employed by the neuroanesthesiologist in addition to maintaining an adequate cerebral perfusion pressure. These recommendations are based on only low-level evidence.

Management of patients undergoing vessel to vessel bypass requires careful control of hemodynamics with induced hypertension or hypotension at different points of the procedure. The need to administer sedative infusions, fluid and blood products, and vasoactive drugs, along with the necessity of monitoring central venous pressure in some patients or procedures, is an indication for central venous catheterization. The catheter must not be inserted at a site that might interfere with the surgical bypass procedure (usually avoiding the ipsilateral neck is prudent). Invasive monitoring of systemic arterial blood pressure during induction is ideal, and is essential throughout the procedure.

Suppression of cerebral electrical activity by administering drugs to produce burst suppression on encephalography (EEG) results in an approximately 50% reduction in the cerebral metabolic rate ($CMRO_2$) [65, 66]. This requires continuous EEG monitoring (the bispectral index monitor or other depth of consciousness monitor may be used for this purpose if the raw EEG waveform can be displayed). Burst suppression can be achieved by administration of potent inhaled anesthetic agents like isoflurane, or more typically, intravenous anesthetics such as propofol. Barbiturates can also be used to provide burst suppression but emergence from anesthesia can be delayed for hours or days. The advantage of using propofol for this purpose is that it can be discontinued after restoration of cerebral blood flow and most patients will emerge and be ready for extubation at the end of the procedure. Although burst suppression with anesthetic agents has been shown in preclinical models to reduce focal ischemic brain injury, it also has been shown that doses of anesthetics substantially less than those required to cause electroencephalographic burst suppression are equally protective [65, 66]. Optimal human dosing is therefore unknown.

The decision to induce burst suppression relies on theoretical evidence; there are no data to guide a preference for barbiturate versus propofol therapy and no human outcome data. Clinical practice and recommendations are based on expert opinion. One suggested practice is to administer a 1- to 2-mg/kg bolus of propofol followed by 150- to 200-μg/kg/min continuous infusion. If, on rare occasion, the neurosurgeon requests prolonged sedation postoperatively (usually to facilitate tight hemodynamic control in a fragile vascular bypass patient), then pentobarbital is administered.

Therapeutic hypothermia can be used as a neuroprotective maneuver in patients who require prolonged intraoperative ischemic times, for example, common carotid to posterior cerebral artery bypass with a saphenous vein graft. A target temperature of 32-34°C is achieved with passive cooling and administration of cold intravenous fluids. Endovascular or surface cooling with commercially available devices may also be employed for induction or maintenance of hypothermia. Evidence for the effectiveness of therapeutic hypothermia in adults exists only for the cardiac arrest patient population [67] in whom it is currently standard of care to initiate therapeutic hypothermia for 24 hours in comatose survivors. The IHAST trial demonstrated no benefit of therapeutic hypothermia in patients undergoing intracranial aneurysm surgery, even in those who received temporary clipping [68], but therapeutic hypothermia also caused no discernable injury. Therefore, high-level evidence exists for lack of benefit or harm of hypothermia in routine cerebral aneurysm surgery. Therapeutic hypothermia can be used along with pharmacologic burst suppression for major cerebral vascular bypass operations during which prolonged temporary vessel occlusion is expected that would place considerable regions of cerebral cortex at risk for infarction. This is our current practice but is justified only on the basis of expert opinion.

ENDOVASCULAR THERAPY FOR ACUTE ISCHEMIC STROKE

Acute ischemic stroke is a leading cause of disability and death worldwide. Acute therapy is predicated on the time from onset (ictus) of the stroke. It is clear that neurologic injury and outcome progressively worsens as the time to restore cerebral blood flow (reperfusion) to ischemic brain increases [69]. Administration of intravenous thrombolytics is the standard of care in patients who have had symptoms for less than 4.5 hours [69]. The use of intra-arterial therapy (thrombolytics, angioplasty, or clot removal) varies from center to center depending on availability and surgical preference. The window during which these therapies may be used is also time limited: 6 hours for intra-arterial thrombolytic therapy in the anterior circulation, 12 hours in the vertebrobasilar vessels, and 8 hours for clot extraction devices (e.g., the Solitaire, Merci, or PENUMBRA devices).

The choice of general anesthesia for endovascular therapy in the setting acute ischemic stroke is a subject of debate amongst endovascular neurointerventionalists [70]. The overall preference in the endovascular community is, however,

for the use of general anesthesia. There are currently three retrospective studies that correlate the use of general anesthesia with worse outcome for acute ischemic stroke interventions [71, 72]. There is no high level evidence for cause and effect at this time and prospective trial data are needed. However, retrospective data suggest that hypotension/hypoperfusion (SBP less than 140 mm Hg) may be a factor [73].

The major concern for the neuroanesthesiologist is to avoid any delay in starting the interventional stroke procedure and restoring blood flow to the ischemic area. These cases should be treated as "level 1" emergencies (i.e., time is brain). Rapid sequence induction is usually indicated with special attention to maintaining moderate systemic hypertension throughout (and hence cerebral blood flow to oligemic penumbral regions around the area of frank ischemia). Some patients will have already received intravenous thrombolytic therapy, also known as "bridging therapy," and caution must be exercised when instrumenting the airway and vasculature due to risk of hemorrhage.

Craniectomy. A discussion of occlusive cerebrovascular disease would be incomplete without the mention of decompressive craniectomy for malignant MCA infarction. Neuroanesthesiologists should know that the use of hemicraniectomy is increasing in patients with malignant middle cerebral artery stroke and traumatic brain injury. Decompressive craniectomy is usually performed within 48 hours of onset of the stroke but may be used sooner or later depending on the individual patient. The purpose of this procedure is to prevent a fatal herniation syndrome in patients who have progressive unilateral hemispheric edema. This procedure should be considered early in the hospital course and in younger patients (aged less than 60 years as a general rule). Older patients often have enough cerebral atrophy to accomodate cerebral edema without herniation. High level evidence exists for the efficacy of hemicraniectomy in reducing mortality and increasing the number of patients with good neurologic outcome, but with an increased risk of survival with severe disability [74]. The optimal use of decompressive craniectomy in traumatic brain injury is less clear (DECRA Trial) but beyond the scope of this chapter [75].

The role of the neuroanesthesiologist is to deliver the patient to the operating room and procedure as expediently as possible while maintaining cerebral perfusion pressure and controlling intracranial pressure. Significant hypotension may occur with removal of the skull plate, as with decompression of any intracerebral lesion causing acute mass effect (i.e., subdural and epidural hematomas).

URGENT ENDOVASCULAR THERAPY FOR CEREBRAL VASOSPASM

The most common cause of symptomatic cerebral vasospasm is subarachnoid hemorrhage, although it may also occur in other disease states such as severe traumatic brain injury (Figure 27.3). Vasospasm usually occurs several days after the initial hemorrhage and frequently becomes symptomatic due to focal cerebral oligemia. Initial treatment is with intravenous fluids and vasopressors (i.e., hypertensive euvolemia). Refractory cases require acute endovascular therapy with angioplasty and/or intra-arterial vasodilators. The interventional procedure may be done under mild sedation or general anesthesia depending on the preference of the endovascular neurosurgeon. These patients are usually being treated with vasopressors to maintain cerebral perfusion, and utmost care must be taken by the neuroanesthesiologist to maintain hypertensive euvolemia throughout the procedure.

CONCLUSION

Occlusive cerebrovascular disease is one of the greatest challenges for the neuroanesthesiologist. Patients often have various other comorbidities, including significant vascular disease in other organ systems. Each patient's individual neurovascular anatomy, neurologic function, and planned procedure must be understood by the neuroanesthesiologist. These patients are at high risk of intraoperative injury from either cerebral hypoperfusion or hyperperfusion at different points in the procedure, depending on the disease state, nature of the occlusive lesions, and type of corrective interventional procedure. Goals for hemodynamic management should be mutually agreed on by the neuroanesthesia and neurosurgical teams. Neuroprotective interventions are not based on high-level evidence but must be considered in appropriate cases to avoid cerebral infarction.

Patients must be carefully managed in the postoperative period in order to avoid cerebral hypoperfusion from "uncorrected" lesions, cerebral hyperperfusion injury into newly revascularized regions, or hemorrhage from new vascular anastomoses. Reocclusion of an angioplastied lesion, intracranial stent, or vascular anastomosis must be recognized immediately and emergently investigated, usually with CT/CTA or conventional angiography, to maximize the likelihood for rescue and good outcome. As we look to the future, intraoperative MRI and CT coupled with biplanar angiography will allow greater diagnostic and interventional capabilities. Neuroanesthesiologists should familiarize themselves not only with traditional electrophysiologic monitoring modalities, but also with ultrasonography, near-infrared spectroscopy, and neuroradiographic technologies while keeping an eye toward the future and the ultimate development of bedside cerebral blood flow monitors!

REFERENCES

1. Sacco RL, Kargman DE, Gu Q, et al. Race-ethnicity and determinants of intracranial atherosclerotic cerebral infarction. The Northern Manhattan Stroke Study. *Stroke.* 1995;26:14–20.

2. Wityk RJ, Lehman D, Klag M, et al. Race and sex differences in the distribution of cerebral atherosclerosis. *Stroke.* 1996;27:1974–1980.

3. North American Symptomatic Carotid Endarterectomy Trial (NASCET) Investigators. Clinical alert: benefit of carotid endarterectomy for patients with high-grade stenosis of the internal carotid artery. National Institute of Neurological Disorders and Stroke, Stroke and Trauma Division. *Stroke.* 1991;22:816–817.

4. European Carotid Surgery Trialists' Collaborative Group. Randomized trial of endarterectomy for recently symptomatic carotid stenosis: final results of the MRC European Carotid Surgery Trial (ECST). *Lancet.* 1998;351:1379–1387.

5. Hobson RW 2nd, Weiss DG, Fields WS, et al. Efficacy of carotid endarterectomy for asymptomatic carotid stenosis. *N Engl J Med.* 1993;328:221–227.

6. Halliday A, Mansfield A, Marro J, et al. Prevention of disabling and fatal strokes by successful carotid endarterectomy in patients without recent neurological symptoms: randomized controlled trial. *Lancet.* 2004;363:1491–1502.

7. Brott TG, Hobson RW 2nd, Howard G, et al; CREST Investigators. Stenting versus endarterectomy for treatment of carotid-artery stenosis. *N Engl J Med.* 2010;363:11–23.

8. Hopkins LN, Roubin GS, Chakhtoura EY, et al. The Carotid Revascularization Endarterectomy versus Stenting Trial: credentialing of interventionalists and final results of lead-in phase. *J Stroke Cerebrovasc Dis.* 2010;19:153–162.

9. Ringelb PA, Allenberg J, Bruckmann H, et al. 30 Day results from SPACE trial of stent-protected angioplasty versus carotid endarterectomy in symptomatic patients: a randomised non-inferiority trial. *Lancet.* 2006;368:1239–1247.

10. Ederle J, Dobson J, Featherstone RL, et al. Carotid artery stenting compared with endarterectomy in patients with symptomatic carotid stenosis (International Carotid Stenting Study): an interim analysis of a randomised controlled trial. *Lancet.* 2010;375:985–987.

11. Stingele R, Berger J, Alfke K, et al. Clinical and angiographic risk factors for stroke and death within 30 days after carotid endarterectomy and stent-protected angioplasty: a subanalysis of the SPACE study. *Lancet Neurol.* 2008;7:216–222.

12. Chiam PT, Roubin GS, Iyer SS, et al. Carotid artery stenting in elderly patients: importance of case selection. *Cathet Cardiovasc Interv.* 2008;72:318–324.

13. Rothwell PM, Eliasziw M, Gutnikov SA, et al. Endarterectomy for symptomatic carotid stenosis in relation to clinical subgroups and timing of surgery. *Lancet.* 2004;363:915–924.

14. Brott TG, Halperin JL, Abbara S, et al; American College of Cardiology Foundation/American Heart Association Task Force on Practice Guidelines; American Stroke Association; American Association of Neuroscience Nurses; American Association of Neurological Surgeons; American College of Radiology; American Society of Neuroradiology; Congress of Neurological Surgeons; Society of Atherosclerosis Imaging and Prevention; Society for Cardiovascular Angiography and Interventions; Society of Interventional Radiology; Society of NeuroInterventional Surgery; Society for Vascular Medicine; Society for Vascular Surgery. 2011 ASA/ACCF/AHA/AANN/AANS/ACR/ASNR/CNS/SAIP/SCAI/SIR/SNIS/SVM/SVS guideline on the management of patients with extracranial carotid and vertebral artery disease: executive summary: a report of the American College of Cardiology Foundation/American Heart Association Task Force on Practice Guidelines, and the American Stroke Association, American Association of Neuroscience Nurses, American Association of Neurological Surgeons, American College of Radiology, American Society of Neuroradiology, Congress of Neurological Surgeons, Society of Atherosclerosis Imaging and Prevention, Society for Cardiovascular Angiography and Interventions, Society of Interventional Radiology, Society of NeuroInterventional Surgery, Society for Vascular Medicine, and Society for Vascular Surgery. *Vasc Med.* 2011;16:35–77.

15. Sloan MA, Alexandrov AV, Tegeler CH, et al. Transcranial Doppler ultrasonography in 2004: a comprehensive evidence based update. *Neurology*. 2004;62:1468–1481.
16. Chimowitz MI, Lynn MJ, Derdeyn CP, et al; the SAMMPRIS Trial Investigators. Stenting versus aggressive medical therapy for intracranial arterial stenosis. *N Engl J Med*. 2011;365:993–1003.
17. Zaidat OO, Klucznik R, Alexander MJ, et al. The NIH registry on the use of Wingspan stent for symptomatic 70-99% intracranial arterial stenosis. *Neurology*. 2008;70:1518–1524.
18. Feldmann E, Wilterdink JL, Kosinski A, et al. The Stroke Outcomes and Neuroimaging of Intracranial Atherosclerosis (SONIA) trial. *Neurology*. 2007;68:2099–2106.
19. Kasner SE, Lynn MJ, Chimowitz MI, et al. Warfarin vs aspirin for symptomatic intracranial stenosis: subgroup analyses from WASID. *Neurology*. 2006;67:1275–1278.
20. Kasner SE, Chimowitz MI, Lynn MJ, et al. Predictors of ischemic stroke in the territory of a symptomatic intracranial arterial stenosis. *Circulation*. 2006;113:555–563.
21. Marquardt L, Kuker W, Chandratheva A, et al. Incidence and prognosis of _50% symptomatic vertebral or basilar artery stenosis: prospective population-based study. *Brain*. 2009;132:982–988.
22. Eckert B. Acute vertebrobasilar occlusion: current treatment strategies. *Neurol Res*. 2005;27(Suppl 1):S36–S41.
23. Savitz SI, Caplan LR. Vertebrobasilar disease. *N Engl J Med*. 2005;352: 2618–2626.
24. Caplan LR. Atherosclerotic vertebral artery disease in the neck. Curr Treat Options Cardiovasc Med. 2003;5:251–256.
25. Canyigit M, Arat A, Cil BE, et al. Management of vertebral stenosis complicated by presence of acute thrombus. *Cardiovasc Intervent Radiol*. 2007;30:317–320.
26. Benesch CG, Chimowitz MI. Best treatment for intracranial arterial stenosis? 50 years of uncertainty. The WASID Investigators. *Neurology*. 2000;55:465–466.
27. Slovut DP, Olin JW. Fibromuscular dysplasia. *N Engl J Med*. 2004;350:1862–1871.
28. Olin JW. Recognizing and managing fibromuscular dysplasia. *Cleve Clin J Med*. 2007;74:273–282.
29. Zhou W, Bush RL, Lin PL, et al. Fibromuscular dysplasia of the carotid artery. *J Am Coll Surg*. 2005;200:807.
30. Laskowitz DT, Kolls BJ. Neuroprotection in subarachnoid hemorrhage. *Stroke*. 2010;41(Suppl 10):S79–S84.
31. Parray T, Martin TW, Siddiqui S. Moyamoya disease: a review of the disease and anesthetic management. *J Neurosurg Anesthesiol*. 2011;23:100–109.
32. Davies KN, Humphrey PR. Complications of cerebral angiography in patients with symptomatic carotid territory ischaemia screened by carotid ultrasound. *J Neurol Neurosurg Psychiatry*. 1993;56:967–972.
33. Leonardi M, Cenni P, Simonetti L, et al. Retrospective study of complications arising during cerebral and spinal diagnostic angiography from 1998 to 2003. *Interv Neuroradiol*. 2005;11:213–221.
34. Fisher M, Paganini-Hill A, Martin A, et al. Carotid plaque pathology: thrombosis, ulceration, and stroke pathogenesis. *Stroke*. 2005;36:253–257.
35. Lal BK, Hobson RW, Pappas PJ, et al. Pixel distribution analysis of B-mode ultrasound scan images predicts histologic features of atherosclerotic carotid plaques. *J Vasc Surg*. 2002;35:1210–1217.
36. Tegos TJ, Sabetai MM, Nicolaides AN, et al. Patterns of brain computed tomography infarction and carotid plaque echogenicity. *J Vasc Surg*. 2001;33:334–339.
37. Zhu CZ, Norris JW. Role of carotid stenosis in ischemic stroke. *Stroke*. 1990;21:1131–1134.
38. Grant EG, Benson CB, Moneta GL, et al. Carotid artery stenosis: gray-scale and Doppler US diagnosis–Society of Radiologists in Ultrasound Consensus Conference. *Radiology*. 2003;229:340–346.
39. Saqqur M, Zygun D, Demchuk A. Role of transcranial Doppler in neurocritical care. *Crit Care Med*. 2007;35(Suppl):S216–S223.
40. Khan S, Rich P, Clifton A, et al. Non-invasive detection of vertebral artery stenosis: a comparison of contrast-enhanced MR angiography, CT angiography, and ultrasound. *Stroke*. 2009;40:3499–3503.
41. Rutt BK, Clarke SE, Fayad ZA. Atherosclerotic plaque characterization by MR imaging. *Curr Drug Targets Cardiovasc Haematol Disord*. 2004;4:147–159.
42. Sadowski EA, Bennett LK, Chan MR, et al. Nephrogenic systemic fibrosis: risk factors and incidence estimation. *Radiology*. 2007;243:148–157.
43. Information for healthcare professionals: gadolinium-based contrast agents for magnetic resonance imaging (marketed as Magnevist, MultiHance, Omniscan, OptiMARK, ProHance). US Food and Drug Administration Web site (accessed August 10, 2011). http://www.fda.gov/Drugs/DrugSafety/PostmarketDrug SafetyInformationforPatientsandProviders/ucm142884.htm
44. Bond R, Rerkasem K, Cuffe R, et al. A systematic review of the associations between age and sex and the operative risks of carotid endarterectomy. *Cerebrovasc Dis*. 2005;20:69–77.
45. Bond R, Rerkasem K, Shearman CP, et al. Time trends in the published risks of stroke and death due to endarterectomy for symptomatic carotid stenosis. *Cerebrovasc Dis*. 2004;18:37–46.
46. Bond R, Rerkasem K, Naylor AR, et al. Systematic review of randomized controlled trials of patch angioplasty versus primary closure and different types of patch materials during carotid endarterectomy. *J Vasc Surg*. 2004;40:1126–1135.
47. Ferguson GG, Eliasziw M, Barr HW, et al. The North American Symptomatic Carotid Endarterectomy Trial: surgical results in 1415 patients. Stroke. 1999;30:1751–1758.
48. Furie KL, Kasner SE, Adams RJ, et al; American Heart Association Stroke Council, Council on Cardiovascular Nursing, Council on Clinical Cardiology, and Interdisciplinary Council on Quality of Care and Outcomes Research. Guidelines for the prevention of stroke in patients with stroke or transient ischemic attack: a guideline for healthcare professionals from the American Heart Association/American Stroke Association. *Stroke*. 2011;42:227–276.
49. PROGRESS Collaborative Group. Randomised trial of a perindopril based blood-pressure-lowering regimen among 6,105 individuals with previous stroke or transient ischaemic attack. *Lancet*. 2001;358:1033–1041.
50. Lawes CM, Bennett DA, Feigin VL, et al. Blood pressure and stroke: an overview of published reviews. *Stroke*. 2004;35:776–785.
51. Karapanayiotides T, Piechowski-Jozwiak B, van Melle G, et al. Stroke patterns, etiology, and prognosis in patients with diabetes mellitus. *Neurology*. 2004;62:1558–1562.
52. van den Berg JC. The nature and management of complications in carotid artery stenting. *Acta Chir Belg*. 2004;104:60–64.
53. Taylor DW, Barnett HJ, Haynes RB, et al. Low-dose and high-dose acetylsalicylic acid for patients undergoing carotid endarterectomy: a randomised controlled trial. *Lancet*. 1999;353:2179–2184.
54. Holt PJ, Poloniecki JD, Loftus IM, et al. Meta-analysis and systematic review of the relationship between hospital volume and outcome following carotid endarterectomy. *Eur J Vasc Endovasc Surg*. 2007;33:645–651.
55. Kennedy J, Quan H, Buchan AM, et al. Statins are associated with better outcomes after carotid endarterectomy in symptomatic patients. *Stroke*. 2005;36:2072–2076.
56. McGirt MJ, Perler BA, Brooke BS, et al. 3-Hydroxy-3-methylglutaryl coenzyme A reductase inhibitors reduce the risk of perioperative stroke and mortality after carotid endarterectomy. *J Vasc Surg*. 2005;42:829–836.
57. GALA Trial Collaborative Group, Lewis SC, Warlow CP, Bodenham AR, et al. General anaesthesia versus local anaesthesia for carotid surgery (GALA): a multicentre, randomised controlled trial. *Lancet*. 2008;372:2132–2142.
58. Rerkasem K, Rothwell PM. Local versus general anesthetic for carotid endarterectomy. *Stroke*. 2009;40:e584–e585.

59. Halsey JH Jr. Risks and benefits of shunting in carotid endarterectomy. The International Transcranial Doppler Collaborators. *Stroke*. 1992;23:1583–1587.

60. Tang TY, Walsh SR, Gillard JH, et al. Carotid sinus nerve blockade to reduce blood pressure instability following carotid endarterectomy: a systematic review and meta-analysis. *Eur J Vasc Endovasc Surg*. 2007;34:304–311.

61. Medel R, Crowley RW, Dumont AS. Hyperperfusion syndrome following endovascular cerebral revascularization. *Neurosurg Focus*. 2009;26:E4.

62. Young WL. Anesthesia for endovascular neurosurgery and interventional neuroradiology. *Anesthesiol Clin*. 2007;25:391–412.

63. Matsushima Y, Suzuki R, Ohno K, et al. Angiographic revascularization of the brain after encephaloduroarteriosynangiosis: a case report. *Neurosurgery*. 1987;21:928–934.

64. Garrett MC, Komotar RJ, Merkow MB, et al. The Extracranial–Intracranial Bypass Trial: implications for future investigations. *Neurosurg Focus*. 2008;24:E4.

65. Warner DS, Takaoka S, Wu B, et al. Electroencephalographic burst suppression is not required to elicit maximal neuroprotection from pentobarbital in a rat model of focal cerebral ischemia. *Anesthesiology*. 1996;84:1475–1484.

66. Sakai H, Sheng H, Yates RB, et al. Isoflurane provides long-term protection against focal cerebral ischemia in the rat. *Anesthesiology*. 2007;106:92–99.

67. Bernard SA, Gray TW, Buist MD, et al. Treatment of comatose survivors of out-of-hospital cardiac arrest with induced hypothermia. *N Engl J Med*. 2002;346:557–563.

68. Todd MM, Hindman BJ, Clarke WR, et al. Mild intraoperative hypothermia during surgery for intracranial aneurysm. *N Engl J Med*. 2005;352:135–145.

69. Lees KR, Bluhmki E, von Kummer R, et al; ECASS, ATLANTIS, NINDS and EPITHET rt-PA Study Group. Time to treatment with intravenous alteplase and outcome in stroke: an updated pooled analysis of ECASS, ATLANTIS, NINDS, and EPITHET trials. *Lancet*. 2010;375:1695–1703.

70. McDonagh DL, Olson DM, Kalia JS, et al. Anesthesia and sedation practices among neurointerventionalists during acute ischemic stroke endovascular therapy. *Front Neurol*. 2010;1:118.

71. Abou-Chebl A, Lin R, Hussain MS, et al. Conscious sedation versus general anesthesia during endovascular therapy for acute anterior circulation stroke: Preliminary results from a retrospective multi-center study. *Stroke*. 2010;41:1175–1179.

72. Jumaa MA, Zhang F, Ruiz-Ares G, et al. Comparison of safety and clinical and radiographic outcomes in endovascular acute stroke therapy for proximal middle cerebral artery occlusion with intubation and general anesthesia versus the nonintubated state. *Stroke*. 2010;41:1180–1184.

73. Davis MJ, Menon BK, Baghirzada LB, et al. Anesthetic management and outcome in patients during endovascular therapy for acute stroke. *Anesthesiology*. 2012;116:396–405.

74. Subramaniam S, Hill MD. Decompressive hemicraniectomy for malignant cerebral artery infarction: an update. *Neurologist*. 2009;15:178–184.

75. Cooper DJ, Rosenfeld JV, Murray L, et al; DECRA Trial Investigators; Australian and New Zealand Intensive Care Society Clinical Trials Group. Decompressive craniectomy in diffuse traumatic brain injury. *N Engl J Med*. 2011;364:1493–1502.

28.

NEUROSURGICAL CRITICAL CARE

Ryan Hebert and Veronica Chiang

INTRODUCTION

The care of patients in neuroscience intensive care units (NICUs) is in many ways similar to that of other ICUs. Many of the multisystem complications associated with NICU care are also identical to those of other ICUs. The purpose of this chapter is to highlight some of the more common clinical situations that are unique to neurosurgical patients in the ICU.

GENERAL CONSIDERATIONS

The majority of NICU admissions are patients with acute vascular events or traumatic injury or for postoperative monitoring after elective surgery. Ropper et al. [1] reported the breakdown of their most common NICU admissions (see Table 28.1).

The remaining diagnoses can vary widely and include intracranial hematomas requiring surgical management, spine and cerebral trauma, intracerebral infections, brain tumors, and neurologic diseases such as Guillain-Barre syndrome and myasthenia gravis [1]. Patients with neurologic conditions are admitted to the ICU to monitor neurologic status or because of instability of other organ systems. Although specific monitoring techniques and management strategies are dictated by the underlying reason for ICU admission, it is important to recognize also that systemic illnesses can exacerbate the underlying neurologic condition, so neurologic monitoring remains an essential component of ICU care.

MONITORING

- General—Hourly measurement of vital signs (including pain level, temperature, heart rate, blood pressure, respiratory rate, oxygen saturation and urine output) are essential in the care of the neurologic ICU patient.

Central venous pressure is frequently used to monitor fluid status. The subclavian vein is the preferred access to the central venous circulation because jugular venous thrombosis may increase intracranial pressure in the neurologically compromised patient. End-tidal CO_2 may be used to monitor ventilation in the intubated patient; this should periodically be validated by arterial blood gases.

- Laboratory studies should include daily complete blood counts and metabolic panels. Daily chest radiographs are also usually performed as neurologically injured patients often manifest symptoms and signs of pneumonia very late in its course. In particular it is important to monitor the white cell count for occult infections, and BUN and creatinine for evidence of nephrotoxicity in patients receiving contrast dye for imaging studies. [2–5] As oxygen carrying capacity is important for brain oxygenation, hematocrits need to be followed closely and blood transfusions administered if hematocrit levels fall significantly below 30%.

- The neurologic specialties are heavily dependent upon imaging for diagnosis and management. Neurologic imaging (e.g., CT or MRI) is obtained as required.

- Neurologic Examination—The specific strategy used for monitoring the patient's neurologic function varies with the patient's level of consciousness. The most important element of neurologic monitoring is the serial neurologic examination. Changes that occur between one examination and the next are often more concerning than a one-time finding of a neurologic deficit. The neurologic examination should be conducted initially at least once every hour. Long-term hourly examinations are impractical for a variety of reasons (e.g., staffing limitations and sleep deprivation) and should be reserved for use during periods when the patient is at high risk for neurologic deterioration. Intracranial pressure (ICP) or electroencephalogram (EEG) monitoring may also be used as part of a neurologic assessment, but do not replace a methodical neurologic examination.

Table 28.1 MOST COMMON NEURO-ICU ADMISSION DIAGNOSES

• Postoperative tumor	• 20%
• Stroke or TIA	• 15%
• SAH	• 12%
• ICH	• 11%

THE NEUROLOGIC EXAMINATION

The purpose of the comprehensive neurologic examination obtained at the time of admission is to find deficits and also to serve as a basis for comparison for subsequent examinations. The hourly examination is more focused and used to detect progressive neurologic deterioration [6]. Each examination's findings should be compared to those of the examination performed at admission as well as to each subsequent exam in order to identify new deficits. The patient is at highest risk for undetected neurologic decline around shift changes if a clear neurologic examination is not communicated and new findings may not be recognized by the oncoming team. It is therefore vital that all members of the patient care team are familiar with the baseline examination and the elements of that examination that may change because of the patient's disease. Although the elements of a comprehensive neurologic examination are beyond the scope of this chapter, a brief discussion of the abbreviated neurologic examination is relevant.

The abbreviated neurologic examination includes evaluation of:

- Level of consciousness (LOC)
- Orientation and insight
- Verbal and cognitive abilities
- Cranial nerve function
- Motor function, reflexes and coordination
- Sensory function

LEVEL OF CONSCIOUSNESS

Any evaluation of the patient's LOC must take into account the degree of sedation and analgesics that have been administered (see Table 28.2). Patients with neurologic injury are particularly susceptible to the effect of sedating medications. Level of consciousness may also be altered by systemic dysfunction such as sepsis, pulmonary, renal or hepatic failure.

LOC is typically quantified using the Richmond Agitation Sedation Scale (RASS), which include the levels:

1. Awake and alert
2. Somnolent
3. Lethargic
4. Diminished responsiveness—responsive to voice, light/deep noxious.

Response to noxious stimulus is commonly documented in an unresponsive patient with the Glasgow Coma Score (GCS)[7]. Reason for endotracheal intubation should be considered. If intubation was performed for a GCS of 3 to 8 then this level of impairment implies an inability to protect the airway.

ORIENTATION AND INSIGHT

Although orientation to time, place and person is sufficient in a patient who is awake and alert and does not have an underlying neurologic problem, this test alone may not detect subtle changes in the neurologic patient. For this reason, patients in the neuroscience ICU should be tested for specific details such as orientation to others (e.g., family and health care providers) and the reason for hospitalization.

SPEECH AND COGNITIVE FUNCTION

Speech fluency and prosody (rhythm of speech), object naming, and phrase repetition should be examined along with the ability to follow simple and complex commands. Simple commands need to be divided into those that cross the midline versus those that are lateralized to one side. Complex commands are those that contain a series of simple commands.

Table 28.2 GLASGOW COMA SCALE

Score	Eye opening	Verbal	Motor
1	Does not open eyes	Makes no sounds	no movements
2	Opens eyes to painful stimuli	Incomprehensible sounds	decerebrate posturing to noxious
3	opens eyes to voice	Inappropriate words	decorticate posturing to noxious
4	opens spontaneously	confused	Withdraws to pain
5	n/a	oriented	localizes painful stimuli
6	n/a	n/a	obeys commands

CRANIAL NERVE FUNCTION

The cranial nerve (CN) examination should include pupil size, symmetry and reaction to light. Other nerves may be evaluated as indicated by reason for admission to the NICU and the patient's baseline neurologic examination. It is impossible to test olfaction, visual fields and acuity, extraocular movements, facial sensation and symmetry and tongue movement in a patient who is unresponsive. Facial symmetry and tongue movement cannot be tested in the intubated patient. In the unresponsive patient, then, the Doll's eye response combined with the corneal reflex, the gag reflex and the pupillary exam may serve as gross indicators of brain stem function at the level of the pons, medulla and midbrain respectively. The gag reflex in an intubated patient is secondary to laryngeal/tracheal irritation and does not trigger a CN IX/ X reflex loop, but rather a CN X, X reflex loop. The doll's eye response requires rotation of the cervical spine, so cold caloric testing should be substituted for the Doll's eye response in patients with suspected cervical spine injury. Cold calories must not be performed however if there is concern for tympanic membrane injury as evidenced by hemotympanum or CSF leak from the ear.

CN VI palsy is one of the earliest findings in patient with intracranial hypertension. CN VII palsy can also indicate an evolving posterior fossa mass[8]. Hearing in both ears should be tested when appropriate (e.g., in a patient who has just undergone resection of vestibular schwannoma). CNs IX and X are tested together as part of the gag reflex. CN IX innervates the sensation of the posterior pharyngeal wall whereas CN X innervates motor. The gag reflex should be tested on both sides (left and right) given the crossover at the midline. The appropriate response to unilateral stimulation is symmetric, bilateral palatal elevation and pharyngeal constriction. Sensory innervation to the soft palate is provided by CN V, so inadvertently touching the soft palate while trying to elicit the gag reflex may produce misleading results.

MOTOR FUNCTION, REFLEXES AND COORDINATION

Motor strength and coordination in both upper extremities is often tested at the same time by asking the patient to hold his or her arms extended in supination. Motor weakness in distal muscle groups will result in the pronation of the forearm and weakness in the proximal groups will cause downward drift of the arm. Cerebellar dysfunction will cause upward or lateral drift of the arm. Coordination in the lower extremities is rarely tested specifically in the hourly exam but both proximal and distal motor groups should be tested by asking the patient to lift the leg against gravity and to dorsiflex the foot against resistance. ICU patients have limited mobility, which makes subtle motor weakness difficult to detect. Asymmetry of the motor exam is often the easiest way to reveal subtle motor changes. Motor strength is typically documented using the 5 point scale[9]:

1 = Evidence of muscle contraction but no movement

2 = Movement but not against gravity

3 = Movement against gravity but not against resistance

4 = Movement against some resistance

5 = Normal strength

Muscle strength and coordination cannot be assessed in the comatose patient. Motor response to noxious stimuli and examination of the triceps, biceps, brachioradialis, patellar and ankle reflexes are therefore used as substitutes. The motor response to a noxious stimulus can be purposeful, semipurposeful or reflexive. The presence of hyperreflexia can suggest injury above the level of the spinal cord.

SENSORY FUNCTION

Sensory testing during the hourly neurologic exam includes testing for light touch and response to noxious stimuli. Testing should be performed on each side separately, and then on both sides simultaneously to look for sensory inattention (as seen in parietal lobe syndromes). As with the motor examination it is important to be aware of any asymmetry. A more detailed examination of proprioception, sharp–dull discrimination and temperature sensation should be performed as needed and when new neurologic changes have been identified.

ICP/CPP MONITORING

Measurement of ICP and calculation of cerebral perfusion pressure (CPP) are required in many patients in the NICU. Specific values should be obtained at hourly intervals to facilitate identification of acute changes and abnormal trends. Alarms should be programmed to alert the care team to potentially dangerous pressures, which may lead to or indicate potential herniation. Urgent action is necessary in the setting of intracranial hypertension and will be discussed later in this chapter.

EEG MONITORING

Continuous EEG monitoring is valuable in patients who are receiving barbiturates and in patients who are seizing. Rapid three lead EEG can be used to ascertain the presence of burst suppression patients who are in a barbiturate-induced coma for management of intracranial hypertension. Patients who are in *status epilepticus* or who have frequent seizures also benefit from EEG monitoring. EEG is particularly valuable in the diagnosis and management of subclinical seizures, that is, seizures that cause the patient to be unresponsive but do not produce motor effects. Periodic EEGs therefore may be helpful in diagnosing seizure in patients who have an unexplained change in mental status [10, 11].

NEUROSURGICAL EMERGENCIES

ACUTE CHANGE IN MENTAL STATUS

Mental status changes can present as an acute event or can be insidious in onset. A clear understanding of the patient's baseline neurologic examination is critical when examining a patient with a change in mental status. The most common causes of decreased alertness in the immediate postoperative period include delayed recovery from anesthesia, administration of sedatives (e.g., narcotics, benzodiazepines, anticonvulsants), hypoglycemia, metabolic derangements, sepsis, adrenal insufficiency and subclinical seizures. Intracranial hemorrhage is potentially life threatening and must always be considered as a causal factor. The patient should be rapidly intubated and mechanical ventilation initiated if the patient is unable to protect his or her airway. Laboratory tests should include a complete blood count, electrolytes, coagulation studies and divalent electrolytes including calcium, magnesium and phosphates. A CT scan of the head should be scheduled immediately. New intracranial hemorrhages seen on CT may necessitate urgent surgical intervention.

ANISOCORIA—UNILATERAL DILATED PUPIL

Anisocoria is often a harbinger of a devastating neurologic insult in the poorly responsive or comatose patient and should be treated as a neurosurgical emergency. Anisocoria of 0.5mm can be normal. It becomes more prominent on examination in a darkened room and occurs in 8% to 18% of the population [8, 12]. It is therefore important to have a baseline examination with which to compare.

The differential diagnosis of unilateral pupillary dilation includes pharmacologic causes (e.g., atropine), seizure, direct trauma to eye causing paralysis of the ciliary muscle, and enlargement of a posterior communicating artery aneurysm compressing the third nerve. Unilateral pupillary dilatation (which may then become bilateral) may also be caused by third nerve compression that results from herniation of the temporal uncus into the brainstem. If the patient has risk factors for intracranial hypertension, anisocoria may signal the development of critically high pressures requiring rapid intervention. Pharmacologic and other causes of anisocoria should only be considered after raised ICP has been excluded.

WOUND COMPLICATIONS

Wound complications may also constitute a neurosurgical emergency. Conditions that may require immediate treatment include large surgical site hematomas, CSF leak, and wound dehiscence.

Surgical site hematomas can vary in depth below the skin. Hematomas outside the skull are almost never an emergency unless they reflect concurrent hemorrhage intracranially. Intracranial hemorrhage is most commonly found in the postoperative cavity, and a hematoma that is larger than expected may be the cause of new mental status changes or a focal neurologic deficit in a patient who has just had surgery. There may be no visible external signs of bleeding if the scalp closure is watertight. Patients who bleed after a craniotomy can present with new hemiparesis or sensory changes. A frontal hematoma may, however, only cause worsening headache, nausea, vomiting and agitation. A posterior fossa hematoma may produce sudden respiratory arrest that may or may not follow the development of diplopia and facial paresis. Patients who have undergone a transsphenoidal hypophysectomy may present with sudden vision loss. In a patient who has had a carotid endarterectomy, there may be no blood in the drain and the patient usually develops agitation and confusion long before respiratory distress. In the patient who has undergone spinal surgery, a hematoma should be suspected if sensory and motor changes occur below the level of the surgery.

If an intracranial hematoma is suspected, the airway should be secured immediately. A CT scan of the head should be obtained as soon as possible, ideally on the way to the operating room. If a neck hematoma is suspected in a patient who has had a carotid endarterectomy, the trachea may already be compressed even if the patient does not have overt respiratory distress. The airway must therefore be secured before further imaging is obtained or the wound is explored. Patients with a spinal hematoma should be taken back to the operating room immediately for reexploration and relief of the cord compression.

Serosanguinous drainage from the wound in the postoperative cranial or spine patient is not uncommon. This can usually be treated by applying pressure to the surgical site or by changing the dressing. The surgical wound should, however, be carefully inspected for thin, clear, continuously dripping fluid from a craniotomy site or from a spinal incision that may be indicative of CSF leak. Diagnosis of a CSF leak in patients who have undergone surgery using a transsphenoidal or transoral approach or that have compromised a sinus may be much more difficult. The patient may complain of a salty taste in the back of the throat. Asking the patient to lean forward may elicit evidence of rhinorrhea. Asking the patient with a suspected CSF leak to perform a Valsalva maneuver may also increase the amount of fluid leakage and confirm the diagnosis.

To confirm that the fluid is CSF, the fluid in question is dripped onto a piece of filter paper. CSF will form an inner circle of pink or red blood that is surrounded by a larger ring of clear CSF. If is it possible to send the fluid for laboratory analysis, a glucose concentration of greater than 30 mg/deciliter is generally consistent with CSF. The concentration of glucose in mucus and lacrimal secretions is generally less than 5 mg/deciliter [8, 9]. The most specific laboratory test for CSF is beta transferrin. Although this test is highly specific, it is not available at many institutions and the results may not be available for several days. Serial noncontrast CT scans of the head showing increasing pneumocephalus are also suggestive of CSF leak. If the situation is still unclear, injecting a colored dye or injecting a radionuclide and then obtaining an image can sometimes confirm the diagnosis and reveal the site of CSF leakage.

A wound with a visible CSF leak should be reinforced immediately along its entire length with a continuous suture. Prophylactic antibiotics such as vancomycin and/or a third generation cephalosporin (e.g., ceftriaxone or ceftazidime) should be administered [9, 13, 14]. While there is very little evidence to support the use of antibiotics in this situation, meningitis in the postoperative neurosurgical patient may be devastating. If the leak stops, antibiotics can be discontinued. If, however, the leak continues, a second line treatment such as acetazolomide (250 mg po QID in an adult patient) may be started. Insertion of a lumbar drain to relieve the pressure may also be considered[9]. Persistent CSF leak in postoperative posterior fossa wounds may reflect intracranial hypertension and require CSF diversion through a shunt. If second line management fails, the patient may require reoperation to close the CSF leak.

STATUS EPILEPTICUS

Status epilepticus is defined either as a seizure that is longer than 30 minutes in duration or as recurrent seizures without recovery of consciousness between episodes [1, 8, 9]. Seizures may occur without physical manifestations, however and as discussed previously, should be suspected in patients with altered consciousness without clear etiology. The prevalence of nonconvulsive status epilepticus in the neurologic intensive care unit [10] has been estimated to be as high as 34%.

The management of status epilepticus consists of airway management, a metabolic workup to determine the cause, and treatment with drugs that raise the seizure threshold. [9, 15, 16]. Supplemental oxygen should be administered to seizing patients. Endotracheal intubation and initiation of mechanical ventilation should be considered if the patient is unable to protect his or her airway. Two peripheral intravenous catheters should be inserted because some medications (e.g., phenytoin and benzodiazipines) cannot be administered through the same tubing. Blood chemistry studies that include a metabolic panel, calcium, magnesium and liver function tests may identify the etiology—of the seizures. A fingerstick blood glucose level will rule out hypoglycemia. Lorazepam 0.03 mg/kg (4 mg in an adult patient of average size) IV over 2 minutes may stop the seizure; this dose may be repeated after 5 minutes. If the patient is not yet on an antiepileptic agent, a loading dose of phenytoin (15 mg/kg) may be given. If seizures continue, IV phenobarbital can be tried. Single doses of 120 mg IV repeated to a maximum of 1400 mg can be used. Patients who receive large doses of a barbiturate may become hypotensive and require vasopressors to maintain an adequate blood pressure. Persistent seizure activity may be treated with further pentobarbital, other anticovulsants, midazolam infusion or propofol infusion. The neurology service should be consulted to facilitate ongoing management and EEG monitoring. Seizures that persist despite comprehensive management suggest a poor prognosis for neurologic recovery.

INTRACRANIAL HYPERTENSION

The physiology of intracranial hypertension has been discussed earlier but is summarized here. Intracranial hypertension results in two deleterious consequences:

- A progressive compression of the cerebral vasculature that decreases blood flow

- Brain herniation into abnormal compartments or into the spinal canal

In the normal brain, CBF is closely coupled to the metabolic demands of the brain. Unlike other tissues, such as muscle, the brain does not store metabolic substrates and therefore the brain relies on blood flow for the continuous delivery of glucose and oxygen [1]. Blood flow in normal brain remains constant as long as mean arterial blood pressures (MAPs) remain within a normal range (70 to 100 mm Hg). In some pathologic states such as cerebral trauma, however, autoregulation is disrupted and CBF can parallel MAP [17]. In these patients, ICP increases with blood pressure because cerebral blood volume is increased.

CPP is defined as the difference between the force pushing the blood through the brain (i.e., MAP) and the intracranial resistance to blood flow (i.e., ICP). Therefore:

$$CPP = MAP - ICP$$

ICP measured in a supine person is usually less than 10 mm Hg when measured at the external auditory canal (approximating the foramen of Monroe) [1]. The Brain Trauma Foundation defines intracranial hypertension as an ICP greater than 20 mm Hg [18]. Therefore CPP is considered normal in the 50– to 100–mm Hg range. Although ICP is the only measured parameter monitored in patients with most disease processes, there is increasing interest in measuring CPP and studying its role in improved outcomes for patients with CNS disease.

HERNIATION SYNDROMES

As ICP rises brain tissues can undergo shifts. These shifts depend on the location of the etiology of the elevated ICP and can produce specific clinical syndromes [1, 9, 12]. Four main types of herniation syndromes have been commonly described—uncal, transtentorial, subfalcine, and tonsillar. Subfalcine is rarely seen as an independent clinical entity in the NICU, although it is often commented upon by radiologists.

Uncal herniation occurs when the medial aspect of the temporal lobe (the *uncus*) is displaced medially until it is compressed between the brainstem and the medial edge of the tentorium. This can be caused by a rapidly expanding hematoma from trauma or surgery or temporal lobe edema caused by a tumor, stroke or infection. The first sign is worsening mental status followed by ipsilateral pupillary dilation secondary to compression of cranial nerve III (oculomotor) against the tentorial edge. This can then be associated with a marked contralateral hemiplegia caused by compression of the ipsilateral brainstem. The contralateral brainstem may occasionally be paradoxically compressed against the contralateral tentorial edge, causing ipsilateral weakness. Further progression leads to central herniation.

Transtentorial (central) herniation occurs when the diencephalon is displaced caudally through the tentorial incisura. This is caused by increased pressure in the supratentorial compartment that may be due to a variety of etiologies. The initial presentation again is worsening mental status followed by the development of decorticate posturing that may still be reversible if the patient is treated quickly. The next stage is marked by continuous tachypnea, midposition fixed pupils and decerebrate posturing and is caused by injury to the upper pons. These findings are irreversible and indicate a poor prognosis. Further progression leads to medullary failure and death.

Tonsillar herniation is the herniation of the cerebellar tonsils through the foramen magnum. The tonsils compress the medulla anteriorly against the bone leading to the development of a clinical triad of hypertension, bradycardia and shallow, irregular breathing known as the *Cushing reflex*. Respiratory arrest occurs unless the patient is treated quickly and death ensues rapidly. Unlike many supratentorial causes of herniation where the etiology is diffuse and management is predominantly medical, surgical decompression is often the most effective treatment in infratentorial herniation cases.

MEASUREMENT OF ICP

Measurement of ICP is a poor substitute for the neurologic examination but is useful when the neurologic examination is unavailable or limited to elicitation of reflex responses. Examples include trauma patients with a GCS less than 9 or requiring paralytic agent use for pulmonary or abdominal trauma management, patients with a subarachnoid hemorrhage of Hunt and Hess grade 3 or greater, patients with a complete MCA territory infarct, or patients with hepatic encephalopathy.

ICP is usually measured in the NICU using an intraventricular catheter or an intraparenchymal monitor. The intraventricular fluid-coupled strain gauge catheter system (commonly referred to as an external ventricular drain [EVD] or ventriculostomy) is the preferred method for ICP monitoring [1] (see Figure 28.1). The advantages of this system are (1) the added ability to drain CSF as a means of treating elevated ICP and (2) the lack of drift within the system because it can be rezeroed at any time. Disadvantages of EVD placement include difficulty of placement (especially when ventricles are small), the risk of iatrogenic intracerebral hemorrhage, and a risk of infection that increases with

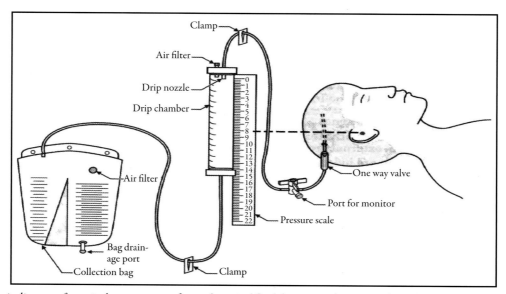

Figure 28.1   Schematic diagram of ventriculostomy system for cerebrospinal fluid drainage and intracranial pressure monitoring.
(From Greenberg, Mark. *Handbook of neurosurgery*. 7th ed. Theime. 2010. Reprinted with permission from Mark Greenberg.)

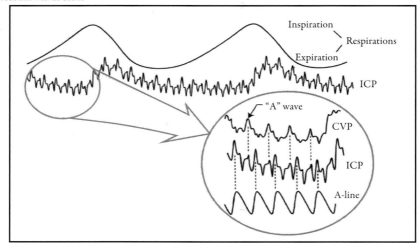

Figure 28.2 Intracranial pressure waveforms and their relationship to cardiopulmonary waveforms. (From Greenberg, Mark. *Handbook of neurosurgery.* 7th ed. Theime. 2010. Reprinted with permission from Mark Greenberg.)

duration of use [19–21]. In situations where a ventriculostomy catheter cannot be inserted, an intraparenchymal monitor is a good alternative.

The pressure recorded from the ICP monitor is a mean value and the "normal" ICP waveform consists of primarily two components (Figure 28.2). The larger peak containing the dicrotic notch corresponds to the arterial systolic pressure wave. The second peak corresponds to the central venous pulsation. The ICP waveform varies with respiration, increasing with inspiration and decreasing with expiration [1, 9].

The ICP in a normal individual in the supine position is less than 10 mm Hg. In pathologic states, an ICP of up to 20 mm Hg may be considered normal. A pathologic state is indicated by sustained rise in the ICP level that may also be associated with loss of the respiratory variation of the waveform or changes in the heights of the vascular peaks. If ICP continues to increase, patients can develop Lundberg plateau waves which are persistently markedly elevated ICP levels in the 50- to 60–mm Hg range that last between 5 and 20 minutes. Lundberg waves indicate impending herniation and intracranial hypertension should be treated quickly.

MANAGEMENT OF RAISED ICP

Management of ICP in the intensive care unit can be divided into first, second and third line treatment options and adjunctive therapies [9, 22] (see Table 28.3).

Additional prophylactic treatments that should be instituted to avoid exacerbation of intracranial hypertension include anticonvulsants, antipyretics, blood glucose and blood pressure homeostasis.

Ventilation—The most important factor in the management of intracranial hypertension is control of

Table 28.3 TREATMENT OPTIONS FOR RAISED INTRACRANIAL PRESSURE

FIRST LINE	SECOND LINE	THIRD LINE
Raise the patient's head	Osmotic therapy	Decompressive craniectomy
Maximize venous outflow	Diuretics	Barbiturate coma
Control of ventilation	Propofol	
Sedation and analgesics	CSF drainage	
	Neuromuscular blockade	

oxygenation and ventilation. There is a linear relationship between $Paco_2$ and CBF when $Paco_2$ is between 20 mm Hg and 80 mm Hg [1]. As $Paco_2$ rises, cerebral resistance arterioles dilate, increasing cerebral blood flow and blood volume, thereby increasing ICP. Acute hyperventilation in the setting of intracranial hypertension increases CSF pH, which causes cerebral vasoconstriction. This acutely decreases CBF, and lowers ICP [23–25], but only for a few hours. With more long term maintenance of hyperventilation, however, renal excretion of bicarbonate begins to return CSF pH to its normal value within several hours, after which, normalizing the $Paco_2$ will cause cerebral vasodilation. Hyperventilation is therefore used in the acute setting but only as a bridge to definitive management. The $Paco_2$ should be allowed to return to the normal range of 35 to 40 mm Hg within a few hours. If ICP remains difficult to control, $Paco_2$ can be decreased slowly, but should kept above 30 to 33 mm Hg to minimize the risk of cerebral ischemia due to excessive vasoconstriction.

Hypoxia can also exacerbate intracranial hypertension. When PaO_2 falls below 50 mm Hg, cerebral vasodilation causes an increase in CBF. This effect is exacerbated by anemia.

Positive end-expiratory pressure (PEEP) may also increase ICP. PEEP elevates intrathoracic pressure, which decreases venous return and cardiac output. This in turn causes a decrease in MAP and CPP. In practice, there is little evidence that less than 10 mm Hg of PEEP causes any significant increase in ICP and any theoretical disadvantages are outweighed by improvements in alveolar ventilation and therefore gas exchange. Moreover, the effect of PEEP on ICP is dependent on contributory factors such as lung and brain compliance. The patient should be monitored for changes in ICP if PEEP is initiated [26–29].

HOB elevation—Raising the patient's head improves venous drainage, which in turn reduces ICP. This effect seems to peak at approximately 30 to 40 degrees of elevation. The patient's head should be kept in a neutral position (i.e., midline) to prevent jugular venous drainage from being obstructed. Neck compression may occlude jugular venous outflow and compromise venous return. Items such as straps that are used to secure the endotracheal tube or tracheostomy should therefore be avoided when possible. For the same reason, internal jugular venous catheters should be avoided.

Sedation and analgesia—Sedation is often an effective component of ICP management when agitation or anxiety are the cause of intracranial hypertension. Short-acting benzodiazepines (e.g., midazolam or lorazepam) and propofol are the most commonly used agents. Benzodiazepines can be easily reversed to allow a neurologic examination and both propofol and benzodiazepines have the added benefit of suppressing epileptiform activity. Propofol has been shown to decrease cerebral metabolic rate and may offer additional neuro protection [30]. Side effects of propofol include hypertriglyceridemia, liver toxicity, metabolic acidosis and zinc depletion (secondary to EDTA chelation). *Propofol infusion syndrome* is a rare complication of sedation with propofol that is characterized by bradycardia, heart failure, lactic acidosis, rhabdomyolysis and hyperlipidemia. Its presentation is similar to septic shock, but can be distinguished by the identification of hyperlipidemia and rhabdomyolysis. Mortality is estimated to be approximately 80% despite intervention but may be reduced by keeping the infusion rate below 4 mg/kg/hr [31].

Benzodiazepines and propofol lack analgesic properties, so narcotics may also be necessary for pain management. Fentanyl and morphine are the most commonly used opiates in the NICU. Fentanyl is a pure *mu* receptor agonist that is roughly 100 times more potent than morphine and is often used in the neuro ICU setting because of its rapid clearance facilitating frequent neurologic examination. Fentanyl also does not cause histamine release that is sometimes associated with morphine administration. Adversely,

sedatives and narcotics can decrease blood pressure which may reduce cerebral perfusion and act synergistically to produce respiratory depression. Neurologically injured patients may be especially susceptible to these agents. It is therefore necessary to continually assess patients receiving sedatives or analgesics for airway protection as well as titrate drug levels to the neurologic exam.

Fluid management, Osmotic therapy and Diuresis—In the past, neurosurgical patients were once maintained in hypovolemic and hyperosmolar states, but repeated studies have demonstrated that euvolemia promotes systemic homeostasis and thus improved brain perfusion. It has been estimated that a 3% drop in plasma osmolality can lead to an increase in ICP by 15 mm Hg [32], so plasma hyperosmolarity helps to reduce cerebral edema. For these reasons, 5% dextrose in 0.9%NaCl is the most commonly used maintenance fluid in the NICU. Measurement of serum sodium levels and osmolarity are obtained as frequently as every four to six hours so that maintenance fluid composition can be changed as needed. Serum sodium should be kept greater than 138mEq/L. Serum osmolarity of more than 320mmol/L does not further decrease ICP, but is associated with acute tubular necrosis [33, 34]. Hyperglycemia should be managed with insulin infusions.

Mannitol is a hypertonic solution that is frequently used as an adjunct to management of intracranial hypertension. While its actual mechanism of action is unknown, it is believed to cause movement of extracellular fluid into the intravascular space which then causes an efflux of intracellular fluid to maintain extracellular homeostasis. The effects of mannitol on ICP are usually observed within 20 minutes of bolus administration and occur before visible diuresis. The recommended dose of mannitol ranges between 0.25 and 1.5 g/kg administered as a bolus over 20 minutes and then 0.25 to 0.5 g/kg every 6 hours as needed for intracranial hypertension. Prolonged use of mannitol can cause hypernatremia and hyperosmolality, although paradoxical hyponatremia has also been documented. In patients who are hyperosmolar, cessation of mannitol may cause a rebound effect that may exacerbate cerebral edema. This rebound effect can be minimized by tapering the dose of mannitol over several days if it has been used for more than 3 days. Because mannitol produces hypovolemia, it should be used with caution and may be contraindicated in hypotensive patients.

Hypertonic saline (23.4%) solution is also used in some facilities to control intracranial hypertension. Hypertonic saline offers the added benefit that it does not cause hypotension, making it a safer choice in hypotensive patients. Hypertonic saline solution is used to resuscitate hypovolemic trauma patients and is commonly given as a 0.5- to 1-mL/kg bolus over 15 to 30 minutes. Furosemide augments the effects of mannitol and hypertonic saline on ICP. The starting dose of furosemide is a bolus dose of 20 mg in an adult of normal size and can be repeated if diuresis is not seen.

CSF drainage—Removing CSF is a rapid and effective method of lowering ICP. Unless the patient has hydrocephalus, this intervention is usually limited by the amount of CSF volume that can be drained. In patients with TBI, SAH and hydrocephalus, the preferred method of CSF withdrawal is through an intraventricular catheter. As described in a previous section, this catheter is usually placed into the nondominant frontal horn. Collapse of the ipsilateral ventricle around the ventriculostomy will occasionally necessitate insertion of a contralateral catheter. ICP should be transduced at the level of the external auditory meatus (EAM), which approximates the foramen of Monroe. In many cases, either intermittent or continuous drainage will be required to manage ICP. Intermittent drainage requires continuous monitoring of ICP and opening of the drain above a defined threshold. An alternative method of CSF drainage is to leave the fluid coupled system open and to place the collection chamber at an appropriate distance above the EAM. When ICP exceeds the pressure exerted by the column of fluid leading to the collection system, CSF will passively drain into the collection bag. This method does not require constant monitoring of ICP but the disadvantage of this method is that the system may become occluded or overdrainage may occur unnoticed.

In some cases when it is clear that communicating hydrocephalus is the cause for intracranial hypertension a lumbar drain may be used in place of an intraventricular catheter. This method does not, however, permit reliable measurement of ICP. A lumbar drain must never be used in patients with obstructive hydrocephalus or in the presence of an intracranial mass as lumbar drainage of CSF may cause downward herniation of the brain.

Neuromuscular Blocking Agents (NMBAs)—NMBAs are rarely used in the management of patients with intracranial hypertension because use of these drugs precludes frequent neurologic examinations. Sedation and mechanical ventilation are required components of the management of patients who are receiving NMBAs. NMBAs decrease ICP by decreasing neuromuscular tone and may therefore be helpful because they abolish coughing and gagging in response to airway instrumentation. A nerve stimulator should be attached to the patient to measure the extent of neuromuscular blockade. Use of NMBAs is thought to be associated with higher rates of pneumonia and deep venous thrombosis due to the abolition of all spontaneous movements by the patient.

PROPHYLACTIC ADJUVANT TREATMENTS

(1) Blood pressure—Many of the interventions used to control ICP, including sedatives, mannitol and IV antiepileptics, can adversely affect blood pressure. Because systemic hypotension can decrease CPP, decreases in blood pressure should be counteracted with vasopressors (e.g., phenylephrine) and treatment of any underlying cause such as hypovolemia, cardiac dysfunction or sepsis. Blood pressure interventions should be titrated to maintain CPP greater than 60 mm Hg [35, 36].

(2) Antipyretics—Fever has been shown to be an independent predictor of poor outcomes in patients with ischemic stroke and subarachnoid hemorrhage [37–39]. $Paco_2$ and cerebral metabolism (and therefore CBF) have been shown to increase during hyperthermia, potentially exacerbating intracranial hypertension. Treatment of the cause of fever, which usually involves the detection and treatment of infection, is essential. Regular administration of acetominophen is common but is not always an effective first line treatment of fever. Cooling blankets are of limited efficacy because they induce secondary shivering that can complicate management of ICP. Newer methods of body cooling, including both conductive and intravascular devices, may be more effective in reducing temperature in the future.

Induced hypothermia has been shown to reduce mortality in the patients experiencing cardiac arrest [40] and is currently being used in some ICUs to treat refractory intracranial hypertension in patients with TBI. The presumed mechanism is that hypothermia decreases cerebral metabolic rate [41]. A recent Cochrane review analyzed 23 trials of induced hypothermia to a maximum of 35 degrees C for a minimum of 12 hours. The use of induced hypothermia trended toward reducing mortality and unfavorable outcomes, but did not reach statistical significance [42].

(3) Anticonvulsants—Seizures produce a significant increase in cerebral metabolism, CBF and CBV, which exacerbates ICP. In patients at risk for intracranial hypertension, seizure prophylaxis in the acute settings carries few risks but may potentially prevent seizure-induced increases in ICP. Recent studies suggest that nonconvulsive (or subclinical) status epilepticus is more common than previously thought [10, 11]. Seizures should therefore be considered as a causative factor in the setting of increased ICP without an obvious cause. Antiepileptics are often administered to patients with subarachnoid hemorrhage or intracerebral hematoma (including tumors) or in any setting where cortical irritation might occur, such as subdural hematomas. Current "first-line" anticonvulsant agents of choice include phenytoin and levetiracetam. Phenytoin is administered as a loading dose of 15 to 20 mg/kg followed by an initial maintenance dose of 300 mg/day that is adjusted to maintain a serum concentration of 10 to 20 μg/mL. Levetiracetam does not require a loading dose; the initial recommended dose is 750 mg every 12 hours, which can be increased to a maximum dosage of 3000 mg/day. While its ease of administration, relative lack of side effects and no need for serum level monitoring has made levetiracetam popular for the initial management of seizures, it is a newer agent and its efficacy is less well tested.

(4) Blood Glucose—Serum glucose control in the ICU setting is known to reduce the possibility of poor

outcome. Recent observations in patients with TBI have associated glucose levels of less than 160 mg/dL in the first 24 hours with increased survival rate [43]. Another NICU study associated decreased variability in the glucose level with improved outcomes [44]. In the past, low blood glucose levels were maintained by removing dextrose from the maintenance fluids. It is now recognized, however, that glucose is the sole energy source for brain cells and therefore should be included in the maintenance fluid, but avoided in fluids that are administered as a bolus. To avoid hyperglycemia an insulin infusion should be instituted in all patients with a target serum glucose level of 80 to 140 mg/dL [22].

Decompressive Craniectomy and Barbiturate Coma— Decompressive craniectomy and barbiturate coma are considered to be interventions of last resort. There is conflicting data regarding the efficacy of both interventions in the management of intracranial hypertension of a variety of etiologies[45, 46]. Decompressive craniectomy is usually reserved for patients with focal areas of cerebral abnormality such as a partial MCA stroke or large frontal hypertensive hemorrhage and who have a good likelihood for recovery if the ICP can be controlled. The decision to proceed with decompressive craniectomy is complex and beyond the scope of this chapter.

The goal of inducing a barbiturate coma is to suppress cerebral metabolism in order to protect the normal brain against the effects of intracranial hypertension [1, 9, 22]. Patients must be euvolemic and normotensive before initiation of this treatment. Barbiturates are titrated to burst suppression on the EEG, so this monitor must be available to monitor cerebral electrical activity. The most commonly used agent is pentobarbital, but thiopental has also been used. A loading dose of pentobarbital 5 to 10 mg/kg every 15 to 20 minutes up to 4 doses is administered while watching for changes in EEG and a decrease in ICP. A continuous infusion of 1 to 8 mg/kg/hr is then initiated and the infusion rate is titrated to EEG burst suppression. Profound hypotension always occurs and is caused by cardiosuppression and peripheral vasodilatation that often responds to vasopressors. Another disadvantage of barbiturate coma is that the neurologic examination is lost, with the possible exception of pupillary response, which may be preserved for a short period of time. More prolonged use of barbiturates however will also cause dilatation of the pupils and produce a neurologic examination that resembles that of brain death. Patients therefore cannot be evaluated for brain death until the serum pentobarbital level falls below 10 ug/mL. The ICU course of patients who survive is often complicated by ileus, pancreatitis and sepsis.

This chapter now turns to the discussion of a few common clinical diagnoses requiring specific management expertise. These include patients with neurovascular disorders, those undergoing pituitary surgery, those with posterior fossa lesions and those with spinal cord injury.

SUBARACHNOID HEMORRHAGE (SAH)

SAH is defined as bleeding into the space between the arachnoid and pial layers that line the brain's surface. The etiologies of SAH include trauma (75%), aneurysms (20%), and less common diagnoses such as arteriovenous malformations, vasculitis, carotid or vertebral dissection, and tumors. The underlying cause of bleeding is never found in 15% of patients with nontraumatic SAH despite repeated imaging of the brain and vasculature. Patients with aneurysmal SAH have a mortality rate of 50% to 80% before reaching medical care [1, 9, 47, 48]. The acute management of SAH depends upon the patient's presentation.

The patient with SAH can present with a neurologic status that varies from being completely intact with a diffuse headache to being comatose and requiring intubation and ventilation. Patients who are neurologically intact or awake with only focal neurologic deficits (Hunt and Hess grades 1 and 2) must be admitted to the NICU for observation because the risk of rebleeding, which is highest in the first 24 hours, can be decreased by the strict control of blood pressure [49–52]. Patients may receive mild sedation and kept in a quiet room with frequent monitoring of vital signs. It is widely believed that maintenance of the SBP below 140 mm Hg results in a lower incidence of rebleeding. Although there is no data proving or discounting this belief, it is universally accepted that the blood pressure should be kept below 140 mm Hg while making preparations for operative or endovascular treatment. Oral nimodipine is also routinely administered for the purpose of preventing vasospasm and often helps with blood pressure management [53]. Prophylactic anticonvulsants should be administered carefully at this time as the addition of this agent can cause hypotension.

CT angiography with intravenous contrast or conventional angiographic images may be required before surgery and it is essential that patients remain well hydrated. A baseline creatinine and creatinine clearance is required before exposing patients to contrast media. Intravenous hydration with 150 mEq solution of $NaHCO_3$ decreases the incidence of contrast induced nephropathy [54, 55]. This protocol usually includes administration of *N*-acetyl-cysteine 600 mg, 2 doses before and 2 doses after contrast administration [54–56]. The administration of contrast nephropathy prophylaxis is currently recommended in patients with a baseline creatinine of 1.2 or patients with a lower creatinine who are receiving multiple dye loads in a 24-hour period. In preparation for aneurysm treatment, a routine set of preoperative laboratory studies are required including CBC, serum electrolytes, and coagulation studies.

Patients whose level of consciousness is impaired (Hunt and Hess grades 3–5) should be intubated and mechanically ventilated. A nasogastric tube should be inserted so that drugs that require oral administration (e.g., nimodipine) may be given. If the patient is not already receiving an anticonvulsant, one should be initiated. Systemic blood pressure should be monitored with an intra-arterial catheter. The incidence of acute hydrocephalus in the setting of a ruptured cerebral aneurysm approaches 20% [57–59]. A depressed level of consciousness may be caused by obstructive hydrocephalus resulting from rupture of the aneurysm into the third ventricle. Treatment consists of urgent insertion of a ventriculostomy catheter. Ongoing management of hydrocephalus should be predominantly by constant slow drainage of CSF to maintain an ICP of approximately 20 mm Hg. Rapid removal of CSF after ventriculostomy may cause a sudden decrease in transmural pressure that may cause the aneurysm to rupture again and should be avoided.

During the first 24 hours after SAH, roughly 50% of patients will have abnormal electrocardiography changes that are attributed to neurogenic stunned myocardium, cardiac dysrythmias and subendocardial ischemia. The mechanism is thought to be a catecholamine surge that is caused by the sudden rise in ICP at the time of SAH. Stunned myocardium is characterized by significant left ventricular dysfunction following SAH that usually returns to normal within 5 days. Hypotension related to stunned myocardium should be treated with inotropic drugs and not vasopressors [60]. Patient presenting with SAH who have cardiac dysrhythmias or other ECG changes should undergo an echocardiogram. Serial echocardiograms can help monitor myocardial function and facilitate changes in management.

Pulmonary complications associated with SAH are expected. Aspiration pneumonia is common in patients with SAH (especially high grade SAH) who have lost consciousness. Neurogenic pulmonary edema is sometimes observed after SAH [61–63]. Although the precise mechanism of neurogenic pulmonary edema is controversial, it has also been attributed to the catecholamine surge that occurs after SAH. Animal studies have revealed left ventricular dysfunction and pulmonary arteriolar vasoconstriction [64], both of which could be an etiology of neurogenic pulmonary edema. Treatment is supportive and consists of prevention of hypoxia and may require endotracheal intubation and mechanical ventilation with high FiO_2. Diuretics and PEEP should be used with caution because they may exacerbate hypovolemia and hypotension, which may exacerbate cerebral ischemic injury.

Gastrointestinal bleeding after SAH is estimated to occur in up to 4% of patients and stress ulcers are a common complication in the ICU. Patients should therefore receive sucralfate, H_2 antagonists, and/or proton pump inhibitors as a preventative measure.

The goal of surgical management is to secure the source of bleeding within the first 72 hours if the patient will tolerate the procedure. After the first 72 hours, the risk of SAH-induced vasospasm increases and persists for up to 14 days after the bleed. Prolonged vasospasm can cause cerebral ischemia, but the risk of this complication may sometimes be averted by the early institution of intra-arterial therapies such as intra-arterial administration of nicardipine or balloon angioplasty. The patient at risk for vasospasm should be carefully observed for the development of any new neurologic deficits. Prophylaxis against vasospasm includes keeping the patient well hydrated with intravenous fluid. Administration of diuretics and antihypertensive agents should be avoided while the patient is at risk for vasospasm. If the patient develops a new neurologic deficit, which can include confusion, a depressed level of consciousness or a focal motor/sensory abnormality, Triple H therapy (hypertension, hypervolemia and hemodilution) should be instituted aggressively regardless of whether the aneurysm has been secured. Vasopressors are often used to maintain the systolic blood pressure above 180 mm Hg, and nimodipine should be discontinued because this drug may make it difficult to raise the blood pressure to an appropriate level. It is often helpful to insert a central venous catheter to guide fluid administration. The patient should be positioned head of bed flat to maximize cerebral perfusion, while intravenous fluid boluses are used to maintain a CVP of 8 to 12 mm Hg. Fluid intake should be kept equal to fluid output over each 8 hour period. In the young patient with normal cardiac and renal function, it may be difficult to maintain fluid balance. Some centers have therefore advocated the use of 5% albumin to maintain intravascular volume in these patients. Patients may develop hyponatremia, which should not be treated with diuretic agents unless pulmonary edema develops. Hyponatremia should instead be treated with 1.5% or 3% hypertonic saline. Because HHH therapy will induce a significant diuresis, it is important to monitor serum levels of potassium, calcium, magnesium and phosphorus and replete them as necessary. The patient's hematocrit should be kept between 30% and 35% to maximize cerebral blood flow and oxygen delivery [1, 9] by transfusion if necessary. Transfusions will also help to expand intravascular volume. If the patient's neurologic examination does not improve to baseline within 1 to 2 hours of instituting triple H therapy then intra-arterial management options should be considered.

THE NEUROENDOVASCULAR PATIENT

Neuroendovascular procedures offer a less invasive approach to the management of vascular lesions, but require specific training and expertise and can have devastating complications. The ICU clinician must have a clear understanding of the rationale for treatment, details of the procedure and the postoperative management. Patients receive care in conjunction with the neurointerventionalist just as a postoperative patient should be managed in conjunction with his or her neurosurgeon. Indications for interventional treatment include coiling of cerebral aneurysms, embolization of cerebral AVMs and highly vascularized tumors before resection, and transvenous instillation of tissue plasminogen activator (tPA) for patients with venous sinus thrombosis. Most neuroendovascular procedures are performed through the femoral artery. It is, however, not uncommon for the neurointerventionalist to choose another site such as the brachial artery or rarely the carotid artery if femoral access is difficult due to atherosclerotic disease. After the procedure, it is important to evaluate the extremity downstream of the arterial puncture for ischemia, embolic events, sensation and movement. Patients are frequently started on antiplatelet therapy or intravenous heparin after the procedure because the materials used to coil or stent intracranial vessels are thrombogenic. The use of anticoagulants may, however, be hazardous in patients who have had a recent intracranial hemorrhage. Patients must be monitored closely for any signs of neurologic deterioration that may be caused by the development of hemorrhage or hydrocephalus. A hemorrhage may also occur near the puncture site, possibly causing a retroperitoneal hematoma if the femoral artery was used. Unexplained hypotension is unlikely to be due to an intracranial cause and should therefore trigger a rapid search for this extracranial source of hemorrhage.

PITUITARY SURGERY

Patients with pituitary tumors may be admitted to the Neuro ICU after resection of a tumor or they may present de novo with a hemorrhage into their pituitary tumor (*pituitary apoplexy*).

Apart from standard cardiopulmonary resuscitation of the patient with hypotension following apoplexy, there needs to be treatment for the associated failure of the pituitary hormonal axis. Addisonian crisis should be considered part of the differential diagnosis in the hypotensive patient, hydrocortisone 100 mg should be given intravenously every six hours and an endocrinology consultation should be requested. Methylprednisolone may offer neural protection in patients who have compromised vision or a depressed level of consciousness, but should not be substituted for hydrocortisone because it has no mineralocorticoid activity. Other hormonal deficiencies, including hypothyroidism, may also be present.

Examination of vision and extraocular movements should be followed in patients who have undergone transphenoidal pituitary surgery, as should motor function. Diplopia or hemiparesis may suggest injury to the cavernous carotid artery and should be ruled out immediately. Close observation of fluid balance is also essential within the first 24 hours because of the possibility of developing diabetes insipidus (DI). Surgically induced diabetes insipidus (DI) should be suspected if urine has a persistent specific gravity of <1.005 and output is greater than 300cc per hour for 2 consecutive hours [65]. Serum sodium and osmolarity can

differentiate DI from normal postoperative fluid mobilization. If the serum sodium and osmolarity are low, the patient is most likely mobilizing fluids; if the serum sodium level is above 145mmol/l, the patient should be presumed to have DI. Given that surgically induced DI can be transient, if the patient can take oral fluids, he or she should be allowed to drink to thirst but must be closely observed. If the patient becomes tired or is unable to take oral fluids, urine output should be replaced with 0.45% saline solution at the rate of 1/2cc of fluid per cc lost through the urine until a diagnosis of DI is made. At that time, 1 mcg of IV DDAVP should be administered. Urine output is then followed and the DDAVP can be repeated as long as the DI continues. Transient DI usually resolves within 48 hours, but if the posterior pituitary is significantly injured, there may be a triphasic response. These patients may develop DI followed by hyponatremia caused by to a massive release of ADH from the injured neurohypophysis. This can be treated with diuresis while observing the patient for signs of DI that returns when all remaining ADH has been released. The patient will then likely require chronic treatment with DDAVP, which can be given intranasally once the nasal packing from the surgery has been removed.

Patients with secretory pituitary adenomas, in particular those with Cushing's syndrome, are at high risk for mortality from myocardial infarction and its complications[66]. Postoperative management should include telemetry as well as hormonal replacement as required. Close monitoring of blood pressure and initiation of beta-blockers is also a critical component of pre- and postoperative management. Serum potassium and divalent levels should be brought into the normal range as quickly as possible and monitored frequently. Unexplained dysrhythmias, new ECG abnormalities, or symptoms of cardiac ischemia should be investigated with cardiac enzymes and by requesting an urgent cardiology consultation. Aspirin and heparin cannot be used in the early postoperative period.

Postoperative patients can have an occult CSF leak that may be revealed when the nasal packing is removed. A CSF leak is sometimes difficult to diagnose because the fluid drips into the back of the throat, but may present as rhinorrhea that is accentuated by leaning the head forward or performing a Valsalva maneuver. The initial management of a CSF leak includes elevation of the head, empiric initiation of broad-spectrum antibiotics (e.g., vancomycin and ceftriaxone) and insertion of a lumbar drain to divert CSF to allow healing of the dural defect. If the rhinorrhea resolves with continuous CSF diversion, antibiotics can be changed to cover skin organisms (i.e., cefazolin) while the lumbar drain is in place. A CT of the head should be obtained within 24 hours of initiating CSF drainage and then daily, or sooner if new neurologic deficits including loss of vision are noted, to look for pneumocephalus or subdural hematoma. Pneumocephalus is caused by negative pressure drawing air into the head through the surgical wound. If pneumocephalus or a subdural hematoma are seen, lumbar drainage must be discontinued immediately and the patient should be taken to the operating room for surgical management.

POSTERIOR FOSSA MASS

A posterior fossa mass can produce rapid neurologic deterioration caused by compression of the brainstem. The first signs of an expanding mass may be acute loss of consciousness followed rapidly by cardiopulmonary arrest. Minimal amounts of anxiolytics and sedatives should be administered judiciously and only in a monitored setting. Careful observation for CN VI and VII dysfunction is critical and development of these cranial neuropathies indicates impending herniation. These patients should be taken to the operating room emergently for decompression. Very rarely, a supratentorial ventriculostomy may be appropriate for management of hydrocephalus caused by a deep focal posterior fossa mass. Given a theoretical risk that decompression of the supratentorial compartment could precipitate upward herniation of the posterior fossa contents through the incisura, CSF drainage needs to be done slowly and carefully.

SPINAL CORD INJURY

Patients with cervical spine injuries are among those most commonly admitted to a NICU. Many of these patients have coexisting multiorgan trauma and the detection of a cervical spinal cord injury may be difficult. They may also have been intubated for airway protection or respiratory failure that could be due a variety of causes such as pneumothorax or pulmonary contusions. A cervical cord injury should be suspected if there is evidence of a cervical spine fracture, if there is flaccid paralysis of all four extremities and if there is persistent hypotension despite adequate fluid resuscitation associated with inappropriate bradycardia.

After fluid resuscitation, hypotension should be treated with vasopressors, which cause peripheral vasoconstriction and improve venous return. It may be necessary to support ventilation with intubation (or tracheostomy) and mechanical ventilation for an extended period of time. If spinal cord injury is suspected within 8 hours of the event, high dose steroids can be administered in an attempt to maximize functional recovery. Current recommendations call for a bolus of methylprednisolone 30 mg/kg IV followed by an infusion of 5.4 mg/kg/hr over the next 23 hours [67].

A bladder catheter should be inserted initially and a regular bowel regimen must be instituted for these individuals because bladder or bowel distention can precipitate significant hypotension and bradycardia.

REHABILITATION OF THE NEUROLOGICALLY INJURED PATIENT

While rehabilitation is not the primary goal of the Neuro ICU, initial steps can help to maximize the possibility of a good recovery.

(1) Tracheostomy—Comatose patients are unable to protect the airway. They are therefore susceptible to recurrent aspiration pneumonia that is associated with significant morbidity. Early tracheostomy is advisable in those patients in whom rapid recovery of consciousness is not expected [68, 69].

(2) Enteral feeding—Given the high risk of gastric reflux and subsequent aspiration in the neurologically injured patient, enteral feeding into the jejunum either by nasojejunal tube or gastrojejunal tube is ideal. Neurologically injured patients are highly catabolic, which mandates initiation of enteral feeding as early as possible to maintain muscle mass [70, 71]. The protein needs of the neurologically injured patient are at least 1.5 times higher than other ICU patients.

(3) Deep Vein Thrombosis and Pulmonary Emboli— Neurologically injured patients are at extremely high risk for DVT and PE development [72, 73]. As early as day 1 after injury or surgery, if coagulation study parameters are normal, subcutaneous heparin at a dose of 5000U three times a day can be instituted. Inflating compression boots should be used at all times while the patient remains bed-ridden and screening Doppler ultrasound of the lower extremities should be performed at least weekly. Unfortunately Doppler ultrasound remains poor at detecting pelvic vein clots and therefore, it is important to maintain a high index of suspicion for the development of pulmonary emboli. New onset arrhythmias including atrial fibrillation or cardiogenic pulmonary edema, or unexplained transient hypoxia should precipitate a workup for pulmonary embolus. If a clot is found, the options of management using an IVC filter versus anticoagulation are individualized to the patient.

(4) Pressure sores—The neurologically injured patient is at very high risk for development of pressure sores caused by prolonged immobility and a catabolic state [74]. Specialized beds have been developed that constantly rotate the patient to limit the time spent on any particular area of skin. Skin should be visually checked each day by the NICU nursing staff and skin care initiated early if areas at risk are identified.

REFERENCES

1. Ropper A, et al. *Neurological and neurosurgical intensive care.* 4th ed. Philadelphia: Lippincott Williams and Wilkins; 2004.

2. Broome DR. Nephrogenic systemic fibrosis associated with gadolinium based contrast agents: a summary of the medical literature reporting. *Eur J Radiol*. 2008;66:230–234.
3. Lakhal K, et al. Acute Kidney Injury Network definition of contrast-induced nephropathy in the critically ill: incidence and outcome. *J Crit Care*. 2011.
4. McCullough PA, Soman SS. Contrast-induced nephropathy. *Crit Care Clin*. 2005;21:261–280.
5. Prince MR, et al. Incidence of nephrogenic systemic fibrosis at two large medical centers. *Radiology*. 2008; 248:807–816.
6. Goldstein JN, Greer DM. Rapid focused neurological assessment in the emergency department and ICU. *Emerg Med Clin North Am*. 2009;27:1–16, vii.
7. Teasdale G, Jennett B. Assessment of coma and impaired consciousness. A practical scale. *Lancet*. 1974;2:81–84.
8. Blumenfeld H. *Neuroanatomy through clinical cases*. Sinauer; 2002.
9. Greenberg M. *Handbook of neurosurgery*. 6th ed. New York: Thieme; 2006.
10. Jordan KG. Continuous EEG and evoked potential monitoring in the neuroscience intensive care unit. *J Clin Neurophysiol*. 1993;10:445–475.
11. Mirski MA, Varelas PN. Seizures and status epilepticus in the critically ill. *Crit Care Clin*. 2008;24:115–147, ix.
12. Posner JB, Plum F, Saper CB. *Plum and Posner's diagnosis of stupor and coma*. Oxford University Press; 2007.
13. Eftekhar B, et al. Prophylactic administration of ceftriaxone for the prevention of meningitis after traumatic pneumocephalus: results of a clinical trial. *J Neurosurg*. 2004;101:757–761.
14. van de Beek D, Drake JM, Tunkel AR. Nosocomial bacterial meningitis. *N Engl J Med*. 2010;362:146–154.
15. Lowenstein DH, Alldredge BK. Status epilepticus. *N Engl J Med*. 1998;338:970–976.
16. Marik PE, Varon J. The management of status epilepticus. *Chest*. 2004;126:582–591.
17. Czosnyka M, et al. Cerebral autoregulation following head injury. *J Neurosurg*. 2001;95:756–763.
18. Bratton SL, et al. Guidelines for the management of severe traumatic brain injury. VIII. Intracranial pressure thresholds. *J Neurotrauma*. 2007;24(Suppl 1):S55–S58.
19. Beer R, et al. Nosocomial ventriculitis and meningitis in neurocritical care patients. *J Neurol*. 2008;255:1617–1624.
20. Hoefnagel D, et al. Risk factors for infections related to external ventricular drainage. *Acta Neurochir (Wien)*. 2008;150:209–214; discussion 214.
21. Park P, et al. Risk of infection with prolonged ventricular catheterization. *Neurosurgery*. 2004;55:594–599; discussion 599–601.
22. Latorre JG, Greer DM. Management of acute intracranial hypertension: a review. *Neurologist*. 2009;15:193–207.
23. Hyperventilation. *J Neurotrauma*. 2000;17:513–520.
24. Diringer MN, et al. Regional cerebrovascular and metabolic effects of hyperventilation after severe traumatic brain injury. *J Neurosurg*. 2002;96:103–108.
25. Rangel-Castilla L, et al. Cerebral hemodynamic effects of acute hyperoxia and hyperventilation after severe traumatic brain injury. *J Neurotrauma*. 2010;27:1853–1863.
26. Caricato A, et al. Effects of PEEP on the intracranial system of patients with head injury and subarachnoid hemorrhage: the role of respiratory system compliance. *J Trauma*. 2005;58:571–576.
27. Cooper KR, Boswell PA, Choi SC. Safe use of PEEP in patients with severe head injury. *J Neurosurg*. 1985;63:552–555.
28. Muench E, et al. Effects of positive end-expiratory pressure on regional cerebral blood flow, intracranial pressure, and brain tissue oxygenation. *Crit Care Med*. 2005;33:2367–2372.
29. Zhang XY, Wang QX, Fan HR. Impact of positive end-expiratory pressure on cerebral injury patients with hypoxemia. *Am J Emerg Med*. 2010;
30. Schlunzen L, et al. Regional cerebral blood flow and glucose metabolism during propofol anaesthesia in healthy subjects studied with positron emission tomography. *Acta Anaesthesiol Scand*. 2012;56:248–255.
31. Marino PL, Sutin KM. *The ICU book*. Philadelphia: Lippincott Williams & Wilkins; 2007.
32. Zander R. Intracranial pressure and hypotonic infusion solutions. *Anaesthesist*. 2009;58:405–409.
33. Feig PU, McCurdy DK. The hypertonic state. *N Engl J Med*. 1977;297:1444–1454.
34. Mendelow AD, et al. Effect of mannitol on cerebral blood flow and cerebral perfusion pressure in human head injury. *J Neurosurg*. 1985;63:43–48.
35. Bratton SL, et al. Guidelines for the management of severe traumatic brain injury. IX. Cerebral perfusion thresholds. *J Neurotrauma*. 2007;24(Suppl 1):S59–S64.
36. Clifton GL, et al. Fluid thresholds and outcome from severe brain injury. *Crit Care Med*. 2002;30:739–745.
37. Badjatia N. Hyperthermia and fever control in brain injury. *Crit Care Med*. 2009;37(Suppl):S250–S257.
38. Oliveira-Filho J, et al. Fever in subarachnoid hemorrhage: relationship to vasospasm and outcome. *Neurology*. 2001;56:1299–1304.
39. Tokutomi T, et al. Optimal temperature for the management of severe traumatic brain injury: effect of hypothermia on intracranial pressure, systemic and intracranial hemodynamics, and metabolism. *Neurosurgery*. 2003;52:102–111; discussion 111–112.
40. Mild therapeutic hypothermia to improve the neurologic outcome after cardiac arrest. *N Engl J Med*. 2002;346:549–556.
41. Sinclair HL, Andrews PJ. Bench-to-bedside review: hypothermia in traumatic brain injury. *Crit Care*. 2010;14:204.
42. Sydenham E, Roberts I, Alderson P. Hypothermia for traumatic head injury. *Cochrane Database Syst Rev*. 2009;CD001048.
43. Griesdale DE, et al. Glucose control and mortality in patients with severe traumatic brain injury. *Neurocrit Care*. 2009;11:311–316.
44. Liu-DeRyke X, et al. Clinical impact of early hyperglycemia during acute phase of traumatic brain injury. *Neurocrit Care*. 2009;11:151–157.
45. Arnaout OM, et al. Decompressive hemicraniectomy after malignant middle cerebral artery infarction: rationale and controversies. *Neurosurg Focus*. 2011;30:E18.
46. Blissitt PA. Controversies in the management of adults with severe traumatic brain injury. *A-ACN Adv Crit Care*. 2012;23:188–203.
47. Hop JW, et al. Case-fatality rates and functional outcome after subarachnoid hemorrhage: a systematic review. *Stroke*. 1997;28:660–664.
48. Rinkel GJ, Algra A. Long-term outcomes of patients with aneurysmal subarachnoid haemorrhage. *Lancet Neurol*. 2011;10:349–356.
49. Broderick JP, et al. Initial and recurrent bleeding are the major causes of death following subarachnoid hemorrhage. *Stroke*. 1994;25:1342–1347.
50. Hashiguchi A, et al. Rebleeding of ruptured cerebral aneurysms during three-dimensional computed tomographic angiography: report of two cases and literature review. *Neurosurg Rev*. 2007;30:151–154.
51. Inagawa T, et al. Rebleeding of ruptured intracranial aneurysms in the acute stage. *Surg Neurol*. 1987;28:93–99.
52. McIver JI, et al. Preoperative ventriculostomy and rebleeding after aneurysmal subarachnoid hemorrhage. *J Neurosurg*. 2002;97:1042–1044.
53. Pickard JD, et al. Effect of oral nimodipine on cerebral infarction and outcome after subarachnoid haemorrhage: British aneurysm nimodipine trial. *BMJ*. 1989;298:636–642.
54. Briguori C, et al. Renal Insufficiency Following Contrast Media Administration Trial (REMEDIAL): a randomized comparison of 3 preventive strategies. *Circulation*. 2007;115:1211–1217.
55. Recio-Mayoral A, et al. The reno-protective effect of hydration with sodium bicarbonate plus N-acetylcysteine in patients undergoing emergency percutaneous coronary intervention: the RENO Study. *J Am Coll Cardiol*. 2007;49:1283–1288.
56. Brown JR, et al. Sodium bicarbonate plus N-acetylcysteine prophylaxis: a meta-analysis. *JACC Cardiovasc Interv*. 2009;2:1116–1124.

57. Graff-Radford NR, et al. Factors associated with hydrocephalus after subarachnoid hemorrhage. A report of the Cooperative Aneurysm Study. *Arch Neurol.* 1989;46:744–752.

58. Hasan D, et al. Management problems in acute hydrocephalus after subarachnoid hemorrhage. *Stroke.* 1989;20:747–753.

59. Vermeij FH, et al. Predictive factors for deterioration from hydrocephalus after subarachnoid hemorrhage. *Neurology.* 1994;44:1851–1855.

60. Lee VH, et al. Mechanisms in neurogenic stress cardiomyopathy after aneurysmal subarachnoid hemorrhage. *Neurocrit Care.* 2006;5:243–249.

61. Bruder N, Rabinstein A. Cardiovascular and pulmonary complications of aneurysmal subarachnoid hemorrhage. *Neurocrit Care.* 2011.

62. Mayer SA, et al. Cardiac injury associated with neurogenic pulmonary edema following subarachnoid hemorrhage. *Neurology.* 1994;44:815–820.

63. Smith WS, Matthay MA. Evidence for a hydrostatic mechanism in human neurogenic pulmonary edema. *Chest.* 1997;111:1326–1333.

64. Maron MB. Pulmonary vasoconstriction in a canine model of neurogenic pulmonary edema. *J Appl Physiol.* 1990; 68:912–918.

65. Singer PA, Sevilla LJ. Postoperative endocrine management of pituitary tumors. *Neurosurg Clin N Am.* 2003;14:123–138.

66. De Leo M, et al. Cardiovascular disease in Cushing's syndrome: heart versus vasculature. *Neuroendocrinology.* 2010;92(Suppl 1):50–54.

67. Bracken MB. Pharmacological interventions for acute spinal cord injury. *Cochrane Database Syst Rev.* 2000:CD001046.

68. Ahmed N, Kuo YH. Early versus late tracheostomy in patients with severe traumatic head injury. *Surg Infect (Larchmt).* 2007;8:343–347.

69. Arabi Y, et al. Early tracheostomy in intensive care trauma patients improves resource utilization: a cohort study and literature review. *Crit Care.* 2004;8:R347–R352.

70. Hartl R, et al. Effect of early nutrition on deaths due to severe traumatic brain injury. *J Neurosurg.* 2008;109:50–56.

71. Zarbock SD, et al. Successful enteral nutritional support in the neurocritical care unit. *Neurocrit Care.* 2008; 9:210–216.

72. Black PM, Baker MF, Snook CP. Experience with external pneumatic calf compression in neurology and neurosurgery. *Neurosurgery.* 1986;18:440–444.

73. Epstein NE. A review of the risks and benefits of differing prophylaxis regimens for the treatment of deep venous thrombosis and pulmonary embolism in neurosurgery. *Surg Neurol.* 2005;64:295–301; discussion 302.

74. Ek AC, Boman G. A descriptive study of pressure sores: the prevalence of pressure sores and the characteristics of patients. *J Adv Nurs.* 1982;7:51–57.

29.
ETHICAL CONSIDERATIONS AND BRAIN DEATH

Adrian A. Maung and Stanley H. Rosenbaum

INTRODUCTION

Throughout our history, humankind has been preoccupied with death. We have extensively contemplated, discussed, and described not only the religious and ethical but also the medical and scientific aspects of death. Until relatively recently, the dividing moment between life and death was the cessation of cardiopulmonary function. However, by the mid twentieth century, numerous advances in medicine made the defining moment of death less clear. Cardiopulmonary resuscitation, mechanical ventilation, and mechanical and pharmacological support of the heart could now maintain and preserve cardiopulmonary function. An alternative definition of death, brain death, was first published in 1959 [1] and has since become an ethical, legal, and medical equivalent to cardiac death in most cases. Practitioners who provide for patients with severe neurological injuries either in the critical care unit or in the operating room need to understand the concept of brain death, the process of declaring a patient brain dead, and the impact that brain death has on human physiology. In this chapter, the authors will review the history of brain death and the ethical, legal, and religious implications; discuss the algorithm for brain death declaration; and conclude with the critical and intraoperative care of the brain-dead organ donor.

HISTORICAL PERSPECTIVE

For most of humankind's history, death was defined by the absence of a pulse and respiration. The common law standard for determining death was the cessation of all vital functions, traditionally demonstrated by "an absence of spontaneous respiratory and cardiac functions" [2]. With the development of the electrocardiogram, the time of death became associated with the onset of asystole. However, in the 1940s and 1950s, clinicians increasingly more frequently provided care to patients supported by machines but who were considered from a neurologically standpoint "hopelessly unconscious" [3]. At the same time, the first successful renal transplant was performed in 1954 and ushered the era of solid organ transplantation with a subsequent demand for viable organs. Although not the first to consider brain death, the report of the Ad Hoc Committee of the Harvard Medical School to Examine the Definition of Brain Death published in 1968 [3] was the first formal attempt to establish the definition of brain death. The committee defined "brain death" as loss of function of the brain and spinal cord. In 1970, Kansas became the first state to incorporate the concept of brain death into law.

In 1980, the Uniform Determination of Death Act (UDDA) [2] was drafted and approved by the American Medical Association and the American Bar Association. The UDDA stated that "an individual who has sustained either: (1) irreversible cessation of circulatory and respiratory functions, or (2) irreversible cessation of all functions of the entire brain, including the brain stem, is dead." However, the UDDA, which was adopted by all 50 states, although with variations, did not provide any specific clinical tests, criteria, or standards that would establish the diagnosis of brain death.

The following year, the President's Commission for the Study of Ethical Problems in Medicine and Biomedical and Behavioral Research published the report "Defining Death: A Report on the Medical, Legal and Ethical Issues in the Determination of Death" [4]. The report, which included and expanded on the UDDA, provided some clinical guidelines on brain death declaration. The most commonly used guidelines for determining brain death in adults are from the American Academy of Neurology, first published in1995 [5] and subsequently updated in 2010 [6].

LEGAL, ETHICAL, AND RELIGIOUS PERSPECTIVES

Although the concept of brain death is legally accepted by statute or judicial ruling in all 50 states, as well as in many other countries, there are no national or international standards for declaring brain death. Although the fundamental principles are similar, the specific procedure can vary across jurisdictions, from state to state and even among hospitals within a state. For example, the Alaska statute specifies that a physician or a registered nurse can declare a patient brain dead, while Virginia mandates two physicians, one of whom is a specialist in neurology, neurosurgery, or electroencephalography [7]. In the United States and in most other countries, the concept of "whole brain death" is accepted, while in the United Kingdom and India, only the loss of brainstem function is required [8]. Individual practitioners must therefore familiarize themselves with the local policies at their own institution and jurisdiction.

Brain death has also been accepted by all major religious groups with notable exceptions of some Orthodox Jewish sects, the Roma ("gypsies"), certain Japanese religions, and some Native American groups. New York and New Jersey have changed their legal statutes to accommodate such religious objections. New Jersey specifically bars the declaration of death by neurological criteria if "there is a reason to believe that the patient's religious beliefs would be violated" by such declaration [9].

From a formal philosophical standpoint, the concept of brain death is not uniformly accepted and is close to a somewhat arbitrary socially derived viewpoint. The distinction between life and death can be ambiguous; clearly tissue and organs, such as a kidney in place in a functioning body, can be alive although the organism might be defined as "brain dead." Brain death can be accepted as a permanent loss of all aspects of personhood. This relates to the conception of humanness as a conscious, thinking, self-aware organism. The absence alone of just consciousness and spontaneous breathing would seem to justify the minimalist "brainstem death" criterion. The use of a whole brain criterion then seems an extra restriction, perhaps useful only to reduce potential ambiguity. The history of the brain death concept suggests that there was a need to have a scheme for declaring the legal death of bodies and yet preserving some physiological reserve to allow for transplantation. The permanent cessation of both personhood and all brain function seems to satisfy most Western intuitions as equivalent to death, even if much of the remaining body is still functioning.

DIAGNOSIS OF BRAIN DEATH

As discussed earlier, the criteria for declaration of brain death may vary depending on the location. Individual practitioners must therefore familiarize themselves with the policy in their own state and institution. The following discussion of brain death evaluation is based on published general criteria [6]. Brain death evaluation can be divided into three sections: appropriate history and clinical setting; complete neurological examination including apnea testing; and, optional, confirmatory testing.

PREREQUISITES

Brain death should be suspected only in an appropriate clinical setting after certain prerequisites are met. The patient should have clinical and/or radiological evidence of catastrophic brain pathology with a known cause of irreversible coma. The most common causes of brain death in adults are traumatic brain injury, subarachnoid hemorrhage, ischemic stroke, and anoxic brain injury [10]. Potential other diagnoses that may mimic brain death include drug intoxication, hypothermia, locked-in syndrome, and Guillain-Barre syndrome.

The patient's core temperature should be greater than 36°C (96.8°F) [6, 10] in order to exclude hypothermia. Brain death can cause loss of the hypothalamic thermoregulatory function with subsequent ambient (poikilothermic) body temperature in some patients, which may necessitate warming blankets and warmed intravenous fluid to reach the goal core temperature. Complicating medical conditions such as acute metabolic derangements (severe electrolyte, acid base or endocrine disturbances) should also be excluded and/or corrected.

The possibility of drug intoxication must be eliminated. If the ingested or administered drug is known, an antidote (if available) should be given. Common antidotes include naloxone for opiates, flumazenil for benzodiazepines, or neostigmine for nondepolarizing paralytics. Another option is to check serial drug levels until they become subtherapeutic. Screening tests for drugs may be helpful, but for many medications the critical levels at which brain death examination is impaired are unknown. The recommended approach is therefore to wait at least four times the elimination half-life of that drug provided that the drug metabolism is not affected by concomitant organ failure or other medications [11]. Electrical nerve stimulation with train-of-four can be used to assess the degree of paralysis. For suspected but unknown drugs, a 48-hour observation period can be used along with a confirmatory test such as cerebral blood flow. Systolic blood pressure should be maintained greater than 100 mm Hg or, if an intracranial pressure monitor is present, cerebral perfusion pressure should be maintained at greater than 60 mm Hg.

CLINICAL EXAMINATION

The standard for the diagnosis of brain death is the clinical neurologic examination, which should demonstrate three cardinal features: coma, absence of brainstem reflexes, and apnea. Coma can be assessed by documenting the absence of brain-mediated responses (decorticate or decerebrate posturing, dyskinesias, or epileptic seizures) or eye opening to verbal or noxious stimuli. Standard noxious stimuli include pressure on the supraorbital nerve, temporomandibular joint or finger nail bed as well as central pain at the sternal notch. Nipple twisting should be avoided because it can cause partial eye lid elevation through sympathetic innervation [12]. Movements originating from spinal cord or peripheral nerves commonly persist in brain death patients. These include deep tendon reflexes, plantar reflexes, finger flexor movements, triple flexion of the legs, superficial abdominal reflexes, and reaction of the blood pressure to noxious stimulation.

Absence of brainstem reflexes can be demonstrated by a cranial nerve examination. Caution is warranted in interpreting the results of a single cranial nerve examination as peripheral nerve trauma, lesions, or other conditions can confound the examination. Multiple cranial nerves should be examined as detailed later. Pupils should be nonreactive to light and mid-size or larger. Unless contraindicated by the presence or suspicion of cervical spine injury, oculocephalic (doll's eye) reflexes should tested by turning the head quickly from side to side and noting any eye movements with each turn. The normal response is deviation of the eyes to the opposite side of head turning. A brain-dead patient will have an absent oculocephalic reflex with no eye movements relative to the head movement during this maneuver. Oculovestibular (ice water caloric) reflex should also be absent. During this test, the patient's head should be 30 degrees above the horizontal and the tympanum should be irrigated with at least 50 mL of ice water. Normal intact reflex is movement of the eye toward the cold stimulus. The reflex is absent if there is no deviation of the eye. There should be no cough response to suctioning and absent gag reflex. Facial motor responses to the corneal reflex (touching the cornea with a cotton swab) or nasal tickle reflex (touching the nostrils with a cotton swab induces a head torn toward the opposite side) should also be absent.

The third and last component of the clinical examination is the apnea test. The test should be carefully performed only after the other criteria for brain death are met as it can lead to hemodynamic instability. The patient should be hemodynamically stable before the examination and core temperature should be at least 97°F. The pH and $PaCO_2$ should be normalized to 7.35 to 7.45 and 35 to 45 mm Hg, respectively. In patients who are known retainers of carbon dioxide, some authors recommend that the starting goal $PaCO_2$ be the patient's baseline [10]. Patient should be pre-oxygenated with 100% oxygen for at least 10 minutes and the blood pressure maintained at greater than 90 mm Hg. The patient should then be discontinued from the ventilator and an oxygen source of 100% FIO_2 is provided. This can be done via a T-piece or a thin cannula to the level of the carina. The patient should be visually observed to detect respiratory movement. The standard observation therapy is 8 to 10 minutes; however, some practitioners will extend the period to 12 to 15 minutes to ensure appropriate CO_2 rise as long as the patient remains stable during the test. An ABG is tested at beginning and conclusion of the test. If hemodynamic instability prevents full completion of the test, an ABG should be drawn before placing patient back on mechanical ventilation to see if the criteria were met. The apnea test is considered positive if there is no respiratory effort with an absolute $PaCO_2$ greater than 60 mm Hg or a rise in $PaCO_2$ of 20 mm Hg from the pretest value.

The apnea test cannot be completed in 10% to 26% of individuals secondary to hypotension, hypoxemia, or cardiac arrhythmias [13]. In these patients, an ancillary test should be performed to finalize the brain death diagnosis.

OBSERVATION PERIOD

In the early brain death diagnosis protocols, a repeat evaluation was required after 24 hours. In the United States, the required observation period was subsequently made age dependent. A 48-hour evaluation for an infant 7 days to 2 months old, 24 hours for 2 months to 1 year old, and 12 hours for those between 1 and 18 years. The American Academy of Neurology has concluded that there is insufficient evidence to determine a minimally acceptable observation period for adults [6], although 6 hours is commonly used. Some countries mandate longer observation times (Switzerland, 48 hours; Iran, 36 hours).

ANCILLARY TESTS

In the United States, the diagnosis of brain death in an adult patient is based on a complete clinical examination as described earlier. However, some countries as well as certain circumstances warrant additional ancillary testing to confirm the diagnosis. These circumstances include, for example, the inability to perform or complete the apnea test, inadequate examination of cranial nerves (e.g., secondary to extensive facial trauma), or multiple organ failure that renders clinical examination and/or drug metabolism unreliable. Multiple ancillary tests are available however none is perfect and studies examining their utility are limited. Different clinical situations as well as local practice and availability may guide their selection. The ancillary tests can be broadly divided into two categories: brain blood flow and electrophysiology.

Cerebral Angiography

Four-vessel cerebral angiography was previously held as the gold standard for confirming complete brain circulatory arrest. In brain-dead patients, two injections of contrast spaced 20 minutes apart should demonstrate absence of flow within the intracranial vessels (internal carotid and vertebral arteries). The blood flow within the external carotid system should be preserved. Angiography is an invasive test that requires special, in-house expertise and may not be available in all institutions. In addition, false negative angiograms have been reported in the literature.

Transcranial Doppler

Transcranial Doppler (TCD) can also demonstrate the absence of intracranial blood flow with preservation of extracranial flow. Two examinations 30 minutes apart are required to evaluate both the anterior and posterior circulations at 11 controlled points. Findings consistent with arrest of brain blood flow include oscillating flow or sharp systolic spikes without diastolic flow. TCD has the advantage of being noninvasive, safe and portable. A meta-analysis published in 2006 demonstrated a sensitivity of 89% and a specificity of 99% [14]. Nevertheless, TCD requires special expertise and may be influenced by technical limitations and operator/interpreter experience. For example, 10% to 15% of patients may have temporal bone thickening that precludes insonation of 6 of the 11 arteries. Two false positive results have also been reported in the literature [14].

Computed Tomography Angiography

Computed tomography (CT) angiography (CTA) is emerging as a possible alternative to conventional angiography. Its advantages include that is readily available in many hospitals, more rapidly performed, and less invasive and does not require an onsite specialist to perform or interpret. Although CTA has been adopted as a valid ancillary test by groups such as the French Society of Neuroradiology [15] and the Canadian Expert Consensus Meeting sponsored by the Canadian Council for Donation and Transplantation [16], there are concerns that CTA may have inadequate sensitivity for the diagnosis brain death as there are several reports that CTA showed persistent although significantly diminished brain blood flow in otherwise clinically brain-dead patients [17]. It is unclear what these findings imply about the clinical diagnosis of brain death.

Brain Scintigraphy

One of the most commonly used ancillary tests is single-photon emission CT (SPECT) brain scintigraphy [18] after the injection of a radionuclide tracer (^{99m}Tc-labeled hexamethylpropyleneamineoxime). The tracer penetrates brain parenchyma proportional to brain blood flow and persists for several hours. Brain-dead patients will have absence of isotope parenchymal uptake demonstrated by the "hollow skull phenomenon." Secondary to preserved external carotid perfusion, there may, however, be uptake in the meninges and face. Brain scintigraphy has been demonstrated to have good sensitivity and specificity compared with conventional angiography and clinical examination [19]. Portable scanners are available that can facilitate bedside ICU testing. However, a recent, nationwide shortage of the radionuclide tracer has made the test less readily obtainable.

Electroencephalography

Although electrocerebral silence or a flat electroencephalogram (EEG) was a component of the first brain death declaration guidelines, it has recently been replaced in many instances in adult patients by brain blood flow studies. EEG monitors potentials from the cerebral neocortex and therefore does not reflect brainstem or thalamic function. It is also affected by confounders such as medications or drug intoxication, hypothermia, and metabolic derangements. In addition, the electric "noise" of multiple electronic devices in the intensive care unit can produce artifacts that can be mistaken for cortical activity.

DECLARATION OF DEATH

In most jurisdictions in the United States, the patient is legally dead at the time of brain death declaration. The family should be informed of the patient's death and medical support can be stopped at this time. In the states of New York and New Jersey, laws do not permit declaration of death by neurological criteria if the family or the patient previously objected to the concept of brain death based on religious beliefs. In most other instances, however, the physician has no moral or legal obligation to continue medical interventions. Occasionally, the family may not accept the brain death declaration right away and may need more time to fully comprehend the difficult situation. Although there is no obligation, many physicians try to accommodate the family for a reasonable period of time.

In the United States, the Centers for Medicare and Medicaid Services require that hospitals notify their local organ-procurement organization in a timely manner of an impending death. The family can then be approached regarding organ donation after the declaration of brain death. Most authors recommend that any requests for donation are done by persons trained specifically in this matter and should be separate from the brain death discussion.

CRITICAL CARE OF THE BRAIN-DEAD PATIENT

If a decision is made to proceed toward organ donation, the potential deceased donor must be supported during the donation evaluation until the time of organ procurement. Brain death causes a number of physiologic derangements that lead to multisystem organ failure and ultimately cardiopulmonary arrest. Despite full medical support, 10% to 30% of potential donors are lost secondary to progressive hemodynamics instability [20, 21]. It is not well defined how long a brain-dead patient can be supported. Most patients are supported for few days until organ procurement or withdrawal of support. There are several case reports of longer survival including a pregnant patient who was supported for 107 days until the delivery of a viable fetus [22]. Donor management requires complex resuscitation that balances preserving viability of all organs. For example, renal graft function is optimized by a well-hydrated, diuresing donor but this strategy may worsen lung graft function. Ideally, the potentially harvestable organs should be identified as early as possible and their function favored.

CARDIOVASCULAR

The systemic effects of brain death develop as the ischemia progresses from cranial to caudal. Shortly preceding medullary-level brain death, a sympathetic surge causes massive release of catecholamines from postganglionic sympathetic nerve endings in a last ditch effort to maintain cerebral perfusion pressure. The surge can produce increased systemic vascular resistance, hypertension, left ventricular dysfunction, arrhythmias, neurogenic pulmonary edema, and cardiac stunning [20]. Brainstem herniation subsequently leads to spinal cord infarction and loss of sympathetic tone with resultant hypotension. Brain death can also lead to loss of pituitary function and a pan-hypopituitary state with low cortisol, T_3, T_4, insulin, and ADH levels. The resultant diabetes insipitus–induced hypovolemia can further worsen hypotension.

Hemodynamic instability in the brain-dead patients requires multisystem support. Adequate volume resuscitation is the first step but may not correct instability in 10% to 30% of patients [23, 24]. Actively bleeding patients or patients with hemoglobin less than 7 g/dL should given blood products; otherwise, crystalloid resuscitation is adequate with lactated Ringer's solution or 0.45% normal saline with the addition of sodium bicarbonate [23]. Hypotonic solution can be used after the plasma volume expansion to correct hypernatremia. The fluid therapy should be balanced between competing organ requirements as discussed earlier. Pulmonary artery catheters or less invasive means of monitoring cardiac function that use stroke volume variation or pulse contour analysis (LiDCO Ltd, London, England; Vigileo, Irvine, CA; PiCCO, Pulsion Medical Systems AG, Munich, Germany) may be helpful. Common targets are mean arterial pressure greater than 60 mm Hg, central venous pressure 4 to 12 mm Hg, pulmonary capillary wedge pressure 8 to 12 mm Hg, and cardiac index less than 2.4 L/min/m² [25].

Inotropic or pressor support is often required secondary to the loss of vascular tone. Dopamine has been traditionally used as a first-line agent; however, doses above 10 µg/kg/min may require addition of other agents such as norepinephrine, phenylephrine, dobutamine, or vasopressin. Combination therapy that avoids high doses of a single agent that has predominantly alpha-adrenergic or vasoconstrictor properties may be advantageous and may also have beneficial immunomodulatory effects [23, 26].

ENDOCRINE

Brain death can be associated with a pan-hypopituitary state that can result in adrenal insufficiency, central diabetes insipidus, hyperglycemia, and sick euthyroid syndrome. The posterior pituitary hormone (ADH) levels generally decrease from baseline, while the anterior pituitary hormone levels are more variable [27]. Diabetes insipidus is caused by inadequate antidiuretic hormone production, results in excessive loss of free water, and contributes to hypovolemia, hyperosmolarity, and electrolyte abnormalities (hypernatremia, hypokalemia, hypocalcemia, hypophosphatemia, and hypomagnesemia). Clinically, it is marked by excessive hypotonic urine production that can exceed 1000 mL/h and should be differentiated from mannitol-, drug-, or hyperglycemia-induced diuresis. Treatment is with urine output replacement with a 5% dextrose in water solution as well as hormone replacement therapy with vasopressin infusion or DDAVP administration. Vasopressin infusion acts on V1 and V2 receptors and produces both vasoconstrictive and antidiuretic effects. In contrast, DDAVP is specific for the V2 receptor only but has a longer duration of action (6 to 20 hours) and be administered by multiple routes (subcutaneously, intranasally, intramuscularly, or intravenously). However, it is less titratable and does not add hemodynamic support. With either medication, serum electrolytes should be monitored frequently.

Hyperglycemia, which is often multifactorial, is common in the donor. Physical stress, increase in counterregulatory hormones, peripheral insulin resistance, and infusion of dextrose containing fluids all contribute to elevated blood glucose levels. Treatment is with insulin infusion adjusted to maintain glucose less than 180 mg/dL. Many institutions now have established nurse-driven protocols for glucose management. Adrenal insufficiency is also common following brain death. In a recent study of 31 patients, the incidence of adrenal insufficiency was 87% and hydrocortisone infusion improved hemodynamic status in 59% [28].

The administration of "triple hormonal therapy" with desmopressin/vasopressin, methylprednisolone, and levothyroxine to counteract the endocrine dysfunction has gradually gained acceptance in the transplant community. The initial literature had mixed results [29], but a consensus conference in 2001 recommended its use along with insulin for donors with left ventricular ejection fraction less than 45% and/or hemodynamic instability [30]. The United Network for Organ Sharing (UNOS) has implanted this recommendation and data from that organization have demonstrated a 22.5% greater number of organs transplanted from donors that received the therapy [31] as well as improved recipient survival (89.9% versus 83.9%) [32]. Solumedrol and insulin are commonly administered early after the diagnosis of brain death, but there is still controversy whether levothyroxine and/or vasopressin should be administered in hemodynamically stable patients without evidence of diabetes insipidus [20].

PULMONARY

Pulmonary management of the brain-dead patient consists mainly of mechanical ventilation and fluid management. Adequate end-organ perfusion should be maintained while minimizing volume overload. Previous ventilator strategies included high tidal volume and high PEEP in an effort to minimize atelectasis and hypoxemia. Although not specifically validated in this population, many practitioners have now extrapolated from the studies of acute lung injury patients and started to use lung protected ventilation in order to minimize lung-induced inflammation. These strategies include low tidal volume ventilation, low plateau pressures, and moderate PEEP. Other supportive measures include aggressive pulmonary toilet with chest physiotherapy, direct suctioning, bronchoscopy, and nebulizer therapy to prevent mucus plugging.

SUPPORTIVE CARE

Additional complications that commonly occur in brain-dead patients include hypothermia, coagulopathy, and electrolyte imbalances. Hypothermia occurs in approximately 50% of patients from hypothalamic injury with loss of the ability to increase metabolism, vasoconstriction, or shiver. Administration of cold intravenous fluids and blood products as well as peripheral vasodilation further exacerbates hypothermia. To maintain normothermia, all administered fluids should be appropriately warmed and forced air rewarming can be utilized. Coagulopathy and thrombocytopenia can occur secondary to the patient's illness, but brain injury and brain death can also cause primary coagulopathy; possibly secondary to cerebral ganglioside release into the circulation [33]. Electrolyte abnormalities should be aggressively managed. Specifically, hypernatremia ($Na^+ >$ 155) should be corrected as it has been associated with poor renal and liver graft function [34].

INTRAOPERATIVE MANAGEMENT OF THE BRAIN-DEAD PATIENT

Management of the brain-dead patient in the operating room is continuation of the care provided in the intensive care unit. In most cases, the patient is in the operating room for organ recovery, although there are case reports of viable fetal delivery after maternal brain death [35]. The organ recovery operation consists of preliminary dissection and isolation of the harvested organs, aortic cross-clamp,

and rapid cooling with an ice slurry. Intraoperative support should include analgesia, anesthesia, and muscle relaxation to abrogate autonomic and spinal cord reflexes. Heparin bolus is also commonly administered before aortic cross-clamping. Medical support should be continued until the time of aortic cross-clamp but can be terminated soon after.

CONCLUSION

In the six decades since it was first described, brain death has become in most cases a medical, religious, legal, and ethical alternative to cardiopulmonary death. The concept of brain death has abrogated the futile cardiopulmonary support of the "hopelessly unconscious" and expanded the field of organ transplantation. However, the ethical implications, diagnostic algorithms, and medical support of the brain-dead patient continue to evolve and practitioners must be aware of the ongoing changes.

REFERENCES

1. Mollaret P, Goulon M. The depassed coma (preliminary memoir). *Rev Neurol (Paris)*. 1959;101:3–15.
2. Uniform Determination of Death Act. In *12*, Uniform Laws Annotated, West 1993 and West supp. 1997.
3. Report of the Ad Hoc Committee of the Harvard Medical School to Examine the Definition of Brain Death. A definition of irreversible coma. *JAMA*. 1968;205:337–340.
4. Report of the Medical Consultants on the Diagnosis of Death to the President's Commission for the Study of Ethical Problems in Medicine and Biomedical and Behavioral Research. Guidelines for the determination of death. *JAMA*. 1981;246:2184–2186.
5. The Quality Standards Subcommittee of the American Academy of Neurology. Practice parameters for determining brain death in adults (summary statement). *Neurology*. 1995;**45**:1012–1014.
6. Wijdicks EF, Varelas PN, Gronseth GS, et al. Evidence-based guideline update: determining brain death in adults: report of the Quality Standards Subcommittee of the American Academy of Neurology. *Neurology*. 2010;74:1911–1918.
7. Choi E, Fredland V, Zachodni C, et al. Brain death revisited: the case for a national standard. *J Law Med Ethics*. 2008;36:824–836, 611.
8. Manno EM, Wijdicks EF. The declaration of death and the withdrawal of care in the neurologic patient. *Neurol Clin*. 2006;24:159–169.
9. Olick R. Brain death, religious freedom, and public policy: New Jersey's landmark legislative initiative. *Kennedy Inst Ethics J*. 1991;1: 275–292.
10. Nathan S, Greer DM. Brain death. *Semin Anesth Perioperat Med Pain*. 2006;25:225–231.
11. Wijdicks EF. The diagnosis of brain death. *N Engl J Med*. 2001;344:1215–1221.
12. Varelas PN, Abdelhak T, Hacein-Bey L. Withdrawal of life-sustaining therapies and brain death in the intensive care unit. *Semin Neurol*. 2008;28:726–735.
13. Wijdicks EF, Rabinstein AA, Manno EM, et al. Pronouncing brain death: contemporary practice and safety of the apnea test. *Neurology*. 2008;71:1240–1244.
14. Monteiro LM, Bollen CW, van Huffelen AC, et al. Transcranial Doppler ultrasonography to confirm brain death: a meta-analysis. *Intensive Care Med*. 2006;32:1937–1944.

15. Leclerc X. CT angiography for the diagnosis of brain death: recommendations of the French Society of Neuroradiology (SFNR). *J Neuroradiol.* 2007;34:217–219.

16. Shemie SD, Lee D, Sharpe M, et al. Brain blood flow in the neurological determination of death: Canadian expert report. *Can J Neurol Sci.* 2008;35:140–145.

17. Combes JC, Chomel A, Ricolfi F, et al. Reliability of computed tomographic angiography in the diagnosis of brain death. *Transplant Proc.* 2007;39:16–20; Leclerc X, Taschner CA, Vidal A, et al. The role of spiral CT for the assessment of the intracranial circulation in suspected brain-death. *J Neuroradiol.* 2006;33:90–95; Quesnel C, Fulgencio JP, Adrie C, et al. Limitations of computed tomographic angiography in the diagnosis of brain death. *Intensive Care Med.* 2007;33:2129–2135.

18. Boissy A, Provencio J, Smith C, Diringer M. Neurointensivists' opinions about death by neurological criteria and organ donation. *Neurocrit Care.* 2005;3:115–121.

19. Facco E, Zucchetta P, Munari M, et al. 99mTc-HMPAO SPECT in the diagnosis of brain death. *Intensive Care Med.* 1998;24:911–917; Munari M, Zucchetta P, Carollo C, et al. Confirmatory tests in the diagnosis of brain death: comparison between SPECT and contrast angiography. *Crit Care Med.* 2005;33:2068–2073; Bonetti MG, Ciritella P, Valle G, et al. 99mTc HM-PAO brain perfusion SPECT in brain death. *Neuroradiology.* 1995;37:365–369; de la Riva A, González F, Llamas-Elvira J, et al. Diagnosis of brain death: superiority of perfusion studies with 99Tcm-HMPAO over conventional radionuclide cerebral angiography. *Br J Radiol.* 1992;65:289–294.

20. Frontera J, Kalb T. How I manage the adult potential organ donor: donation after neurological death (part 1). *Neurocrit Care.* 2010;12:103–110.

21. Grossman MD, Reilly PM, McMahon D, et al. Who pays for failed organ procurement and what is the cost of altruism? *Transplantation.* 1996;62:1828–1831.

22. Bernstein IM, Watson M, Simmons GM, et al. Maternal brain death and prolonged fetal survival. *Obstet Gynecol.* 1989;74:434–437.

23. Wood K, Becker B, McCartney J, et al. Care of the potential organ donor. *N Engl J Med.* 2004;351:2730–2739.

24. Wheeldon DR, Potter CD, Oduro A, et al. Transforming the "unacceptable" donor: outcomes from the adoption of a standardized donor management technique. *J Heart Lung Transplant.* 1995;14:734–742.

25. Zaroff JG, Rosengard BR, Armstrong WF, et al. Consensus conference report: maximizing use of organs recovered from the cadaver donor: cardiac recommendations, March 28-29, 2001, Crystal City, Va. *Circulation.* 2002;106:836–841.

26. Schnuelle P, Lorenz D, Mueller A, et al. Donor catecholamine use reduces acute allograft rejection and improves graft survival after cadaveric renal transplantation. *Kidney Int.* 1999;56:738–746.

27. Subramanian A, Brown DR. Management of the brain-dead organ donor. *Contemp Crit Care.* 2010;8:1–12.

28. Nicolas-Robin A, Barouk JD, Amour J, et al. Hydrocortisone supplementation enhances hemodynamic stability in brain-dead patients. *Anesthesiology.* 2010;112:1204–1210.

29. Novitzky D, Cooper DK, Rosendale JD, et al. Hormonal therapy of the brain-dead organ donor: experimental and clinical studies. *Transplantation.* 2006;82:1396–1401.

30. Rosengard B, Feng S, Alfrey E, et al. Report of the Crystal City meeting to maximize the use of organs recovered from the cadaver donor. *Am J Transplant.* 2002;2:701–711.

31. Rosendale JD, Kauffman HM, McBride MA, et al. Aggressive pharmacologic donor management results in more transplanted organs. *Transplantation.* 2003;75:482–487.

32. Cooper DK. Hormonal resuscitation therapy in the management of the brain-dead potential organ donor. *Int J Surg.* 2008;6:3–4.

33. Jenkins DH, Reilly PM, Schwab CW. Improving the approach to organ donation: a review. *World J Surg.* 1999;23:644–649.

34. Kazemeyni SM, Esfahani F. Influence of hypernatremia and polyuria of brain-dead donors before organ procurement on kidney allograft function. *Urol J.* 2008;5:173–177.

35. Catlin AJ, Volat D. When the fetus is alive but the mother is not: critical care somatic support as an accepted model of care in the twenty-first century? *Crit Care Nurs Clin North Am.* 2009;21:267–276.

30.

QUALITY MANAGEMENT AND PERIOPERATIVE SAFETY

Robert Lagasse

INTRODUCTION

Quality management (QM), total quality management (TQM), quality improvement (QI), continuous quality improvement (CQI), and performance improvement (PI) all describe processes for data collection and collation. Effective programs also include a peer review process that makes the data more relevant to current practices and a remedial process to improve patient care.

The American Society of Anesthesiologists (ASA) was one of the first medical specialty societies to endorse a structured peer review process [1] and offers current practice parameters to anesthesiologists looking to improve care in targeted areas [2]. For example, the ASA *Manual for Anesthesia Department Organization and Management* (*MADOM*) contains relevant clinical practice parameters and tips for organizing a QM program within a department of anesthesiology [3]. Additional informational sources on the principles of QM and peer review, as well as tools for data collection and collation, are also distributed through the Anesthesia Quality Institute via the World Wide Web [4].

Participation in a QM program is not just the "right thing to do"; it is now required by most health care organization accrediting bodies. For example, the mission of The Joint Commission (TJC), formerly the Joint Commission on Accreditation of Healthcare Organizations (JCAHO), is to continuously improve the safety and quality of care provided to the public through the provision of health care accreditation and related services that support performance improvement in health care organizations. To achieve accreditation, a health care organization must comply with TJC's standards, which include requirements for improving organizational performance and demonstrating leadership within the institution. TJC requires hospitals to collect data that must be systematically aggregated and analyzed

to identify undesirable patterns or trends in performance. Information from the data analyses must then be used to make changes that improve performance and patient safety, while reducing the risk of sentinel events. TJC defines sentinel events as unexpected occurrences involving death or serious physical or psychological injury, or the risk thereof. The phrase "or the risk thereof" includes any process variation for which a recurrence would carry a significant chance of a serious adverse outcome [5]. Needless to say, compliance with these criteria requires a large amount of data collection. TJC's leadership standards also require each organization to have an organization-wide, patient safety program.

Although TJC accredits more than 80% of U.S. hospitals, the American Osteopathic Association Healthcare Facilities Accreditation Program (HFAC) and Det Norske Veritas (DNV) Healthcare also offer accreditation for hospitals in the United States. These alternative accrediting agencies are considered to be less prescriptive in terms of accreditation requirements. For example, DNV focuses on continual improvement that is prioritized by the organization, while TJC standards are very specific in their requirements. For instance, the express requirements, which TJC calls Elements of Performance (EP), for their standard requiring hospitals to collect data to monitor performance specify exactly what data should be collected. These data include performance improvement priorities identified by hospital leaders. TJC defines hospital leaders as the governing body, senior managers, and the organized medical staff. In addition, TJC requires hospitals to monitor outcomes of operative or other procedures that place patients at risk of disability or death, all significant discrepancies between preoperative and postoperative diagnoses, adverse events related to moderate or deep sedation or anesthesia, problems related to use of blood and components, confirmed transfusion reactions, the results of resuscitation, significant medication errors, significant adverse drug reactions,

Table 30.1 ELEMENTS OF PERFORMANCE FOR TJC STANDARD PI.01.01.01

1. The leaders set priorities for data collection
2. Hospital identifies the frequency for data collection

The hospital collects data on the following:

3. Performance improvement priorities identified by leaders
4. Operative or other procedures that place patients at risk of disability or death
5. All significant discrepancies between preoperative and postoperative diagnoses
6. Adverse events related to using moderate or deep sedation or anesthesia
7. Use of blood and components
8. All confirmed transfusion reactions
11. The results of resuscitation
12. Behavior management and treatment
14. Significant medication errors
15. Significant adverse drug reactions
16. Patient perception of safety and quality

and patient perception of safety and quality (Table 30.1). Many of these measures relate directly to the practice of anesthesiology.

REGULATORY INITIATIVES

All hospitals in the United States are subject to a set of regulations called the *Medicare Conditions of Participation* (CoPs). Under the Social Security Act, The Centers for Medicare and Medicaid (CMS) may recognize national accrediting organizations as having "deeming authority" if they demonstrate that their health and safety standards, and their survey and oversight processes, meet or exceed those used by CMS for the CoPs. Hospitals accredited by TJC, DMV, or HFAC are deemed to have met most of the requirements set forth in the CoPs for Medicare. CMS regulations also provide a financial incentive for hospitals to report quality of care data for release to health care consumers. There were originally 10 measures for three medical conditions that included myocardial infarction, congestive heart failure, and pneumonia. Reporting was voluntary, but if the hospital did not report, their annual payment from Medicare was reduced by 0.4%, which encouraged over 99% of U.S. hospitals to participate. Subsequent changes in these rules in 2007 increased the incentive from 0.4% to 2% of their annual update. CMS also established procedures for making the reported data available to the public through the U.S. Department of Health and Human Services. After October 1, 2008, hospitals could no longer receive additional payment for certain high-cost, high-volume diagnoses

if they represented adverse conditions that were not present on admission (*Federal Register*, 2007). In other words, hospitals are now paid as if the acquired secondary diagnosis is not present, even though it must be reported. According to the federal government, these so-called *never events* should not occur, and include catheter-associated urinary tract infections, decubitus ulcers, foreign object retained after surgery, venous air embolism, blood incompatibility, and staphylococcus aureus septicemia. In the near future, the federal government's move toward value-based purchasing in health care is likely to include a performance assessment model that is used to score a hospital's performance on a specified set of measures. That score will then be translated into a positive, or negative, financial incentive [6].

The Physicians Quality Reporting Initiative (PQRI), which was established by the Tax Relief and Health Care Act of 2006, is a program that pays physicians to report compliance with specific quality measures. In 2007, eligible professionals who successfully reported a designated set of quality measures earned an additional payment from Medicare of up to 1.5% of total allowed charges. Few physicians participated, however, because the bonus payment did not offset the burden imposed by data collection. Many physicians who did participate did not earn their bonus because of the idiosyncratic accounting methodology used by CMS. The Patient Protection and Affordable Care Act (often called the Affordable Care Act) transitioned PQRI incentives to payment withholds, as had been done to hospitals. The new system, referred to as the Physician Quality Reporting System (PQRS), will reduce payments by 2% to physicians who do not report by 2016. This transition to PQRS may push more physicians to participate. In 2007, PQRI had 74 quality measures and by 2010, this number had more than doubled for PQRS. At the time of this printing, three measures are applicable to anesthesiologists: antibiotic timing, central venous catheter insertion protocols, and normothermia. Additionally, the American Board of Anesthesiologists (ABA) has proposed that Maintenance of Certification in Anesthesiology be included as a PQRS measure.

BOARD CERTIFICATION AND QUALITY MEASUREMENT

The ABA requires anesthesiologists who became board-certified after 1999 to maintain ongoing certification through participation in their Maintenance of Certification in Anesthesiology (MOCA) program. Anesthesiologists who entered the MOCA program after January 2008 are required to participate in Practice Performance Assessment and Improvement (PPAI) unless they hold a non time-limited certificate. PPAI is a three-part program that includes simulation education, patient safety education, and case evaluation.

MOCA case evaluation is a four-step process that involves data collection, comparison to community benchmarks, formulation and implementation of a performance improvement plan, and subsequent reevaluation of the data. The performance data must be a "meaningful sample" that is collected over an extended period of time, and may include outcome data or feedback from patients that relates to the quality of clinical care that was provided. The diplomate must then compare the performance data with evidence-based clinical practice guidelines that have been created by professional societies such as the ASA, publications such as *Cochrane Reviews*, or derived from meta-analyses. If evidence-based clinical practice guidelines are not available, individual outcomes may be compared with consensus opinion or peer data to determine areas for improvement. The diplomate must then design and implement a plan to improve outcomes in one of the identified areas through data collection and comparison. This plan should include clinical reminders, personal education, system changes, or standardization of a clinical care pathway. The development and implementation of a practice improvement plan may be an individual or a group effort, but it must be possible to extract the individual diplomate's performance data from the group data. The final step involves reevaluation of the data to assess changes in practice that have occurred since the original assessment. The goal is for the diplomate to improve performance or maintain a high standard of practice in comparison to established benchmarks [7].

QUALITY MANAGEMENT

Unfortunately, benchmarks have not yet been established for most clinical performance measures. Creating meaningful benchmarks is complicated because few clinical outcome measures have standardized definitions, meaningful risk adjustment, and consistent reporting mechanisms. One review of 23 anesthesia-related mortality studies conducted between 1955 and 1992 showed wide-ranging perioperative mortality (1 death in 53 anesthetics to 1 in 5417 anesthetics) and anesthesia-related mortality (1 in 1388 anesthetics to 1 in 85,708 anesthetics) with no clear trend due to differences in operational definitions, patient populations, and data capture [8]. Despite the warnings accompanying this literature review, investigators continue to make bold claims of improved anesthesia-related outcomes based on faulty comparisons [9–15]. Even if outcome measures were to be standardized, they may still lack validity. A review of performance measurement in anesthesia revealed that 60% of clinical measures relied on expert opinion alone as a source of validation [10]. This is unacceptable in an environment where performance measures are being developed and promoted by professional organizations, governmental agencies, and payers who are using them to guide reimbursement or for value-based purchasing in health care.

The Physician Consortium for Performance Improvement (PCPI) was convened by the American Medical Association (AMA) to develop and implement evidence-based performance measures for individual health care providers participating in PQRS. Most of the performance measures developed for individual providers are clinical process measures that determine the rates at which health care providers adhere to evidence-based guidelines. In general, risk adjustment is not necessary for process measures if the rate is based upon a specific patient population to which the guideline applies. Process measures can be developed in parallel with clinical practice guidelines because the evidence that validates a clinical process measure (*i.e.*, that connects the process being measured to a desired outcome) is the same evidence used to make an evidence-based care recommendation. Clinical outcome measures examine the results of clinical care that depend upon multiple factors including concurrent disease and concurrent care. Adjusting these factors to allow comparison of performance between individual providers is time consuming and costly, and may be impossible. Table 30.2 lists two process measures, and one combined process and outcome measure, relevant to anesthesia care that were developed by the AMA PCPI and subsequently adopted by CMS for PQRS.

Most health care institutions have developed entire departments that manage compliance with the performance improvement standards imposed by TJC and performance reporting required by CMS. Individual departments are,

Table 30.2 **PERFORMANCE MEASURES RELEVANT TO ANESTHESIA CARE**

Timing of Prophylactic Antibiotics—Administering Physician©
Percentage of surgical patients aged 18 years and older undergoing procedures with the indications for prophylactic parenteral antibiotics who have an order for an antibiotic to be given within one hour (if fluoroquinolone or vancomycin, two hours) before the surgical incision (or start of procedure when no incision is required)
Prevention of Catheter-Related Bloodstream Infections (CRBSI)—Catheter Insertion Protocol©
Percentage of patients who undergo CVC insertion for whom CVC was inserted with all elements of maximal sterile barrier technique (cap AND mask AND sterile gown AND sterile gloves AND a large sterile sheet AND hand hygiene AND 2% chlorhexidine for cutaneous antisepsis [or acceptable alternative antiseptics, per current guideline]) followed
Perioperative Temperature Management©
Percentage of patients, regardless of age, undergoing surgical or therapeutic procedures under general or neuraxial anesthesia of 60 minutes duration or longer for whom *either* active warming was used intraoperatively for the purpose of maintaining normothermia, OR at least one body temperature equal to or greater than 36 degrees Centigrade (or 96.8 degrees Fahrenheit) was recorded within the 30 minutes immediately before or the 15 minutes immediately after anesthesia end time

©Measures copyrighted by the AMA Physician Consortium for Performance Improvement.

however, ultimately responsible for the safety of all patients and staff and are required by TJC to implement a safety management program. The personnel responsible for planning these programs include the governing body, the chief executive officer and other senior managers, departmental leaders, the elected and appointed leaders of the medical staff, and the clinical departments and other medical staff members in organizational administrative positions. This group is responsible for creating a process to continually measure and assess the effectiveness of performance improvement and safety activities. Leaders must also assess the adequacy of the human, information, physical, and financial resources allocated to support performance improvement and safety activities [5].

Clinical departments can support performance improvement activities by establishing a QM program that integrates with the hospital performance improvement activities and feeds a national outcomes database to facilitate comparative benchmarking. Effective QM programs include processes for data collection and collation, peer review, and data-driven performance improvement. The typical flow of data through a QM program within a department of anesthesiology is shown below in Figure 30.1.

Data collection is a necessary process for any QM program, but there is little agreement on what data should be collected. The Anesthesia Quality Institute (AQI) is a nonprofit corporation that was established by the American Society of Anesthesiologists and maintains the National Anesthesia Clinical Outcomes Registry (NACOR). The AQI was created to provide benchmarks for performance improvement. As a part of this initiative, the ASA's Committee on Performance and Outcomes Measurement (CPOM) developed of a list of measures that have been included in NACOR (Table 30.3). This list is a compilation of perioperative adverse events solicited from anesthesia subspecialty societies such as the Society for Ambulatory Anesthesia, Society for Pediatric Anesthesia, Anesthesia Society for Regional Anesthesia and Pain Management, Society for Obstetric Anesthesia and Perinatology, and the Society for Cardiovascular Anesthesiologists. Additionally, CPOM considered the adverse perioperative events collected by the Anesthesia Business Group, a coalition of several large anesthesia practices in the United States, and the American College of Surgeons' National Surgical Quality Improvement Program. Notably absent from this list of contributors was the Society for Neurosurgical Anesthesia and Critical Care [11].

Because the purpose of data collection is to identify elements of patient care that require improvement, adverse events are frequently used as indicators. That does not mean, however, that occurrence of an event designated as a quality indicator signifies substandard care. Occurrence

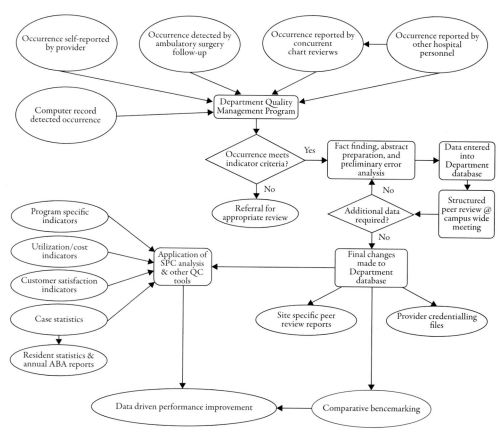

Figure 30.1 The typical data flow through a QM program within a department of anesthesiology.

Death
Cardiac arrest
Perioperative myocardial infarction
Anaphylaxis
Malignant hyperthermia
Transfusion reaction
Stroke, cerebral vascular accident, or coma following anesthesia
Visual loss
Operation on incorrect site
Operation on incorrect patient
Medication error
Unplanned ICU admission
Intraoperative awareness
Unrecognized difficult airway
Reintubation
Dental trauma
Perioperative aspiration
Vascular access complication, including vascular injury or pneumothorax
Infection following epidural or spinal anesthesia
High spinal
Postdural puncture headache
Major systemic local anesthetic toxicity
Peripheral neurologic deficit following regional anesthesia
Infection following peripheral nerve block

of an indicator simply means that the circumstances surrounding the event should be subjected to a structured peer review process that examines faults in the system as well as human errors. In fact, systemic faults may offer more opportunities for performance improvement than does correction of human errors [12]. Indicator data can either be expressed as a rate and trended over time within an institution or compared to benchmark data from outside of the institution. Meaningful comparison to outside benchmarks requires standardized definitions of outcomes and may require risk adjustment, especially for patients undergoing complex procedures such as neuorosurgery. Standardizing definitions for outcomes as easily recognized as anesthesia-related mortality can be fraught with difficulty [8], and complex risk-adjustment methodology is beyond the scope of this chapter. Trending indicator data, however, can be accomplished by referring to statistical process control (SPC) charts.

SPC charts use statistical criteria to distinguish "common cause variation" from "special cause variation." *Common cause variation* is a source of random variation that is inherent in the process itself or the tool used to measure the process. *Special cause variation* is a source of variation that is unpredictable or intermittent, and is caused by an individual or some special event. The type of action required to reduce special cause variation is different from that required to reduce variation inherent in the system, and confusing the two sources can result in increased variability [12]. For example (in a subspecialty other than neurosurgical anesthesia), placement of epidural catheters for analgesia by an anesthesia group is associated with a certain rate of accidental dural puncture. In a stable system, this rate is predictable and related to system components that include the loss of resistance technique, type of needle, and type of syringe used. If a provider with a higher rate of accidental dural puncture due to an improper technique entered the practice, and the group responded to their overall increased rate by requiring all practitioners to use ultrasound for lumbar catheter use, they might cause a further increase in their overall accidental dural puncture rate. Control charts ensure that the appropriate action is taken only when there is clear evidence that it is required and they lessen the possibility of precipitating trouble by reacting to normal sampling variation.

Several statistical software applications offer SPC charts that can be applied to attributes (e.g., postdural puncture headaches per neuraxial anesthetics) or continuous variables (e.g., scores from patient satisfaction surveys). A sample attribute SPC chart for case cancellations related to problems with patient assessment is shown in Figure 30.2. In this example, an anesthesiologist may be able to reduce special cause variation, but cannot improve a stable system by individual action. Improving a stable system is the responsibility of management (health care leaders) and requires changing the underlying health care processes.

When all special causes of variation have been eliminated and only common cause variation remains, the system is said to be stable or in statistical control. A system that is in control has a statistically definable "process capability." In other words, the system's performance is predictable and has a measurable, communicable capability [12]. This is not meant to imply that statistical control is the end goal of performance improvement efforts. A system can certainly be stable and still be of poor quality (i.e., an increased mean occurrence rate of adverse outcomes with minimal variation). The attribute SPC chart in Figure 30.2 shows that the system responsible for case cancellations related to patient assessment went out of control in December of 1997, and then stabilized again at a level of lesser quality related to this indicator (i.e., there was a higher mean number of case cancellations per month). In fact, this system experienced special cause variation when the staffing of the preanesthesia patient evaluation unit was decreased and fewer patients were evaluated before the day of surgery. SPC charts are an excellent way to monitor quality, and to demonstrate that monitoring activity to accrediting agencies. Systems that

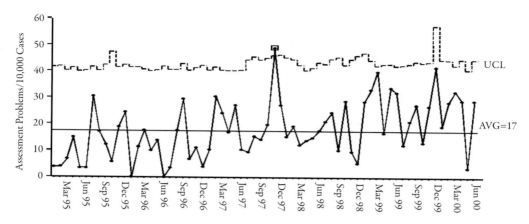

Figure 30.2   SPC chart for case cancellations related to problems with patient assessment.

are out of control or functioning at an unacceptable level of quality should be subjected to data-driven performance improvement initiatives.

Peer review is a more common method of determining the need for performance improvement. An important feature of peer review is that system errors be evaluated as critically as human errors, which permits anesthesiologists to share responsibility with managers for delivering quality health care. Quality control through peer review then becomes less threatening, encouraging broader participation and honest self-evaluation. Suggestions for improving the interrater reliability of peer review include the use of multiple reviewers who discuss the case, making outcome data available, and adding structure to the review process [13]. Structured peer review (SPR) focuses the reviewers' efforts on particular aspects of care and increases agreement among multiple reviewers by limiting reviewers' choices of a standardized list of contributing factors. As noted above this list must include both human and system errors (Table 30.4). Typically, system factors contribute to adverse outcomes about 90% to 95% of the time, while human errors by anesthesia providers contribute to only 5% to 10% of adverse perioperative outcomes [12]. Therefore, in addition to control charts showing systems that are out of control or functioning at an unacceptable level of quality, the need for performance improvement may be indicated by adverse outcomes with a high frequency of contribution from human factors, or system factors such as limitations of resources, communication failures, equipment failures, inadequacies in supervision, or a lack of professionalism by non-anesthesia personnel. Once the need for performance improvement has been identified, quality managers can then initiate a remedial process.

Although accrediting agencies like TJC require changes that improve system performance and patient safety, determination and implementation are not specified. For some, it may be as simple as choosing an already published practice guideline to reduce human error or improve outcomes in a specific area of clinical practice. For others, there may

be a more formal process of problem solving as suggested by the Shewart Cycle shown in Figure 30.3.

The Shewart cycle simply applies the scientific method of problem solving, which is familiar to all physicians, to quality improvement. In performing the steps in the Shewart cycle, quality managers often apply various problem-solving and graphical tools [15]. These include flow charts, run charts, cause and effect diagrams, and Pareto charts. Many of these techniques are familiar to physicians, and descriptions can be found in several handbooks and pocket manuals on the subject [16, 17] or posted on the AQI website [4]. Interestingly, many anesthesiologists appear hesitant to initiate the Shewart cycle for performance improvement but may have completed the cycle without even knowing it.

Quality management as an integral part of perioperative neurosurgical care is an emerging trend. An international "Conference on Risk Control and Quality Management in Neurosurgery" was held in Munich, Germany, during 2000. The purpose of the meeting was to bring together safety experts from around the world to discuss risk reduction and quality management principles applicable to neurosurgery [18]. In addition to basic principles of quality management and perioperative safety, the presenters discussed standards of care specific to neurosurgical patients [19–21]. Organizers of the conference described their experience with internally developed surgical and nursing standards. Steiger described written descriptions for common neurosurgical procedures that included the "standard part of a procedure" defined as positioning, opening, and closure. The "central or variable part of a procedure," as described by Steiger, was not described in the standards in detail because it was often "left to the discretion of the usually very experienced surgeon performing this part of surgery." In other words, these standards were limited to those parts of an operation performed by residents in training at their university practice and included typical indications for the procedures, important anatomical landmarks, positioning and skin incisions, craniotomy approach, procedure goals, closure, and management of potential complications.

Table 30.4 **FACTORS CONTRIBUTING TO ADVERSE EVENTS IN STRUCTURED PEER REVIEW MODEL**

FACTORS	EXAMPLES
Human	
Operator error	Failing to perform a proper preanesthesia machine check results in inability to ventilate
Improper technique	Leaving a short intravenous catheter in an external jugular vein leads to infiltration and airway compromise
Communication error	Improper sign-out during transfer of care results in patient mismanagement
Inadequate data sought	Failure to check appropriate extubation criteria results in reintubation
Data disregarded	Giving a patient a known allergen results in anaphylaxis
Inadequate knowledge	E.g, incorrect interpretation of hemodynamic variables obtained from a pulmonary artery catheter results in fluid overload and pulmonary edema
Supervision of resident/CRNA	Not fulfilling supervisory requirements contributes to mismanagement of a patient and subsequent adverse event
Lack of professionalism	Being unresponsiveness to changes in a clinical situation, such as a patient in a post-anesthesia care unit, results in further deterioration of the patient's condition
System	
Equipment failure	An adverse event is caused by equipment failure despite appropriate maintenance and checks
Technical/accidental	An adverse event occurs during a procedure despite appropriate technique, such as a dural puncture during loss of resistance technique for epidural catheter placement
Communication failure	Communication failure despite following the proper lines of communication, such as a case delay caused by missing lab data due to facsimile transmission error
Limitation of therapeutic standards	An adverse event that is not preventable by current standards of care, such as a child hit by a motor vehicle and is not resuscitatable despite appropriate efforts
Limitation of diagnostic standards	An adverse event that could be preventable if all preexisting conditions were known, but current standards of care do not supply this information, such as reaction to administration of a previously unknown allergen
Limitation of resources available	An adverse event that occurs as a result of limited resources such as appropriately trained personnel, fiberoptic equipment, blood products, etc.
Supervision of resident/CRNA	Fulfilling all supervisory requirements contributes to mismanagement of a patient and subsequent adverse event because of responsibilities in multiple locations at the same time
Lack of professionalism	Lack of professionalism on the part of a non-anesthesia provider is considered to be a part of the system, such as a surgeon who cannot be contacted for emergency care despite well delineated call responsibilities

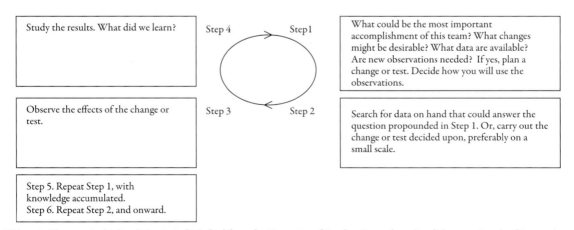

Figure 30.3   Walter A. Shewart, in his book *Statistical Method from the Viewpoint of Quality Control,* outlined the steps involved in continuous quality improvement. As you go through the steps, you'll notice a striking resemblance to the scientific method of problem solving. Basically, one formulates a hypothesis, tests the hypothesis, looks at the results, and then formulates a conclusion with plans for further experimentation.

These standard procedure descriptions were supplemented by intraoperative checklists executed before induction of anesthesia, before opening dura, before closing dura, while writing postoperative orders, and during emergencies due to complications [20]. Uhl and Heinlein described standardized nursing care plans for neurosurgical procedures including angiographies, myelographies, neurovascular procedures, surgery for pain and stereotactic biopsies. The nursing care plans deal with general problems of neurosurgical patients, such as reduced mobility, as well as special care problems related to a specific procedure or patient disease [21]. These procedure descriptions and care plans might be better defined as clinical pathways, or process management, for common neurosurgical procedures, and not minimal standards of care. Regardless of the nomenclature, both Steiger and Uhl concluded that quality of neurosurgical care was improved by implementation of these standardized processes at their institution.

At the same conference in 2000, Arthur Lam, from the Departments of Anesthesiology and Neurological Surgery at the University of Washington in Seattle, offered "standards of neuroanesthesia" care in the areas of premedication, intraoperative algorithms, emergency algorithms, and postoperative care of the neurosurgical patient [19]. Although there were "no published standards of neuroanesthesia," Lam believed that there were accepted guidelines, primarily based on consensus of expert opinions. His description of these "guidelines" was an overview of the current practice and knowledge of neuroanesthesiology at the time. Such an overview is unlikely to meet the requirement for becoming an ASA standard or guideline, however.

According to the ASA Policy Statement on Practice Parameters [22], standards and guidelines are evidence-based practice parameters that are developed by a rigorous process that combines scientific and consensus-based evidence. This process uses a systematic and standardized approach to the collection, assessment, analysis and reporting of the current scientific literature, expert opinion, surveys of ASA members, feasibility data and open forum commentary. Standards provide rules or minimum requirements for clinical practice that are supported by meta-analyses of findings from multiple clinical trials. All or nearly all expert consultants and surveyed ASA members are expected to agree with the recommendations found in evidence-based practice standards. Guidelines, on the other hand, are not intended to be minimum requirements, but rather recommendations for patient care that describe basic management strategies. Evidence-based practice guidelines contain recommendations that are supported by meta-analyses of findings from multiple clinical trials. A majority of expert consultants and surveyed ASA members are expected to agree with guideline recommendations and areas of divergent opinion are clearly indicated in the guidelines. Unfortunately, there are still no ASA-defined, evidence-based standards or practice guidelines for neuroanesthesia care.

The existence of a few related practice advisories [23, 24] suggests that anesthesiologists would like to identify best practices related to neuroanesthesia care. Practice advisories provide statements to assist decision-making in areas of patient care where there are not a sufficient number of adequately controlled studies to permit meta-analysis. Evidence-based practice advisories are, therefore, supported by a descriptive summary of the available literature. Areas of controversy may exist, so practice advisories are not intended as minimum requirements and do not carry the weight of guidelines with regard to directing care. In 1999, the ASA Committee on Professional Liability established the ASA Postoperative Visual Loss (POVL) Registry. In 2006, the American Society of Anesthesiologists Task Force on Perioperative Blindness published the Practice Advisory for Perioperative Visual Loss Associated with Spine Surgery [23]. The purposes of this advisory were to enhance awareness of perioperative visual loss and reduce its frequency in patients who undergo spine procedures while they are positioned prone and receiving general anesthesia. The task force identified patients who undergo prolonged procedures, have substantial blood loss, or both, as being at increased risk for ischemic optic neuropathy. Although this risk is small and unpredictable, the task force recommended that anesthesia providers consider informing patients who might be at increased risk of perioperative visual loss. Intraoperative management should include continual blood pressure monitoring, consideration of central venous pressure monitoring, and periodic determinations of hematocrit if there is substantial blood loss. Patients should be positioned so that the head is level with or higher than their heart when possible, and vision should be assessed as soon as the patient is alert. The practice advisory also recommends that surgeons give consideration to the use of staged spine procedures in these higher risk patients. In 2009, the American Society of Anesthesiologists Task Force on Anesthetic Care for Magnetic Resonance Imaging also published a practice advisory that was highly relevant to neuroanesthesia care, but by no means exclusive to neuroanesthesiologists [24]. The advisory makes several recommendations with regard to anesthesia provider education, screening providers and patients for the presence of ferromagnetic materials, preparation for anesthetics management, patient management during the MRI, management of emergencies, and postoperative care. These practice advisories might have risen to the level of practice guidelines had there been more controlled studies to support their recommendations

The American Association of Neurological Surgeons (AANS) has had slightly more success in the development of evidence-based guidelines applicable to the clinical care of neurosurgical patient. Its most notable safety initiatives include guidelines for the management of severe traumatic brain injury, which were developed collaboratively with the Brain Trauma Foundation (BTF) and Congress of Neurological Surgeons (CONS). These evidence-based guidelines include recommendations for prehospital management [25], medical management [26], surgical management [27], and prognosis [28] of patients suffering from severe traumatic brain injury. These guidelines offer Level 1, Level 2, and Level 3 recommendations based on Class 1, Class 2, and Class 3 evidence, respectively.

Level 1 recommendations are based on the strongest evidence for effectiveness and can be applied to patient management with a high degree of clinical certainty. Level II recommendations have only a moderate degree of certainty regarding clinical effectiveness; and for Level III recommendations, the certainty of clinical effectiveness has not been determined [28]. Unfortunately, the evidence for surgical management of traumatic brain injury is not nearly as strong as that for medical management. In fact, a review of more than 700 scientific manuscripts for the preparation of the guideline for the surgical management of traumatic brain injury revealed no controlled clinical trials to support specific types of surgical management, or support surgical management over medical management. Therefore, the guideline for the surgical management of traumatic brain injury contains no Level 1 recommendations. Similarly, the AANS and CONS developed guidelines for the management of acute cervical spine and spinal cord injuries, but found that the scientific evidence was insufficient to support standards or guidelines for the majority of the clinical management.

In an attempt to fill the void created by the paucity of efficacy studies for neurosurgical interventions, the AANS has formed NeuroPoint Alliance (NPA). NPA is a data management organization dedicated to collecting and analyzing data relevant to neurosurgical practice. Like the AQI for anesthesiologists, the NPA promises to benefit neurosurgeons by assisting with Maintenance of Certification, participation in federal and other pay for performance programs, and permitting benchmarking for identification of best practices. The National Neurosurgery Quality and Outcomes Database (N2QOD) is currently a pilot registry with 20 participating practice groups from academic, private, rural, and urban settings. This pilot is focusing on data from low back surgery and aims to demonstrate the feasibility and validity of data collection. By 2015, N2QOD aims to have half of all practicing neurosurgeons reporting data. The challenge for N2QOD, and NCOR, will be to offer enough value to justify the costs of data collection, risk adjustment, and measure maintenance associated with successful centralized performance data registries.

CONCLUSIONS

In summary, quality management is required by accrediting agencies for health care organizations, the American Board of Anesthesiology's Maintenance of Certification in Anesthesiology program, and emerging federal initiatives aimed at value-based purchasing of health care. One way for leaders of clinical departments to support performance improvement activities is to establish a quality program at the department level that integrates with the hospital performance improvement activities, and feeds a national outcomes database like the Anesthesia Quality Institute for comparative benchmarking. Effective QM programs include processes for data collection and collation, peer review, and data-driven performance improvement. Performance improvement may be as simple as choosing an already published practice guideline to reduce human error or improve outcomes in a specific area of clinical practice. For others, performance improvement may be a more scientific process of problem solving. Although there are tools available for establishing quality management programs and participating in data registries, neurosurgical anesthesiologists need to take a more aggressive role in the development of evidence-based clinical practice guidelines and performance measures specific to their practice.

REFERENCES

1. Vitez T. *Judging clinical competence.* Park Ridge, IL: American Society of Anesthesiologists; 1989.
2. Standards, guidelines, statements and other documents. American Society of Anesthesiologists, 2011. https://www.asahq.org/For-Members/Standards-Guidelines-and-Statements.aspx.
3. American Society of Anesthesiologists. *2010 Manual for anesthesia department organization and management.* Park Ridge, IL: American Society of Anesthesiologists; 2010.
4. Anesthesia Quality Institute, home of the National Anesthesia Clinical Outcomes Registry (NACOR). http://www.aqihq.org/
5. *Comprehensive Accreditation Manual for Hospitals: CAMH 2013.* Park Ridge, IL: Joint Commission Resources; 2012.
6. Hospital quality initiatives—overview. Centers for Medicare and Medicaid Services, 2011. http://www.cms.gov/HospitalQualityInits/
7. *Booklet of Information: certification and maintenance of certification.* Raleigh, NC: American Board of Anesthesiology; 2011.
8. Lagasse RS. Anesthesia safety: model or myth? A review of the published literature and analysis of current original data. *Anesthesiology.* 2002;97:1609–1617.
9. Sprung J, Warner ME, Contreras MG, et al. Predictors of survival following cardiac arrest in patients undergoing noncardiac surgery: a study of 518,294 patients at a tertiary referral center. *Anesthesiology.* 2003;99:259–269.
10. Haller G, Stoelwinder J, Myles PS, et al. Quality and safety indicators in anesthesia: a systematic review. *Anesthesiology.* 2009;110:1158–1175.
11. *Development of the ASA critical incidents reporting system.* Park Ridge, IL: American Society of Anesthesiologists; 2009.
12. Lagasse RS, Steinberg ES, Katz RI, et al. Defining quality of perioperative care by statistical process control of adverse outcomes. *Anesthesiology.* 1995;82:1181–1188.
13. Goldman R. The reliability of peer assessments of quality of care. *JAMA.* 1992;267:958–960.
14. Shewart WA. Statistical method from the viewpoint of quality control. Dover: Dover Publications; 1986.
15. Deming WE. *Out of crisis.* Cambridge, MA: Massachusetts Institute for Technology, Center for Advanced Engineering; 1986.

16. Walton M. *The Deming management method*: New York, NY: Berkley Publishing Group; 1986.

17. Brassard M RD. The memory jogger II. Salem, NH: GOAL QPC; 1994.

18. Proceedings of the International Conference on Risk Control and Quality Management in Neurosurgery. Munich, Germany, October 15–18, 2000. *Acta Neurochir Suppl.* 2001;78:1–223.

19. Lam AM. Standards of neuroanesthesia. *Acta Neurochir Suppl.* 2001;78:93–96.

20. Steiger HJ. Standards of neurosurgical procedures. *Acta Neurochir Suppl.* 2001;78:89–92.

21. Uhl E, Heinlein M. Quality management in neurosurgical nursing. *Acta Neurochir Suppl.* 2001;78:111–114.

22. American Society of Anesthesiologists I. Policy statement on practice parameters. In: ASA House of Delegates; 2007.

23. Perioperative ASoATFo, Blindness. Practice advisory for perioperative visual loss associated with spine surgery. *Anesthesiology.* 2006;104:1319–1328.

24. Anesthetic ASoATFo, Imaging CfMR. Practice advisory on anesthetic care for magnetic resonance imaging. *Anesthesiology.* 2009;110:459–479.

25. Foundation BT. Guidelines for prehospital management of traumatic brain injury, 2nd edition. *Prehosp Emerg Care.* 2007;12: S1–S53.

26. Foundation TB. *Guidelines for the management of severe traumatic brain injury.* New York: Mary Ann Liebert; 2007:1–116.

27. Foundation BT. Surgical management of traumatic brain injury. *Neurosurgery,* 2006;58:S2-1–S2-3.

28. Early indicators of prognosis in severe traumatic brain injury. 2000. https://www.braintrauma.org/pdf/protected/prognosis_guidelines.pdf

INDEX

Figures and tables are indicated by an italic *"f"* or *"t"* following the page number.